CONELY BRANCH LIBRARY
4600 MARTIN
DETROIT, MI 48210
(313) 224-6461

'02

Low

THE ENCYCLOPEDIA OF

MENTAL HEALTH

Second Edition

THE ENCYCLOPEDIA OF

MENTAL HEALTH

Second Edition

Ada P. Kahn, Ph.D.

Jan Fawcett, M.D.

☑®
Facts On File, Inc.

The Encyclopedia of Mental Health, Second Edition

Copyright © 2001, 1993 by Ada P. Kahn, Ph.D.

Facts On File, Inc.
132 West 31st Street
New York, NY 10001

Library of Congress Cataloging-in-Publication Data

Kahn, Ada P.
Encyclopedia of mental health / Ada P. Kahn and Jan Fawcett—2nd ed.
p.cm.
Includes bibliographical references and index.
ISBN 0-8160-4062-1 (alk. paper)
1. Psychiatry—Encyclopedias. 2. Mental health—Encyclopedias. I. Fawcett, Jan, 1934–   . II. Title.
RC437 .K34 2001
616.89'003—dc21   00-069511

Text and cover design by Cathy Rincon

Printed in the United States of America

VB FOF 10 9 8 7 6 5 4 3 2 1

This book is printed on acid-free paper.

CONTENTS

ACKNOWLEDGMENTS

We thank the following for providing information and materials useful in preparation of this work: Linda Hughey Holt, M.D.; Dorothy Riess, M.D.; Ray Ulmer, Ph.D.; Marlene Wilson and H. Michael Zal, D.O. We also thank Lenore Opasinski for production assistance.

—Ada P. Kahn, Ph.D., Evanston, Ill.
—Jan Fawcett, M.D., Chicago, Ill.

INTRODUCTION

In this second edition of *The Encyclopedia of Mental Health*, we have added many articles relating to contemporary challenges to good mental health, including the workplace, family and marital relationships, domestic violence, sexual concerns, lifestyle choices, everyday sources of stress, coping with chronic illness and aging. We have also considered cultural differences in the presentation of symptoms, and we included an extensive article about the cross-cultural influences on mental health.

Good mental health includes a balance between mind, body and spirit. Physical illness influences mental health, and both affect the human spirit. Increasingly, health professionals acknowledge these important links and look at the individual with a total perspective. Recognizing this trend, we have included many sections on complementary medicine, coping with stress and useful relaxation techniques, as well as entries on mind/body connections, the role of neurotransmitters, psychoneuroimmunology and contemporary psychology. We have tried to achieve a balance between psychodynamic theories relating to symptoms of mental distress as an expression of underlying conflicts, behavioral theories centered on conditioned learning and vicarious learning models and cognitive theories focusing on how people interpret or think about anxiety-producing situations.

Mental health is the successful performance of mental function, which results in productive activities, fulfilling relationships with other people and an ability to cope with adversity and adapt to change. The term *mental illness*, as described in a 1999 report by the surgeon general of the United States, refers collectively to all mental disorders—health conditions that are characterized by alterations in thinking, mood, behavior or some combination associated with distress and/or impaired functioning.

Mental outlook can directly affect physical health. Research has shown that an optimistic attitude can affect the immune system and increase killer cells, which attack malignant tumors. In contrast, depression can lower immune system activity and possibly invite physical illness. Being in excellent physical condition because of regular exercise is good for the cardiovascular system as well as for one's self-image and sense of self-mastery, both essential components of good mental health.

A good mental outlook gives one a sense of optimism that can help in dealing with disappointments, rebuffs, unfair treatment or failures, all of which are stressors. The avenue to good mental health is the ability to place these factors in perspective, realize that they are usually transitory rather than permanent and learn not to base generalizations about one's whole life on one adverse event. In other words, keep the big picture in mind, maintain your sense of humor and avoid letting unimportant things get to you.

Many people discover that physical symptoms can be related to their mental attitudes. Some who visit their primary care physicians really have psychosocial problems rather than strictly medical ones, and for many, the underlying cause is stress. Symptoms of stress can be varied, confusing and frustrating. Often, when the psychological aspects are uncovered, and can then be described and discussed, physical symptoms improve as a result. This book includes many examples of such sources of stress.

For most people, good physical health means feeling well. Good mental well-being includes an ability to get through the interactions of daily life without experiencing excessive emotional or behavioral incapacity. We all have good and bad days, experience stress brought on by particular situations and have moods that seem better on some days than others. Sometimes we experience anger, frustration, fears and "the blues." Good mental well-being means we are able to be flexible and adaptive, with a good sense of humor and positive self-esteem. We view mental health as a continuum, and we want to stay on the positive side.

Mental and physical health can be improved with individual lifestyle changes, such as not smoking, moderate or no alcohol consumption, planned exercise and recreation, maintenance of a moderate weight, healthy choices of nutritional foods, sufficient and restorative sleep and satisfaction with one's chosen career, school or life track. Additionally, feeling related to a social group is important as our society becomes increasingly mobile and fragmented and fewer people are able to rely on their families for guidance and emotional support.

In addition to the countless millions of people who experience occasional emotional upheaval simply because of the human condition, more than 20 percent of our population at any time is affected with some form of a specifically diagnosable mental health concern. These disorders range from anxiety, alcoholism and substance abuse, to depression and schizophrenia, and some are life-threatening. Help is necessary and available.

All age groups face mental health concerns. Recent studies have estimated that 50 million Americans suffer from some form of mental illness during their lives. Many young people under the age of 18 suffer from hyperactivity and autism. Among teenagers and young adults, suicide is an increasing cause of death. Among all age groups, more than 15 million Americans have serious depression each year; statistics show that about two of every 10 Americans have at least one episode of major depression during their lifetimes. Among all age groups, alcohol and other substance abuse is prevalent. Among the elderly, about 25 percent of those who were once labeled "senile," really have some form of mental illness that can be effectively treated. Among all age groups, 1.4 million Americans suffer from schizophrenic disorders; about 300,000 cases occur each year.

At the end of 1999, national attention was focused on mental health with the release of the U.S. surgeon general's Report on Mental Health. The high prevalence of anxiety disorders was noted, and emphasis was placed on encouraging treatment for these disorders. The report emphasized that anxiety disorders are often accompanied by a mood disorder and/or substance abuse disorder in both adults and children. According to the report, the more psychoanalytically oriented approaches have given way over the last several decades to cognitive and behavioral assessments and newer types of interventions that address symptoms directly and are more focused and time-limited.

Many scientists now agree that some mental health disorders are caused by a variety of factors, such as outside stressors, genetic defects, organic diseases or by degrees of imbalances among neurotransmitters, the brain chemicals that take messages between nerve cells. Such imbalances may be linked with depression and schizophrenia. Because of the great strides in understanding the physiological as well as chemical processes leading to good mental health in the past four decades, more accurate diagnosis and better treatment of many mental health disorders is now possible.

An increasing number of people now seek professional assistance. The surgeon general's report emphasized that mental health conditions are serious and impact individuals and families. The stigma of asking for help and therapy has lessened with the dissemination of information on mental health in the media and through the Internet. With more knowledge about their conditions, people can now develop better understanding of what type of health professional to seek out, feel comfortable consulting and working with a professional and be able to realize their potential toward a better quality of life while enjoying a better sense of mental health. This book can help in achieving that end.

Many people suffering from a condition affecting their emotions and behavior can be treated effectively and lead fuller lives. In response to these needs, those in the "helping" professions have developed a wide menu of therapies in an attempt to educate, counsel and assist struggling people to cope better. A wide and varied range of treatments exists for most mental disorders, including pharmacological therapies as well as "talking," or cognitive, therapies. Help is available through the medical profession and its subspecialty, psychiatry, those trained in the science of behavior, such as psychologists, and social workers. All these developments have resulted in an extensive and perhaps confusing array of terms describing symptoms, theories, belief systems and therapies, ranging from the names of medications prescribed by physicians to tested self-help techniques.

The Encyclopedia of Mental Health, Second Edition will be useful for readers to develop a better understanding of terms, theories, beliefs, causes and treatments. We have selected terms to provide the most factual and accurate definitions relating to many emotional, mental and behavioral situations facing individuals. As contemporary problems arise, such as environmentally caused illnesses, and a significantly large population of baby boomers ages within a youth-oriented society, language evolves and new words are created to describe situations and the various strategies individuals use to stay mentally fit. While this is not intended as a self-help book, it may help readers put terminology into better perspective and be more empowered to sort through the vast language explosion in this area. However, suggestions in this encyclopedia are not meant to take the place of professional advice.

A major step in coping with any problem is to obtain and understand accurate information. Curious readers who have heard mental health terms can use this volume as a reference to orient themselves, perhaps explore certain areas further, and more importantly, dismiss a term as not relevant to them. We hope this volume will provide a good, solid first step on the path toward understanding what some individuals and their loved ones face. In the interest of producing a book of manageable size, we intentionally omitted many terms because they are well-described in other reference books and texts.

We encourage readers to make use of the list of resources and the extensive bibliography at the back of this volume in search of information on mental health, the ongoing research in the relative roles of brain chemistry, environment and genetics.

—Ada P. Kahn, Ph.D., Evanston, Ill.
—Jan Fawcett, M.D., Chicago, Ill.

aberration Any behavior considered a deviation from the normal or typical in a particular culture. Aberrations are defined differently in different cultures. In some societies, for example, any sexual practice that is not related to reproduction (including any act from autoeroticism to voyeurism) is considered an aberration. In a sexually restricted culture, the strict "nonreproductive behavior" norm could apply. In a more liberal, sexually free culture, any type of sexual behavior occurring between or among consenting adults might be considered quite acceptable; in such a culture, the term "aberrant" might apply only to behavior in which there is victimization (for example, child abuse or the threat of violence) or adverse social consequences.

abnormal Applied to behavior, the term relates to any deviation from what is considered normal in the culture. Abnormal behavior is usually considered evidence of a mental disturbance that could range from a minor adjustment problem to a severe mental disorder. Abnormal psychology is the branch of psychology that studies mental and emotional disorders. Applied to statistics, the term indicates scores that are outside the expected range or normal range.

abortion Interruption or loss of any pregnancy before the fetus is capable of living. The term *abortion* usually refers to induced or intentional termination of a pregnancy, while *spontaneous abortion,* the natural loss of a pregnancy, is usually referred to as a miscarriage.

Considering and undergoing an abortion causes anxiety for many women. For example, some mourn the loss of their fetus, while others, years later, fantasize about how old the child would have been. Women who have the least anxiety surrounding an abortion are those who undergo mental health counseling before and after the procedure. The subject of abortion is also a source of anxiety for the men who may share in the decision-making process regarding the continuation of the pregnancy.

Throughout history, many women have attempted self-abortion and tried innumerable "abortifacients" without success, and indeed, in many cases, caused themselves injuries, requiring emergency medical care, and incurred permanent damage. These methods, including concentrated soap solutions and the ingestion of quinine pills, castor oil or other strong laxatives, can endanger a woman's physical health and are not necessarily effective as abortifacients.

Women who find themselves with an unwanted pregnancy should seek counseling to determine their options and help relieve the stresses of the situation.

Selecting the Safest Method

To minimize anxieties and fears, a woman should get information and counseling before seeking an abortion. Once the decision is made, women should have a medical examination before undergoing an abortion to detect possible cardiac conditions or bleeding disorders. In the United States, Planned Parenthood maintains offices in many large cities that can provide information on clinics and services. Local health departments can provide names of services that meet acceptable health standards. Women may feel less stressed and more confident if they have a recommendation from a trusted physician or a member of a local hospital gynecology staff.

See also PREGNANCY.

Holt, Linda Hughey, and Melva Weber. *AMA Book of Woman Care.* New York: Random House, 1982.

Kahn, Ada P., and Linda Hughey Holt. *The A to Z of Women's Sexuality.* Alameda, Calif.: Hunter House, 1992.

Abraham, Karl (1877–1925)   German psychoanalyst and one of Sigmund Freud's early disciples. As the first German psychoanalyst, he made significant contributions to the study of manic depression, schizophrenia, the relation between symbolism in dreams and myths and the formation of the oral and anal characters through pregenital fixation.

See also ANAL CHARACTER; DREAMING; ORAL CHARACTER; SCHIZOPHRENIA; FREUD, SIGMUND.

abreaction   A therapeutic process originated by Josef Breuer, in which a patient discharges repressed emotions by reviving and reliving painful experiences buried in the unconscious. The desired result of abreaction is catharsis (the discharge of tension).

See also CATHARSIS.

abstract thought   An ability to appreciate ideas from multiple frames of reference. It is often associated with high intelligence. Abstract thinking is usually part of a mental status examination given by mental health professionals. An individual's capacity to think abstractly can be assessed in various ways, including interpreting proverbs or identifying commonalities between two items. Some answers may indicate a disturbance in the form of thinking, such as loose associations (no logical connection discernible), incoherence, illogicality, clanging (repeating words with similar sound and different meanings) or flight of thought (jumping from one somewhat related thought to another with no conclusion of the main idea).

abuse   See ADDICTION; DOMESTIC VIOLENCE.

acceptance   An attitude on the part of a psychotherapist toward the individual under treatment for a mental health concern. A nonjudgmental attitude is considered a necessary aspect in therapy.

The therapist conveys respect and regard for the individual, without implying approval of specific behaviors or an emotional attachment toward the client. Acceptance was defined by Carl Rogers (1902–1987), an American psychologist, as "valuing or prizing all aspects of the client including the parts that are hateful to himself or appear wrong in the eyes of society." The term "acceptance" is used interchangeably with unconditional positive regard by client-centered therapists ascribing to the ideas of Carl Rogers.

See also BEHAVIORAL THERAPY; CLIENT-CENTERED THERAPY.

access to care   A term that refers to the health care system in terms of both geographic accessibility of physicians and facilities and financial accessibility. Many individuals who are uninsured and underinsured do not have access to good mental health care because they cannot pay the costs themselves. Co-payments for individuals who are insured for health care also have an effect of reducing access to health care. In general, people in rural areas in the United States have less access to mental health care than those in metropolitan areas in which major teaching institutions are located.

Recent decisions to exclude insurance coverage or drastically reduce coverage for "mental disorders" in order to save money greatly remove patients' access to care.

accommodation   Adaptation of language and specific therapeutic techniques to meet needs of each individual under treatment. With accommodation, the therapist enhances trust and rapport and helps promote change for the individual or family.

See also PSYCHOTHERAPIES.

acculturation   A process associated with increased anxieties and fears, in situations where there are linguistic or cultural communication barriers or an individual's expectations are not congruent with actual events. As reported in an editorial in *Canadian Family Physician,* (October 1995) the anxieties of the immigration experience are compounded particularly for individuals whose future residency status is in question. Behavioral changes, such as an increase in alcohol and tobacco consumption, may follow immigration. When different family members become accustomed to a new culture at different rates, conflicts can arise between the generations, adding to the overall anxiety.

Increasingly, mental health workers see immigrant patients from ethnic backgrounds that do not use the Western medical model. Some of these patients see Western medicine as one of many healing systems, or hold cultural beliefs that clash with standard medical procedures. Cultural expectations can cause anxieties for both physicians and patients. For example, some East Indian women cannot allow a pelvic examination by male physicians, even by those from their own culture. Because such an examination can be used as grounds for divorce, the relatively simple procedure becomes both a cultural and a medical issue.

Practitioners of biomedicine should address the clinical issues surrounding folk beliefs and behaviors in a culturally sensitive manner, according to an article in *The Journal of the American Medical Association* (March 1, 1994). Lee M. Pachter, D.O., associate director of Inpatient Pediatrics, St. Francis Hospital and Medical Center, Hartford, Connecticut, wrote: "A culturally sensitive health care system is one that is not only accessible, but also respects the beliefs, attitudes and cultural lifestyles of its patients. It is a system that is flexible and acknowledges that health and illness are in large part molded by variables such as ethnic values, cultural orientation, religious beliefs and linguistic considerations."

Dr. Pachter explained that most medical folk beliefs and practices are not harmful and do not interfere with biomedical therapy. Under these circumstances, the clinician should not attempt to dissuade the patient from these beliefs but instead should discuss the importance of the biomedical therapy in addition to the patient-held belief. However, any ethnomedical practice that has the potential for serious negative outcome needs to be discouraged. This must be done in a sensitive and respectful way, possibly by replacing dangerous practices with alternatives that fit into the patient's ethnocultural belief system and are thus easier to accept.

Reducing Anxieties Involved in Interactions Between Mental Health Workers and Patients

Pachter recommended the following strategies for physicians treating ethnic populations:

- Become aware of the commonly held folk medical beliefs and behaviors of the patient's community.
- Assess the likelihood of a particular patient or family acting on these beliefs during a specific illness episode.
- Arrive at a way to successfully negotiate between the two belief systems.

Following a study conducted in Canada, researchers drew up a list of recommendations to reduce anxieties on the part of the physician as well as the patient:

- Be aware of your own cultural biases.
- Determine whether language will be an issue during office visits.
- Develop an office guide for immigrant patients including typical questions asked during an examination, needs for disrobing and types of examinations and testing procedures and their importance.
- Prepare a list of local agencies that are available to help with multicultural issues.
- Train the nurse or receptionist to explain the preliminary aspects of routine examination procedures.
- Encourage patients to share their culture and lifestyle with you. Explain that you are not trying to pry into their lives but need the information for accurate diagnoses and appropriate therapy.
- Ask before going ahead with any procedures. Seeking permission and explaining the procedures removes the mystery, and patients become partners in the activity rather than objects of scrutiny. Compliance improves with understanding.
- Take advantage of opportunities for cross-cultural learning in group discussions with other professionals from different cultural backgrounds.

See also COMPLEMENTARY THERAPIES; CROSS-CUL-
TURAL INFLUENCES; MIGRATION; PERSONAL SPACE.

Cave, Andrew et al. "Physicians and immigrant
    patients." *Canadian Family Physician* 41 (October
    1995): 1685–90.
Pachter, Lee M. "Physicians should not ignore folk med-
    icine beliefs and remedies." *The Journal of the Ameri-
    can Medical Association* (March 1, 1994).

acetylcholine   A naturally occurring substance in
many body tissues that functions as a neurotransmitter to facilitate transfer of nerve impulses
between nerve cells. Acetylcholine plays an important role in memory storage and retrieval. Individuals who have Alzheimer's disease show losses of
acetylcholine. Dysregulation in the acetylcholine
system has been suggested as a possible neurochemical mechanism for the symptoms of depression. Many medications such as antihistamines
(antiallergy) and antidepressant medications can
temporarily block acetylcholine function, resulting
in dry mouth, constipation and sometimes short-
term memory loss and blurred near vision.

See also ALZHEIMER'S DISEASE; DEPRESSION.

acquaintance rape   See RAPE.

acquired immunodeficiency syndrome (AIDS)
One of the most feared, complicated and devastating diseases ever identified. New therapies are
developed each year, but as of the early 2000s, no
cure or vaccine exists. Study of AIDS at the basic
and clinical levels calls upon biomedical techniques
that did not even exist before the 1990s. It is a
debilitating disease that leaves the body vulnerable
to many opportunistic infections, many types of
cancer and, in many cases, death. It is caused by
the HIV (HUMAN IMMUNODEFICIENCY VIRUS) virus.

The epidemic was first recognized between 1981
and 1984. Many people discovered their illness for
the first time in the emergency room when an
AIDS-defining condition was diagnosed. Before
1986, HIV testing was not generally available
except to a few people enrolled in research studies.
Since then both knowledge of AIDS and screening
tests have become widespread. The drug AZT has
been available since 1987 to combat the disease,
and other new and powerful treatments for opportunistic infections have subsequently been
approved. Thus the treatment of infections and
cancers became more sophisticated and more effective during the latter part of the 1980s, and during
the 1990s, contributed to a more positive outlook
for people with AIDS.

According to a report by the Centers for Disease
Control, in 1996 there were 235,470 diagnosed
cases of AIDS in the United States. During 1996,
AIDS and opportunistic infections resulting from
the infection were diagnosed in an estimated
56,730 persons, a decline of six percent compared
with 1995. This marked the first calendar year during which AIDS incidence overall did not increase
in the United States. Deaths among persons
reported with AIDS declined 23 percent in 1996
compared with 1995.

According to a 1997 report from UNAIDS, the
United Nations agency, there were 30 million cases
of AIDS worldwide, with 16,000 people being
infected every day. Among those infected, only one
in 10 knows, the UNAIDS report said. "The main
message of our report is that the AIDS epidemic is
far from over," said UNAIDS director general Peter
Piot. In Washington, D.C., a World Bank report said
AIDS is having a devastating effect in the developing world, where 90 percent of victims live. "AIDS
is reversing decades of progress of improving the
quality of life in developing countries," said Martha
Ainsworth, a senior economist at the World Bank.
The disease has trimmed years off life expectancy
in Brazil, Thailand, Zimbabwe and other countries.

Worldwide Distribution of AIDS Patients

There is a growing gap between the developed and
the developing world with respect to the scale of
HIV spread, as well as morbidity and mortality from
AIDS. In North America, Western Europe, Aus-
tralia and New Zealand, newly available antiretro-
viral drugs are reducing the speed at which
HIV-infected people develop AIDS, according to
Peter O. Way, Bernard Schwartlander and Peter
Piot in "The Global Epidemiology of HIV and
AIDS," published in *Sexually Transmitted Diseases*. In
most of these countries, substantial decreases in
AIDS incidence have been observed since 1996.
Additionally, early and targeted prevention pro-

grams were successful in reducing the number of HIV infections, especially in the high-risk groups in the mid to late 1980s, which further limited the impact of the disease.

In less developed areas of the world, the number of new infections has reached dramatic levels and is still increasing in many regions. However, because of the long latency period between infection and the development of HIV-related diseases, the major impact of the disease is still to come, even if new infections could be reduced in the near future. Way, Schwartlander and Piot report that nine out of 10 HIV-infected persons in underdeveloped countries do not know about their HIV infection and very often do not have a chance to learn about it through testing and counseling.

How AIDS Affects Mental Health

Because people may be infected and not know it, and because symptoms may lie dormant for years, it is especially easy for a person to worry that he or she might have AIDS. Some individuals, especially hypochondriacs, homosexual men and needle users, may experience anxiety or panic attacks, and even some minor, superficial symptoms that mimic AIDS. They may feel certain that they are dying and become obsessed with details of the disease or the thought of having to face the stigma it still carries as of the late 1990s. Furthermore, obsessional worries are common in populations at risk (which include women) and sometimes even more so in non-risk people who fear contracting the disease unknowingly.

People who fear AIDS may reduce their sexual contacts, have less interest in sexual activity or have sexual difficulties; may stop participating in activities of the gay community; may feel depressed or anxious for no obvious reason and may have sleeplessness, nightmares or loss of appetite. They may feel guilty for their past lifestyle of high-risk activity. To alleviate anxiety, individuals should know that they are not alone with these fears, get a complete medical check-up, practice safe sex and if they are a drug user, be sure to use clean needles. Educational materials, available from health clinics and civic health departments, can also be helpful.

Because AIDS is transmitted through the exchange of bodily fluids, including blood, drug users who share needles, persons receiving or donating blood and health-care workers have all been subject to anxiety surrounding the disease. With proper precautions, risk to health-care workers, hemophiliacs and persons receiving blood transfusion are minimal, and risks to blood donors are virtually nonexistent.

Psychological Reactions to Diagnosis

Individuals may experience intense grief, heartbreak and uncertainty when they learn that they have AIDS. They feel the loss of their health, loss of freedom to live each day without the threat of sudden illness and loss of desire to make plans for the future. Individuals may experience these feelings long before physical symptoms begin. In the early stages of the disease, the infected person may wonder how long it will take to become ill, whether he or she will experience pain, what treatments will be available, who will take care of him or her and how to maintain hope in the face of such great uncertainty.

Anger is often a major reaction to the discovery that one is HIV-positive. According to Judith G. Rabkin, Robert H. Remien and Christopher R. Wilson in *Good Doctors, Good Patients: Partners in HIV Treatment,* the anger may be directed at possible sources of infection, such as blood banks, past sexual partners or needle sharing friends, or it may be directed at oneself for not having acted responsibly in past behavior. However, anger can also contribute to the "fighting spirit" that some people with AIDS consider the explanation for their continued psychological and physical survival.

Complementary Therapies and HIV Infection

AIDS patients may be motivated to explore alternatives when traditional therapies do not relieve illness and its symptoms. An increasing number of therapies is available to supplement treatment recommendations. As researchers continue to study the mechanisms and efficacy of various therapies, acceptance of complementary modalities is growing among patients, health care providers and even some managed care programs and insurance companies.

According to Benjamin Evans, writing in the *American Journal of Nursing* (February 1999), patients with HIV disease have sought care from modern Western medicine and from complementary therapies, including Ayurvedic medicine, traditional Chinese medicine, naturopathy, nutritional approaches, homeopathy and mind/body methods. At the 12th World AIDS Conference in 1998 in Geneva, multiple studies on complementary therapies were reported.

Relationship with Mental Health Professionals

The primary doctor-patient relationship can provide constancy and comfort, as well as uncertainty. For people with AIDS ("PWAs"), the association with a caring physician may constitute one of the patient's most enduring and emotionally intimate connections. Rabkin, Remien and Wilson suggest that a successful relationship can mean shared expectations, good communication and satisfaction about their collaboration at all stages of illness up to and including the patient's death, should that occur.

Physicians and patients constantly face crises. Demands upon both require flexibility, initiative and courage to make difficult decisions that make sense to both. Physicians and patients have considerably different attitudes in the 1990s than in earlier years about prospects of health and survival after diagnosis. Before 1987, many patients were told that they had only six months to a year to live. At the end of the 1990s, an AIDS diagnosis no longer means imminent demise, although many people continue to equate HIV with death. Many infected persons now lead reasonably healthy lives when using medications available since 1987.

Family and Friends: Disclosure and Support

For people who discover they are HIV-positive through an antibody or blood test, there is usually no urgency about disclosure (except to sex or needle-sharing partners). However, if one is hospitalized for any of the infections associated with AIDS, family and friends find out. Disclosure is usually a highly charged topic. When family members and friends learn about one's HIV status, they may react with varying degrees of shock and disbelief. Many people do not know how they should act or what they should say. Some people may avoid the infected person, or they may become overly solicitous. Unsuspecting parents may feel guilt and anger. Most relatives and friends need time to adjust to the news. Family and friends are understandably upset, sad, angry and distraught when they learn a loved one has HIV. However, it is important for friends to express reassurance that the relationship will remain unchanged. Confidentiality is an important issue; one who is close enough to the infected individual to be informed of his or her HIV-positive status should not betray that trust and not gossip with mutual friends.

During acute illness, after hospital discharge or when the illness becomes chronic, the question of providing practical assistance arises. People may truly need help but do not want to acknowledge or accept it. Friends can be most helpful by making it clear that they are not "taking over," but merely doing whatever the ill person indicates is important to him or her. Friends can let it be known that they are available for specific tasks, such as providing transportation for medical attention, shopping, delivering meals or cooking.

For information: National AIDS Hotline: (800) 342-2437

See also ANXIETY; COMPLEMENTARY THERAPIES; ELISA TEST; EPIDEMIC; HOMEOPATHY; NATUROPATHY; PANIC ATTACKS; SEXUALLY TRANSMITTED DISEASES.

Centers for Disease Control. *Update: Trends in AIDS Incidence, Deaths, and Prevalence—United States 1996.* 46 MMWR (1997): 165–73.

Centers for Disease Control. *HIV/AIDS surveillance report.* Atlanta: U.S. Department of Health and Human Services, Public Health Service 8, no. 2 (1996).

Evans, Benjamin M. "Complementary Therapies and HIV Infection." *American Journal of Nursing* 99, no. 2 (February 1999).

Holmes, King K. et al. *Sexually Transmitted Diseases,* 3rd ed. New York: McGraw-Hill, 1999.

Leary, W. E., "U.S. Offers Guide for Doctors on Care of Those With HIV," *New York Times,* 21 January 1994, 21(A).

Over, Mead. "The Public Interest in a Private Disease: An Economic Perspective on the Government Role in STD and HIV Control." In *Sexually Transmitted Diseases,* 3rd ed., edited by King K. Holmes et al. New York: McGraw-Hill, 1999.

Perry, S. L. et al. "Severity of Psychiatric Symptoms After HIV Testing." *American Journal of Psychiatry* 150 (1993): 775–79.

Rabkin, Judith G., Robert H. Remien, and Christopher R. Wilson. *Good Doctors, Good Patients: Partners in HIV Treatment.* New York: NCM Publishers, 1994.

Ungvarski, P. J., and J. H. Flaskerud. *HIV/AIDS: A Guide to Primary Care Management,* 4th ed. Philadelphia: Saunders, 1999.

Way, Peter O., Bernard Schwartlander, and Peter Piot. "The Global Epidemiology of HIV and AIDS." In *Sexually Transmitted Diseases,* 3rd ed., edited by King K. Holmes et al. New York: McGraw-Hill, 1999.

WHO, UNAIDS: HIV/AIDS. "The Current Global Situation of the HIV/AIDS Pandemic." *Weekly Epidemiol. Rec.* 72 (1997): 357–58.

acrophobia   Fear of heights, one of the most common phobias. Individuals who have acrophobia fear being on the tops of mountains or on high floors of buildings. They usually feel a high level of anxiety when approaching overlooks or rooftops. Some fear falling or being injured. Fears of elevators, escalators, being on a balcony or on the steps of a ladder are related to acrophobia.

See also ANXIETY DISORDERS; PHOBIA.

ACTH   See ADRENOCORTICOTROPHIC HORMONE.

acting out   An uncontrolled release of aggressive, violent or sexual impulses to relieve anxiety or tension through acting on impulses. The term is sometimes applied to antisocial or delinquent behavior. Acting out is often more common in individuals who cannot express feelings verbally (alexithymia) or cannot stop and fantasize or anticipate the outcome of acting on impulses. These behaviors are often seen in patients diagnosed as having antisocial personality disorder as adults or conduct disorders as children. For example, children who are abused and beaten at home by a parent may "act out" in school, bully others or show signs of extreme, uncontrolled aggressiveness.

Recent research findings have shown that men with low breakdown metabolites of serotonin (5H IAA) in their spinal fluid have a higher risk for violent, impulsive behavior, drug or alcohol abuse and violent suicide.

actualization   The process of bringing together an individual's potentialities and expressing them in concrete form. Actualization (also known as self-actualization) is the ability to transform one's potentials into accomplishments. In a world preoccupied with intellectual and artistic potential, it is common to see pressured young people fear failure, avoid hard work and thus fail to reach their potential. Actualization is also known as actualization therapy.

See also PSYCHOTHERAPIES.

acupressure   Sometimes referred to as acupuncture without needles, acupressure embraces the same concepts of energy flow and point stimulation as the original science but uses the pressure of the therapist's fingers for point stimulation. Acupressure is used by many people for relief of physical symptoms as well as anxieties. Acupressure is thought to combine the science of acupuncture with the power of the healing touch and has been most widely used for pain control.

In Eastern medicine, acupressure is helpful in conditions where the body's energy balance has been upset by a variety of physical and/or emotional stresses. Because it is an extremely gentle technique, acupressure is sometimes used by those individuals fearful of needles.

See also ACUPUNCTURE; COMPLEMENTARY THERAPIES; SHIATSU.

acupuncture   A technique used to relieve anxieties and pain. It has been used for thousands of years as a component of Chinese medicine, and it is based on theories about the body's "vital energy" (*chi*) which is said to circulate through "meridians" along the surfaces of the body. The ancient theory holds that illness and disease result from imbalances in vital energy that can be remedied when therapy is applied to "acupuncture points" located along the meridians.

The goal of acupuncture is to rebalance the flow of energy, promoting health and preventing future imbalance. The points are believed to have certain electrical properties, which, when stimulated, can alter chemical neurotransmitters in the body and bring about a healing response. Practitioners of acupuncture insert hair-thin stainless steel needles into body surfaces at acupuncture points.

In addition to the reduction of anxieties and relaxation, many people have used acupuncture for many conditions, including osteoporosis, asthma, back pain, painful menstrual cycles and migraine headaches.

Increasing Acceptance of Acupuncturists

In the mid-1990s, acupuncture was permitted in all 50 states. In some states, only physicians are permitted to practice acupuncture, while other states allow the procedure to be performed by acupuncturists under medical supervision or by unsupervised lay persons. In the United States, an estimated 3,000 medical doctors and osteopaths have studied acupuncture and use it in practice, up from 500 practitioners a decade before. Additionally, some 7,000 nonphysicians use acupuncture for a wide array of problems, sometimes in conjunction with massage, herbal therapies and other traditional Eastern techniques.

Choosing an Acupuncturist

Individuals choosing a therapist to perform acupuncture should be examined by their physician first. Some conditions are beyond the scope of acupuncture treatment and demand immediate medical attention. Discuss your expectations with the acupuncturist. Ask how long it takes to see a change in your condition. Be suspicious of promises of a quick cure, especially if you have had your problem for some time. If you don't see progress after six to eight treatments, reevaluate your choice of treatment and the practitioner.

Check the credentials of the acupuncturist you are considering. Ask whether he or she is certified by the National Commission for the Certification of Acupuncturists. Discuss the costs of the procedure. Depending on the area of the country, and whether or not the acupuncturist is a physician, fees vary. Usually the first visit is considerably higher than subsequent visits.

See also ACUPRESSURE; ADDICTION; COMPLEMENTARY THERAPIES.

A. Campbell. "A Doctor's View of Acupuncture: Traditional Chinese Theories are Unnecessary." *Complementary Therapies in Medicine* 6 (1998): 152–55.

Helms, Joseph M. "An Overview of Medical Acupuncture." *Alternative Therapies* 4, no. 3 (1998): 35–45.

James, R. "There is More to Acupuncture than the Weekend Course." *Complementary Therapies in Medicine* 6 (1998): 203–7.

acute dystonia   See DYSTONIC REACTION.

Adapin   Trade name for the generic drug doxepin, a tricyclic antidepressant.

See also ANTIDEPRESSANT MEDICATIONS.

adaptation   The process by which an individual combines personal changes with alterations of the external environment. For example, a newcomer to a country learns to alter patterns of socialization, based on the need to learn a new language. Individuals who are better able to adapt have fewer episodes of depression and anxiety.

Since we all face severe stress and adversity at times, the ability to adapt is important in regard to how life turns out. It has been shown that individuals who demonstrate the ability to adapt well have qualities of being able to suppress worry about ongoing stress while addressing immediate issues and being able to maintain a sense of humor or perspective under stress. Self-esteem also helps one to adapt.

See also SELF-ESTEEM; STRESS.

adaptive behavior scale   A test developed by the American Association of Mental Deficiency for assessing the effectiveness of mental retardates in coping with environmental demands. Observers provide information on ten behavior factors, such as independent functioning, language development, physical development and socialization, as well as maladaptive behaviors such as withdrawal, hyperactivity and destructive behavior.

See also MENTAL RETARDATION.

addiction   Psychological dependence on the use of a chemical substance or activity. Some individuals develop addictions to alcohol, caffeine, tobacco, narcotics and some sedatives, many of which are prescribed by physicians. Other individuals develop addictions to gambling, stealing or sexual activity.

The term "substance abuse" or "substance dependence" has largely replaced the word "addiction" when referring to drug dependence.

Criteria for addiction are a compulsive craving leading to persistent use or repeated actions, a need to increase the dose or level of activity due to increasing tolerance, and possibly acute withdrawal symptoms if the drug is reduced or withdrawn abruptly, depending on the drug involved (e.g., alcohol, narcotics, barbiturates). Withdrawal symptoms alone do not necessarily imply addiction. However, physical dependence can develop with prolonged use of a drug (e.g., morphine for pain). Psychological dependence can involve a loss of control of the substance use and a tendency to orient behavior or life priorities toward obtaining the drug or pursuing the addictive behavior.

For information:

American Society of Addiction Medicine
4601 North Park Avenue, Arcade Suite 101
Chevy Chase, MD 20815
Phone: (301) 656-3950
Web site: www.asam.org

See also ALCOHOL DEPENDENCE; ANXIETY; NARCOTIC DRUGS; SEDATIVE DRUG; SUBSTANCE ABUSE.

Bugelski, B. Richard, and Anthony M. Graziano, *Handbook of Practical Psychology.* Englewood Cliffs, N.J.: Prentice-Hall, 1980.
Hofler, Dagmar Zimmer, and Martien Kooyman. "Attachment Transition, Addiction and Therapeutic Bonding: An Integrative Approach." *Journal of Substance Abuse Treatment* 13, no. 6 (Nov.–Dec. 1996): 511–519.

addictive personality   A personality pattern characterized by strong tendencies to become psychologically and physically dependent on one or more substances, such as alcohol and tobacco, or activities, such as sexual encounters. The existence of this as a specific personality type or disorder has been questionable, and it is not an officially accepted diagnostic term in the *Diagnostic and Statistical Manual of Mental Disorders,* (4th ed., rev.).

See also DIAGNOSTIC AND STATISTICAL MANUAL OF MENTAL DISORDERS.

additive effect   A term used when two drugs are taken together and the result is equal to the sum of the two separate effects. Two drugs given for different purposes may have additive side effects, such as taking a tricyclic antidepressant from one doctor and an antihistamine drug for allergies from another. Both have additive anticholinergic side effects.

See also ACETYLCHOLINE.

Roesch, Roberta. *The Encyclopedia of Depression.* New York: Facts On File, 1991.

ADHD   See ATTENTION-DEFICIT HYPERACTIVITY DISORDER.

adjustment disorders   Clinically significant emotional or behavioral symptoms in response to an identifiable psychosocial stressor or stressors. The stressor may be a single event, such as ending a romantic relationship, or multiple stressors, such as marked business problems as well as marital problems. Symptoms develop within three months after the onset of the stressor or stressors. The significance of the reaction is in excess of what would be expected given the nature of the stressor, or by significant impairment in social, occupation or academic functioning.

Stressors may be recurrent, such as seasonal business crises or continuous, such as living in a crime-ridden area. Stressors may affect one individual, an entire family, or a larger community, in the case of a natural disaster.

The American Psychiatric Association characterizes adjustment disorders according to the predominant symptoms:

Adjustment disorder with depressed mood
Adjustment disorder with anxiety
Adjustment disorder with mixed anxiety and depressed mood
Adjustment disorder with disturbance of conduct
Adjustment disorder with disturbance of emotions and conduct
Adjustment disorder: unspecified

Symptoms of adjustment disorder may be either acute or chronic. If symptoms of adjustment disorders last more than six months, they may meet the criteria for other disorders, such as major depression, dysthymia or generalized anxiety disorder.

See also ANXIETY DISORDER; DEPRESSION; DYSTHYMIC DISORDER; GENERAL ANXIETY DISORDER.

American Psychiatric Association. *Diagnostic and Statistical Manual of Mental Disorders,* 4th ed., rev. Washington, D.C., 1994.

Adler, Alfred (1870–1937)   An Austrian psychiatrist and the first disciple of Sigmund Freud to break away and form his own school. Known as individual psychology, Adler's theory is based on the idea that human beings are governed by a conscious drive to express and fulfill themselves. It also included concepts such as striving for superiority, feelings of inferiority, the inferiority complex, compensation and overcompensation and the creative development of an individual style incorporating both personal and social goals.

See also FREUD, SIGMUND; INFERIORITY COMPLEX; PSYCHOLOGY.

adolescent depression   See DEPRESSION.

adolescent suicide   See SUICIDE.

adoption   A legal proceeding that permits individuals to take a child into their family and raise him or her as their own child. At one time parents tried to keep their adopted children's origins a secret, but this rarely happens now. Most parents first tell their children of their adoption when they begin to question where babies come from. As adopted children grow older, they usually begin to dwell on the fact that they are not like other children, not related by blood to their adoptive families, and they become curious about the fact that their birth parents did not want them. The turbulence of adolescence may be more difficult for adopted children, who have additional problems added to the almost inevitable conflicts with their parents.

It is usually in adulthood that an adoptee will take steps to contact birth parents. Although most states have sealed adoption records, adoptees can sometimes go through the courts or contact their birth parents with the assistance of agencies that often act as go-betweens to determine if birth parents wish to make contact with their children. Although there are exceptions, many adoptive parents are distressed and feel threatened when their grown children wish to make contact with their birth parents.

Open adoption, a practice that is not new but is becoming more common, is a system that gives the birth mother access to her child although the child is placed with an adoptive family. Open adoption is a solution for mothers who are unable to care for their child but are distressed by the idea of complete separation. The mother may participate in the process of selecting adoptive parents and visits the child, who is eventually spared the shock of being told that he is adopted and the lack of knowledge of his true origin. Open adoption is controversial and may create uncertainty for adoptive parents; but with a dwindling supply of adoptable children, a birth mother who wants this arrangement will be more likely to get her way.

In 1991 there were approximately 3 million adopted persons in the United States. The National Committee for Adoption estimates that there will be about 60,000 adoptions in the United States per year. Despite what appears to be a high number of adoptions, many prospective parents who want an infant with no known physical or mental defects may expect a long wait. Because of improved birth control methods and legal abortions and because it has become acceptable for an unwed mother to keep and raise her child, the supply of infants who will match the typical prospective adoptive parents (financially secure white couples) is low. Some couples turn to the gray or black market in babies, through which an infant may be literally sold through a doctor, lawyer or other intermediary.

Because of difficulties of adopting a child, many couples are turning to children from abroad, frequently Asian, who need homes. These couples encounter a unique set of concerns ranging from adapting a child's eating habits from a diet high in rice or beans to American meat and potatoes to responding to questions and dealing with double takes from strangers because of the child's different appearance. Ironically, while approximately 10,000 children are being adopted from abroad per year, a 1989 study showed that 34,000 children, 51 percent minority and others with physical or mental problems, were awaiting adoption in the United States. White prospective parents who are willing and eager to adopt a black infant frequently find it frustrating that many agencies have adopted the objections of the National Association of Black Social Workers to placing black children in white homes. Basing their opinions on the outcomes of freer black-white adoptions before 1972, the social workers objected that black children were growing up in white communities where they were out of touch with their roots and might encounter racism for which their idealistic parents had not prepared them.

Still another difficult-to-place group of adoptive children are older children who have memories and scars from earlier experiences. These children are the most likely to be among the 20 to 25 percent of adopted children who develop mental health needs that require professional help.

An extremely difficult situation arises when adoptive parents feel that they must return a child to the adoption agency because of behavior or physical problems that manifest themselves after the adoption that they cannot handle. Approximately 1,000 children per year are returned to agencies for these reasons. Some parents have accused agencies of hiding factors from them that, if known, would have kept them from adopting.

Qualities that agencies look for in adoptive parents are stability, a positive attitude toward adoption and a good marital relationship. Adoption agencies try to guard against parents who are adopting to solve their own personal problems, have unrealistic attitudes about adoption or negative feelings about illegitimacy.

See also INFERTILITY.

Reynolds, Nancy Thalia. *Adopting Your Child: Options, Answers, and Actions.* Bellingham, Wash.: Self-Counsel Press, 1993.

adoption studies   Researchers interested in the nature versus nurture question like to study adoptive children's characteristics in relation to their adoptive and biological parents. One study, undertaken by a group of American and European scholars, compared criminal records from 14,000 adopted children with those of their adoptive and biological parents from 1927 to 1947. The study showed a stronger relation between criminal behavior of the children and that of their biological parents than between criminal behavior of the children and that of their adoptive parents. A study at the University of Colorado, which consisted of testing the intelligence of adoptive children and their biological parents over a period of years, showed a higher correlation with the biological than with the adoptive parents. Although such studies are controversial, this was considered to be particularly significant because the children were not matched to adoptive parents by educational or socioeconomic level.

Several adoption studies of alcoholism were conducted during the 1970s in Denmark. Sons of alcoholics raised by unrelated, nonalcoholic adoptive parents were four times more likely to become alcoholic by an early age than were adopted-out sons of nonalcoholics, but were no more likely to have other forms of psychopathology and no more likely to be classified as heavy drinkers.

Daughters of alcoholics raised by nonalcoholic adoptive parents and daughters raised by their own alcoholic parents were also studied in Denmark. The adopted-out daughters had a higher rate of alcoholism than exists in the general population (4 percent versus 0.1 percent), but adopted-out controls also had a high rate of alcoholism and the findings were equivocal. Daughters raised by the alcoholic parent or parents also had an alcoholism rate of 4 percent, but this rate contrasted with no alcoholism in matched controls.

Later, two other adoption studies were performed in Sweden and in Iowa. Both produced the same results as the Danish studies. There was an increased prevalence of alcoholism in adopted-out children of alcoholics, with no evidence of an increased prevalence of other disorders. The Iowa study recently produced evidence that adopted-out daughters as well as sons of alcoholics have increased rates of alcoholism when compared with controls.

In adoption studies of schizophrenia, it has been found that congenital factors (genetic or intrauterine environmental) may play a role in the development of chronic schizophrenia.

See also ALCOHOLISM; SCHIZOPHRENIA.

adrenal cortex The outer layer of the adrenal gland. The adrenal cortex is the source of several hormones, including androgens, glucocorticoids and mineral corticoids. Functions of the adrenal cortex are controlled by ACTH, a hormone secreted by the pituitary gland especially under conditions of physiological and extreme psychological stress. Excessive production of one or more of the hormones of the adrenal cortex is known as adrenal-cortical hyperfunction. Some types of severe depression, including those that may result in suicide if not treated, show evidence of adrenal hyperfunction.

Recently, animal studies have shown evidence that prolonged stress-related adrenal hyperfunction can be associated with cell death in an area of the brain called the hippocampus, which regulates adrenal stress response and is essential for recent memory and learning. There is suggestive evidence that this process might occur in humans under conditions of prolonged severe stress (e.g., torture and severe depression).

adrenal gland A small organ above the kidney that secretes several hormones. The medulla and the cortex are the two important parts of the gland. The adrenal medulla secretes two hormones, epinephrine (or adrenaline) and norepinephrine (or noradrenaline). The adrenal gland is also known as suprarenal gland.

See also ADRENAL CORTEX.

adrenaline A hormone (also known as epinephrine) secreted by the central, or medullary, portion of the adrenal gland that produces an increase in heart rate, a rise in blood pressure and a contraction of abdominal blood vessels. These sympathetic changes can be reversed by activation of the parasympathetic system.

See also ADRENAL GLAND; EPINEPHRINE; NEURO-TRANSMITTERS.

adrenergic blocking agents Agents that inhibit some responses to adrenergic, or adrenaline-like

(energizing), nerve activity. The term "adrenergic blocking agent" (a.b.a.) also applies to drugs that block action of the neurotransmitters epinephrine and norepinephrine. A.b.a.s are selective in action and are classed as alpha a.b.a.s (alpha blockers or alpha-receptor blocking agents) and beta a.b.a.s (beta blockers or beta-receptor blocking agents), depending on which types of adrenergic receptors they affect. Medications for some mental disorders may involve both alpha blockers and beta blockers, although the beta blockers are used primarily for certain forms of anxieties, such as test taking, performance and public speaking. Some beta blockers may produce depression as a side effect.

See also ADRENERGIC DRUGS; ADRENERGIC SYSTEM.

adrenergic drugs Substances that stimulate activity of adrenaline (epinephrine) or mimic its functions and produce stimulation of the central nervous system. Adrenergic agents are produced naturally in plants and animals but can also be developed synthetically. Adrenergic drugs (a.d.s) are part of a group of sympathomimetic amines that includes ephedrine, amphetamines and isoproterenol.

See also ADRENERGIC BLOCKING AGENTS; ADRENERGIC SYSTEM.

adrenergic system Part of the autonomic nervous system, including receptor sites, that is influenced by adrenergic drugs, which stimulate the activity of epinephrine or mimic its functions.

See also ADRENERGIC BLOCKING AGENTS; ADRENERGIC DRUGS.

adrenocorticotrophic hormone (ACTH) A substance secreted by the pituitary gland to control the release of steroid hormones from the adrenal cortex; ACTH is also known as corticotropin.

See also PITUITARY GLAND.

adultery Sexual intercourse between a married individual and another person who is not the legal spouse; adultery is also known as extramarital sex. Historically, in many countries, adultery has been considered a taboo and major (and sometimes the only) grounds for divorce. Since the early 1990s, adultery and extramarital affairs carry the strong threat of acquiring a sexually transmitted disease. In the United States, adultery is a challenge to mental health within marriages and in many cases; even when participants in an affair try to keep it a secret, it can produce anxieties, conflict and guilt feelings on the part of one involved in the affair and emotions ranging from ANGER to DEPRESSION in the other partner left behind.

See also ANGER; DEPRESSION; MARRIAGE; SEXUALLY TRANSMITTED DISEASE.

Kahn, Ada P., and Linda Hughey Holt. *The A to Z of Women's Sexuality.* Alameda, Calif.: Hunter House, 1992.

advantage by illness   The benefit or relative satisfaction a sick person gains from being ill. Sigmund Freud differentiated between primary and secondary advantages, or gains, of illness. In primary advantage, the psychic mechanism is preserved because inaction and withdrawal lower anxiety and avoid the emergence of possibly destructive impulses. In secondary advantage, the individual consciously or unconsciously perceives an environmental gain, such as sympathy and attention from family members, removal of responsibilities or possible failures and avoidance of frightening situations.

See also ANXIETY; FREUD, SIGMUND; SECONDARY GAIN.

affect   Mood, or inner feelings at a particular moment. The word "affect" is often used to describe the mood as perceived by another person. One whose mood does not change, is not excited or angered by any stimuli, is said to have flattened affect (affective flattening).

See also AFFECTIVE DISORDERS.

affective disorders   Affective disorders (also known as mood disorders) involve changes in affect, a term that means mood or emotion. An affective disorder usually is a mood disturbance intense enough to warrant professional attention. One who has an affective disorder may have feelings of extreme sadness or intense, unrealistic ela-

tion with the disturbances in mood that are not due to any other physical or mental disorder.

A disorder of the thought processes is not commonly associated with affective disorders; however, if the affective disorder becomes intense, there may be changes in thought patterns that will be somewhat appropriate to the extremes of emotion the person perceives.

Affective disorders differ from thought disorders, as schizophrenic and paranoid disorders are primarily disturbances of thought, although individuals who have those disorders may also have some distortion of affect.

Death rates for depressed individuals seem to be about 30 times as high as in the general population because of the higher incidence of suicide. Manic individuals also have a high risk of death, because of physical exhaustion, neglect of proper precautions to safeguard health or accidents (with or without alcohol as a contributing factor).

Historically, there have been descriptions of mood disorders in the early writings of the Egyptians, Greeks, Hebrews and Chinese. Descriptions of mood disorders appear in the works of Shakespeare, Dostoyevsky, Poe and Hemingway. Many historical figures have suffered from recurrent depression, including Churchill, Freud, Dostoyevsky, Moses, Queen Victoria, Lincoln and Tchaikovsky.

Affective disorders, or mood disorders, can be subcategorized as major depression and bipolar disorders. These disorders can be acute or chronic, and both show symptoms by changes in the biologic, psychological and sociological functioning of the individual. In some individuals, bipolar disorders and depressive disorders occur according to a seasonal pattern, with a regular cyclic relationship between the onset of the mood episodes and particular seasons.

A mood syndrome (depressive or manic) is a group of associated symptoms that occur together over a short duration. For example, major depressive syndrome is defined as a depressed mood or loss of interest, of at least two weeks' duration, along with several associated symptoms, such as difficulty concentrating and sleeping, fatigue, hopelessness, loss of pleasure and weight loss or gain with suicidal thoughts sometimes present.

A mood episode (major depressive, manic or hypomanic) is a mood syndrome not due to a known organic factor and not part of a nonmood psychotic disorder such as schizophrenia, schizoaffective disorder or delusional disorder. Psychiatrists diagnose a mood disorder by the pattern of mood episodes. For example, the diagnosis of major depression, recurrent type, is made when an individual has had one or more major depressive episodes without a history of a manic or hypomanic episode.

Manic Episodes

Manic episodes are distinct periods during which the individual experiences a predominant mood that is either elevated, expansive or irritable. Such individuals may have inflated self-esteem, increased energy, accelerated and loud speech, flight of ideas, distractibility, grandiose delusions and decreased need for sleep. The disturbance may cause marked impairment in working, social activities or relationships; an episode may require hospitalization to prevent harm to themselves or others. There may be rapid shifts of mood, with sudden changes to depression or anger. The mean age for the onset of manic episodes is in the early twenties, but many new cases appear after age 50.

Hypomanic Episodes

These are mood disturbances less severe than mania but sometimes severe enough to cause marked impairment in judgment, financial, social or work activities. Such episodes may be associated with increased energy and activity, exaggerated self-confidence, hypertalkativeness, euphoria and increased sense of humor. Hypomanic episodes may be followed by depressions of moderate to great severity.

Major Depressive Episodes

Major depression affects approximately 10 percent of the adult population. A major depressive episode includes either depressed mood (in children or adolescents, irritable mood) or loss of interest or pleasure in all, or almost all, activities for at least two weeks. Symptoms persist in that they occur for most of the day, nearly every day, during at least a two-week period. Associated symptoms may include feelings of worthlessness or excessive or inappropriate guilt, difficulty concentrating, restlessness, inability to sit still, pacing, handwringing, appetite disturbance, change in weight, sleep disturbance, decreased energy and recurrent thoughts of death or of attempting suicide.

Depressive episodes are more common among females than among males. The average age of onset of depressive episodes is in the late twenties, but a major depressive episode may begin at any age. Studies of depression show an earlier age at onset of depression among younger people, suggesting the rate of depressive disorders may be rising in successively younger-aged groups.

Bipolar Disorders

Bipolar disorders (episodes of mania and depression) are equally common in males and females. Bipolar disorder seems to occur at much higher rates in first-degree biologic relatives of people with bipolar disorder than in the general population.

Cyclothymia

In this condition, there are numerous periods of hypomanic episodes and numerous periods of depressed mood or loss of interest or pleasure that are not severe enough to meet the criteria for a bipolar disorder or a major depressive episode.

Dysthymia

In dysthymia, there is a history of a depressed mood for at least two years that is not severe enough to meet the criteria for a major depressive episode. This is a common form of depression, and one who has this condition may have periods of major depressive episodes as well.

Causes of Affective Disorders

There are many explanations for affective disorders, including psychoanalytic theory, interpersonal theory, cognitive theory, behavioral theory, learned helplessness theory and genetic theory. These theories have common points of focus that can be roughly categorized as biologic, psychosocial and sociocultural.

Personality characteristics of some individuals predispose them to affective disorders, such as lack of self-esteem and negative views of themselves and of the future. A stressful life event for some individuals activates previously dormant negative thoughts. Individuals who become manic are generally ambitious, outgoing and energetic, care what others think about them and are sociable before their episodes and after remission. However, depressive individuals appear to be more anxious, obsessive and self-deprecatory. They often are prone to feelings of self-blame and guilt. Depressed individuals tend to interact with others differently than manics do. For example, some manic individuals dislike relying on others and try to establish social roles in which they can dominate others. On the other hand, depressed individuals take on a role of dependency and look to others to provide support and care.

Feelings of a loss of hope and helplessness are central to most depressive reactions. In severe depression, "learned helplessness" may occur, in which the individual sees no hope and gives up trying to cope with his or her situation.

There seems to be a hereditary predisposition, because incidence of affective disorders is higher among relatives of individuals with clinically diagnosed affective disorders than in the general population. There has been considerable research during the 1970s and 1980s to explore the view that depression and manic episodes both may arise from disruptions in the balance of levels of brain chemicals called biogenic amines. Biogenic amines serve as neural transmitters or modulators to regulate the movement of nerve impulses across the synapses from one neuron to the next. Two such amines involved in affective disorders are norepinephrine and 5-hydroxytryptamine (serotonin). Some drugs are known to have antidepressant properties and biochemically increase concentrations of one or the other (or both) of these transmitters.

In many individuals, psychosocial and biochemical factors work together to cause affective disorders. For example, stress has been considered as a possible causative factor in many cases. Stress may also affect the biochemical balance in the brain, at least in some predisposed individuals. Some individuals experience mild depressions following significant life stresses, such as the death of a family member. Other major life events may precipitate changes in mood, such as those involving reduced self-esteem, physical disease or abnormality or deteriorating physical condition.

Treatment

A variety of treatments, including behavioral therapy and drugs, are used to treat affective disorders. Some behavioral approaches, known as cognitive and cognitive-behavioral therapies, include efforts to improve the individual's thoughts and beliefs (implicit and explicit) that underly the depressed state. Therapy includes attention to unusual stressors and unfavorable life situations and observing recurrences of depression.

See also AGORAPHOBIA; ALCOHOLISM; ANTIDEPRESSANT MEDICATIONS; BIPOLAR DISORDER; DEPRESSION; LEARNED HELPLESSNESS; LEARNED OPTIMISM; MANIC-DEPRESSIVE ILLNESS; PHOBIA; SEASONAL AFFECTIVE DISORDER; SUICIDE.

American Psychiatric Association. *Diagnostic and Statistical Manual of Mental Disorders,* 4th ed., Washington, D.C.: 1994.

Fawcett, Jan, Bernard Goldin, and Nancy Rosenfeld. *New Hope for People with Bipolar Disorder.* Roseville, Calif.: Prima Publishing, 2000.

McFarland, Gertrude K., and Mary Durand Thomas. *Psychiatric Mental Health Nursing.* Philadelphia: J. B. Lippincott, 1991.

affective flattening (blunting) A behavior pattern involving a lack of emotional expression, reactivity and feeling. The individual may fail to smile or laugh when prompted, fails to show normal vocal emphasis patterns, acts "wooden" and does not use hand gestures or body position as an aid to expressing ideas. Such behavior is also seen in the neurologic disorder Parkinson's disease. It can also be a symptom of severe hypothyroidism (myxedema).

Affective flattening can be evaluated by a mental health professional by observation of the individual's behavior and responsiveness during a routine interview. Some aspects of behavior may be affected by drugs, because side effects of some neuroleptics may lead to a masklike facial expression and diminished movements (pseudo-Parkinsonism). However, other aspects of mood, such as responsivity and appropriateness, are usually not so affected. Affective flattening is sometimes referred to as blunting. Affective flattening may develop in the psychiatric disorder schizophrenia or major depression.

See also AFFECTIVE DISORDERS; DEPRESSION.

affirmation   An affirmation (self-affirmation) is a positive self-statement. Affirmations help many individuals change negative feelings to more positive ones. They help the individual break the stress-tension cycle. Affirmations are stated in a positive framework, such as "I feel great after exercising" or "I have a lot to offer" rather than "I won't just sit around so much." These are stated in the present tense, rather than future tense, and are repeated three to five times during daily relaxation practice sessions or other times frequently throughout the day. Individuals who benefit from affirmations imagine doing what they say in as much detail and with as much pleasure as possible. Affirmation statements often include the words "I can" or "I am" and are used by individuals to improve self-esteem and self-confidence, break the cycle of codependency and overcome addictions.

See also SELF-ESTEEM.

McFarland, Gertrude K., and Mary Durand Thomas. *Psychiatric Mental Health Nursing.* Philadelphia: J. B. Lippincott, 1991.

agape (agapism)   In psychoanalytic terms, agape involves the practice of erotic love of the body and also feelings of tenderness and protectiveness for the traits, gestures or speech of another person.

The term is derived from the Greek word *agape,* referring to unselfish, spiritual love of one person for another with no sexual implications. In Christian tradition, agape also encompasses the love of God for humankind, as well as the love of humankind for God.

See also EROS.

Kahn, Ada P., and Linda Hughey Holt. *The A to Z of Women's Sexuality.* Alameda, Calif.: Hunter House, 1992

age associated memory impairment   See FORGETTING; MEMORY.

age discrimination   Older adults from 55 to 65 years and older are often the first workers fired in business downsizings and mergers and overlooked as potential employees when applying for new jobs. Both of these factors constitute age discrimination, a major challenge to mental health. Age discrimination is usually defined by negative stereotypes depicting older adults as less productive than younger workers and unable to be trained in new technology. According to Patricia O'Toole in the May 1992 issue of *Lear's* magazine, during 1990 and 1991, the ranks of unemployed men and women between the ages of 45 and 54 grew by more than 50 percent to almost 1 million. Much too young to retire, they are finding that employers consider them too old and too expensive to hire.

There are increasing numbers of unemployed older adults. Polls conducted by the Commonwealth Fund, a New York-based foundation, showed that there are 6 million unemployed Americans older than 55, half of whom are women who want to continue working. Traditionally, women have been subject to both age and sex discrimination. Those with jobs were slow in getting the recognition their male counterparts have. They were the first to be forced out of work because of layoffs or cutbacks; employers often used the excuse that women did not really have to work, or did not really need the money. And though everyone knew that women were often the backbones of the organizations in which they worked, they were made to feel incompetent and thus forced out or "encouraged" to take early retirement.

Despite the fact that there has been much research to disprove the stereotypes attributed to aging, they continue to influence judgments made concerning employment. Statistics have shown that workers age 40 and older take less time off than any other age group and are less accident-prone than younger workers. This age group has also experienced more massive changes in technology over their lifetimes than any past generation and are no less—if not more—adept at learning and using technology than those who are younger.

Middle-aged, mid-career adults in the 40- to 55-year-old range who lose their jobs experience loss of income and benefits at a time when their families may still be young and in need of their support and protection. They are often the most rooted in their communities and unwilling to move. Even when they are willing to leave, they can have the most difficulty in breaking even on heavily mortgaged homes.

For those older adults in the 55- to 65-year-and-older range, loss of work may mean loss of health insurance and/or pension benefits at a time when they need them most.

In *Coping with Job Loss,* authors Carrie R. Leana and Daniel C. Feldman report these comments from workers laid off from the aerospace industry:

"Age and salary had a great deal to do with my job loss. My job was not eliminated—myself, along with several others, were replaced by people half our age. Simple economics."

"I felt tossed aside, like an old shoe."

"Old age is most definitely a drawback in seeking employment, no matter what the law says."

Corporations who have ignored the stereotypes and made a point of hiring older workers have said it pays. For a decade, Travelers Corporation, an insurance company, has operated an in-house temporary service staffed mainly by its retirees who need little training and are highly productive because of their knowledge of the company. At Days Inn, the over-50 recruits stay longer and learn faster than younger workers. Many other companies report huge savings when employing older adults.

age factors   There is a significant rise in the rate of depression among adolescents, teenagers and young people. In the 1970s, mental health facilities reported more cases of young individuals who were depressed than the textbook description of depressed persons as middle-aged.

Today depression appears to occur more in the 20-to-40 age range than in older persons. As depression affects more people under the age of 45 and fewer over age 65, 25 to 44 may be the most susceptible age range. Until the last decade, depression in children and infants was underidentified. Now it is estimated that from 3 million to more than 6 million American children suffer from depression, much of it unrecognized and untreated.

Under age 65, twice as many women as men are treated for depressive disorders, with the exception of bipolar disorder (manic-depression), which occurs equally in both sexes. Although fewer people over age 65 are affected by depression, it is still common among the elderly. In elderly people, depression may occur because of loneliness, physical deterioration, poor health, death of loved ones and friends and an awareness of their own mortality. By contrast, schizophrenia has an early onset, in the late teens and twenties, and tends to be chronic. Panic disorders, which may accompany depression or occur by themselves, may have onsets from the late teens to the forties and tend to be recurrent. Agoraphobia often occurs in people in their twenties, and social phobias often originate in the teen years.

See also AGORAPHOBIA; DEPRESSION; PANIC DISORDER; PHOBIA; SCHIZOPHRENIA.

Roesch, Roberta. *The Encyclopedia of Depression.* New York: Facts On File, 1991.

ageism (agism)   Discrimination against someone on the grounds of age, particularly middle-aged or elderly people. Victims of ageism experience challenges to good mental health because of this unwarranted prejudice.

See also AGE DISCRIMINATION.

aggression   A general term for a variety of behaviors that appear outside the range of what is socially and culturally acceptable. Aggression includes extreme self-assertiveness, social dominance to the point of producing resentment in others and a tendency toward hostility. Individuals who show aggression may do so for many reasons, including frustration, as a compensatory mechanism for low self-esteem, lack of affection, hormonal changes or illness. Aggression may be motivated by anger, over competitiveness, or directed toward harming or defeating others.

An individual with aggressive personality may behave unpredictably at times. For example, such an individual may start arguments inappropriately with friends or members of the family and may harangue them angrily. The individual may write letters of an angry nature to government officials or others with whom he has some quarrel.

Hormonal differences account for some aggression because excessive androgens, the male sex hormones, seem to promote aggression (e.g., the use of androgenic steroids to promote development of muscle mass in athletes).

Some psychiatric conditions occasionally are associated with aggression. These include antisocial personality disorder, schizophrenia and mania. The abuse of amphetamines, alcohol, PCP ("Angel dust"), cocaine and androgenic steroids (such as weight lifters use) is even more frequently associated with violent behavior. Other medical causes include temporal lobe epilepsy, hypoglycemia and confusion due to illness.

Individuals who are continuously aggressive may show changes in brain-wave patterns in electroencephalograms (EEG).

The opposite of aggression is passivity. The term "passive aggression" relates to behavior that seems to be compliant but in which "errors, mistakes or accidents" for which no direct responsibility is assumed result in difficulties or harm to others. (A passive-aggressive person might say, "Gee, I'm sorry, I didn't mean to ruin all your work.") Patterns of behavior such as making "mistakes" that harm others are considered "passive aggressive."

See also PASSIVE-AGGRESSIVE PERSONALITY DISORDER.

aggressive behavior See AGGRESSION; PASSIVE-AGGRESSIVE PERSONALITY DISORDER.

aging Growing older is a lifelong concern. The aging process begins the day one is born, but concern mounts as the years go by. Anxieties about health status, financial capabilities, standard of living and surviving loved ones mount as one grows older. In 1990, according to the National Council on the Aging, there were 36 million Americans (one out of every seven persons) over the age of 60.

People have always been preoccupied with longevity and have dreaded old age. There have been three major categories of theories on achieving old age. One is the biblical theory, which holds that the righteous are granted long life. Second is the theory that there are special places in the world where people live long. Third, the modern theory, is that to some extent, people have an influence on the length as well as the quality of their lives. One's genetic makeup also influences one's life, but that is a situation over which one has no control. The object of successful aging is to make the best use of what one has.

SUCCESSFUL AGING

Eat a proper diet with a reasonable amount of fiber
Reduce intake of salt and cholesterol
Do a reasonable amount of exercise
Avoid smoking and excessive alcohol intake
Wear a seat belt in cars
Protect skin from the sun
Keep physically and intellectually active
Make constructive use of time
Undergo periodic health examinations
Examine risk factors; determine necessary lifestyle changes
Maintain friendships and relationships with others

During the first half of the 20th century, life expectancy was increased by reducing neonatal, infant and maternal deaths. Since the 1980s, there has been an increase in life expectancy even after the age of 60 that is probably due in part to the decreasing incidence of cardiovascular risk factors. Now there seems to be consensus by geriatricians that certain lifestyle components can help one age successfully.

Characteristics of aging can be slowed down by regular exercise programs. Exercise strengthens the body, improves one's outlook and widens one's social contacts. Older adults are now jogging, walking, bicycling and swimming. These exercises improve the condition of the heart and lungs, aid in weight control and decrease many aspects of stress.

Many older adults skip meals or seem to have a reduced appetite. Eating well is important to keep up vitality in old age. Even people who come from families with a history of heart disease can lower their own risk of becoming ill by following a low-fat diet, eliminating smoking, controlling their weight and exercising regularly.

One of the sad effects of aging is the loss of loved ones and treasured relationships. A nine-year study of 7,000 Alameda County (California) residents indicated that people with few relationships died at rates two to five times higher than those with more friendships. Another study, done in England, of females who had suffered severe depression revealed that women who experienced severe stress and did not have a confidante were approximately 10 times more likely to be depressed than women who did. Even caring for pets has a beneficial effect on aging; being responsible for something other than oneself is a morale booster.

Planning for retirement helps one stay active. In a study by the American Association of Retired Persons, members ranked boredom as one of the most serious problems of retirement.

Many healthy people move into retirement communities or buildings during their later years so that they will have companionship as well as available health care nearby. Among the fears of the aging population are concerns over ability to continue to manage one's own affairs, remaining independent and not being a burden to children or society and the dread of living out one's last years in a nursing home.

See also ELDERLY PARENTS; RETIREMENT.

aging parents   See ELDERLY PARENTS.

agitation   Behavior that is tense and excited, with rapidly fluctuating levels of physical activity. It may be evidenced by pacing, loud and rapid speech, tense facial expression, cursing, wringing of hands, perspiration, short attention span and inability to concentrate or purposeless, potentially injurious movements.

Agitation may be a reaction to stressful events or relationships or an untoward response to psychotropic medications (akathisia). Agitation can occur in some mental disorders, such as schizophrenia, bipolar disorder, major depression, delirium and dementia. Agitation has been observed in otherwise normal individuals when exposed to a crisis situation, such as bereavement or natural disasters, in which they often experience extreme fear, isolation and sleep deprivation.

See also AKATHISIA; ANXIETY; FEAR.

agnosia   A failure or impairment of the ability to recognize objects, grasp the meaning of words and other symbols or interpret sensory stimuli. The condition may be due to organic brain damage (strokes, brain tumors, brain injury) or to emotional factors, seen rarely in schizophrenia. Visual agnosia refers to an inability to respond appropriately to visually presented material. Color agnosia refers to an impaired ability to select colors of the same hue, name colors or give the color of a specifically colored object, such as the sky. Prosopagnosia refers to the inability to recognize faces of people well known or newly introduced to the individual. Spatial agnosia includes disorders of spatial perception and loss of topographical memory. Auditory agnosia is an impairment in recognition of nonverbal sound stimuli in the presence of adequate hearing. Agnosia for music includes tone deafness, melody deafness and disorders in perception of rhythm. Tactile agnosia is apparent in the individual who is unable to recognize objects by handling the objects without seeing them. Verbal agnosia implies the recognition of a word or object but the inability to verbalize its name (often as a result of strokes).

See also STROKE.

agonist   A drug that affects a nerve receptor by binding to its surface and producing a physiological change. Such a change might involve stimulation of a neuron, causing a nerve impulse to be fired, or it could provide the mediation needed to inhibit a nerve-cell discharge. The term also refers to a contracting muscle whose action is opposed by another muscle. L-dopa is a dopamine-receptor agonist used to treat Parkinson's disease.

See also PHARMACOLOGICAL APPROACH.

agoraphobia   A complex syndrome characterized by a fear of being in public places where escape may be blocked or help unavailable in the event that embarrassing or incapacitating symptoms develop. Agoraphobia involves a combination of fears, such as being without help in stores, public transportation and crowds. Agoraphobia involves fear of losing control of oneself, as in fainting or "going crazy." Agoraphobia usually occurs in adults; the ratio of women with agoraphobia versus men is three to one.

Agoraphobia frequently results from panic attacks or panic disorder. Panic attacks are either "out-of-the-blue attacks" or those that occur in a setting of anticipatory anxiety related to previous panic attacks. They are attacks of overwhelming anxiety, leading the victim to fear death from a heart attack, or loss of mental control. After repeated panic attacks, victims frequently develop a fear of crowds, enclosed places (e.g., tunnels, airplanes) and even leaving home; they are afraid that a repeat panic attack might occur. Panic anxiety is the most severe form of anxiety, and individuals suffering from panic attacks may exhibit suicidal impulses as an escape from this torment. There are successful pharmacologic and psychotherapeutic treatments for panic attacks and agoraphobia, which develops after panic attacks.

Many agoraphobics are socially disabled because they cannot travel to visit friends, work or shop. Many refuse invitations and often make excuses for not going out. Thus adjustments are necessary to compensate for the agoraphobic's lack of participation in family life and activities outside the home.

Anxious, shy women are the group of individuals most prone to agoraphobia. Some agoraphobics tend to be indecisive, have little initiative, are guilty and self-demeaning and feel they should be able to get out of their situation themselves. They may become increasingly withdrawn into their restricted life. There is some evidence that dependency and perfectionism are associated with a subgroup of people who develop agoraphobia. There is also substantial clinical evidence that emotional suppression is strongly associated with development of agoraphobia.

Most agoraphobics are married at the time they come for treatment. In most research projects involving agoraphobics, spouses seem well adjusted and integrated individuals. In some cases, therapists use the Maudsley Marital Questionnaire to assess the individual's perception of his or her marriage before and after treatment. Questions relate to categories of marital and sexual adjust-

ment, orgasmic frequency, work and social adjustment and "warmth" items. When agoraphobia improves with treatment, marriages usually remain stable or improve.

Agoraphobia may strain a marriage because the agoraphobic person may ask the spouse to take over chores that require going out, such as shopping or picking up children; spouses often must fulfill social obligations without the companionship of their mates. Spouses are additionally stressed by having to be "on call" in case anxiety attacks occur that require communication or a trip home to soothe the agoraphobic. Thus a couple that may have been happy may be driven apart by the disorder, with each blaming the other for a lack of understanding. The husband may think that the wife is not trying to overcome her phobic feelings, and the agoraphobic wife may think that her husband does not understand her suffering. The wife may become so preoccupied with fighting her daily terrors that she focuses little attention on their marital relationship and her husband's needs. However, in cases in which the agoraphobic has an understanding, patient and loving spouse, this support can be an asset in overcoming the agoraphobic condition. The spouse can attend training sessions with the therapist and group therapy sessions and act as the "understanding companion" when the agoraphobic is ready to venture out.

When agoraphobics seek treatment, they are often in a constant state of alertness and have a passive, dependent attitude and a tendency toward sexual inhibition. Typically, the agoraphobic admits to being generally anxious and often expresses feelings of helplessness and discouragement. However, many agoraphobics were formerly active, sociable, outgoing persons. Some agoraphobics abuse alcohol and drugs, and researchers are beginning to uncover the extent of such abuse. Some current estimates place 30 percent of alcoholics as having a primary anxiety disorder that leads to the chronic use of alcohol.

Symptoms

Symptoms may include fear of dizziness or falling, loss of bladder or bowel control, vomiting, palpitations and chest pain. There may be a fear of having a heart attack because of the rapid heart action, of fainting if the anxiety becomes too intense and of being surrounded by unsympathetic onlookers. The individual then develops a fear of the fear that brings about anxiety in anticipation of a panic reaction, resulting in avoidance of the feared situation.

A common characteristic of agoraphobia is a history of panic attacks in which the individual experiences many symptoms including an overwhelming sense of imminent catastrophe and fear of loss of control or of public humiliation. However, agoraphobia may occur with or without a history of panic attacks. Many women report that generalized anxiety and panic in agoraphobia tend to be worse just prior to and during menstruation.

Broader symptoms include general anxiety, spontaneous panic attacks and occasional depersonalization—a change in the perception or experience of the self so that the feeling of one's own reality is temporarily lost. For some individuals, anxiety in agoraphobia may be aggravated by certain predictable situations, such as arguments between marital partners and general stress. For some, the anxiety is nearly always relieved somewhat in the presence of a trusted companion, a pet or an inanimate object such as an umbrella or shopping cart.

Some agoraphobics develop ways to live more comfortably with their disorder. For example, those who go to churches or movie theaters may be less frightened in an aisle seat so that they can make a fast exit if they experience a panic attack. Having a telephone nearby is another comfort.

Many agoraphobics have episodes of depression. The first episode may occur within weeks or months of the first panic attack. Individuals complain of feeling "blue," have crying spells, feel hopeless and irritable, suffer from a lack of interest in work and have difficulty in sleeping. Agoraphobia is often aggravated during a depressive episode. The increased anxiety may make individuals less motivated to work hard at tasks (such as going out) that they previously did with difficulty.

Some agoraphobics are also claustrophobic. Claustrophobia is usually present before the agoraphobia develops. The common factor between the two phobias is that escape is blocked, at least temporarily. Symptoms of the phobic anxiety in agoraphobia may include many physical sensations that accompany other anxiety states, such as dry mouth, sweating, rapid heart beat, hyperventilation, faintness and dizziness.

Panic Attacks and Agoraphobia

Panic attacks are defined, discrete episodes of unpredictable, intense fearfulness, terror or extreme apprehensiveness, along with feelings of impending doom. An individual may experience symptoms such as difficulty in breathing (hyperventilation), palpitations, chest pain or discomfort, choking or smothering sensations and fear of going crazy or losing control. Attacks may last from minutes to hours. Diagnosticians use three panic attacks within a two-week span of time to characterize the panic "syndrome." Panic attacks often precede the agoraphobic state, although some individuals have agoraphobia without panic attacks.

In panic disorder with agoraphobia, the individual meets the criteria for panic disorder and additionally has a fear of public places from which escape might be difficult or embarrassing or where help might not be available.

Obsessions

Many agoraphobics experience obsessions, which are persistent and recurrent ideas, thoughts, impulses or images that occur involuntarily as ideas that invade consciousness. Obsessional behavior is usually present before an individual develops agoraphobia. Individuals may develop obsessional thinking about certain places, situations or objects that might cause them to experience their fear reaction. Obsessional thinking is difficult to control, often distorts or exaggerates reality and causes much anticipatory anxiety. Individuals may develop compulsive behavior in an attempt to reduce obsessional thoughts and resultant anxiety. Some agoraphobics often have obsessive symptoms, such as ritual checking or thoughts of harming others or themselves.

Causes

For some individuals, learned experiences condition them to regard the world as a dangerous place. Many agoraphobics have had at least one agoraphobic parent, and many have had at least one parent who is somewhat fearful. In some cases, they received mixed messages from their parents; while they were encouraged to achieve, they were not well prepared to deal with the world, either because they were overprotected—taught that home is the only safe place—or underprotected, having to take on too much responsibility at an early age.

Recent studies have suggested evidence for a genetic predisposition to panic disorder. Family history studies have found panic disorder to be as much as 10 times more frequent in the biologic relatives of those with panic disorder as among normal control subjects.

The biologic basis for panic attacks and resultant agoraphobia is being researched, and theories abound. Symptoms of panic attacks, such as palpitations, sweating and tremulousness, lead to a theory that they are the result of massive discharges from the adrenergic nervous system. (Some studies suggest that beta-blocking agents such as propranolol may ameliorate panic attacks.)

The triazolobenzodiazepine drug alprazolam (trade name: Xanax) has been approved by the Food and Drug Administration for the treatment of panic attacks or panic disorder. Imipramine or monoamine oxidase inhibitors (MAOIs) such as phenelzine (trade name: Nardil) are helpful in suppressing panic attacks.

Another hypothesis is that panic attacks result from increased discharge in the locus coeruleus and increased central noradrenergic turnover. While electrical stimulation of this structure in the brains of animals has been shown to produce fear and anxiety, relevance of these animal studies to anxiety disorders in humans is unclear.

Researchers have found that intravenous infusion of sodium lactate will provoke a panic attack in most panic disorder sufferers, but not in normal subjects. The mechanism by which this occurs is not clear; further study may lead to an understanding of the biochemical factors in the etiology of panic attacks.

Treatment

Treatment is usually targeted toward several aspects of the agoraphobic syndrome: agoraphobia, panic attacks and anticipatory anxiety. A variety of treatments are used, sometimes in sequence or in combination. Treatment of agoraphobia is more complicated than treatment of simple phobias because panic attacks themselves seem to be the basis of the disorder.

Many treatments are based on exposure therapy. A major component of treatment involves exposing the agoraphobic to situations that are commonly avoided and frightening in order to demonstrate that there is no actual danger. Treatment may include direct exposure, such as having the individual walk or drive away from a safe place or a safe person or enter a crowded shopping center. Indirect exposure is also used; this may involve use of films with fear-arousing cues. Systematic desensitization is included in this category, as this procedure is characterized by exposure (either in imagination or in vivo) to the least reactive elements of a situation or object until the anxiety response no longer occurs. Then a slightly more reactive element or item is presented and so on until the individual can be exposed to the most critical aspect without a strong anxiety response. Another imaginal procedure for anxiety treatment includes flooding or continuous presentation of the most reactive elements of a situation until anxiety reduction occurs.

Behavior therapy is used to treat many agoraphobics. This includes educating individuals about their reactions to anxiety-producing situations, explaining the physiology and genetics involved (where applicable) and teaching breathing exercises to help overcome hyperventilation. In many cases, three to six months of behavior therapy is effective, and subsequent supportive and behavioral techniques reduce the anxiety level and help individuals master their fear of recurrent attacks in specific situations.

Also known as in vivo therapy, exposure therapy uses real-life exposure to the threat. Facing the fearful situation with appropriate reinforcement may help an individual undo the learned fear. Some therapists set specific goals for the sufferer for each week, such as walking one block from home, then two and three, taking a bus and progressing after each session. Particularly in the early stages of treatment, many therapists accompany agoraphobic individuals as they venture into public places. In some cases, spouses or family members are trained to accompany the agoraphobic individual; other therapists recommend structured group therapy with defined goals and social skill training for the agoraphobic and their families.

Psychotherapy

With psychotherapy, agoraphobics learn to resolve past conflicts that may have contributed to their agoraphobic state. Psychotherapy is often used in conjunction with an attempt to relieve symptoms with behavioral therapies and possibly drug therapy.

Drug Therapy

The treatment of choice today for agoraphobia involves the use of behavioral exposure therapy and careful use of medication, with the latter withdrawn as progress is made in behavioral therapy. Particularly for those who have panic attacks, drug therapy initially seems to enhance results of exposure-based treatments. In many cases, drugs are used for three to six months and then discontinued once the individual has some control over bodily sensations. Some individuals never experience recurrence of attacks, while attacks return months or years later for others. When attacks recur, a second course of drug therapy is often successful.

A variety of drugs are used in the treatment of panic attacks associated with agoraphobia. These include the tricyclic antidepressants and the MAOIs (which are also used to treat severe depression) and alprazolam, an antianxiety drug. For many individuals, panic attacks are successfully controlled with use of particular tricyclic antidepressants (imipramine, desipramine or clomipramine). MAOIs are often used as second-line medications when patients do not respond to a tricyclic.

Free-floating or anticipatory anxiety is often treated with selective use of a benzodiazepine (for example, oxazepam) or alprazolam (Xanax) alone, because it both reduces anticipatory anxiety and blocks panic attacks. Xanax has recently been approved by the Food and Drug Administration to treat symptoms of panic attacks. Clonazepam (trade name: Klonopin) is a newer benzodiazepine that is also thought to have antipanic properties, but it has not yet been well studied. Buspirone (trade name: Buspar), a nonbenzodiazepine antianxiety agent, is less sedating and less prone to be abused than the benzodiazepines, but its efficacy in panic disorder is still under study.

Involvement of spouses and family members usually produces more continuing improvement with better results than treatment involving the agoraphobic alone. Greater improvement occurs because of the motivation for continued "practice" in facing feared situations both between sessions and after treatment is completed. Home-based treatment, where individuals proceed at their own pace within a structured treatment program, produces fewer dropouts than the more intensive, prolonged exposure or pharmacologic treatments.

Self-help

Self-help groups for agoraphobic people encourage participants to offer one another mutual support in going out. As recovery from agoraphobia is a long-term process, self-help groups can provide valuable support. Individuals share common experiences and coping tips and have an additional social outlet. Some agoraphobics get together for outings, help take children to and from school, arrange programs and retrain themselves out of their fears and anxieties.

Alcoholism and Agoraphobia

Because alcohol is somewhat effective in relieving chronic anticipatory anxiety, some agoraphobics move toward alcoholism in an unsuccessful attempt to prevent panic. However, alcohol may even exacerbate panic by bringing about a feeling of loss of control and causing strange body sensations. Moreover, the use of alcohol may interfere with effective treatment of the agoraphobia, as central nervous system depressants reduce the efficacy of exposure treatment. However, some agoraphobic men avoid social situations in which alcohol is not served and believe that alcohol helps to calm them before they venture out into public.

Agoraphobics who abuse alcohol and nonalcoholic agoraphobics may both have histories of disturbed childhoods. Disturbed childhoods of alcoholic agoraphobics frequently include familial alcoholism and depression. In addition, children whose early attachments to caretakers are characterized by lack of consistent support as well as frightening and dangerous interactions may fail to develop a sense of trust and security. Such individuals may be particularly vulnerable to later psychopathology, such as panic attacks and agoraphobia; alcoholism may be one mode of coping for such individuals.

The clinical picture of both agoraphobia and alcoholism often involves depression. Agoraphobics who are alcohol abusers may also be more socially anxious than their nonalcoholic peers. High rates of social phobia have been noted among inpatient alcoholics, and major depression has been found to increase both the likelihood and intensity of agoraphobia and social anxieties.

For more information:

American Psychiatric Association
1400 K Street, NW
Washington, D.C. 20005
Phone: (888) 357-7924
Web site: www.psych.org

American Psychological Association
750 First Street, NE
Washington, D.C. 20002-4242
Phone: (202) 336-5500 or (800) 374-3120
Web site: www.apa.org

Anxiety Disorders Association of America
11900 Parklawn Drive, Suite 100
Rockville, MD 20852
Phone: (301) 231-9350
Fax: (301) 231-7392
Web site: www.adaa.org

National Alliance for the Mentally Ill
2107 Wilson Boulevard, Suite 300
Arlington, VA 22201
Phone: (800) 950-NAMI (6264)
Fax: (703) 524-9094
Web site: www.nami.org

National Mental Health Association
1201 Prince Street
Alexandria, VA 22314-2971
Phone: (800) 969-6642
Fax: (703) 684-5968
Web site: www.nmha.org

See also ALCOHOLISM; ANTIDEPRESSANT MEDICATIONS; ANXIETY; BEHAVIORAL THERAPY; CLAUSTROPHOBIA; DEPRESSION; ANXIETIES AND ANXIETY DISORDERS in bibliography.

Doctor, Ronald M., and Ada P. Kahn. *Encyclopedia of Phobias, Fears, and Anxieties.* 2nd ed. New York: Facts On File, 2000.

Frampton, Muriel. *Agoraphobia: Coping with the World Outside.* Wellingstorough, Northamptonshire, England: Turnstone Press, 1984.

Kahn, Ada P. "Panic Attacks." *Chicago Tribune,* June 23, 1991.

Magee, William J. et al. "Agoraphobia, Simple Phobia, and Social Phobia in the National Comorbidity Survey." *Archives of General Psychiatry* 53 (Feb. 1996) 159–168.

Marks, Isaac M. *Fears, Phobias and Rituals.* New York: Oxford University Press, 1987.

McFarland, Gertrude K., and Mary Durand Thomas. *Psychiatric Mental Health Nursing.* Philadelphia: J. B. Lippincott, 1991.

Waldinger, Robert J. *Psychiatry for Medical Students.* Washington, D.C.: American Psychiatric Press, 1990.

aha experience   A descriptive term for the emotional reaction that typically occurs at a moment of sudden insight after a long process of problem solving, learning or psychotherapy; it is the moment when various elements of a problem situation come together and seem to make sense.

See also PSYCHOTHERAPIES.

AIDS   See ACQUIRED IMMUNODEFICIENCY SYNDROME; HUMAN IMMUNODEFICIENCY VIRUS.

AIDS-related complex (ARC)   A condition affecting some persons with HIV infection. Common symptoms include fatigue, weight loss, diarrhea and oral candidiasis. Some symptoms become severe enough to cause disability. Some persons in this group will suffer further damage to their immune system and will ultimately be diagnosed as having AIDS (acquired immunodeficiency syndrome). Persons who have been diagnosed as having ARC have a high level of anxiety related to their health status and may have depression related to changes in their lifestyle and possible impending death, fears related to loss of control, pain and suffering, powerlessness related to feelings of stigmatization and possible guilt related to having caused HIV infection through behavior (for example, needle sharing or sexual practices).

See also ACQUIRED IMMUNODEFICIENCY SYNDROME.

akathisia   An inability to sit still, which sometimes occurs as a side effect of a neuroleptic medication. Akathisia also occurs as a rare complication of Parkinson's disease.

Al-Anon   An organization for the families of alcoholics who belong to Alcoholics Anonymous, formed as a support system for those who want to cope better with the problems of living with an alcoholic. Spouses, children and parents meet with others who have similar concerns.

See also ALATEEN; ALCOHOLICS ANONYMOUS; ALCOHOLISM.

Alateen   An organization for teenagers from 12 to 20 who have been affected by someone, usually a parent, with a drinking problem. Alateen was started in 1957 by a boy in California whose father was an alcoholic in Alcoholics Anonymous (AA) and whose mother was in Al-Anon. Alateen was patterned after Al-Anon and shares with it the same Twelve Steps and Twelve Traditions. Alateen meetings are conducted by teenagers with an adult member of Al-Anon as a sponsor.

See also AL-ANON; ALCOHOLICS ANONYMOUS; ALCOHOLISM.

alcohol amnestic disorder   See ALCOHOLISM.

Alcoholics Anonymous   See ALCOHOLISM.

alcoholism and alcohol dependence   A chronic disorder associated with excessive consumption of alcohol over a period of time. Most authorities recognize alcoholism as a disease, although some say that it is a self-inflicted condition and cannot properly be designated a disease. Nevertheless, it is a physiological and psychological dependence on alcohol and therefore an addiction. Alcohol exerts mental and physical effects and becomes a major part of the dependent person's life.

Many people become dependent on alcohol for relief of symptoms ranging from loneliness to anxiety and panic attacks. Some agoraphobics become alcoholics as a way of coping with their fears. Because agoraphobic individuals do not go out, it is fairly easy for them to conceal their habit.

Estimates indicate that there are approximately 5 million alcohol-dependent persons in the United States. According to the American Psychiatric Association's *Diagnostic and Statistical Manual of Mental Disorders*, 4th ed. as many as 90 percent of adults in the United States have had some experience with alcohol, and a substantial number (60 percent of males and 30 percent of females) have had one or more alcohol-related adverse life events, such as driving after consuming too much alcohol or missing school or work due to a hangover.

Factors that lead many individuals to alcohol dependence include fears, personality, environment and the addictive nature of the drug alcohol. Many people become dependent on alcohol for relief of symptoms ranging from loneliness to anxiety and panic attacks. Some agoraphobics become alcoholic as a way of coping with their fears. Because agoraphobic individuals do not go out, it is fairly easy for them to conceal their habit.

The term "alcoholism" was coined by Magnus Huss, a Swedish scientist, in 1852, when he identified a condition involving abuse of alcohol and labeled it "alkoholismus chronicus." However, references to the problem are found in earlier works of Benjamin Rush, an 18th century American physician, considered the "father of American psychiatry," and the Roman philosopher Seneca. In 1956 the American Medical Association and the American Bar Association officially recognized alcoholism as a disease, an action which affected the legal status of alcoholics, alcoholism-related state and federal laws, program financing, insurance coverage and hospital admissions.

How Alcohol Affects the Body

Contrary to popular belief, alcohol is a depressant, not a stimulant. The effects of alcohol are felt most noticeably in the central nervous system. As sensitivity is reduced in the nervous system, the higher functions of the brain are dulled, leading to impulsive actions, loud speech and lack of physical control. The drinker's face may turn red or pale. While drinking, the alcoholic loses any sense of guilt or embarrassment, gains more self-confidence and loses inhibitions as the alcohol deadens the restraining influences of the brain. Large quantities impair physical reflexes, coordination and mental acuteness.

Symptoms and Stages of Alcoholism

In the first phase of dependence on alcohol, the heavy social drinker may feel no effects from alcohol. In the second phase, the drinker experiences memory lapses relating to events that happen during drinking episodes. In the third phase, there is lack of control over alcohol, and the drinker cannot be certain of discontinuing to drink by choice. The final phase begins with long binges of intoxication, and there are observable mental or physical complications.

Behavioral symptoms may include hiding bottles, aggressive or grandiose behavior, irritability, jealousy, uncontrolled anger, frequent change of jobs, repeated promises to self or others to give up drinking and neglect of proper eating habits and personal appearance. Physical symptoms may include unsteadiness, confusion, poor memory, nausea, vomiting, shaking, weakness in the legs and hands, irregular pulse and redness and enlarged capillaries in the face. Alcohol dependent persons are more susceptible than others to a variety of physical and mental disorders.

Treatment for Alcoholism

Medical help for alcohol dependence includes detoxification (assistance in overcoming withdrawal symptoms) and psychological, social and physical treatments. Psychotherapy is usually done in groups, using a variety of techniques. Therapists for alcoholic dependent persons may be psychiatrists, psychologists or social workers. Social treatments involve family members in the treatment process. Many alcohol dependent persons benefit from involvement in self-help groups such as Alcoholics Anonymous.

Life Expectancy May Increase with Abstinence

Life expectancy may be improved by alcoholics who go dry, according to a study published in the *Journal of the American Medical Association* (Jan. 4, 1992). Results of the study supported the notion that achievement of stable abstinence reduces the risk of premature death among alcoholics. Kim D. Bullock, Psychiatry and Research Services, Veterans Affairs Medical Center, San Diego, and col-

leagues reported on 199 men who had histories of at least five years of drinking at alcoholic levels. All were current or former patients of the V.A. Alcoholism Treatment Program and/or members of Alcoholics Anonymous. The men were recruited from 1976 to 1987. Follow-up on relapse and mortality was obtained; 101 men had relapsed, and 98 were abstinent. A control group of 92 nonalcoholics equated for age, education and sex were also studied for mortality. There were 19 deaths among the relapsed alcoholics compared with the expected number of 3.83. Among abstinent alcoholics there were four deaths. Alcoholic men who achieved stable abstinence did not differ from nonalcoholic men in mortality experience. However, alcoholics who relapsed died at a rate 4.96 times that of an age-, sex- and race-matched representative sample.

Alcoholics Anonymous and Self-help

Alcoholics Anonymous is an international organization, founded in 1935, devoted to maintaining the sobriety of its members and helping them control the compulsive urge to drink through self-help, mutual support, fellowship and understanding. Medical treatment is not used. The program includes the individual's admission that he or she cannot control his or her drinking, the sharing of experiences, problems, and concerns at meetings, and helping others who are in need of support.

At the core of the program is the "desire to stop drinking." Members follow a 12 step program, which stresses faith, disavowal of personal responsibility, passivity in the hands of God or a higher power, confession of wrongdoing and response to spiritual awakening by sharing with others.

See also ADDICTIONS; AGORAPHOBIA; ANXIETY; CODEPENDENCY; CONTROL; EMPLOYEE ASSISTANCE PROGRAMS; PANIC ATTACKS.

Allan, Carole A. "Alcohol problems and anxiety disorders: a critical review." *Alcohol and Alcoholism* 30, no. 2 (1995) 145–151.

American Psychiatric Association. *Diagnostic and Statistical Manual of Mental Disorders,* 4th Edition. Washington, D.C.: 1994.

Caldwell, Paul Elliott, and Henry S. Cutter. "Alcoholics Anonymous Affiliation During Early Recovery." *Jour-*

nal of Substance Abuse Treatment. 15, no. 3 (May–June 1998) 221–228.
Eliason, Michele J. "Identification of Alcohol-Related Problems in Older Women." *Journal of Gerontological Nursing* (October 1998) 8–15.

Alexander technique   A technique developed by the Australian actor F. Matthias Alexander (1869–1955). It is a practical method of education/reintegration, which uses observation, awareness and attention to the performance of simple activities to explore the relationship between the mind and body. Stress, tension headaches and anxiety states, including performance anxiety and panic attacks, have been responsive to the technique for many people.

See also BODY THERAPIES; COMPLEMENTARY THERAPIES; MIND/BODY CONNECTIONS.

alexithymia   An inability to express emotion.

algolagnia   A psychiatric term for a disorder in which an individual derives sexual excitement by inflicting pain on his or her partner (sadism), experiencing pain (masochism) or both (sadomasochism).

See also MASOCHISM; SADOMASOCHISM.

alienation   A term that relates to withdrawal or separation of one's affections from an object or position of former attachment or from the values of one's family and culture. The term also refers to estrangement from one's own feelings. Alienation causes an individual to feel powerless and isolated. Boredom and depression may follow.

Alienation is a characteristic of obsessive-compulsive disorder and also occurs in extreme forms of schizophrenia.

See also DEPERSONALIZATION; OBSESSIVE-COMPULSIVE DISORDER; SCHIZOPHRENIA.

alogia   A general term referring to impoverished thought processes that often occur in individuals who have schizophrenia. Persons with alogia have thinking processes that seem slow or empty. Because thinking cannot be seen, it is inferred from the individual's speech.

alpha adrenergic blockers   See ADRENERGIC BLOCKING AGENTS; ADRENERGIC MEDICATIONS.

alpha adrenergic function   See ADRENERGIC SYSTEM.

alprazolam   Generic name for a pharmaceutical product marketed as Xanax. It is in a class of drugs known as triazolobenzodiazepine compounds with antianxiety and sedative-hypnotic actions. It is efficacious in agoraphobia and panic disorders and is also used to treat generalized anxiety disorder. Studies suggest that alprazolam also has antidepressant properties.

Drowsiness is the most commonly reported side effect. Caution should be observed when other drugs possessing sedative actions are given with alprazolam. Physical and psychological dependence is likely when larger than usual doses are prescribed or therapy is prolonged. As with all benzodiazepines, treatment should be terminated by gradually reducing the dose.

See also PHARMACEUTICAL APPROACH.

Fawcett, Jan A., and Howard M. Kravitz. "Alprazolam: Pharmacokinetics, Clinical Efficacy and Mechanism of Action." *Pharmacotherapy* 2, no. 5 (Sept.–Oct. 1982).

alternative therapies   See COMPLEMENTARY THERAPIES.

Alzheimer's disease   A progressive, irreversible, neurological disorder. Many people fear developing the disease as they age, and families of Alzheimer's disease sufferers cope with the anxieties of caregiving, as well as the fears involved in watching the disease advance. Sufferers aware of the disease's progress face increasing challenges to their mental health.

The disease was named in 1907 by Alois Alzheimer (1864–1915), after diagnosing a 51-year-old patient. Although there is currently no cure (in the early 2000s), there are many research projects underway worldwide, and researchers increasingly understand more about the disease.

Symptoms

Symptoms of Alzheimer's disease vary in rate of change from person to person. However, they generally include gradual loss of memory, particularly for recent events; dwindling powers of judgment, reasoning and understanding; disorientation; personality changes; an inability to perform normal activities of daily living; difficulty in learning; loss of language skills and general intellectual deterioration. The dementia is progressive, degenerative and irreversible, and eventually, patients become totally incapable of caring for themselves. For caregivers of Alzheimer's sufferers, it is a very frustrating and dehumanizing condition to witness. It has been referred to as "Old Timer's disease," although it may occur as early as age 40. More commonly, it occurs in those 65 years of age and older. It is the fourth leading cause of death for people over age 65. More women than men are affected, but that may be because women statistically outlive men. Alzheimer's disease is a major cause for admission to long-term care facilities and nursing homes.

Symptoms of Alzheimer's should not be confused with age-associated memory impairment (AAMI), a term health care professionals use to describe minor memory difficulties that come with age. According to the Alzheimer's Disease and Related Disorders Association, Inc., there are some differences between AAMI and Alzheimer's.

SOME DIFFERENCES BETWEEN AGE ASSOCIATED MEMORY IMPAIRMENT AND ALZHEIMER'S DISEASE

Activity	Alzheimer Patient	AAMI
Forgets	Whole experience	Part of an experience
Remembers later	Rarely	Often
Follows written or spoken directions	Gradually unable	Usually able
Able to use notes, reminders	Gradually unable	Usually able
Able to care for self	Gradually unable	Usually able

Diagnosis

Before a diagnosis of Alzheimer's disease is made, the physician will want to rule out other conditions, such as potentially reversible depression, adverse drug reactions, metabolic changes, nutritional deficiencies, head injuries and stroke. Before technologically sophisticated testing procedures became available, many sufferers were misdiagnosed and consequently mistreated. For example, screen star Rita Hayworth was misdiagnosed with alcoholic dementia in the 1970s; later she was diagnosed as suffering from Alzheimer's, and she died from the disease in 1987. Her stage career ended when she could not remember her lines. Former president Ronald Reagan's diagnosis of Alzheimer's disease was made public in 1994.

Caregivers of Alzheimer's Patients

The following guidelines, which may help reduce anxieties and stresses for caregivers, were compiled by the Pennsylvania Hospital, Philadelphia:

- Take one day at a time, tackling each problem as it arises. One cannot predict how an Alzheimer's patient will behave.

- Try to put yourself in the patient's shoes. You will feel less annoyed the tenth time you are asked what day it is if you imagine how unsettling it must be not to be oriented in time and space.

- Maintain a sense of humor. This is especially valuable in getting through potentially embarrassing situations.

- Arrange for time for yourself. Get another family member or friend to relieve you for an hour or two each day. Hire a part-time caretaker. Arrange for the patient to spend time at a senior day-care facility.

- Pay attention to your own needs. Be sure to maintain good nutrition and get regular exercise; develop hobbies and outside interests. Find people you can talk to such as family members, friends or, if needed, professional counselors.

Writing in *The Quill*, a publication of the Pennsylvania Hospital, Todd Iscovitz advised those who give care to AD patients to keep in mind that the elderly and afflicted never outgrow their need for love and affection. Being honest with yourself is most important when caring for a loved one. Know your limitations, and recognize when the burden of caregiving is too much. If your own health starts to fail, or if you are feeling overwhelmed, consider other care alternatives. These guidelines for caregivers also apply to caregivers of patients with other disorders as well.

Information Line and Support Groups

The Alzheimer's Association has a national, toll-free information and referral service telephone number. The 800 line offers callers the most current information available on Alzheimer's disease and support services through the association. The number is: (800) 272-3900.

The Alzheimer's Disease and Related Disorders Association (ARDRA) is a privately funded national voluntary health organization, founded in 1980 and headquartered in Chicago. ARDRA has more than 1,000 support groups and 160 chapters and affiliates nationwide. ARDRA's board of directors is comprised of business leaders, health professionals and family members. A medical and scientific advisory board consults on and monitors related issues.

To contact ADRA:

Alzheimer's Disease and Related Disorders
  Association
70 East Lake Street
Chicago, IL 60601
Phone: (312) 853-3060

The nationwide hot line number is (800) 621-0379.

See also DEPRESSION; MUSIC THERAPY; SUPPORT GROUPS.

Kahn, Ada P. *Stress A to Z: A Sourcebook for Facing Everyday Challenges.* New York: Facts On File, 1998.
O'Rourke, Norm. "Alzheimer's Disease as a Metaphor for Contemporary Fears of Aging." *Journal of the American Geriatrics Society.* 44, no. 2 (Feb. 1996): 220–21.
Reekum, Robert Van, Martine Simard, and Karl Farcnik. "Diagnosis of Dementia and Treatment of Alzheimer's Disease." *Canadian Family Physician* 45 (April 1999): 945–952.

Ambien   Trade name for zolpidem, a non-benzodiazepine hypnotic for treatment of insomnia.

ambisexuality   Sexual behavior related to erotic interest in both males and females. The term was introduced by Sandor Ferenczi (1873–1933), a Hungarian psychoanalyst and an associate and follower of Sigmund Freud, to identify the psychological aspects of bisexuality. Ambisexuality also refers to the possession of sexual characteristics that are both male and female, such as pubic hair.

See also TRANSSEXUALISM.

ambivalence   The existence of two sometimes contradictory feelings, attitudes, values or goals at the same time. For example, some individuals have feelings of ambivalence toward a mate whom they love but who abuses them. Other individuals are ambivalent about work and other major life issues. The term was introduced by Eugen Bleuler, a Swiss psychiatrist (1857–1939), to refer to the simultaneous feelings of antagonistic emotions, such as approach or avoidance of the same activity or goal. Ambivalence is a characteristic of some individuals who have schizophrenia.

See also AGORAPHOBIA; SCHIZOPHRENIA.

amentia   Subnormal development of the mind, particularly the intellectual capacities; a type of severe mental retardation.

See MENTAL RETARDATION.

American Association of Suicidology (AAS)   A not-for-profit, tax-exempt organization whose goal is to understand and prevent suicide and to help suicide prevention centers throughout the United States and Canada. The work of AAS includes promoting research, public awareness and training for professionals and volunteers. Membership includes mental health professionals, researchers, suicide prevention and crisis intervention centers, school districts, survivors of suicide and lay persons interested in suicide prevention. The AAS has developed standards for the certification of suicide prevention centers.

Contact:

American Association of Suicidology
4201 Connecticut Avenue NW, Suite 408
Washington, D.C. 20008
Phone: (202) 237-2280

Fax (202) 237-2282
Web site: www.suicidology.org

American Board of Medical Psychotherapists (ABMP)   An organization that provides training and certification to professionals who practice psychotherapy. The purpose of the ABMP is to apply high standards to the professional credentialing procedure and to encourage interdisciplinary excellence in medical psychotherapy and related methods of behavioral assessment and change. The ABMP was founded in 1982.

For information:

American Board of Medical Psychotherapists
Physicians' Park B, Suite 11
300 Twenty-first Avenue North
Nashville, TN 37203
Phone: (615) 327-2984

See also PSYCHOTHERAPY.

American Council for Drug Education   (CDE)
The purpose of the CDE is to educate the public about health hazards associated with use of psychoactive drugs and drug abuse, including persons suffering from serious underlying depression. The CDE promotes scientific findings, organizes conferences and seminars, provides media resources and publishes educational materials. The CDE was established in 1977 as the American Council on Marijuana and Other Psychoactive Drugs (ACM); the name was changed in 1983.

For information:

American Council for Drug Education
204 Monroe Street, Suite 110
Rockville, MD 20850
(310) 294-0600

American Medical Association (AMA)   An association of physicians and surgeons that keeps the medical profession abreast of progress in clinical medicine, pertinent research and developments. Its primary function is to promote the art and science of medicine, improve public health and provide advisory, interpretative and referral information on medicine and health care.

The association publishes the *Journal of the American Medical Association,* in which articles on mental

health frequently appear. The AMA is a source for statistics on mental health as well as other aspects of health, including brochures, pamphlets and library searches. A publication list is available.

Contact:

American Medical Association
515 N. State Street
Chicago, IL 60610
Phone: (312) 464-5000

American Psychiatric Association (APA)   A medical organization whose members specialize in psychiatry in the United States and Canada. The purposes of the APA include: (1) improving treatment, rehabilitation and care of the mentally ill; (2) promoting research; (3) advancing standards of all psychiatric services and facilities; and (4) educating medical professionals, scientists and the general public.

Founded in 1844 as the Association of Medical Superintendents of American Institutions for the Insane, it became the American Medico-Psychological Association in 1891 and adopted its present name in 1921.

The APA provides many services, including advisory, analytic, bibliographic and historical services and referrals and technical information on psychiatric care, psychiatric insurance and mental illness. The APA holds an annual meeting and publishes advance and postconvention news releases and articles on the proceedings. The American Psychiatric Association also publishes a regular tabloid-size newspaper for its members and many books and other publications that can be purchased by the public.

Contact:

American Psychiatric Association
1400 K Street NW
Washington, D.C. 20005
Phone: (888) 357-7924
Fax: (202) 682-6850
Web site: www.apa.psych.org

See also PSYCHOTHERAPIES.

American Psychological Association (APA)   A professional organization to which psychologists belong. The purpose, functions and services of the APA correspond to those of the American Psychiatric Association. The APA is a source of information and referrals on mental health concerns for professionals as well as the general public.

Contact:

American Psychological Association
750 First Street NE
Washington, D.C. 20002
Phone: (202) 336-5700 or (800) 374-3120
Web site: www.apa.org

amine A chemical produced by the central nervous system involved in the functioning of the brain. Some researchers indicate that depression may result from decreased levels of amines. Amines are technically known as biogenic amines or neurotransmitters and are chemical transmitters that nerves use to send messages to each other. Amines include norepinephrine, dopamine and serotonin.

See also BRAIN; CENTRAL NERVOUS SYSTEM; DOPAMINE; SEROTONIN.

amineptine An antidepressant drug not used in the United States.

See also ANTIDEPRESSANT MEDICATIONS.

aminobutyric acid, gamma See GAMMA-AMINOBUTYRIC ACID.

Amitid Trade name for amitriptyline, an antidepressant medication.

See also AMITRIPTYLINE; ANTIDEPRESSANT MEDICATIONS.

amitriptyline (amitriptyline hydrochloride)
One of the antidepressant drugs known as tricyclic antidepressants (one of two major classes of antidepressants). It is prescribed in the treatment of depressive episodes of major depression, bipolar disorder, dysthymic disorder and atypical depression. It has moderate to marked sedative action. However, because the sedative effect of amitriptyline interacts additively with the sedative effect of alcohol, alcohol consumption should be avoided by individuals taking amitriptyline, particularly if they drive a car or work in a hazardous occupation. Amitriptyline is sometimes prescribed for eating disorders in bulimic individuals and headaches associated with depression that are the result of nonorganic causes.

Amitriptyline is known by many trade names, such as: Endep, Elavil, Amitid, Domical, Lentizol, Triptafen and Triptizol.

See also ANTIDEPRESSANT MEDICATIONS; DEPRESSION; HEADACHES; TRICYCLIC ANTIDEPRESSANT MEDICATIONS.

American Medical Association. *AMA Drug Evaluations Annual, 1991.* Chicago: AMA, 1991.

amnesia Loss of memory; an inability to recall past experience. Amnesia may be due to many factors, including organic factors, such as a head injury, alcoholic intoxication, epileptic seizure, stroke or senile dementia, or psychological factors, such as the unconscious repression of painful experiences, in which the memory loss serves as a defense against anxiety.

One type of amnesia is an inability to remember recent happenings since the onset of amnesia (anterograde amnesia); the individual does not consolidate what is perceived into permanent memory storage or cannot retrieve recent memories from storage. Another type is a loss of remembrances before the memory disturbance began (retrograde amnesia). Episodic amnesia refers to a particular event or period from the individual's life that is forgotten. Fear of having amnesia is known as amnesiophobia.

Amnesic confabulation is a term applied to imagined occurrences unconsciously made up to fill gaps in memory; this occurs in Korsakoff's syndrome and other organic psychoses. Amnesic-confabulatory syndrome is another name for Korsakoff's syndrome.

See also ALZHEIMER'S DISEASE; REPRESSION.

amoxapine An antidepressant drug of the tricyclic class. It is generally more effective in major depression than in dysthymic or atypical depression. It has relatively weak sedative and anticholinergic activities compared with imipramine or amitriptyline. Amoxapine has a more rapid onset of action, but this finding has not been consistently observed in all patients. Amoxapine is known under the trade name Asendin.

See also ANTIDEPRESSANT MEDICATIONS.

amphetamine drugs Amphetamines and several chemically related drugs are central nervous system (CNS) stimulants that in small doses may give the user a feeling of increased mental alertness and a sense of well-being. As doses are increased, however, decreased appetite, excitement and tremor may occur, and tolerance and psychological dependence can develop with large doses. Thus amphetamines and other stimulants should be prescribed for specific purposes and only for a limited time. Rarely, amphetamines are used to treat adult attention-deficit hyperactivity disorder or to potentiate antidepressant medications in conditions resistant to conventional treatment.

Amphetamines are sometimes associated with dependence that can produce one or more organic mental disorders, including intoxication, delirium, delusional syndrome or withdrawal syndrome. Because of the possibility of developing dependency on amphetamines, many physicians no longer prescribe them.

Some individuals may take amphetamines in combination with alcohol in an attempt to counteract the depressant effects of alcohol. Although there may be some possible antagonism of the depressant effects of alcohol of the CNS, there is no improvement of impaired motor coordination, and the combination may produce a dangerous sense of false security. High levels of amphetamines and alcohol may produce gastrointestinal upsets. If amphetamines are taken with foods or beverages containing tyramine, an excessive rise in blood pressure may occur.

Amphetamine psychosis occurs in a more chronic form after prolonged use of the drugs. The psychotic symptoms can be difficult to distinguish from schizophrenia. Symptoms may include talkativeness, hyperactivity, repetitive behavior, grinding the teeth, suspiciousness and, in more severe cases, paranoia, hallucinations and delusions.

Crashing is the term used to denote the symptoms that occur with sudden withdrawal of amphetamines, including drowsiness, fatigue, apathy and severe depression. Individuals who "crash" need sleep as well as physical and emotional support.

Amphetamines are popularly referred to as "speed." They include dextroamphetamines, methamphetamines and methylphenidates.

See also ADDICTION; DEPRESSION.

Waldinger, Robert J. *Psychiatry for Medical Students.* Washington, D.C.: American Psychiatric Press, 1990.

amphetamine psychosis See AMPHETAMINE DRUGS.

amygdala A small, almond-shaped organ within the brain located below the cerebral cortex. Part of the limbic system, the amygdala is thought to be involved in memory and a wide range of internal activities including digestion and excretion, heart rate, arterial blood pressure, muscle tone, sexual activity and aggression and may also be involved in reactions to fear and avoidance.

See also BRAIN; LIMBIC SYSTEM.

anabolic steroids Steroids are chemical derivatives of, or structurally similar to, testosterone, the major male hormone. Some steroids have legitimate purposes. For example, they are used to treat certain kinds of anemia and specific cancers. When used for these purposes, doses are carefully controlled and administered by injection, often in three- to six-week intervals. However, anabolic steroids have been used illegally by athletes to build muscle mass. In these cases, the drug is administered orally and often on a daily basis, sometimes exceeding legitimate dosage levels by as much as 20 times.

Steroids can cause mental health problems. These drugs have been reported to cause changes in brain wave activity and to increase moodiness, depression, listlessness and the violent, aggressive behavior sometimes known as "body builders' psychosis."

See also HORMONES; SUBSTANCE ABUSE; TESTOSTERONE.

Media Resource Guide on Common Drugs of Abuse. Public Relations Society of America, National Capital Chapter, Fairfax, Va., September 1990.

Anafranil Trade name of clomipramine, a tricyclic antidepressant that is also used to induce remission of symptoms in some individuals who have obsessive-compulsive disorder.

See also ANTIDEPRESSANT MEDICATIONS; OBSESSIVE-COMPULSIVE DISORDER; TRICYCLIC ANTIDEPRESSANT DRUGS.

anal character In psychoanalysis, a pattern of personality traits believed to stem from the anal phase of psychosexual development, when defecation was a primary source of pleasure. The theory holds that a child who derives satisfaction from retention of feces tends to develop personality traits of frugality, obstinacy and orderliness. As an adult, such an individual may be compulsive, meticulous, rigid and very conscientious.

See also PERSONALITY; PERSONALITY DISORDERS.

anal fantasy A fantasy of anal intercourse or anal pregnancy and childbirth, sometimes reported by children. Psychoanalytic theory suggests that such fantasies may manifest themselves as gastrointestinal symptoms in later years. Some adults also fantasize about anal sexually related activities.

anal stage According to Sigmund Freud's psychosexual development theory, the anal stage is the second stage of development (the first is the oral stage). Maturation continues, with one area of the body maturing before the child is aware of the next. Around the first birthday, the anal zone becomes the source of interest to the infant and the parents. The infant becomes aware of a full rectum and later develops control over the innate urges. During this stage, the child may consider producing feces as a gift to the parents and social environment or as something to withhold with stubbornness. Thus the anal area and associated activities become a means of interacting with the child's environment. Subsequent stages of development are the phallic stage, latency stage, and genital stage.

See also FREUD, SIGMUND; GENITAL STAGE; LATENCY; PHALLIC STAGE.

analgesia Absence of sensitivity to pain. This can be produced by medications given for the relief of pain and can also occur in some rare emotional and physical disorders such as conversion hysteria. In this disorder, part of the body may develop analgesia not related to known patterns of neurological pain perception. Analgesia can also sometimes be achieved with hypnosis, which was used to reduce pain of surgery before the discovery of other anesthesia.

An analgesic is a drug or other agent that relieves pain without causing loss of consciousness. Analgesic drugs act on the central nervous system to reduce the ability of the body to feel pain. The most widely used drugs are aspirin and related compounds that provide inexpensive and fast relief for many everyday aches and pain, such as minor headaches and cold symptoms. In addition to relieving pain, aspirin and related medications combat fever and reduce inflammation that leads to pain. These drugs are not addictive, but for some people they are irritating to the lining of the digestive tract. Some people are allergic to aspirin and must take aspirin substitutes for pain.

For severe pain, morphine and chemically related drugs provide relief. Such drugs also produce a mild sensation of freedom from anxiety, which somewhat reduces the psychological reaction to pain. However, drugs in this group have disadvantages of depressing breathing in high doses and creating drug dependence or addiction when used without close supervision.

In some disease conditions, such as tabes dorsalis, the pain pathways on the spinal cord become affected. In the nerves, the fibers for pain, pressure, touch and temperature are usually combined. When they reach the spinal cord, the fibers are separated. As pain and temperature are nearly always in the same pathway, both senses can be lost at the same time.

See also PAIN.

analysand The individual undergoing psychoanalysis.

See also ANALYST; PSYCHOANALYSIS.

analysis See PSYCHOANALYSIS.

analyst The term usually refers to therapists who follow the teachings of psychoanalysis as outlined by Sigmund Freud (1856–1939) to help restore mental health. However, the term also applies to analysts who adhere to the ideas of Heinz Kohut (1913–1981) and also Adolf Meyer (1866–1950), who coined the term "psychobiologist" for psychiatrists who consider both psychological and biological (medical) factors. Other analysts who follow fundamentals of Carl Jung (1875–1961) are known as analytical psychologists; those who follow Alfred Adler (1870–1937) are individual psychologists.

See also FREUD, SIGMUND; KOHUT, HEINZ; PSYCHO-ANALYSIS; SELF PSYCHOLOGY.

Anatomy of Melancholy An early volume on physical and mental health, compiled by Robert Burton (1577–1640), an English clergyman and writer. The work concerns the historical background of mental health, and it contains sections on causes, symptoms and treatment of melancholy (depression). The book indicates early connections between mental disorders and environmental conditions. Burton recommended special hospitals, pensions for the elderly and free housing for the poor; he also believed in witches and thought that witches could cure melancholy.

See also DEPRESSION; MIND/BODY CONNECTIONS.

Cox, Maksimov. "Burton's Anatomy of Melancholy: Philosophically, Medically and Historically: Part 2." *History of Psychiatry* no. 27 (Sept. 1996): 343–360.

androgens See HORMONES.

anger An intense emotional state in which one feels a high level of displeasure and frustration. The spectrum of anger may range from slight irritation to explosive hostility. Anger is a source of energy that is discharged on others, objects or oneself. Anger is sometimes related to and involved with agitation and aggression.

Physiological changes occur when one feels angry. Anger increases the heart rate, blood pressure and flow of adrenaline. Suppressed anger may result in hypertension, skin rashes and headaches.

Some typical characteristics of anger include frowning, gritting the teeth, pacing and clenching the hands. There may be changes in vocal tone. One may yell or shout, or the person may speak in short, clipped sentences. During anger, some people may attempt to gain control of a situation or clearly demonstrate that they have lost control themselves.

Most people at times are caught between two attitudes with regard to anger. According to psychological and medical opinion, suppressed anger is physically and psychologically damaging, yet there are social pressures that at different levels label angry behavior destructive, illegal or unsophisticated. Further limiting expression of anger is the feeling that such behavior may bring regrets later.

Anger seems to be most directly related to frustration and feelings of inferiority. Bigotry or generally negative thinking appears to be anger turned against specific groups or humanity as a whole. Some mental health professionals believe, as Sigmund Freud observed in "Mourning and Melancholia," that feelings of depression are actually anger turned inward, directed at the self. Adults who express anger directly with physical violence or verbal abuse usually do so because they model their behavior on others in their environment or because there seems to be a reward for violent behavior. In American frontier society, for example, violent behavior was common and usually considered admirable. Since it is unacceptable in most situations to express anger directly, many people react by becoming sulky or indifferent or by adopting a superior, patronizing attitude toward the person or situation that angered them.

A baby's first cries may be an expression of anger or simply a less focused reaction to the birth experience. Small children do react most directly to situations that make them angry, sometimes by simply screaming or pulling or striking the object or person who has angered them. As children mature, angry behavior becomes focused on retaliation. By the early teens, sulking and impertinence have replaced retaliation. In both children and adults, hunger and fatigue increase the potential for anger. Researchers believe that anger is a product of the most primitive part of the brain that is capable of operating and becomes more dominant when other mental powers are impaired by illness or alcohol.

Constructive Anger

Anger may be constructive. The exercise that an individual chooses to use to work off anger will do him or her good in other ways. Releasing an angry feeling sometimes brings with it a sense of pleasure. Some mental health professionals equate ambition and attempts to improve society with a healthy expression of anger.

Among athletes, anger can have a harmful effect on athletic performance. Anger drains energy and diverts attention from what must be done at the moment. However, professional athletes are trained to recover quickly from events that arouse anger. In some cases, anger may make a player more forceful and positive.

Overcoming Anger

An individual in psychotherapy who expresses extremely angry feelings might be given three goals: first, to identify the feelings of anger; second, to use constructive release of the energy of anger and third, to identify thought and thought processes that lead to anger. For example, to identify feelings of anger, one might keep a diary of angry feelings and learn to recognize anger before losing control. The individual will learn to take responsibility for his or her own emotions and stop blaming others for arousing the anger. In addition, with validation from a therapist, the individual will learn to accept that some anger is justified in certain situations. In learning to use constructive release of the energy of anger, the individual may benefit from assertiveness training and learn to express anger verbally to the appropriate source. Assertive techniques will help the individual increase his or her feelings of self-esteem, demonstrate internal control over behavior and harness energy generated by the anger in a nondestructive manner. One will also learn to use energy through physical activity that involves the large muscles, such as running, walking or playing a racket sport.

Anger and Grief

After a loved one dies, it is common to feel angry. The anger may be directed toward the person who died, for leaving the other person alone. Or the anger may be directed toward the medical care system for not being able to cure a disease or mend a body after an accident. In cases of accidents, often there is anger at a drunk driver or a person who has taken drugs and committed a crime or at the drug dealer who sold the drugs taken by the perpetrator of the loved one's death. Anger is a normal part of the cycle of the grief reaction. However, prolonged anger that leads to depression may indicate a need to consult a mental health professional.

See also AGITATION; AGGRESSION; ANXIETY; DEPRESSION; GRIEF.

Callwood, June. *Love, Hate, Fear, Anger and Other Lively Emotions.* Van Nuys, Calif.: Newcastle Publishing Co., 1964.

Goldstein, A. P. "Aggression." In *Encyclopedia of Psychology,* vol. 1., edited by Raymond J. Corsini. New York: Wiley, 1984.

McFarland, Gertrude K., and Mary Durand Thomas. *Psychiatric Mental Health Nursing.* Philadelphia: J. B. Lippincott, 1991.

angina pectoris   A type of chest pain and discomfort that may be a symptom related to heart problems. Angina pectoris is not a sharp pain but rather a sensation of pressure, squeezing or tightness. Usually it starts in the center of the chest under the breastbone (sternum) and radiates to the throat area. Typically, the pains are along the inside of the left arm, part of the wrist, a few fingers and the shoulder. Symptoms of angina are usually due to muscle fibers of the heart not getting enough blood through the coronary arteries to nourish them.

Chest pains cause some individuals great mental anguish because they fear that they are having a heart attack and they also fear hearing a diagnosis from a physician. However, all chest pains should be carefully diagnosed by a physician as soon as possible. Most chest pains are not angina but are caused by emotional tension, strain of the chest muscles, referred pain from a spinal disk, indigestion, ulcers, lung problems or other disease not directly related to the heart. Knowing the source of a chest pain can reassure an individual and put her mind at rest concerning the condition of her heart.

Typically, an angina symptom appears when a person exerts himself and disappears when he rests. Most attacks last for only two or three minutes, but if they are set off by anger or other emotional tension and the individual cannot relax, they may last 10 minutes or longer.

Individuals who have angina pectoris should become aware of what it is that precedes attacks and learn to avoid those situations. Typically, such individuals are advised to reduce fat in their diet, lose weight, possibly take antianxiety medications when they feel extremely anxious and stop smoking (if they are smokers), as tobacco may provide an angina attack by speeding up the heartbeat, constructing blood vessels and raising blood pressure.

Treatment for angina pectoris includes immediate rest and a nitroglycerin tablet dissolved under the tongue. Some people take this drug as a preventive measure if they are subject to attacks and are going through a period of unusual stress. Amyl nitrite is another drug that can be administered by inhalation. When neither drug is available, a sip of whisky or brandy may be helpful.

See also CHRONIC ILLNESS.

angst   A feeling of anxiety. Angst is a central concept in the existentialist approach to psychology, which interprets the essence of human existence by emphasizing basic human values such as self-awareness, love and free will. The word "angst" is derived from the German term meaning "fear, anxiety, anguish."

See also ANXIETY; FEAR.

anhedonia   A diminished capacity to enjoy or experience pleasure in situations or acts that normally would be pleasurable. Anhedonia is a marker for classic depression states. Anhedonia, also known as dystychia, in extreme forms may be a symptom of schizophrenia or a depressive disorder. The word "anhedonia" was coined by Ribot, a French psychologist, to refer to "an insensibility relating to pleasure alone," in contrast to "analgesia," or the absence of pain. Anhedonia was described as a schizophrenic symptom by Kraepelin and Bleuler, although both psychopathologists viewed anhedonia as only one facet of the deterioration of the emotional life of the individual.

Freud associated loss of capacity for enjoyment with the repression that accompanies neurotic conflict. Behavioral clinicians have suggested that changes in a person's reinforcement schedule or a change of reinforcers may shape depressive behavior, also causing anhedonia.

See also DEPRESSION; SCHIZOPHRENIA.

Fawcett, Jan; David C. Clark; William A. Scheftner; and Robert D. Gibbons. "Assessing Anhedonia in Psychiatric Patients." *Archives of General Psychiatry* 40 (Jan. 1983).

anniversary reaction   Feelings of anxiety or other symptoms that arise around the anniversary of a significant event, such as a divorce or the death of a family member or close friend. The reaction brings anxieties because it may involve the recall and reliving of the events. Some individuals experience dreams or minor illness at the same time each year. Anniversary reactions are often common when an individual has experienced a traumatic event.

See also ANXIETY DISORDERS; GRIEF; POST-TRAUMATIC STRESS DISORDER.

Campbell, Robert Jean. *Psychiatric Dictionary.* New York: Oxford University Press, 1981.

anomaly   Anything that is abnormal or irregular or a deviation from the natural order, such as a structure that varies significantly from the normal. For example, an individual who has an extra X or Y sex chromosome, a female without an external vaginal opening or a male with three testicles is said to be an anomaly. A person whose sexual practices are outside his or her society's usual habits is also referred to as an anomaly.

anomie   Apathy, alienation and personal distress resulting from the loss of previously valued goals.

anorexia nervosa   See EATING DISORDERS.

anorgasmia (anorgasmy)   Inability to achieve orgasm. This term has been replaced with psychosexual dysfunction and refers to lack of orgasm that may be caused by sociocultural attitudes of the partners, anatomical or neurophysiological problems or fear of painful intercourse. Sex therapy is helpful in many such cases.

See also FRIGIDITY; PSYCHOSEXUAL DYSFUNCTIONS; SEX THERAPY.

Antabuse Trade name of the generic drug disulfiram, used to deter consumption of alcohol by individuals being treated for alcoholism. When a person taking Antabuse consumes alcohol, a severe reaction usually follows, including vomiting, breathing difficulty, headache and, occasionally, collapse and coma. Reaction to Antabuse begins within five to 10 minutes after ingesting alcohol and may last from 30 minutes to several hours, depending on the amount of alcohol in the body.

Antabuse works by interfering with the metabolism of alcohol in the liver by causing a toxic buildup of acetaldehyde. Antabuse is prescribed with the individual's full knowledge and consent. It should not be taken by pregnant women.

See also ALCOHOLISM.

O'Brien, Robert, and Morris Chafetz. *The Encyclopedia of Alcoholism.* New York: Facts On File, 1982.

antianxiety medications Also known as anxiolytics, these are medications prescribed to reduce anxiety and tension. They are sometimes referred to as minor tranquilizers. Antianxiety drugs are prescribed for many individuals during times of stress and in treatment of stress-related physical disorders. Antianxiety drugs or anxiolytics include those in the benzodiazepine class, such as alprazolam (Xanax), lorazepam (Ativan), diazepam (Valium) and chlordiazepoxide (Librium). Some are shorter acting because of more rapid body metabolism. While relatively nontoxic when first taken, they can reduce alertness (making driving inadvisable) and cause potentiation of alcohol (multiplying its sedative effects), and individuals prone to abuse drugs and alcohol can become dependent on them. They should not be stopped suddenly if taken regularly over two weeks because of possible withdrawal symptoms (nausea, sweats, tremulous feelings, possibly seizures) but should be gradually tapered or reduced in dose over two to four weeks. These medications are used to treat anxiety disorders or adjustment disorders with anxiety. Alprazolam (Xanax) is approved by the Food and Drug Administration for the treatment

of panic disorder. Non-benzodiazepine anxiolytics such as buspirone have been developed but do not have immediate effects. Meprobamate and phenobarbital were once used but have high toxicity if used in overdose and have more serious addictive properties.

See also ANXIETY.

anticholinergic medications A group of drugs that block effects of acetylcholine, a chemical released from nerve endings in the parasympathetic division of the peripheral autonomic nervous system in the brain. (The parasympathetic nervous system produces relaxation, calmness, digestion and sleep.) Anticholinergic drugs are used in the treatment of irritable bowel syndrome, certain types of urinary incontinence and in nervous system disorders, such as Parkinson's disease.

Well-known natural substances with anticholinergic effects are atropine (used as a drug to dilate the eye) and scopalamine (a plant substance used with morphine to induce sleep). Some antidepressants and antipsychotic drugs have anticholinergic effects; these side effects sometimes include extreme dryness of the mouth, abnormal retention of urine, constipation, blurred near vision, short term memory loss and mental confusion in high doses. All are reversible by changing dosage or stopping the medications.

See also AGORAPHOBIA; ANTIDEPRESSANT MEDICATIONS; DEPRESSION.

anticipatory anxiety The anxiety an individual feels when thinking about an anxiety-producing situation, such as an approaching examination, a visit to the dentist or a difficult interview. Individuals who have phobias experience anticipatory anxiety when the possibility of facing their feared stimulus occurs.

See also ANXIETY; PHOBIA.

anticipatory grief See GRIEF.

anticonvulsant medications A group of prescription drugs that prevent convulsions or limit their frequency or severity; also known as antiepileptics. In high doses, minor tranquilizers and hypnotic drugs may act as anticonvulsants. Many anticonvulsants are central nervous system depressants and also reduce some symptoms of anxiety.

See also MINOR TRANQUILIZERS.

antidepressant medications Prescription drugs used to counteract depression. Antidepressants are available only by prescription, and because depressive symptoms are merely suppressed, not cured, by these drugs, they are usually prescribed for three to six months or more until the symptoms remit on their own. These medications are also frequently used in conjunction with some type of psychotherapy.

Commonly, antidepressant medications take up to two to three weeks before having a full effect (although side effects may begin immediately). The time elapsing before the drug becomes therapeutic varies with the drug. Antidepressants may have to be taken regularly for months, even years in the case of patients with prior depressive episodes, if their gains are to persist. Relapse often occurs upon stopping the drug.

Most drugs used to treat depression either mimic certain neurotransmitters (biochemicals that allow brain cells to communicate with each another) or alter their activity. Antidepressants are thought to reverse the depletion or decrease activity of these neurotransmitters that occurs during depression. Two of the major neurotransmitters involved appear to be norepinephrine and serotonin. The precise pharmacologic mechanisms of antidepressant drugs, as well as the balances of neurotransmitters in individuals who have depression, are still not entirely understood. As newer, more specific antidepressants are developed, understanding of antidepressants and depression evolves.

Antidepressant medications were developed during the 1950s after physicians noticed that tuberculosis patients treated with iproniazid sometimes became extremely cheerful. The notion that this elevated mood might be a side effect of the drug led to the development of a class of antidepressants known as monoamine oxidase inhibitors. They were followed by the tricyclic antidepressants and lithium.

There are five major categories of antidepressants: tricyclic antidepressants (TCAs), monoamine oxidase (MAO) inhibitors, lithium, serotonin specific reuptake inhibitors (SSRI) and novel antidepressants such as trazodone and bupropion.

ANTIDEPRESSANT MEDICATIONS

Trade Name	Generic Name
Tricyclic antidepressants	
Elavil, Endep	amitriptyline
Asendin	amoxapine
Anafranil	clomipramine
Norpramin, Pertofrane	desipramine
Sinequan, Adapin	doxepin
Tofranil, Janimine	imipramine
Ludiomil	maprotiline
Aventyl, Pamelor	nortriptyline
Vivactil	protriptyline
Surmontil	trimipramine
Monoamine oxidase inhibitors (MAOIs)	
Marplan	isocarboxazid
Eutonyl	pargyline
Nardil	phenelzine
Parnate	tranylcypromine
Examples of "Novel" antidepressants	
Wellbutrin	bupropion
Prozac	fluoxetine
Desyrel	trazodone
Zoloft	sertraline
Paxil	paroxetine
Serzone	nefazodone
Effexor	venlafaxine
Remeron	mirtazapine
Celexa	citalopram

Tricyclic Antidepressants

Tricyclic antidepressants are referred to as "tricyclic" because the chemical diagrams for these drugs resemble three rings connected together. An example of a tricyclic antidepressant is imipramine, which was first synthesized in the 1940s.

Tricyclics elevate mood, alertness and mental and physical activity and improve appetite and sleep patterns in depressed individuals. When given to a nondepressed person, tricyclics do not elevate mood or stimulate the person; instead, the effects are likely to increase anxiety and arouse feelings of unhappiness.

Tricyclic antidepressants are generally well tolerated and relatively safe, with minimal side effects. Their antidepressant effects, however, often take several weeks to appear, for reasons not yet well understood. Because of this lag, tricyclics are not prescribed on an "as-needed" basis.

Some depressed individuals may respond well to one tricyclic but not at all to another. Because of the time lag of several weeks before any beneficial effects are apparent, the physician will first try one drug for that time and then, if results are not achieved, prescribe another tricyclic, again for several weeks. Such trials, with their waiting and uncertainty, may lead to some anxiety and frustration for both the individual and the physician.

Some of the more well known tricyclic antidepressants (and their trade names) are shown in the table on page 38.

Side effects. Side effects of tricyclic antidepressants include excessively dry mouth, sweating, blurred vision, headache, urinary hesitation and constipation. Drowsiness and dizziness, as well as vertigo, weakness, rapid heart rate and reduced blood pressure upon standing upright, are likely to occur early on but usually disappear within the first several weeks. Tricyclics should be used cautiously in persons with heart problems and in elderly patients who may not break them down as rapidly as other adults.

Drug interactions and cautions. Tricyclic antidepressants and MAO inhibitors are not recommended to be combined except under unusual circumstances by a physician expert in their use. Although very rare, a severe interaction between the two drugs can occur; in extreme cases, convulsions, seizures and coma can occur. A more common drug interaction involves the combination of tricyclics and alcohol, and possibly other sedatives, as tricyclics increase effects of these substances. Use of other anticholinergic drugs will increase likelihood of anticholinergic side effects.

Monoamine Oxidase (MAO) Inhibitors

MAO inhibitors (or MAOIs) are primarily used for individuals who have not responded adequately to tricyclic antidepressants or serotonin reuptake inhibitors. Because of a wider range of potential, often unpredictable complications, use is limited. However, MAO inhibitors may be prescribed for certain types of depressions, generalized anxiety and phobic disorders and are used to help individuals who have panic attacks.

When a tricyclic antidepressant is tried and discontinued because of ineffectiveness, a gap of ten days is recommended before the monoamine oxidase inhibitor is prescribed. Tricyclic antidepressants and MAO inhibitors may be cautiously combined by physicians experienced in the use of this combination. In the reverse case, where the MAO inhibitor is ineffective and is to be replaced by a tricyclic, a period of two weeks between medications is recommended.

Interactive effects. A drawback of the MAO inhibitors, as a group, is that they may lead to unpredictable and occasionally serious interactions with some foods and drugs. For example, combining MAO inhibitors with a class of drugs called sympathomimetic drugs may lead to serious complications. Common nasal decongestant sprays often include phenylpropanolamine or phenylephrine, both sympathomimetics. Cough and cold preparations or any preparation not specifically recommended by a physician should also be avoided. The pain drug Demerol should not be given with MAOIs, but other pain-relieving drugs, such as morphine, can safely be used.

Individuals taking MAO inhibitors must conform to a special diet that avoids the amino acid tyramine or they may experience a dangerous rise in blood pressure. Tyramine is present in many foods, including alcoholic beverages, aged cheese, liver, fava beans and chocolate.

A side effect of monoamine oxidase inhibitors is that they lower blood pressure, an effect not well understood by researchers.

Lithium

Lithium is effective in individuals who have both depression and mania and in preventing future episodes. It acts without causing sedation but, like the tricyclics and MAO inhibitors, requires a period of use before its actions take effect. Side effects of lithium may rule it out for use as an antidepressant; there may be nausea and vomiting, muscular weakness and confusion.

Other Treatments

Amphetamines and related psychostimulant drugs, such as methylphenidate (a mild central nervous system stimulant), are sometimes used as antidepressants. While they may bring on temporary mood elevation, their prescription for such purposes is controversial, as they are subject to abuse. Some physicians try amphetamines for short-term use in certain patients and may also prescribe amphetamines diagnostically to determine more rapidly the value of moving on to tricyclic antidepressants and rarely to potentiate antidepressant medications in treatment-resistant depression. More recently, stimulants have been added to antidepressants to augment their effects in the case of a partial response.

Alprazolam may lift moderately severe depression, although it is primarily a drug used to treat anxiety. In some individuals, alprazolam has shortened or interfered with panic attacks and also induced sleep. In depressed individuals with a high level of anxiety, alprazolam may be added to tricyclic antidepressants.

New Developments of Antidepressant Medications

The development of innovative antidepressants combined with more precise research approaches holds great promise for the understanding and more effective treatment of affective disorders. In the last several decades, while conventional antidepressants have been helpful for many individuals, limitations of these antidepressants have been noted, namely their lack of specificity of action, delayed onset of action, side-effect profile and potential for lethality in overdose. Approximately 20 to 30 percent of depressed persons do not respond to traditional antidepressants.

Similarly, electroconvulsive therapy has drawbacks, such as the potential for short term cognitive deficits and problems associated with sustaining the antidepressant response. Over the last several years, newer antidepressants have emerged, such as sertraline, paroxetine, fluoxetine and bupropion, that offer the advantages of antidepressants with more favorable side-effect profiles and a decreased potential for lethality in overdose. However, research has shown that while these agents have unique side-effect profiles, their overall efficacy appears to be no greater than conventional antidepressant treatments and they also have a delayed onset of action.

The goal of recently developed antidepressants is to act faster and with more power than previously

used antidepressants, with less frequent and less severe side effects and with more ability to target an individual's specific type of depression. Newer antidepressants are not tricyclic or the monoamine oxidase inhibitors. They are unicyclic, bicyclic or of other molecular configurations. Whereas tricyclics and MAO inhibitors are understood to influence chemicals known as neurotransmitters, the newer antidepressants are technically classified by their preferential influence over individual neurotransmitters—norepinephrine and serotonin.

Selective Serotonin Reuptake Inhibitors

Fluoxetine, sertraline and paroxetine are compounds which are part of a new class of selective serotonin reuptake inhibitors (SSRIs) with low toxicity and free of many side effects attributed to tricyclic antidepressants. They are not sedative, have no anticholinergic side effects and do not promote weight gain.

Like other antidepressant drugs, SSRI medications do not help everyone with depression. They have their own unique side effects, including possible nausea, weight loss—both usually time limited—insomnia and rarely anxious agitation that is dose related.

See also ADVERSE DRUG REACTIONS; AGORAPHOBIA; ANXIOLYTIC MEDICATIONS; BENZODIAZEPINE DRUGS; DEPRESSION; MANIC-DEPRESSIVE ILLNESS; POSTPARTUM DEPRESSION; SEDATIVE DRUG.

Ballenger, James C. "Pharmacotherapy of the Panic Disorders." *Journal of Clinical Psychiatry* 47; no. 6, supplement (June 1986).

Doctor, Ronald M., and Ada P. Kahn. *Encyclopedia of Phobias, Fears, and Anxieties.* 2nd ed. New York: Facts On File, 2000.

Fawcett, Jan, Bernard Golden, and Nancy Rosenfeld. *New Hope for People with Bipolar Disorder.* Roseville, Calif.: Prima, 2000.

Fawcett, Jan et al. "Fluoxetine Versus Amitriptyline in Adult Outpatients with Major Depression." *Current Therapeutic Research* 45, no. 5 (May 1989).

Hollister, Leo E., M.D. "Pharmacotherapeutic Considerations in Anxiety Disorders." *Journal of Clinical Psychiatry* 47, no. 6, supplement (June 1986).

Ostraw, David, M.D. "The New Generation of Antidepressants: Promising Innovations or Disappointments?" *Journal of Clinical Psychiatry* 46, no. 10, Sec. 2 (Oct. 1985).

Zajecka, John M., and Jan Fawcett. "Recent Advances in the Treatment of Depression." *Current Opinion in Psychiatry* 4 (1991).

antimanic medications A group of drugs that reduce symptoms of mania or manic episodes of manic-depressive illness. Antimanics are also used as neuroleptics (major tranquilizers or antipsychotics). The major types of antimanics are butyrophenones, lithium, phenothiazines and anticonvulsants.

Antimanic medications reduce the agitation and lack of control seen in mania but may cause sedation; lithium produces this effect somewhat more slowly (5–10 days) without sedation and is useful in preventing recurrences that are usual without prophylactic treatment.

Certain anticonvulsant medications will reduce mania more rapidly. These include clonazepam (trade name: Klonopin); lorazepam (Ativan), which may be given by injection like some neuroleptics; and carbamazepine (Tegretol) and divalproex sodium (Depakote), which act more rapidly and have long-term effects with sedation or the side effects of neuroleptics.

Each of the types of antimanic drugs produces somewhat different pharmacologic actions. Lithium is particularly effective in preventing relapses in manic-depressive illness. Other drugs with antimanic effects are haloperidol and chlorpromazine.

See also ANTIDEPRESSANT MEDICATIONS; BUTYROPHENONES; LITHIUM CARBONATE; MANIC-DEPRESSIVE ILLNESS; PHENOTHIAZINE DRUGS.

antipsychotic medications Medications used to treat serious psychotic illness sometimes with the risk of homicide or suicide. Although they have side effects and certain serious risks, they are currently the best available treatments for acute and chronic psychoses. Monitored carefully by a physician experienced in their use, they can be beneficial and safely used and often represent the only available treatment in carefully selected patients.

These medications are used to relieve symptoms of psychotic illnesses including thought disorders, hallucinations, delusions, bizarre behavior and agitation. They are useful in chronic schizophrenia because they reduce the rate of exacerbation. While primarily prescribed for schizophrenia and related illnesses (schizophreniform disorder, schizoaffective disorder), antipsychotics are also prescribed to psychotic patients who have mood disorders and organic mental disorders. They are also prescribed usually in lower doses to control behavior in some mentally retarded individuals, as well as individuals with borderline personality disorder, organic disorders and Tourette Syndrome. Antipsychotics are also known as neuroleptics because of their capacity to block dopamine receptors.

How Antipsychotic Drugs Work

Antipsychotic drugs work on receptors in the brain to influence emotional behavior. Although the exact mechanisms of action are not clearly understood, most antipsychotics are known to inhibit transmission of nerve impulses in the central nervous system (CNS) by blocking the action of dopamine, a neurotransmitter, at certain receptor sites.

Antipsychotics have a number of adverse drug reactions. For example, reserpine is no longer used as an antipsychotic because it has been known to produce depression and low blood pressure. Antipsychotic drugs are not usually appropriate for use with anxiety reactions in the absence of severe psychotic symptoms. A new class of "atypical" antipsychotic medications have been introduced and found effective. Clozapine (Clozaril) was found to reduce both negative (lack of initiative, motivation and social interest) as well as cognitive (capacity to think) symptoms in schizophrenia. Since clozapine has significant side effects and can cause aplastic anemia in a small percentage of cases, frequent blood tests to measure white and red blood cells are considered necessary. Since then safer "atypical" antipsychotic medications such as resperidone (Resperdal), olanzapine (Zyprexa), quetiapine (Seroquel) and ziprasidone (Geodon) have been approved for use in schizophrenia.

Side Effects/Adverse Effects

Side effects occur with therapeutic doses; close and critical observation by a physician is essential for therapeutic effects. Side effects include sedation and extrapyramidal effects, such as acute dystonia (a state of abnormal muscle tension), akathisia (restlessness, agitation) and Parkinsonism (rigidity, shuffling gait, hypersalivation and masklike facial appearance), all of which are reversible by dose change or a medication to prevent these effects. Tardive dyskinesia (unwanted movements of the face, jaw, tongue, trunk and extremities and restless movements) can occur with greater likelihood over time (risk increases about 4 percent per year of exposure, and effects can be permanent, especially if medications are not stopped). Clozapine thus far has not been found to have a significant risk of tardive dyskinesia but can produce epileptic seizures and dangerous decrease of white blood cell levels, which can be fatal if not monitored by weekly blood tests.

Individuals taking antipsychotics usually participate in informed-consent procedures. A physician may also wish to inform relatives or other responsible persons of the risks and benefits of treatment as well as the early symptoms of tardive dyskinesia, which are often unnoticed by the patient. Neuroleptic malignant syndrome is a rare but major adverse effect.

See also ADVERSE DRUG REACTIONS; HALLUCINATION; SCHIZOPHRENIA; TARDIVE DYSKINESIA.

American Medical Association. *AMA Drug Evaluations Annual, 1991.* Chicago: AMA, 1991.
Andreason, Nancy D., and Donald W. Black. *Introductory Textbook of Psychiatry.* Washington, D.C.: American Psychiatric Association, 1991.

antisocial personality disorder   Characteristics include a consistent pattern of behavior that is intolerant of the conventional behavioral limitations imposed by a society, an inability to sustain a job over a period of years, disregard for the rights of others (either through exploitiveness or criminal behavior), frequent physical fights and, quite commonly, child or spouse abuse without remorse and a tendency to blame others. There is often a facade of charm and even sophistication that masks disregard, lack of remorse for mistreatment of others and the need to control others.

Although characteristics of this disorder describe criminals, they also may befit some individuals who are prominent in business or politics whose habits of self-centeredness and disregard for the rights of others may be hidden prior to a public scandal.

During the 19th century, this type of personality disorder was referred to as moral insanity. The term described immoral, guiltless behavior that was not accompanied by impairments in reasoning.

According to the classification system used in the *Diagnostic and Statistical Manual of Mental Disorders* 4th ed. antisocial personality disorder is one of the four "dramatic" personality disorders, the others being borderline, histrionic and narcissistic.

See also CONDUCT DISORDER; PERSONALITY; PERSONALITY DISORDERS.

Andreason, Nancy C., and Donald W. Black. *Introductory Textbook of Psychiatry.* Washington, D.C.: American Psychiatric Association, 1991.
Davis, Kenneth; Howard Klar; and Joseph T. Coyle. *Foundations of Psychiatry.* Philadelphia: W. B. Saunders, 1991.

anxiety   Uneasiness, apprehension and tension that stems from anticipating danger, which may be imagined or real. Some definitions of anxiety distinguish it from fear by limiting it to anticipation of a danger from a largely unknown source, whereas fear is a response to a consciously recognized and usually external threat or danger. Others can see or recognize external dangers but not the "internal" threats that an anxious individual experiences. Signs and symptoms of anxiety and fear may seem the same, as they include hyperactivity, apprehension, excitability, irritability and suffering from exaggerated and excessive worry and fearful anticipation. Many abused and psychologically traumatized individuals, such as victims of family violence, have lifelong symptoms of anxiety.

Until 1980, anxiety was considered a one-dimensional condition. Then mental health professionals began to realize that there are several categories of specific symptom clusters, with unique causes, treatments and outlooks for improvement. Following are several of the major categories described in the *Diagnostic and Statistical Manual of Mental Disorders*, 4th ed., published in 1994:

- Generalized anxiety disorder
- Phobias: Specific phobia (formerly simple phobia) and social phobia

- Agoraphobia
- Panic attacks and panic disorder
- Obsessive-compulsive disorder
- Post-traumatic stress disorder

However, according to Sheryle Gallant, Gwendolyn Puryear Keita and Renee Royak-Schaler, in *Health Care for Women: Psychological, Social and Behavioral Influences,* two of the most prevalent categories are generalized anxiety disorder and panic disorder. Primary care physicians have indicated that anxiety disorders are the most common mental health problem in their practice.

In primary care settings, anxiety disorders often are underrecognized because anxious individuals often present doctors with physical symptoms rather than psychological concerns.

Most mentally healthy people experience anxiety in everyday life. For example, many may experience anxiety about getting to a job interview on time, going on a first date or looking just right at an important event. Others become anxious about being held up in traffic because of a bridge raising or a delayed train, while still others become anxious when they hear reports of imminent bad weather conditions. Most people learn to cope with such transient anxieties by taking more time, making additional preparations and facing the fact that the situations are temporary and are not really threatening.

Many individuals who face a threat or change in their health status may become anxious. These anxieties may relate to a fear of the unknown or a fear of unpleasant treatment and possible pain and disability.

Anxieties also occur relating to socioeconomic status. For example, threats of job layoffs cause many people anxieties, while others become anxious over changes in stock market prices and develop constant fears that their fortunes will be wiped out. These situations, if severe enough to interfere with function or sleep in an otherwise well-adjusted individual, would be categorized as adjustment disorder.

Anxious individuals focus on a situation, object or activity that they want to avoid; extreme anxieties and fears of these experiences can become phobias. If the anxiety seems unfocused, it is known as free-floating anxiety. This is a fear of social criticism, diagnosed as a social phobia if it interferes with normal social or occupational function. Other phobias may be more specific, such as fear of public speaking, riding in cars, snakes or mice.

Those who suffer from agoraphobia often experience panic attacks first. Recent studies have shown that about 25 percent of patients with major depression suffer panic attacks. The suicide-attempt rate in patients with panic attacks has been found to be just as high as in those with depressive disorders.

Anxieties may be experienced in specific periods of sudden onset and be accompanied by physical symptoms such as nausea or dizziness. Anxiety focused on physical symptoms that preoccupy individuals to the point that they believe they have a disease can lead to hypochondriasis.

Many people turn to smoking, alcohol or drug use to cope with anxieties. These habits are not considered healthy coping mechanisms, as they can lead to health hazards and dependencies. Physicians may prescribe antianxiety drugs, or anxiolytic drugs, for some individuals who experience temporary anxieties at certain times.

American Psychiatric Association. *Diagnostic and Statistical Manual of Mental Disorders,* 4th ed. rev. Washington, D.C.: 1994.
Gallant, Sheryle J., Gwendolyn Puryear Keita, and Renee Royak-Schaler, eds. *Health Care For Women: Psychological, Social and Behavioral Influences.* Washington, D.C.: American Psychological Association, 1997.
Marks, Isaac. *Fears, Phobias, and Rituals: Panic, Anxiety, and Their Disorders.* New York: Oxford University Press, 1987.

See also ALCOHOLISM; ANXIETY DISORDERS; HYPOCHONDRIASIS; PANIC ATTACK AND PANIC DISORDER; PHOBIA.

anxiety disorders   Disorders in which symptoms of anxiety and avoidance behavior are characteristic features. Anxiety disorders is a categorical term encompassing a group of mental health disorders including generalized anxiety disorder, panic disorder with or without agoraphobia, simple and social phobias, obsessive-compulsive disorder and post-traumatic stress disorder.

Of all mental health problems, anxiety disorders are the most frequently occurring in the general population. Eight out of every 100 Americans suffer from anxiety disorders. A survey by the National Institute of Mental Health showed that the six-month prevalence rate of anxiety disorders among the adult population in the United States was 8.3 percent. Only 23 percent of these individuals had received any form of treatment. This survey showed that anxiety disorders, the most common mental health problem in the community, usually go untreated.

Anxiety disorders are sometimes detected when an individual seeks repeated treatment for a nonexistent medical condition or makes needless visits to emergency rooms. The physical symptoms of anxiety disorders are often so severe that many people are convinced they have serious medical problems. Many victims of anxiety disorders find themselves isolated from the course of daily activity. Some individuals have symptoms so severe that they are almost totally disabled. While simple phobia is the most common anxiety disorder, panic disorder is the most common among people seeking treatment. According to the American Psychiatric Association, panic disorder, phobias and obsessive-compulsive disorder seem to be more common among first-degree biologic relatives of people with each of these disorders than among the general population. People who experience anxiety disorders are usually apprehensive and frequent worriers and anticipate something unfortunate happening to themselves or others. Characteristics may include "edginess," irritability, easy distractibility and impatience. Some have a feeling of impending death or a desire to run and hide.

Causes of Anxiety Disorders

Because anxiety disorders are such an individual matter, causes cannot be generalized. Usually it is not a single situation or condition that causes anxiety disorders for most individuals but rather a combination of physical and environmental factors linked together. Researchers have pinpointed several general theories relating to causes of anxiety disorders that may be applicable to some cases. Theories involve the psychoanalytic approach, the learning approach and the biologic approach. Individual causes may be traced to one or more of these theories. For example, a person may develop or inherit a biologic susceptibility to anxiety disorders, and events in childhood may teach a person certain fears, which then develop over time into a diagnosable anxiety disorder.

According to the psychoanalytic theory, anxiety comes from an unconscious conflict that originated in the individual's past. Such conflicts may have developed during infancy or childhood. Sigmund Freud suggested that one may carry unconscious childhood conflicts regarding sexual desire for the parent of the opposite sex. A person may also have developed conflicts because of an illness or a scare or other emotionally charged event during childhood. According to this theory, anxiety can be resolved after identifying and resolving the unconscious conflict.

According to learning theory, anxiety is a learned behavior that can also be unlearned. People who feel uncomfortable in certain situations or involved in certain events will try to avoid them. However, some individuals, by persistently confronting the feared situation or object, can relearn their responses and relieve anxiety. Behavioral therapy is largely based on learning theory.

Research has also indicated that biochemical changes occur as a result of emotional, psychological or behavioral changes. According to biochemical theory, biochemical imbalances may be responsible for some anxiety disorders, and some anxiety disorders seem to run in families. According to this theory, medical treatment of biochemical imbalances in the central nervous system may relieve symptoms of anxiety.

Changes in Terminology

The language relating to anxiety disorders has changed over the years. For example, anxiety disorder was once termed "anxiety neurosis" but is no longer referred to in that way in psychiatric literature. "Anxiety hysteria" was once used to refer to what is now generally called phobia, phobic disorder or somatoform disorder.

Therapy for Anxiety Disorders

Anxiety disorders are usually treated with a variety or combination of approaches individualized for each person. According to Eric Stake, M.D., Pennsylvania Hospital, Philadelphia, following a comprehensive assessment, treatment is generally administered on an outpatient basis, with most patients showing improvement within five to six sessions.

Techniques include behavioral therapy, psychotherapy, medication and education. For example, phobias, agoraphobia and obsessive-compulsive disorders are often treated with behavioral therapy. According to Victor Malatesta, Ph.D., Pennsylvania Hospital, Philadelphia, behavioral therapy is based on the belief that changing how we approach a given situation can help change how we react toward it. It is crucial that patients actively come to terms with their fears. As part of the behavioral approach, therapists use a step-by-step process of introducing patients to a series of situations progressing from the mildly anxiety-provoking to the highly anxiety-provoking. This continual but graduated exposure helps patients tackle their fears one step at a time, slowly learning to control their anxiety, gain self-confidence and finally master the situation. With this method, many phobic individuals have experienced long-term recovery.

Many who have recovered from anxiety disorders have lived with their disorder for years without being properly diagnosed or offered appropriate and effective therapy.

Individuals with anxiety disorders should seek therapists who are experienced in recognizing and treating mental health problems. Recommendations may be obtained by contacting major medical centers of the Anxiety Disorders Association of America:

11900 Parklawn Drive
Suite 100
Rockville, MD 20852-2624
Phone: (301) 231-9350
Fax: (301) 231-7392
Web site: www.adaa.org

Medications by themselves are not considered adequate treatment for anxiety disorders. However, for many people, the use of antianxiety medications (also known as anxiolytic medications) helps reduce intense symptoms so that they can benefit from behavioral therapy or other psycho-therapeutic techniques. Individuals who are continuously anxious and tense find it difficult to relax sufficiently during a therapy session or to practice relaxation exercises between therapy visits. The use of medications seems to help many individuals do this more efficiently.

Ongoing patient education can help prevent a recurrence of symptoms during or after treatment. People with anxiety disorders learn to understand how and why they developed these problems and learn ways to cope with them. They learn to recognize the signs of an attack, to keep track of their breathing, to use relaxation techniques and to make lifestyle changes. Support groups in which patients help one another overcome fears and learn to relax are also helpful.

Generalized Anxiety Disorder (GAD)

Characteristics of this disorder are a constant feeling of being nervous and on edge without any apparent reason. Or there may be unrealistic or excessive anxiety and worry (apprehensive expectation) about two or more life circumstances, such as needless financial worries and concerns about possible misfortune to one's spouse (who is in no danger) for six months or longer. There may be signs of nervousness, hyperactivity and excitability that interfere only mildly with work or social activities. Individuals may feel shaky, experience trembling or twitching, have muscle aches and soreness and become tired easily. Age of onset is usually between 20 and 40, and the disorder is equally common in men and women. In some cases, generalized anxiety disorder follows a major depressive episode. Generalized anxiety disorder is not an anxiety about having a panic attack (as occurs in panic disorder) or feeling embarrassed in public (as occurs in social phobia) or a fear of being contaminated (as occurs in obsessive-compulsive disorder).

Phobias

According to the American Psychiatric Association, phobias afflict between 6 and 11 percent of all Americans. Phobias are intense, unrealistic fears that usually lead to avoidance of the feared object, situation or event. Phobic individuals feel terror, dread or panic when confronted with their feared situation. Some avoid the source of their fear to the extent that it interferes with their work and social and family life.

Specific phobias are fears of specific objects or situations. Well-known examples are fears of flying, snakes or high places. Specific phobias can begin at any age. When exposed to the sight of the feared object, any one or more anxiety responses occur, including trembling, sweating and feeling faint, nauseated or dizzy. For some phobics, just the thought of, or seeing a picture of, the feared object brings on these responses.

Social phobias are persistent fears of one or more situations in which the person is exposed to possible scrutiny by others and fears that he or she may do something or act in a way that will be humiliating or embarrassing. Social phobias usually begin in late childhood or early adolescence, at a time when the individual normally is keenly aware of comparison with and evaluation by peers. Examples of social phobias range from fears of public speaking to fears of vomiting in a public place.

When faced with the socially phobic situation, such as standing up at a meeting and speaking, the individual will almost invariably have an anxiety response, such as having a fast heartbeat, sweating and having difficulty breathing. Usually a cycle occurs, in which the individual fears a situation, such as going into a room and meeting new people, and then avoids the situation. Social phobias are generally not as disabling as agoraphobia, but social phobias may interfere with one's choice of employment, professional advancement or social life.

Agoraphobia, a fear of fear, includes an extreme fear of any situation in which escape is difficult and help unavailable. It may involve a fear of going outside, being in a public place alone or being in a place with no escape, such as an airplane, train or center aisle in a theater or church. This is the most disabling because many sufferers become housebound. Agoraphobia begins in late childhood or early adolescence and, without appropriate therapy, gets worse as the individual ages.

Agoraphobia occurs with or without panic attacks. Authorities differ on whether the panic attacks come first, leading to agoraphobia, or agoraphobia leads to the panic attacks.

Panic Attacks and Panic Disorder

Panic disorder involves an impending sense of doom marked by a sudden onset of severe anxiety attacks that reach their peak in a matter of minutes and then subside. People who have panic disorders experience intensely overwhelming terror for no apparent reason. Some individuals experiencing a panic attack for the first time rush to the hospital, convinced they are having a heart attack and will die. Although sufferers cannot predict when the attacks will occur, they know that certain situations, such as being in a closed place, might cause them because they recall having experienced a panic attack in such a place.

During an attack, persons feel helpless, out of control and, in some instances, as if they are going crazy. Shortness of breath, dizziness and heart palpitations usually accompany an attack.

Obsessive-Compulsive Disorder

Obsessions are repeated, unwanted thoughts. Compulsive behaviors are rituals that get out of control. For many people, obsessions begin as a coping mechanism for overcoming anxieties. People who experience obsessive disorders do not automatically have compulsive behaviors. However, most people who have compulsive, ritual behaviors also suffer from obsessions.

Obsessive-compulsive disorders often begin during the teens or early adulthood. Generally they are chronic and cause moderate to severe disability. People who have obsessive-compulsive disorders usually have involuntary, recurrent and persistent thoughts or impulses that are distasteful to them. Examples are fears of becoming infected by shaking hands with others or fears of committing a violent act. These thoughts can last for seconds or hours. The most common obsessions focus on hurting others or violating socially acceptable behavioral standards, such as swearing or making inappropriate sexual advances. For some individuals they are focused on religious or philosophical issues.

Compulsive individuals go through repeated, involuntary ritualistic behaviors in the belief that they are preventing an unwanted future event, as in the case of those who worry about infection and develop compulsive hand-washing habits. Hand washing affects more women than men. Compulsives also check and recheck that doors are locked or that electric switches and ovens are turned off. The checking compulsion seems to affect more men than women.

Post-Traumatic Stress Disorder (PTSD)

PTSD is an avoidance of thoughts, feelings, situations or activities that are associated with a shocking or painful experience in the individual's past. This can affect anyone who has survived a severe physical or mental trauma. It is now known that it can affect children as well as adults. For example, children who have witnessed a shooting in a school or restaurant, or violence in the streets, suffer symptoms similar to those of adults who have been through wars, witnessed airplane collisions or been physically attacked. The severity of the disorder seems to increase when the trauma is unanticipated. For that reason, not all war veterans develop post-traumatic stress disorder—despite prolonged and brutal combat—because soldiers expect a certain amount of violence, whereas rape victims may be especially affected by the unexpectedness of the attack.

Individuals who suffer from post-traumatic stress disorder reexperience the traumatizing event through flashbacks of the event, dreams or nightmares. Rarely does the person get into a temporary dislocation from reality, in which the trauma is relived for a period of days. "Psychic numbing," or emotional anesthesia, may occur, in which victims have decreased interest in or involvement with people or activities they once enjoyed. They may experience excessive alertness and a highly sharpened startle reaction. They may have general anxiety, depression, panic attacks, inability to sleep, memory loss, difficulty concentrating or completing tasks and survivors' guilt. There is evidence that neglected and abused children experience PTSD. It is also likely that many anxiety disorders develop as PTSD phenomena.

See also AGORAPHOBIA; DIAGNOSTIC AND STATISTICAL MANUAL OF MENTAL DISORDERS; OBSESSIVE-COMPULSIVE DISORDER; PANIC ATTACKS AND PANIC DISORDER; POST-TRAUMATIC STRESS DISORDER; PHOBIA.

Liebowitz, Michael R. "Anxiety Disorders and Obsessive Compulsive Disorder." *Neuropsychobiology* 37, 2 (March 1998): 69–71.

anxiety disorders of childhood and adolescence

Disorders in which symptoms of anxiety are central characteristics. While major symptoms may seem similar to anxieties in adults, mental health professionals have divided disorders of childhood and adolescence into three major categories. The first two involve anxiety focused on a specific situation (separation anxiety disorder and avoidant disorder of childhood or adolescence), and the third involves generalized anxiety related to a variety of situations (overanxious disorder).

ANXIETY DISORDERS OF CHILDHOOD OR ADOLESCENCE

1. Separation anxiety disorder
2. Avoidance disorder of childhood or adolescence
3. Overanxious disorder

Separation Anxiety Disorder

Diagnosis of excessive anxiety, for at least two weeks, concerning separation from those to whom the child is attached. A diagnosis requires at least three of nine items from the following:

- Unrealistic and persistent worry about possible harm occurring to major attachment figures or fear that they will leave or not return.

- Unrealistic and persistent worry that an untoward calamitous event will separate the child from a major attachment figure (e.g., that the child will be lost, kidnapped or killed or be the victim of an accident).

- Persistent reluctance or refusal to go to school in order to stay with major attachment figures or at home.

- Persistent reluctance or refusal to go to sleep without being near a major attachment figure or to go to sleep away from home.

- Persistent avoidance of being alone, including clinging to and "shadowing" major attachment figures.

- Repeated nightmares involving the theme of separating.

- Complaints of physical symptoms (e.g., headaches, stomachaches, nausea or vomiting) on many school days or on other occasions when anticipating separation from major attachment figures.

- Recurrent signs or complaints of excessive distress in anticipation of separation from home or major attachment figures (e.g., temper tantrums or crying, pleading with parents not to leave).

- Recurrent signs of complaints or excessive distress when separated from home or major attachment figures (e.g., wants to return home, needs to call parents when they are absent or when child is away from home).

Onset must be before age 18. The disturbance must not occur only during the course of a pervasive developmental disorder, schizophrenia or another psychotic disorder. In some cases, school phobia is considered a type of separation anxiety disorder.

Avoidant Disorder of Childhood or Adolescence

Diagnosis of excessive avoidance of contact with unfamiliar people, for at least six months, severe enough to interfere with social functioning in peer relationships. Additionally, there must be a desire for social involvement with familiar people and generally warm and edifying relationships with family or familiar figures. The child must be at least age two and a half. The child may retreat from strangers and seem extremely shy with other children.

Overanxious Disorder

A diagnosis of excessive or unrealistic anxiety or worry for at least six months. The diagnosis requires at least four of seven items from the following:

- Excessive or unrealistic worry about future events.

- Excessive or unrealistic concern about the appropriateness of past behavior.

- Excessive or unrealistic concern about competence in one or more areas (e.g., athletic, academic or social).

- Somatic complaints (such as headaches or stomachaches) for which no physical basis can be established.

- Marked self-consciousness.

- Excessive need for reassurance about a variety of concerns.

- Marked feelings of tension or inability to relax.

The individual must not meet criteria for generalized anxiety disorder if over age 18. The disturbance must not occur only during the course of a pervasive developmental disorder, schizophrenia or another psychotic disorder.

See also ANXIETY; ANXIETIES AND ANXIETY DISORDERS.

anxiogenic   A term referring to activities, drugs or substances that may raise anxiety levels and arouse physical symptoms of anxiety. Examples of anxiogenic agents or activities include hyperventilation, caffeine, yohimbine, sodium lactate or isoproterenol infusion, carbon dioxide inhalation and exercise in some individuals. In phobic individuals, the thought or sight of the phobic object is usually anxiogenic; agoraphobics regard the idea of going outside or on a public bus alone as anxiogenic.

See also CAFFEINE.

apathy   A characteristic of mild boredom and lack of energy and drive. There may be little emotional response to stimuli. Most people become apathetic at some time, depending on their circumstances. However, the situation is usually temporary rather than chronic. Apathy occurs during depression and some types of schizophrenia. People who are apathetic are usually unable to mobilize themselves to get started or complete many different kinds of tasks. Apathy can result from lack of interest or stimulation. For example, a highly trained individual who, because of economic necessity, is forced to take a more menial job in which his training cannot be used may develop characteristics of apathy toward his employer's activities or the other workers around him.

aphasia   A disturbance of the ability to read and write and/or the ability to comprehend and read, when these abilities previously existed. The term "aphasia" usually refers to a complete absence of these communication and comprehension skills, while dysphasia is a disturbance. Related disabilities that may occur as a characteristic of aphasia or, more rarely, by themselves are alexia (word blindness) and agraphia (writing difficulty).

Aphasia occurs as a result of brain damage following a stroke or head injury.

aphonia Total loss of the voice, usually suddenly, caused by emotional stress. The loss of voice occurs because the vocal cords do not meet as they normally do when the individual tries to speak. However, they do come together when the individual coughs. The voice usually returns as suddenly as it disappeared. Reassurance and psychotherapy are frequent treatments.

apraxia Loss of ability to perform purposeful movements such as getting dressed or lifting a simple item. Apraxia may occur when the parietal lobe of the brain is damaged, causing loss of memory for certain acts or series of skills. No paralysis or loss of sensation occurs.

aromatherapy The art and science of using essential oils from plants and flowers to reduce anxieties as well as to enhance mental and physical health. Practitioners of aromatherapy blend essential oils from around the world based on one's current physical, bioenergetic and emotional condition, and then apply them with a specialized massage technique focusing on the nervous and lymphatic system. Aromatherapy massage has been used to treat conditions ranging from job anxieties, muscle soreness, acne and varicose veins to allergies.

The art of aromatherapy is fairly new in the United States, but it has been used for centuries elsewhere in the world, particularly Egypt and Greece. During World War I, Dr. Jean Valnet, a Parisian physician, used essential oils to treat injured soldiers. He also influenced Marguerite Maury, a biochemist, who developed a special way to apply the penetrating oils with massage.

Finding a Practitioner for Aromatherapy

There is no national organization overseeing training standards in this field. Techniques vary from practitioner to practitioner. Many therapists are employed in spas in larger cities or resort areas. If you are seeking this therapy, look for someone who is a licensed, certified massage practitioner and who can show proof of training in the use of essential oils.

See also COMPLEMENTARY THERAPIES.

art therapy Use of artistic activities during psychotherapy and rehabilitation to promote a healthier communication of feelings as well as a way to channel impulses. Activities such as clay modeling or painting offer individuals a nonthreatening emotional release, a means of restoring self-esteem and self-confidence, an opportunity for communicating in a nonverbal way and a means of reestablishing social relationships. In some cases, the therapist may watch for hidden sources of emotional problems. Art therapy with children is particularly useful when they tell their story by drawing a picture or express the feelings they experience when looking at artwork. In some cases, children are asked to draw themselves or their families or depict what they want to be when they grow up. These drawings can then be discussed in individual therapy sessions with the child or in family therapy sessions.

See also ALTERNATIVE THERAPIES.

Asendin Trade name for amoxapine, a tricyclic antidepressant medication.

See also ANTIDEPRESSANT MEDICATIONS; PHARMACEUTICAL APPROACH.

asociality Behavior characteristics that indicate withdrawal from society, a lack of involvement with other people or lack of concern for social values and customs. Asociality is sometimes associated with recluses or hermits. Individuals with asocial characteristics may have few or no interests or hobbies and may show an inability to feel closeness and intimacy of a type appropriate for his or her age, sex and family status.

However, like many other psychological characteristics, asociality represents a continuum, and most individuals fall somewhere along the line between being socially well adjusted to their life circumstances and totally asocial. Social withdrawal is often associated with depression.

assertiveness training   A process through which the individual learns to speak up whenever he or she believes an injustice is done. Assertiveness training helps raise self-esteem and is helpful in treating some anxiety disorders.

See also AGORAPHOBIA; BEHAVIORAL THERAPY.

assignment   A way in which a psychiatrist, psychologist or other mental health professional is compensated for services covered by Medicare (in the United States) when the practitioner wishes to receive direct payment from Medicare and is willing to permit it to determine the amount of payment. Under this system, both the patient and the practitioner agree to accept Medicare's determination of a "reasonable charge" for the services involved. Medicare reimburses the practitioner directly, paying only 80 percent of what is considered the reasonable charge. The individual is usually asked to pay the remaining 20 percent. Alternatively, when a practitioner does not accept assignment, the individual is billed directly and then sends the bill to Medicare for reimbursement of 80 percent of Medicare's predetermined reasonable charge. Not all mental health practitioners accept assignment. Individuals concerned about this aspect of payment should inquire before beginning therapy with a new practitioner.

"assisted" suicide   See SUICIDE.

association, free   A method used by Sigmund Freud that required the patient to speak freely of whatever might come to mind during a therapy visit. This method formed the basis of the therapeutic application of psychoanalysis and of continued study and research into the nature of mental processes.

See also FREUD, SIGMUND; PSYCHOANALYSIS.

assortative mating   The tendency of individuals with a specific mental illness or mental retardation to mate with, or marry, a person who has a similar condition. This may occur as a consequence of simple social convenience, because the partners often meet each other in therapy groups, group living situations or hospitals and may have few friends without mental health problems because of social handicaps produced by these problems. It may occur because people with similar problems (alcoholism, depression, etc.) have a propensity for one another. Assortative mating causes problems for researchers in family and genetic mental health studies, because it results in a double genetic loading, increasing the risk for illness in offspring.

astereognosis   A condition in which one does not recognize objects by touch when they are placed in one hand. Testing for astereognosis is part of an examination of the central nervous system. Astereognosis is either left-sided or right-sided. Astereognosis (and tactile agnosia) are due to a disease or malfunction of parts of the cerebrum (the main mass of the brain) concerned with recognition by touch. This term is not applicable if objects cannot be recognized by touch because of difficulty holding the object or defect of sensation in the fingers.

asthenic personality   A type of personality characteristically lacking energy, chronically fatigued and oversensitive to emotional or physical stress. This type lacks enthusiasm and capacity for enjoyment of life. The term comes from the word *asthenia,* which means a loss of strength and energy.

See also CHRONIC FATIGUE SYNDROME; PERSONALITY.

Ativan   Trade name for the generic drug lorazepam. It is in a class called benzodiazepine drugs.

See also BENZODIAZEPINE DRUGS; PHARMACEUTICAL APPROACH.

attentional impairment   A diagnostic term used by mental health professionals that applies to individuals who have trouble focusing attention or who are able to focus only sporadically and erratically. They may ignore attempts to be conversed with, wander away while in the middle of an activity or task or appear to be inattentive when engaged in formal testing or interviewing. Such individuals may not be aware of their difficulty in focusing attention. In social situations, such an individual seems inattentive, may look away during conversation and may seem to have poor concentration when playing games, reading or watching television. In popular terms, such an individual may seem "out of it."

attention-deficit/hyperactivity disorder (ADHD)

A persistent pattern of inattention and/or hyperactivity-impulsivity that is more frequent and severe than is typically observed in individuals at a comparable level of development. It is a source of anxiety to children, young people, their parents and teachers. Childhood ADHD often sets the stage for adult anxiety, particularly generalized anxiety disorder (GAD).

To make the diagnosis of ADHD, according to the *Diagnostic and Statistical Manual of Mental Disorders*, 4th Ed., some hyperactive-impulsive or inattentive symptoms that cause impairment must have been present before age seven, although many individuals are diagnosed after the symptoms have been present for a number of years. Additionally, there must be clear evidence of interference with developmentally appropriate social, academic or occupational functioning, and the disorder cannot be better accounted for by another mental disorder, such as anxiety disorder, dissociative disorder or personality disorder.

Estimates are that ADHD affects three to five percent of the school age population, and is more common in boys. Data on prevalence in adolescence and adulthood are limited. No precise definition or approach to treatment is universally accepted, although there is extensive literature upon which rational approaches to management of individual cases are based. Symptomatic treatment with stimulant medication in selected patients is effective and safe but not curative. Successful outcome depends on multimodal therapy involving parents, teachers and mental health professionals.

Usually ADHD is noticed before age five; ADHD sufferers are often overactive, impulsive and easily distractible. When young people are untreated in childhood, they often develop very negative attitudes toward school and patterns of failure which can be avoided with prompt diagnosis and treatment. Even with treatment, some develop behavioral and substance abuse problems in later life.

In recent years, diagnosis and management has created public and professional controversy. The definition of ADHD, according to the *Diagnostic and Statistical Manual,* emphasizes the attention deficit as the central feature, and the other symptoms to a variable extent. It also recognizes that ADHD exists as a separate entity from conduct disorder. The essential feature of conduct disorder is a persistent conduct pattern in which rights of others and age-appropriate societal norms or rules are violated. While the two conditions often occur in the same individual, it is not assumed that one is a necessary concomitant of the other. Making the distinction has important implications for outcome. Mental health professionals treating children with ADHD generally agree that individualized management, on a case method, is most effective.

Diagnosing ADHD

Diagnosis is based on descriptions of the child's behavior obtained from parents and teachers as well as observation of behavior in the office. Questions for the child are directed toward features of hyperactivity, impulsiveness and lack of attention. Such children are often restless, particularly while the physician talks with parents.

Many parents look back and report that their child was hyperactive from a very early age, even from one to two years of age. In those with a later onset, the disorder is more likely to be associated with social disruption or specific difficulties at school. However, many parents do not seek medical attention until the child is in first or second grade and presents difficulties.

To determine whether the child has an associated disorder, such as a learning disorder or mild mental retardation, psychological tests are sometimes useful. Biochemical studies have shown statistically significant differences in catecholamine excretion and peptide-containing urinary complexes. However, these findings have not reached diagnostic significance, although they do represent a promising field for further study.

Treating ADHD

Individualized treatment managed on a case by case method is most effective. No one approach to treatment is universally accepted. Successful treatment depends on multimodal therapy involving parents, teachers and mental health professionals.

In an effort to reduce stress levels of both the child and the family, the physician usually explains the nature of ADHD, with the objective to reduce feelings of guilt and blame in the family and at the same time improve the child's self-esteem. When there are disorders of family dynamics or a learning disorder underlying the symptoms, these must also be addressed. Often other health and educational professionals, such as psychologists, special education specialists or social workers become involved in treating the child.

General advice from physicians counseling families with an ADHD child usually addresses behavior management and how to avoid confrontation with the active, restless child. Such a child should be encouraged to channel energy into productive activities, such as doing errands or erasing the blackboard.

Behavior modification and cognitive therapy are used in some cases of ADHD. Other approaches include dietary restrictions of food additives or refined sugar (Feingold diet); supplementation with megavitamins, trace elements, or amino acids; and compensating for vestibular dysfunction. However, best results have been noted with multimodal therapy, including behavior management, special educational intervention and in some cases, use of stimulant drugs—a controversial method supported by some double-blind studies.

A widely used but controversial stimulant medication is methylphenidate (trade name: Ritalin). It is the most commonly prescribed medication for children in the United States. The drug is effective for three to four hours and is often prescribed for use in the morning and afternoon. Individualizing dosage is important because high doses may help hyperactivity but have been found to impair learning. When the dose is too high, some children become excessively quiet, indecisive and cry easily. When symptoms occur only in school, the medication may be given only on school days. A child on stimulant medication should be evaluated by the prescribing physician with some regularity.

Research Results Reported

In June 1995, the issue of the American Medical Association's *Archives of General Psychiatry* contained five articles on ADHD, which gave varying viewpoints on detection and treatment. Joseph Biederman, M.D., and colleagues at Massachusetts General Hospital and Harvard Medical School, Boston, Massachusetts, studied 140 ADHD and 120 control subjects to determine if family-environment risk factors are associated with ADHD. The findings support earlier research that a positive association appears to exist between the risk for ADHD and adversity indicators such as severe marital discord, low social class, large family size, paternal criminality, maternal mental disorder and foster care placement.

Thomas Spencer, M.D., Massachusetts General Hospital, Boston, and colleagues, conducted a study to determine the effectiveness of methylphenidate hydrochloride (Ritalin) in adults with ADHD. The researchers studied 23 adult patients during a seven-week, placebo controlled, crossover study of the drug. They found "a marked therapeutic response for methylphenidate treatment of ADHD symptoms that exceeded the placebo response. Response to methylphenidate was independent of gender, psychiatric comorbidity with anxiety or moderate depression, or family history of psychiatric disorders." They concluded that robust doses of Ritalin are effective in the treatment of ADHD.

Nora D. Volkow, M.D., Brookhaven National Laboratory, Upton, New York, and colleagues conducted a study to investigate the pharmacokinetics of Ritalin in the human brain, to compare them with those of cocaine, and to evaluate whether cocaine and Ritalin compete for the same binding sites. The researchers compared the results of previously obtained positron emission tomography for cocaine with the results from eight healthy males, with and without Ritalin, and with results from baboons given both Ritalin and cocaine.

The study said the regional distribution of Ritalin in the human brainwaves is almost identical to that of cocaine. However, they added that the similarity between cocaine and Ritalin regarding their binding to the dopamine transporter should not be used as an argument against the use of Ritalin because their kinetics in the brain are markedly different, and differences in their kinetics are probably further accentuated by the fact that Ritalin is prescribed orally. They cautioned, however, with a speculation that because of the high associated with the fast uptake of cocaine and Ritalin in the brain, the slow clearance of Ritalin from the brain may serve as a limiting factor in promotion of its frequent self-administration.

Kenneth D. Gadow, Ph.D., State University of New York-Stony Brook, conducted a study to determine the effectiveness of Ritalin for ADHD in children with a tic disorder. The study revealed that findings from case reports and patient questionnaire surveys have been interpreted as indicating that administration of stimulants is ill-advised for the treatment of ADHD in children with tic disorder. The researchers administered placebo and three doses of Ritalin twice daily for two weeks each, to 34 children between the ages of six and 11. The study found that Ritalin appears to be a safe and effective treatment for ADHD in the majority of children with comorbid tic disorder. However, the study said that the data pertaining to Ritalin's effect on the frequency of motor tics are mixed.

Writing in the June 20, 1995 issue of *The Journal of the American Medical Association,* Alan J. Zemetkin, M.D., National Institute of Mental Health, National Institutes of Health, Bethesda, Maryland, commented that within the next quarter of a century, we should have answers to these and other questions:

- Why does ADHD often result in delinquent or oppositional behavior?

- How prevalent is symptomatic ADHD in adults?

- Is there a particular gene linked to the disorder?

- Can pharmacological or gene manipulations lead to a cure?

- Does early treatment with stimulants affect the body?

- Can medications be developed that are effective and safe without having the stigma of being controlled substances?

- Will highly technological brain-imaging techniques prove more useful in providing information for the diagnosis of ADHD.

- What is the incidence of overdiagnosis and misdiagnosis?

In providing an overview of ADHD, Zametkin warned of misdiagnosis of ADHD because there are look-alike syndromes that make it easy to misdiagnose. Stimulants, often prescribed as treatment for ADHD, can also increase the attention of those not suffering from ADHD when administered to them. Individuals misdiagnosed with ADHD may think that due to the improvement in their attention resulting from the medication, the diagnosis was correct, when it wasn't. In some cases, they more effectively treat "negative symptoms" and cognitive dysfunction in schizophrenia. They have a lower occurrence of extrapyramidal side effects and tardive dyskinesia.

Addressing myths about ADHD, Zametkin commented that many think stimulants are no longer useful once a child enters puberty. He dispelled this myth, saying documentation exists showing that teenagers and adults with ADHD continue to benefit from stimulant treatment. He added that people think ADHD is outgrown with maturation but explains that studies show this is not necessarily true. He said the concept that sugar and food additives cause ADHD is also a myth.

Summarizing treatment modes for ADHD, Zametkin wrote that any of the following may be included in a treatment plan:

- Educational material or discussions for child, parents and school personnel

- Behavioral modification techniques for parents and for teachers

- Social skills training if needed, although the literature regarding its effectiveness is inconsistent

- Remedial or special education for children with severe learning disability

- Although not indicated for the treatment of core symptoms of inattention, impulsivity, and hyperactivity, individual counseling may work to alleviate secondary symptoms.

- Stimulant medication

See also RITALIN.

American Medical Association. *Archives of General Psychiatry* 52, no. 66 (June 1995).

American Medical Association, *The Journal of the American Medical Association* 273, no. 23 (June 1995).

American Psychiatric Association. *Diagnostic and Statistical Manual of Mental Disorders,* 4th ed., rev. Washington, D.C., 1994.

attitude   A characteristic of personality that includes a fixed tendency to like or dislike classes of people or things based on one's beliefs and feelings. For example, employers who do not want to hire older workers may be said to have a prejudiced attitude.

Attitudes can also be characterized as positive or negative. A positive attitude can be helpful in performance in school, taking examinations or learning a new skill, whereas a negative attitude can get in one's way of moving ahead. The well-known phrase "power of positive thinking" is an example of positive attitude in play.

Attitude can also make a difference in recovering from disease. An example is the late Norman Cousins (1912–1990), former editor of the *Saturday Review of Literature* and writer, who used a happy mental attitude to overcome a severe, disabling joint disease (ankylosing spondylitis). He spent weeks watching old comedy movies; he believed that laughter and the positive attitudes it aroused in him were vital to his recovery.

See also CHRONIC ILLNESS; LAUGHTER.

"atypical" antipsychotic medications   A class of medications developed to treat schizophrenia and other psychoses. These medications act by a different mechanism than traditional or typical antipsychotic medications.

aura   Sensations that warn an individual that a migraine headache or epileptic attack is approaching. For example, before a migraine headache becomes full-blown, there may be perceptions of colored lights or flashing lights, numbness or stomach distress. Different individuals learn to recognize their own symptoms, sometimes in time to take a medication to ward off the attack. The word comes from the Greek word meaning "breeze."

See also EPILEPSY; HEADACHES.

autism   A condition in which children withdraw from others, either by pretending or experiencing muteness, having a delayed onset of speech or developing strange speaking patterns. Also known as autistic disorder, this occurs in about two to four out of every 10,000 children, affects more boys than girls and is usually evident when the child is about two or two and a half years old. It may be caused by a subtle form of brain damage. Usually autistic infants appear normal for the first few months of life but then become increasingly unresponsive to their parents or caretakers. Autism may be linked to variations from normal patterns of speech control by the hemispheres of the brain. A majority of autistic children are left-handed. Often autistic children show considerable artistic or musical abilities. One in 50 autistic children becomes a fully normal adult, but almost half become moderately well adjusted.

Most autistic children require special schooling. Children and their parents can benefit from counseling. In some cases, medications are given to reduce hyperactivity.

autogenic training   A relaxation and stress management technique developed in 1932 by Johannes Heinrich Schultz (1884–1970), a German neurologist. Dr. Schultz used it successfully for the treatment of high blood pressure, digestive disorders and musculoskeletal problems. Since then its therapeutic applications have expanded to include a wide variety of cardiovascular, respiratory, endocrine, gastrointestinal, metabolic and sleep disorders.

Autogenic training is one of the oldest behavioral techniques known and used for stress management. It seems to be the forerunner of progressive muscle relaxation.

With autogenic training, the individual self induces a hypnotic-like state and achieves relaxation through breathing and muscular decontraction exercises. The technique is often accompanied by meditation and affirmative statements regarding feelings of relaxation, warmth, inner quietness and calm.

A basic assumption behind autogenic training is that people are innately equipped with "self-regulatory brain mechanisms" that maintain a dynamic balance in all our bodily functions. When this balance is disrupted, our self-regulating mechanisms have the capability of restoring a healthy equilibrium, whether by calming an escalated heart rate, lowering elevated blood pressure or healing an ulcer.

See also COMPLEMENTARY THERAPIES; BEHAVIOR THERAPY; BIOFEEDBACK; MEDITATION; PROGRESSIVE MUSCLE RELAXATION.

Kerman, D. Ariel, with Richard Trubo. *The H.A.R.T. Program: Lower Your Blood Pressure Without Drugs.* New York: HarperCollins, 1992.

Lehrer, Paul M., and Robert L. Woolfolk, eds. *Principles and Practice of Stress Management.* New York: The Guilford Press, 1993.

autohypnosis   See AUTOSUGGESTION; HYPNOSIS.

autoimmune disorders   A diverse group of disorders in which the immune system mistakes parts of its own body for the enemy, causing symptoms that can lead to anxieties, fears and symptoms of debilitating and long-term disease. Mental health consequences may follow, including isolation and depression.

The main characteristic of these disorders is inflammation varying from the merely irritating to the potentially deadly, as in diabetes. For example, in Type I diabetes, the immune system has damaged the body's insulin-producing capabilities. Rheumatoid arthritis and systemic lupus erythematosus are also autoimmune diseases. Resulting autoimmune diseases can be either systemwide or specific to a particular body part.

See also COMPLEMENTARY THERAPIES; IMMUNE SYSTEM; MIND/BODY CONNECTIONS; PSYCHONEUROIMMUNOLOGY.

autonomic nervous system (ANS)   The part of the nervous system that controls the automatic activities of organs, blood vessels, glands and many other tissues in the body. The ANS is made up of a network of nerves categorized as the sympathetic nervous system and the parasympathetic nervous system.

The sympathetic nervous system heightens activity in the body, such as causing the breathing rate to increase and making the heart beat faster as though it were preparing the body for a "fight or flight" response. The parasympathetic system has the opposite effect. The two systems work together and usually balance each other, except at times of extreme stress or fear or during exercise, when the sympathetic nervous system takes over. During sleep, the parasympathetic nervous system (PNS) is in control. The PNS slows down heart rate, reduces blood pressure and aids in digestion. In individuals who are blood phobic, there is an intense PNS response, resulting in blood pressure reduction, dizziness and even fainting.

The autonomic nervous system is affected by certain drugs. For example, anticholinergic drugs, those that block the effect of acetylcholine, can reduce painful muscle spasms in the intestine. Beta-adrenergic-blocking drugs block action of epinephrine and norepinephrine on the heart, slowing down the heart rate and reducing situational anxiety.

ANS side effects may result from use of some antipsychotic and antidepressant drugs (tricyclic and monoamine oxidase inhibitors). Such disturbances may benefit ANS functions, such as lowering of blood pressure, but they also cause lightheadedness (dizziness), blurred vision, nasal congestion, dryness of the mouth and constipation.

See also BLOOD PRESSURE; DIZZINESS.

Ost, L.-G.; U. Sterner; and L.I. Lindahl. "Physiological Responses in Blood Phobics." *Behavior Research and Therapy* 22 (1984).

autonomy   A feeling of being in control associated with attitudes of independence and freedom that may take many forms. An individual may express autonomy by making simple decisions for him- or herself. When one loses a sense of autonomy, one may experience anxieties, lose self-esteem and become frustrated.

In developing a sense of autonomy, peer groups play an important role. Children with good peer relationships generally acquire good feelings about themselves and develop confidence that others will like them. They will also develop the ability to realize what others expect of them and to make choices about meeting those expectations in a flexible way without anxieties.

For some individuals, particularly teenagers, peer groups may be destructive to autonomy. This may be the case with teenagers whose experiences with peers have not enabled them to develop self-confidence. Under these circumstances, anxieties and a desire for approval or acceptance may lead to drugs, smoking cigarettes or other destructive behaviors that seems to make the individual feel part of the group.

See also ANGER; CONTROL; FRUSTRATION; SELF-ESTEEM.

Johnson, D. S., and R. T. Johnson. "Peer Influences." In *Encyclopedia of Psychology,* edited by Raymond J. Corsini. New York: Wiley, 1984.

May, Rollo. *Freedom and Destiny.* New York: W. W. Norton, 1981.

Vinack, W. E. "Independent Personalities." In *Encyclopedia of Psychology,* edited by Raymond J. Corsini. New York: Wiley, 1984.

autosome   Chromosomes other than sex chromosomes. Normal human beings normally have 22 pairs of autosomes, plus the sex chromosomes (XX for women and XY for men), which are responsible for determining male or female sexual characteristics.

See also CHROMOSOME.

autosuggestion   Adopting a mental attitude or putting oneself in a mood that makes one more receptive to therapy and improvement of a mental or physical condition. For example, if one suggests to oneself that self-improvement will occur, one will be more receptive to learning.

Autosuggestion is related to the "power of positive thinking." It is useful in controlling anxiety symptoms and phobic reactions. Learned relaxation techniques are a form of autosuggestion; biofeedback is based on autosuggestion, because the individual learns to control certain physical functions, such as muscular tensions, and even temperature and heart rate.

See also HYPNOSIS.

Aventyl   Trade name for nortriptyline, a tricyclic antidepressant medication.

See also ANTIDEPRESSANT MEDICATIONS; PHARMACOLOGICAL APPROACH.

aversion   A term referring to a mild dislike for situations or things. This word is commonly mis-

used in place of phobia, which is a more severe reaction.

See also AVERSION THERAPY; PHOBIA.

aversion (aversive) therapy   Therapy to help a person overcome habits and unwanted behaviors by associating those habits or behaviors with painful experiences or unpleasant feelings. Aversion therapy has been used to treat many conditions, including alcoholism, bedwetting, smoking, sex addiction, nail biting and many other problems. In some cases, it has been useful in treating obsessive-compulsive disorder.

Therapy is designed to help the person connect the habit with the unpleasant reaction, thus reducing the occurrence of the unwanted habit. New behaviors that are more acceptable to the individual have to be developed and reinforced. To create aversions, many techniques have been used. One is electrical therapy in which a trained therapist administers a mildly uncomfortable shock to the individual whenever the unwanted behavior, either real or imagined, is present. The electrical method has been used predominantly in the treatment of sexual disorders. This method of treatment is no longer deemed acceptable and is prohibited by mental health codes of several states. With chemical therapy, the patient receives a drug to induce nausea and is then exposed to smoking, nail biting or other habit that he or she is trying to overcome. The chemical method has been used most widely in the treatment of alcoholism.

A more modern form of aversion therapy is known as covert sensitization. In this form of therapy, the individual is asked to imagine the unwanted habit and then to envision some extremely undesirable consequence, such as nausea or pain.

See also ALCOHOLISM; BEHAVIORAL THERAPY; COGNITIVE THERAPY; SEX ADDICTION.

Blake, B. "The Application of Behavior Therapy to the Treatment of Alcoholism." *Behavioral Research Therapy* 5 (1967).

Cautela, J. "Covert Sensitization." *Psychological Reports* 20 (1967).

avoidant personality disorder   Individuals who have avoidant personality disorder may show a pattern of timidity, anxiety, low self-esteem, social discomfort and fear of rejection. Some individuals develop social phobias or agoraphobia, and others may have depression and feel angry at themselves for failing to adapt better in social ways. Avoidant personality traits may be thought of as a continuum, and many individuals have avoidant personality traits but not to the extreme that they may be categorized as having a personality disorder.

According to the American Psychiatric Association, diagnostic criteria for avoidant personality disorder include:

- Reticence in social situations out of fear of saying something inappropriate or seeming foolish, or of being unable to answer a question

- Fears being embarrassed by blushing, crying or showing signs of anxiety in front of others

- Exaggerates potential difficulties, physical dangers or risks involved in doing ordinary activities outside his or her usual routine

- Easily hurt by disapproval or criticism

- No close friends or confidants (or only one) other than first-degree relatives

- Unwilling to become involved with people unless certain of being liked

- Avoids social or occupational activities involving significant interpersonal contact; for example, refuses a promotion that will increase social demands

See also AGORAPHOBIA; ANXIETY; PERSONALITY DISORDERS; PHOBIA.

American Psychiatric Association. *Diagnostic and Statistical Manual of Mental Disorders,* 4th ed., rev. Washington, D.C., 1994.

avolition An inability to initiate and persist in goal-directed activities. When severe enough to be considered pathological, avolition is pervasive and prevents the person from completing many different types of activities, such as work, intellectual pursuits and self-care.

awareness (self-awareness) In the language of psychotherapy, the consciousness of information and understanding about personal facts that the individual may have repressed or previously refused to acknowledge. Self-awareness is often the first step toward improving a mental health concern.

Ayurveda Derived from the Sanskrit words for "the science of health and knowledge." Over time, Ayurveda has come to mean "the science of life." While Western medicine works on illness, Ayurvedic medicine focuses on the person as a complex, multileveled individual. Many mental health concerns, such as anxiety and fears, can be addressed by Ayurveda diagnosis and treatment.

Ayurvedic treatment is highly individualized. For one who feels well, Ayurvedic activities make the most of one's mental, physical and spiritual well-being, enabling better coping skills against the anxieties of daily life. When fighting illness or coping with specific mental health concerns, Ayurvedic therapy works by enhancing the healing potential within oneself.

In the United States Ayurvedic health care is meant to complement, not replace, advances of modern medicine. Ayurvedic health care is considered a form of complementary therapy. Ayurvedic medicine was first recorded in the holy scriptures of the Vedas of India and is possibly the oldest recorded health science. Currently, Ayurvedic therapy addresses health in terms of body, mind and spirit and may be helpful to some individuals experiencing stress in their lives.

Ayurveda is an art of insight that brings harmony to daily life and relationships. Believers say it can bring a quality of consciousness, such that one can develop insight to deal with one's inner life and the anxieties of one's inner emotions, one's inner hurt, grief and sadness. Ayurvedic beliefs hold that life is a relationship between you and your body, mind and consciousness. These relationships are life, and Ayurveda is a healing art that helps being clarity in relationships. Clarity in relationships brings compassion, and compassion is love and therefore clarity is love. Without this clarity, there is no insight.

A characteristic element of Ayurveda is the determination of one's mind/body type. One's specific type is a combination of three fundamental principles, known as *doshas*, which govern thousands of mental and physical processes. These three principles, *Vata* (movement), *Pitta* (metabolism) and *Kapha* (structure), are the governing agents of nature. Permutations of the *doshas* determine an individual's subtype; through careful history taking and pulse diagnosis, a practitioner can determine imbalances of energy. Disease is diagnosed through questioning, observation, palpation, percussion and listening to the heart, lungs and intestines.

An ancient art of tongue diagnosis also describes characteristic patterns that can reveal the functional status of respective internal organs merely by observing the surface of the tongue. The tongue is the mirror of the viscera and reflects many pathological conditions.

Many factors affect the *doshas.* Disease can result from imbalanced emotions, such as unresolved anger, fear, anxiety, grief or sadness. Ayurveda classifies seven major causative factors in disease: hereditary, congenital, internal, external trauma, seasonal, natural tendencies or habits and supernatural factors. Disease can also result from misuse, overuse and underuse of the senses (hearing, touch, sight, taste, and smell).

Prana, the Ayurvedic term for energy, has counterparts in Eastern medicine (*Qi*) and homeopathy (vital force). Pranic energy is mental and physical and can be changed by diet, exercise, herbs or spiritual practices such as meditation. Pranic energy flows along specific paths, called *nadis*, which converge and cross in energy centers called *chakras* located along the length of the body. During an Ayurvedic examination, *chakras* are studied and *doshas* may be determined to be out of balance, which leads to ill health.

In the United States, physician training in Ayurveda is under the direction of the Maharishi Training Program in Fairfield, Iowa, and directed by Dr. Deepak Chopra, a contemporary writer and practitioner of Ayurvedic medicine.

See also CHOPRA, DEEPAK; COMPLEMENTARY THERAPIES; IMMUNE SYSTEM; MIND/BODY CONNECTIONS; PSYCHONEUROIMMUNOLOGY.

Kahn, Ada P. *Stress A to Z: A Sourcebook for Coping with Everyday Challenges.* New York: Facts On File, 1998.

azidothymidine (AZT)   See ZIDOVUDINE.

AZT   The abbreviation for azidothymidine, the old name for the drug zidovudine, used to treat patients with AIDS (acquired immunodeficiency syndrome). This drug is one of a very few thus far discovered that will in some patients delay the development or progression of AIDS symptoms.

See also ACQUIRED IMMUNODEFICIENCY SYNDROME; ZIDOVUDINE.

"baby blues" A mild form of depression that many women experience after childbirth. It may be caused by a combination of factors, including hormonal changes, the realization that one's life is changed with the addition of another person to care for, and the tiredness that naturally occurs after childbirth. A supportive family can be helpful at this time. Usually the "blues" disappear within a few weeks; if a woman continues to experience depression for an ongoing period—and particularly if her ability to care for her baby is hindered by her moods—professional help should be sought.

See also CHILDBIRTH; DEPRESSION; POSTPARTUM DEPRESSION.

baby boomers The 76 million Americans born between 1946 and 1964. They are products of the population explosion that began during World War II, peaked following the war, and lasted until the mid-1960s. The baby boom has been attributed to several factors, including the wartime prosperity following the Great Depression, increased births as servicemen returned after the war, a lower marriage age than for previous generations and a tendency to have children in quick succession early in marriage.

This generation has experienced many mental health concerns, both individually and collectively. Some, such as anxiety disorders, are influenced by the changing times in which baby boomers have lived. As young adults, their protest against the Vietnam War labeled them hedonistic, rebellious and undisciplined. When they reached college age, they were fighting for civil rights and were active in the women's movement. Improved birth control, more permissive sexual standards and an emphasis on education for both sexes plunged young women

of the baby boom generation into a world of choices. Resulting questions about pursuing careers, entering marriage and having children are issues of anxiety that continue to haunt women into the 21st century.

A good job market and a rapidly expanding economy greeted baby boomers upon graduation from college, and they were soon described as having tendencies toward materialism that included acquiring possessions at an early age and "having it all." In reaction, baby boomers tended to become entrepreneurial and viewed a job as something that should be fulfilling and stimulating rather than simply a means of supporting themselves and their families. However, the sheer numbers of the baby boom generation created a population bulge that increased competition for the remaining corporate and government positions. Facing a changing economy, downsizing, the future of Social Security, rising health care costs and the need for retirement savings, has led to frustrations and additional anxieties for many.

Less Age Discrimination

In 2011, baby boomers will start turning age 65 at the rate of one every 21 seconds. They are likely to represent the most employable group of retirees in U.S. business history because of their educational background and high-tech skills, according to *What's Next? Challenger Workplace Trends Outlook* (2001), published by Challenger, Gray & Christmas, an international outplacement firm that tracks workplace trends.

Baby boomers have doubled the amount of schooling of previous generations. Currently, 9 percent of adults 65 and older hold bachelor's degrees. In contrast, 18 percent of baby boomers hold bachelor's degrees. Additionally, another 18 percent of boomers have had at least some college, compared to 13 percent for adults 65 and older. Baby boomers will also be helped in the job market by their comfort and skill with technology. While they did not grow up with computers in the home as today's children are doing, boomers have mastered computers in the workplace. They are accustomed to the rapid changes that occur in technology as they have experienced the evolution of computers from their earliest form to the present high-speed, Internet-driven technology.

See also BIOLOGICAL CLOCK; COMMUNICATION; HAVING IT ALL; INTERGENERATIONAL CONFLICTS; RETIREMENT.

Light, Paul Charles. *Baby Boomers*. New York: Norton, 1988.
Mills, D. Quinn. *Not Like Our Parents: How the Baby Boom Generation Is Changing America*. New York: William Morrow, 1987.
Silver, Don. *Baby Boomer Retirement: 65 Simple Ways to Protect Your Future*. Los Angeles: Adams-Hall Publishers, 1994.

barbiturate drugs   Medications used to induce sleep and provide sedation for tension and anxiety that act as central nervous system depressants. These medications are legitimately sold by prescription only. Barbiturates slow down the activity of nerves that control many mental and physical functions, such as emotions, heart rate and breathing. The first barbiturate drug, a derivative of barbituric acid, was manufactured and used in medicine in 1882 as barbital and sold under the trade name Veronal. Since then many barbituric acid derivatives have become available as tablets, capsules, suppositories and injectable liquids. Some sleeping pills are "short-acting" barbiturates; their effects last only five or six hours and produce little or no after-effects if used properly. When abused, barbiturates can cause addiction and the sleeping problem can worsen.

Barbiturates have many serious disadvantages that have led to a sharp decline in their use by physicians. They are very toxic, and thus death through overdose—accidental or intended—is a significant danger, particularly if they are combined with alcohol. Regular use can produce physical and psychological dependency and mood changes.

Chronic use at high dosage can produce damage to brain cells.

In recent years, physicians have been prescribing drugs in a class known as benzodiazepines for many anxiety situations in which barbiturates were once prescribed. Benzodiazepines can produce dependency but have not been shown to cause the degree of overdose toxicity, dependency or evidence of cell death associated with barbiturates.

See also BENZODIAZEPINE MEDICATIONS, PHARMACOLOGICAL APPROACH.

Bardet-Biedl syndrome   One of many genetic conditions that can cause moderate to severe mental retardation. Characteristics of an infant born with this syndrome include obesity, retinal abnormalities, small genitals and extra digits on hands and feet (polydactyly).

See also MENTAL RETARDATION.

battered child syndrome   See DOMESTIC VIOLENCE.

battered women   See DOMESTIC VIOLENCE.

Beckwith-Wiedeman syndrome   A form of mild to moderate mental retardation that probably has a genetic cause. Features of the syndrome include hypoglycemia in early infancy, large stature with large muscle mass, large tongue and unusual ear creases.

See also MENTAL RETARDATION.

bedwetting   Unconscious or unintentional wetting by a person over the age of three during sleep, medically known as enuresis. When the child or adult urinates involuntarily during waking hours, the condition is known as incontinence. In both cases, the problem may have emotional as well as physical causes and consequences.

Some children fear having a urinary accident or may have reacted severely to punishment or embarrassment for such an accident in the past. As a result, he or she may have nightmares about the accident or about going to the bathroom, and during the dream urinates in the bed. Punishment and shaming may increase and perpetuate this type of problem. A better solution is to reassure the child and relieve his or her fears. A skilled counselor may be able to help locate and explain the habits and reactions of the child, parents or other caretakers. All concerned should try to reinforce a child's successes and reward good behavior by compliments and possible special privileges.

Some children sleep so heavily that they cannot awaken to normal urinary impulses. This problem may be due to a new schedule, such as a child who is used to napping early and has just begun kindergarten. The new schedule means that the daily nap is postponed until after school. In cases of repeated bedwetting, physical causes such as infection or illness can be ruled out by a physician. If the cause of bedwetting is emotional, try to identify contributing factors and start taking positive steps to correct the situation. Whether the causes are physical or emotional, a child can be retrained regarding toilet habits to help restore coordination of mental, neurological and physical impulses involved. Figure out the approximate times when bedwetting occurs and list contributing factors before bedtime. Give the child less liquid in the few hours before bedtime. Plan on awakening the child a few hours after he has gone to sleep and have him go to the bathroom. Help him train reflexes during waking hours by having him visit the bathroom immediately on feeling the first impulse. Since bedwetting may lead to further shame and problems, other symptomatic treatments have been used. The use of appropriate doses of imipramine, a tricyclic antidepressant, may be appropriate in some cases. This decision should be made by a pediatrician.

behavior therapy (behavior modification) A type of psychotherapy used to treat some mental health problems that emphasizes learned responses. It is often used in conjunction with other types of therapies, including psychopharmacotherapy. Behavioral therapy is used to treat people who have a wide variety of mental health concerns, including anxieties, phobias, agoraphobia, obsessions, compulsions and alcoholism.

Behavioral therapy is also widely used in the treatment of sexual dysfunction. At one time, sex therapists were criticized for using a behavioral approach, as psychoanalytic thinking viewed sexual dysfunctions as originating during childhood. However, as the success rates for behavioral therapy are often quite high in sexual dysfunction, behavioral approaches have gained credibility.

Therapists strive to modify or alter the undesirable or self-defeating behaviors of an individual, such as anxiety and avoidance, instead of working toward changing the "personality" by probing into the individual's "unconscious." Behavioral therapists work on the theory that behavior has a learned component (as well as a biologic component) and thus many unwanted behaviors and reactions can be replaced with more desirable behaviors and reactions.

The focus of behavioral therapy is on observable aspects of specific behaviors, such as the frequency or intensity of a physiological response (e.g., sweating as a reaction to anxiety) or of obsessive hand washing. Reports by the patient and self-rating scales are also often used to describe details of behavior. Specific treatment techniques are tailored by each therapist to the particular needs of each individual.

Goals of treatment are determined by the therapist and the patient and often the patient's family as well. The patient in behavioral therapy views the therapist as a coach and usually makes choices about trying to learn new behaviors and responses. Usually the goal is for the patient to learn self-control of her bad behaviors and increase her number of revised, more acceptable, behaviors.

A variety of learning techniques are used by behavioral therapists. These include classical conditioning, desensitization, flooding, operant conditioning and modeling. In cases of social phobias, for example, therapists may use techniques in which the individual is gradually exposed to the fear-producing situations. The exposure may take place in the patient's imagination first and then in reality. Sometimes the reality never occurs (some situations are easy to imagine but difficult to simulate). However, the key to effective treatment is the gradualness of the exposure combined with the simultaneous use of relaxation training and new physiological and behavioral responses.

Exposure Therapy (Desensitization)

Exposure therapy refers to many behavioral techniques that involve the use of gradual exposure to an anxiety-producing situation. These techniques include systematic desensitization and exposure at full intensity (flooding and implosive therapy).

In systematic desensitization, a technique used by behavioral therapists, patients learn to rank situations that cause anxiety and distress, as well as a variety of deep-muscle-relaxing techniques. For example, an individual who fears the sexual act might place coitus at the top of the list of activities that make him or her anxious; thinking about sitting with a date in a restaurant might rank at the bottom of the list.

The individual is trained in relaxation, both mental and physical. When these techniques are mastered, the person is asked to imagine, in as much detail as possible, the least fear-producing item from the list; when a comfort level is reached in imagining this item, the patient can move up the hierarchy with success. However, when the individual has completed treatment and goes out in the real world to face anxieties and fears, there may be slight regression down the list. For example, an individual who has learned to remain calm while walking into a party and meeting new people may not be comfortable alone with a date. However, the individual will eventually be able to move from nonthreatening group social events to more intimate settings and progress to a desired level of sexual behavior.

Systematic desensitization was explained in 1958 by Joseph Wolpe, an American psychiatrist (1915–1997). His first reports were on adults who had many mental health problems, including obsessive-compulsive disorder, reactive depressions and phobias. He adapted his technique from experiences gained in the 1920s when he worked with children in overcoming phobias of animals.

Flooding and Implosive Therapy

Flooding is another technique used by behavioral therapists. The individual is asked to experience an anxiety-producing situation by imagination or in actuality (in vivo) while experiencing the supportiveness of the therapist. Then the individual is directly exposed to a high-intensity, peak level of the anxiety-producing situation without benefit of a graduated approach, as is the case in the systematic desensitization technique. The therapist controls the content of scenes to be imagined and experiences that reoccur. The therapist describes scenes with great vividness, deliberately making them as disturbing as possible to the anxious individual, who has not been instructed to relax. Prolonged experience with these situations is planned to help the individual to experience "extinction" of the anxiety responses and thus overcome them.

Implosive therapy is another technique used by therapists. The individual is repeatedly encouraged to imagine anxiety-producing situations at maximum intensity and experience an intense anxiety reaction. The anxiety response is not reinforced and thus becomes gradually reduced.

Like desensitization, the techniques of flooding and implosion reduce anxieties and unwanted behaviors in some persons (such as those with simple fears), but desensitization seems to be more effective and to have more permanent results.

Modeling

As a form of behavioral therapy, the individual watches another person—often of the same sex and age as the troubled person—successfully perform a particular feared action, such as entering a room full of strangers or being introduced to members of the opposite sex. The fearful person experiences extinction of the feared responses in a vicarious way. This technique is really social learning or observational learning.

Modeling has another aspect; in "covert modeling" the anxious patient simply imagines that another person faces the same anxieties or concerns without unwanted physiological responses.

Operant Conditioning

This is a theory applied in behavioral therapy work. Because people will either maintain or reduce frequency of certain behaviors because of responses they get from their environment, behaviors that produce reinforcing consequences can be strengthened and behaviors producing unpleasant consequences reduced. Behaviors of avoidance in certain situations are considered under "operant" control and are thus changeable.

Hypnosis and Biofeedback

Hypnosis is considered a behavioral technique and is often used in conjunction with other techniques. Hypnosis can help the individual reach a trancelike state in which he or she becomes extremely receptive to suggestion. Then, through posthypnotic suggestions, the individual may learn to change patterns of behavior, such as having fearful reactions to entering a room full of strangers at a party. By itself, hypnosis is not considered an appropriate treatment for most mental health disorders. It is often used to modify specific, unwanted behaviors, such as smoking cigarettes.

Biofeedback is often used in conjunction with relaxation training and to enhance possibilities for a person's response to treatments. In biofeedback, physiological reactions can be monitored electrically. An anxious person can learn to regulate certain processes, such as breathing or heart rate.

Family Therapy

Behavioral techniques are often used in modifying ways in which an individual interacts with other members of his or her family. It is useful in some cases of childhood behavior problems, school phobia and agoraphobia, in which other members of the family "enable" the agoraphobic to persist in fearful habits.

See also AGORAPHOBIA; PSYCHOTHERAPIES.

behaviorism   A school of thought that holds that learning comes from conditioning, the most important factor in shaping who we are. Behaviorists believe that environment—not heredity—counts and that behavior, rather than experience, is all that can be observed in others. This school of thought was founded by James Broadus Watson (1878–1958), an American psychologist, early in the 20th century. Behavioral therapy techniques are generally based on these tenets.

Benson, Herbert (1935–)   The founding president and associate chief of the Mind/Body Medical Institute, Division of Behavioral Medicine, Harvard Medical School, and chief of the Division of Behavioral Medicine, New England Deaconess Hospital.

He is a cardiologist who discovered and described how the relaxation response is a protective mechanism against overreaction to stress and anxieties. He is the author and coauthor of several books relating to relaxation and stress, including *The Relaxation Response* and *The Mind/Body Effect;* hundreds of his articles have appeared in medical journals and popular magazines.

Dr. Benson discovered the relaxation response while studying people who practiced transcendental meditation. As a specialist in high blood pressure, Dr. Benson's particular interests have included how the relaxation response can help people with high blood pressure and other health concerns. He warns that people with high blood pressure should not just give up their medication. What meditation and the relaxation response do, he maintains, is improve upon the benefit of the medication. He argues that "mindfulness" is needed to be healthy and productive.

For more information:

Mind-Body Medical Institute
New Deaconess Hospital
Harvard Medical School
185 Pilgrim Road
Cambridge, MA 02215
Telephone: (617) 632-9530

See also COMPLEMENTARY THERAPIES; HIGH BLOOD PRESSURE; MEDITATION; RELAXATION; TRANSCENDENTAL MEDITATION.

Benson, Herbert. *The Relaxation Response.* New York: Avon Books, 1975.
———. *Beyond the Relaxation Response.* New York: Berkeley Press, 1985.
———. *The Mind/Body Effect: How Behavioral Medicine Can Show You the Way to Better Health.* New York: Simon and Schuster, 1979.

benzodiazepine drugs   A group of prescription medications widely prescribed to help relieve symptoms of anxiety. They also act as muscle relaxants, sedatives and anticonvulsants. Different drugs in this class are approved for different conditions, such as panic disorder.

Benzodiazepine drugs have less toxicity and fewer drug interaction problems than barbiturates and non-barbiturate sedative-hypnotic drugs. Also, benzodiazepine drugs have a lower risk of cardiovascular and respiratory depression compared with barbiturates and are often used before general anesthesia.

Persons taking benzodiazepine drugs should avoid alcohol because interaction may result in depression of the central nervous system.

See also PANIC ATTACKS AND PANIC DISORDER; PHARMACOLOGIC APPROACH.

BENZODIAZEPINE DRUGS

LONG ACTING

Trade Name	Generic Name
Librium	chlordiazepoxide
Klonopin	clonazepam
Tranxene	clorazepate
Valium	diazepam
Dalmane	flurazepam
Paxipam	halazepam
Centrax	prazepam
Doral	quazepam

SHORT ACTING

Xanax	alprazolam
Ativan	lorazepam
Serax	oxazepam
Restoril	temazepam
Halcion	triazolam

BENZODIAZEPINE DRUGS: GENERIC AND TRADE NAMES

Generic Name	Trade Name
alprazolam	Xanax
chlordiazepoxide	Librium
clonazepam	Klonopin
chorazepat	Tranxene
diazepam	Valium
flurazepam	Dalmane
halazepam	Paxipam
lorazepam	Ativan
oxazepam	Serax
prazepam	Centrax
quazepam	Doral
temazepam	Restoril
triazolam	Halcion

Adapted from *Comprehensive Psychiatric Nursing*, 5th ed. by Judith Haber and Barbara Krainovich-Miller St. Louis: Mosby, 1997.

bereavement A feeling of grief, numbness, emptiness and deprivation, particularly following the death of a loved one. Bereavement may also follow the loss of a pet, a material item or a relationship. In most cases, bereavement is diagnosed as a "normal" response to a situation. However, when signs and symptoms of bereavement become excessive, the condition may be considered a disorder and require professional treatment. In the course of the grieving process, each person progresses at an individual pace. While some people are ready, after a certain period of time, to socialize and resume many former activities, others take longer to feel comfortable in conversation with strangers, in crowds or attending any type of social events.

Many individuals find self-help groups for widowed people helpful after the loss of a spouse. There are also self-help groups for individuals who have lost a child or miscarried a pregnancy.

See also GRIEF.

beta adrenergic-receptor blockers A group of drugs, also called beta blockers, some of which are used to relieve symptoms of anxiety. While beta blockers have been considered effective in treating generalized anxiety disorder (GAD), they are not considered as effective as benzodiazepines, since they seem more effective at blocking peripheral or somatic anxiety symptoms.

Examples of some uses for these drugs are to reduce rapid heart rate, palpitations, sweats and hand or voice tremors rather than to relieve feelings of fear or anxiety.

There is some evidence that beta blockers may increase depressive feelings in some individuals, but they do not characteristically produce drowsiness. They are typically used by people who react to anxiety-producing situations in which somatic anxiety symptoms may impair function, such as addressing a large group. Beta blockers are also used in general medicine to prevent heart arrhythmias, treat high blood pressure and prevent migraine headaches. Examples of beta blocking drugs are propranolol (Inderal) and atenolol (Tenormin). They are not generally associated with the development of physical dependency but should not be discontinued suddenly in patients with atherosclerotic heart disease.

See also HEADACHES.

binge eating See EATING DISORDERS.

binge-purge syndrome See EATING DISORDERS.

bioavailability A means by which the effectiveness of various types of drugs or methods of administration can be compared. Preparations with the same bioavailability are said to be bioequivalent. This term is often used with regard to generic forms of drugs. Bioavailability refers to the amount of a drug that enters the bloodstream and reaches tissues and organs around the body. It is usually expressed as a percentage of the dose given. For example, intravenous administration (injection) produces 100 percent bioavailability as the drug is injected directly into the bloodstream, whereas only a proportion of the drug can be absorbed through the digestive system with drugs taken by mouth. Some drugs are broken down in the liver before getting into the circulatory system. When prescribing antidepressants and tranquilizers, physicians take into account the bioavailability of various preparations and the needs of the individual.

See also ANTIDEPRESSANT MEDICATIONS.

biochemical disturbances See BRAIN CHEMISTRY.

bioenergetics An approach to improving mental health proposed by Wilhelm Reich (1897–1957). Bioenergetics is a method for understanding personality in terms of the body and its energetic processes, as well as a way to relieve the individual's muscular tensions and rigidities resulting from emotional stress and unresolved emotional conflicts. The major techniques used to achieve full aliveness and emotional well-being include respiratory exercises, free expression of feelings and improvement of the body image.

See also BODY IMAGE; REICH, WILHELM.

biofeedback A technique to monitor mental and physical events using electrical feedback. Biofeedback is useful in many approaches to therapy for mental health concerns, such as anxieties and phobias. It provides an anxious or phobic individual with a basis for self-regulation of certain processes, such as autonomic system reactions to fear situations. It establishes a diagnostic baseline by noting physiological reactions to stressful events, enables therapists to relate this information to the individual's self-reports, fills gaps in the individual's history and encourages relaxation in the part of the individual's body to which the biofeedback equipment is applied. Relaxation training is often suggested to assist the individual in control anxiety reactions.

See also BEHAVIOR THERAPY.

Doctor, Ronald M., and Ada P. Kahn. *The Encyclopedia of Phobias, Fears, and Anxieties.* New York: Facts On File, 2000.

biogenic amines Chemicals produced by the central nervous system that are involved in the functioning of the brain. Their role is to assist in the transmission of the electrochemical impulses from one nerve cell to another. Examples of biogenic amines include norepinephrine, dopamine and serotonin.

See also AMINE; NEUROTRANSMITTERS; NOREPINEPHRINE; SEROTONIN.

biological clock A term in contemporary usage referring to the limit on the period of time a woman has in which to bear children. Women in their mid- to late thirties say their "biological clock is running out." For many who desire to become mothers, this is a source of stress and anxiety.

Actually, the central nervous system has been found to have several "biological clocks" such as circadian rhythms and diurnal rhythms, which affect levels of brain chemicals or neurotransmitters and affect preparation of the individual for physical and intellectual response during varying times of the day. This is being increasingly recognized as an important factor in shift workers, especially those who must change shifts and maintain alertness, productivity and a sense of well-being.

biological markers   Genes or genetic characteristics that can be identified and followed from generation to generation. Theories about the causes of affective disorders suggest that a disruption of neurotransmitters occurs, either by blockage of receptors or changes in receptors associated with the hypothalamus. The hypothalamus receives input from almost all regions of the brain. Changes in neurotransmitter patterns in a variety of brain areas alter neurotransmitter patterns in the hypothalamus. The hypothalamus exerts direct control on the anterior pituitary by a process known as neuroendocrine transduction. In this process, electrical signals determine the secretion patterns of hypothalamic neurotransmitters that stimulate specialized hypothalamic cells to secrete certain hormones. The hormones travel throughout the bloodstream to determine the release patterns of anterior pituitary hormones. Thus, changes in the neurotransmitters in the hypothalamus, as evident in an individual with affective disorders, may exhibit changes in the hormonal secretion patterns from the pituitary.

The first disrupted hormonal pattern to be studied was alteration in cortisol production. It was known that acutely depressed individuals showed extremely elevated levels of circulating cortisol. Cortisol (a glucocorticoid) is secreted by the adrenal cortex and regulated by the hypothalamic-pituitary-adrenal axis. Adrenocorticotrophic hormone (ACTH), released from the pituitary, is the major regulator of cortisol production. Release of ACTH is controlled by corticotrophin-releasing factor (CRF) from specialized cells in the hypothalamus. Secretion of CRF is stimulated by serotonin and acetylcholine and inhibited by norepinephrine.

The pituitary gland secretes ACTH in bursts, with the lowest levels secreted in late evening and highest levels in early morning, just after awakening. There are eight to nine secretory bursts during the day, for a total of approximately 16 mg. of cortisol released per day. Feedback loops, to the pituitary and hypothalamus, exist to regulate the release of ACTH and, subsequently, cortisol.

Some individuals who have affective disorders have increased levels of cortisol as measured in the plasma, CSF and urine. The elevated levels of cortisol secretion have been shown in individuals with unipolar depression and bipolar disorder. The secretion pattern is shifted, with the largest increase occurring from six to eight in the morning. In addition to elevated cortisol levels, individuals also have a flattened curve with loss of its normal circadian pattern.

There are two basic tests relating to biological markers. One is the dexamethasone suppression test; the other is the thyroid-releasing hormone challenge test.

Dexamethasone Suppression Test (DST)

The dexamethasone suppression test was the first biological marker for affective disorder. Dexamethasone is a synthetic glucocorticoid that has the effect of turning off the secretion of ACTH and, subsequently, cortisol. In normal persons, a dose of dexamethasone given at 11:00 P.M. reduces cortisol levels for the next 24 hours. In depressed individuals, however, the suppression effect of dexamethasone does not occur. The nonsuppression of cortisol is called a positive dexamethasone suppression test. A positive DST result suggests depression but other illnesses such as alcoholism may show nonsuppression. However, a negative DST result does not rule out the diagnosis of major depression. In addition, studies suggest a positive correlation between the severity of depression and the rate of DST nonsuppression. There is also a correlation between the DST nonsuppression index and risk of suicide.

Individuals identified as nonsuppressors upon testing before antidepressive medication return to a normal suppression pattern when the treatment is successful. Individuals who show no reversal effect after treatment are at increased risk of relapse. The DST test is not considered specific enough for routine clinical use but may be of value in special circumstances.

While DST is considered a biological marker for mood disorders, it identifies only about 30–50 percent of clinically depressed individuals.

Thyroid-releasing Hormone (TRH) Challenge Test

Indications for clinical use of the TRH challenge test are similar to those for DST. It is sometimes used as an aid in diagnosing depression and assessing thyroid status. A positive test result suggests the diagnosis of major depression, but a negative test result does not eliminate the diagnosis. When the two tests are used together, the increased sensitivity rate has been reported as high as 84 percent.

The hypothalamic-pituitary-thyroid (HPT) axis is the thyroid gland link to the central nervous system. The hypothalamus releases thyroid-releasing hormone (TRH) from neurons that stimulate pituitary cells to release thyroid-stimulating hormone (TSH) into the blood. TSH then stimulates release of other chemicals from the thyroid gland. Release of TRH is facilitated by dopamine and norepinephrine and is inhibited by serotonin. Levels of TSH have a circadian rhythm, with the highest levels of secretion from 4:00 A.M. to 8:00 A.M. Some individuals who are depressed have symptoms of hypothyroidism. A TRH test is used to determine if the HPT axis is functioning normally.

See also ANTIDEPRESSANT MEDICATIONS; DOPAMINE; NOREPINEPHRINE; SEROTONIN.

McFarland, Gertrude K., and Mary Durand Thomas. *Psychiatric Mental Health Nursing.* Philadelphia: J. B. Lippincott, 1991.

biorhythms A term that describes all of the body's physiological functions that vary in certain predictable rhythmic ways. An example is the menstrual cycle in women, which is usually about 28 days. On a day-to-day basis, human bodies and their periods of sleepiness and wakefulness are governed by an internal clock regulated by hormones. When the internal clock is upset by long-distance jet travel, a syndrome known as jet lag occurs. This involves becoming sleepy at unusual times of the day, a groggy feeling, becoming hungry at odd hours and waking up during the middle of the night.

See also CIRCADIAN RHYTHMS; HORMONES.

bipolar disorder A group of mood disorders characterized by alternating mood swings of mania and severe depression. The American Psychiatric Association's *Diagnostic and Statistical Manual of Mental Disorders,* 4th ed., breaks bipolar disorders into a variety of types, based on prevalence of symptoms.

During the manic phase, the individual may have an enormous amount of energy and may feel agitated, excited and capable of any undertaking. There may be constant talking, inappropriate degrees of self-confidence, little need for sleep, irritability, aggressiveness and impulsive behavior, such as excessive shopping and spending.

During the depressive phase, the individual suffers from any of the symptoms associated with major depression. They may feel sad, helpless and hopeless.

Bipolar disorder may start in childhood or later, during the 40s and 50s. Often bipolar disorder is first noticed during adolescence. However, as moodiness and crises surrounding personal and school relationships often arise at this time, symptoms of bipolar disorder might be at first incorrectly attributed to normal adolescent problems. Bipolar disorder often runs in families, and evidence from family and twin studies supports genetic transmission of susceptibility. Evidence from biochemical and imaging studies using PET scanning and MRI and CAT studies offers further support for the biologic nature of this illness.

Additional problems of alcohol and substance abuse are common with bipolar disorder. This is called a "co-morbid" condition. Early detection and finding the right medication is crucial in helping people recover. Many people are helped by taking lithium and one of many antidepressant medications, as well as other drugs under the close supervision of their physician.

See also AFFECTIVE DISORDERS; ANTIDEPRESSANT MEDICATIONS; DEPRESSION; LITHIUM CARBONATE; MOOD DISORDERS.

American Psychiatric Association. *Diagnostic and Statistical Manual of Mental Disorders,* 4th ed., rev. Washington, D.C., 1994.
Fawcett, Jan, Bernard Golden, and Nancy Rosenfeld. *New Hope for People with Bipolar Disorder.* Roseville, Calif.: Prima, 2000.

birth control A term referring to controlling the number of children born by preventing or reducing the chance of conception by natural or artificial means. The issue produces anxieties for many people, including those making a choice of birth control methods or those whose religious convictions run counter to using birth control as a practical and economic plan for their families. Furthermore, side effects of birth control medication can lead to anxieties for some individuals.

Methods of Birth Control

Each method of birth control has advantages, disadvantages and sources of anxieties. They should be discussed by couples before they engage in sexual intercourse. Women and men must weigh the factors in a birth control method including effectiveness in preventing unwanted pregnancy, protection from a sexually transmitted disease and freedom from side effects, costs or spontaneity of use.

According to the 1995 National Survey of Family Growth by the National Center for Health Statistics, the most popular method of birth control is female sterilization (29.5 percent), followed by the birth control pill (28.5 percent), male prophylactics (17.7 percent), vasectomy (12.5 percent), the diaphragm (2.8 percent), the IUD (1.4 percent) and all other methods (4.9 percent). The numbers total more than 100 percent because some women use more than one method.

For information:

American College of Obstetricians
   and Gynecologists
409 12th Street SW
Washington, D.C. 20024-2188
Phone: (202) 638-5577

See also CONDOMS; PREGNANCY; SEXUALLY TRANSMITTED DISEASES; UNWED MOTHERS.

Franklin, Deborah. "The Birth Control Bind." *Health* (July/Aug. 1992).
Kahn, Ada P., and Linda Hughey Holt. *The A-Z of Women's Sexuality.* New York: Facts On File, 1990.

birth defects   Also known as congenital anomalies. The birth defects most likely to be lethal include malformations of the brain and spine, heart defects and combinations of several malformations. Defects may be obvious at birth or detectable early in infancy. Infant mortality from congenital anomalies has been declining, although the last decade has seen slight increases in the incidence of some birth defects. In 1985, about 11,000 babies were born with moderate to severe impairments. Congenital anomalies, when they do not result in death, may cause disability. One-fourth of all congenital anomalies are caused by genetic factors, suggesting a need for preconception genetic counseling for both men and women. Environmental hazards and alcohol use during pregnancy are other important factors. Fetal alcohol syndrome (FAS) affects as many as one to three infants per 1,000 live births. In some populations, the incidence is higher. A similar syndrome has been observed in babies born to drug-addicted mothers.

Parents of children born with congenital anomalies can benefit from special counseling.

See also MENTAL RETARDATION.

birth order   Researchers in the area of birth order study personality development and mental health in relation to position in the family constellation. Alfred Adler, a student of Sigmund Freud, began the study of birth order in the early 1900s. Many studies of birth order have been undertaken as data were compiled for other projects. Birth order has been studied in relation to characteristics ranging from alcoholism to affiliation with religious orders. Most researchers believe that it is not a dominant force in personality development but one of the many determining factors in shaping a child's personality.

Studies of birth order have led to some generalizations about how a child's position in relation to his parents and siblings may affect his personality and view of the world.

The older child shares many of the qualities of the only child, as he or she is alone until the birth of a brother or sister. He has the attention and resources of the family for a certain length of time. As a result, older children tend to be more adult in behavior, are more interested in goals and personal achievement and are strongly represented in the ranks of the successful and powerful. Older children tend to score highest on intelligence tests. The arrival of a sibling, even though happily anticipated by the first child, has the ultimate effect of making him feel, in Adler's term, "dethroned." The older child often assumes a certain amount of responsibility for younger children in the family. He may be held responsible for setting a good example, showing younger children how to do things and baby-sitting. Older children are frequently more aware of family difficulties and problems and their own parents' insecurities. As a result, they tend to be more anxious, conservative and responsible than younger brothers and sisters.

The middle child position in the family has more variables attached to it, since the ages and sex of siblings may have a profound effect on the middle child. Middle children usually become good at sharing but also guard their privacy. Because of what they may perceive as a chaotic situation at home in which they are too young for the privileges of the oldest and too old for the coddling of the youngest, the middle child may show off to get attention and may also seek rewarding relationships outside the family. Middle children are team players and are frequently quite popular. The need to belong to a peer group is strong in middle children. To compete with an older sibling, a middle child develops her abilities in an area quite different from the talents of her older brother or sister. Middle children are frequently mavericks and are sensitive to inequities and injustices.

The youngest child of a family never has the experience of having his position usurped by a younger sibling. Younger children tend to preserve and use childish characteristics such as crying, acting cute or emphasizing their dependence and inadequacy to get what they want. Younger children frequently have very positive feelings about themselves because of their position in the family and tend to be charming and popular. They often have the best sense of humor in the family. Younger children are at a disadvantage in that they tend to obtain information and opinions from other children rather than adults and therefore lack the wisdom and realism they might gain from adult contact.

A very specific type of younger child is the "little caboose," often a "change of life" baby who arrives several years after the other siblings. This younger child is really more in the position of being the only child, but with several parents, since usually one or more of his siblings acts as a parent. These children grow up with a great deal of attention and support but may also have a confused sense of themselves, as they get a variety of images and ideas from siblings who are perceived as adult but are, in fact, children.

See also ONLY CHILDREN.

bisexuality   See SEXUAL PREFERENCES.

blocking   An interruption in thought or speech that is abrupt and involuntary, when the individual cannot remember what it was he or she was about to say. This is also referred to as thought deprivation, thought obstruction and emotional blocking. This happens to most people at some time, especially if they are in a state of severe anxiety, grief or anger. In such circumstances it is normal to experience blocking at intermittent times. By itself, blocking is not a symptom of poor mental health. However, some individuals who are mentally disturbed may use blocking to keep distasteful ideas out of their consciousness. In some forms of schizophrenia, thoughts and speech may be blocked for prolonged periods of time.

Blocking should not be confused with "word finding" difficulties or recent memory loss seen in patients with multi-infarct dementia or with medication side effects.

See also SCHIZOPHRENIA.

blood brain barrier   A physiological metabolic system that limits entry into the brain, protecting it from a number of potentially brain-damaging substances throughout the body, as well as from fluctuations in chemicals it needs to function normally.

It is a physiological "barrier" that regulates certain substances' rate of entry or egress in or out of the brain to or from its blood circulation. This is one reason why specific blood tests for mental disorders have not been developed beyond the stage of research findings.

Because of the blood brain barrier, chemicals composed of large molecules generally cannot pass from the blood into the brain as they do into other organs. This is so because in most parts of the body the smallest blood vessels are porous, whereas cells in the brain are tightly joined and adjacent cells are almost fused together. However, substances with small molecules, including oxygen, alcohol and medications that are highly fat soluble—anesthetics, for example—can cross the barrier.

Some substances, such as amino acids, require energy provided by glucose metabolism to cross the blood brain barrier.

See also BRAIN.

blood pressure   The force of the blood against the walls of the arteries, created by the heart as it pumps blood through the body. As the heart pumps or beats, the pressure increases. The pressure decreases as the heart relaxes between beats. High blood pressure, known as hypertension, is the condition in which blood pressure rises too high and stays there. One cannot feel blood circulating through the body; thus one usually does not feel symptoms of high blood pressure. The only effective way to measure blood pressure is to have it checked with specially designed equipment.

Many individuals who are told that they have high blood pressure are advised to change their diet (lower cholesterol, lose weight) and exercise more. For some, medications that lower blood pressure are prescribed. Many individuals have difficulty complying because they cannot "see" or "feel" their disease. For these reasons high blood pressure has been referred to as "the silent killer."

blood tests   Many individuals who are taking medication as part of their treatment for a mental health condition will be asked to have frequent and repeated blood tests. The reason is to determine how much of the medication remains in their bloodstream over a prolonged period of time. Blood tests help the prescriber determine an effective dose for each individual.

One such test is the lithium blood level test that individuals who have manic-depressive disorder undergo. With these measurements, the physician can choose and maintain the most effective dose for the individual and avoid a toxic dose. When a patient stops taking lithium, the blood level drops and symptoms may reappear.

Other tests are used to monitor the function of various organs (e.g., kidneys, liver) or thyroid gland function to ascertain that no medical illness is causing a mental disturbance or that medications are not causing any toxic effects.

Currently, there are no blood tests considered clinically reliable enough to diagnose mental disorders not related to medical illnesses (hypothyroidism, vitamin deficiencies) because the metabolism of the brain is not reliably reflected in blood or urine samples.

See also ANTIDEPRESSANT MEDICATIONS; BLOOD BRAIN BARRIER; DEPRESSION; LITHIUM; MANIC-DEPRESSIVE ILLNESS.

"blues"   When people feel down, they are often referred to as suffering from the "blues." A "blue" mood is considered a sad mood. Most people experience these mood changes from time to time, but this does not necessarily indicate depression. Changes in mood are normal with the ups and downs of daily life, and individuals are able to function normally. It is only when mood characteristics meet the criteria for depression and interfere with daily living that professional help should be sought. The "baby blues" is the feeling of being overwhelmed or helpless after the birth of a baby. If the feeling continues and interferes with function or relationships, this is known as POSTPARTUM DEPRESSION.

See also DEPRESSION; POSTPARTUM DEPRESSION; SEASONAL AFFECTIVE DISORDER.

blunted affect   An affect or mood with a lack of, or significant reduction in, the intensity of emotional expression.

See also AFFECT; AFFECTIVE DISORDERS; DEPRESSION.

boarder babies   A term denoting babies born with HIV infections (human immunodeficiency virus) who remain in the hospital because their mothers are too ill to care for them and they are difficult to place in foster homes.

See also ACQUIRED IMMUNODEFICIENCY SYNDROME.

body builder's psychosis   See ANABOLIC STEROIDS.

body dysmorphic disorder   See BODY IMAGE.

body image The mental picture an individual has of his or her body at any moment. Perception of one's own body often determines one's level of self-esteem and self-confidence. Body image is derived from internal sensations, postural changes, emotional experiences, fantasies and feedback from others. A misperception of one's body image can lead to avoidance of social or sexual activities and eating disorders such as anorexia nervosa or bulimia.

Fear of deformity of one's own body is known as dysmorphophobia.

See also ANOREXIA NERVOSA; BODY DYSMORPHIC DISORDER; BULIMIA; EATING DISORDERS; SEX APPEAL.

Veale, David, Kevin Gournay, Windy Dryden et al. "Body Dysmorphic Disorder: A Cognitive Behavioural Model and Pilot Randomised Controlled Trial." *Behaviour Research and Therapy* 34, no. 9 (Sept. 1996): 717–779.

body language A form of communication through facial expression, posture, gestures or movements, accompanied with or without words. Both the communicator and the listener may employ body language. It can be a device used to express emotion or a reaction to the meaning of communication.

Body language may be an indicator of the anxiety that the communicator and the listener are experiencing. Gay Turback wrote in The *Rotarian* (April 1995) that "without uttering a syllable, it's possible to communicate love, hate, fear, rage, deceit, and virtually every other emotion in the human repertoire." The article goes on to describe how body signals have been around for more than a million years, with some researchers having catalogued 5,000 hand gestures and 1,000 postures, each with its own message. Turback continued, "Although some body language is nearly universal, much of it is an accouterment of one culture or another. Certain actions may have one meaning in Mexico, a different meaning in the United States, and no relevance in Canada." Other examples given in the article that are especially common among North Americans are shown in the following table.

EXAMPLES OF BODY LANGUAGE AS INDICATORS OF ANXIETIES IN THE UNITED STATES

Action	Meaning
Toes pointed outward	Confidence
Toes pointed inward	Submission
A jutting chin	Belligerence
Lip and nail biting	Disappointment
Lip licking	Nervousness
Foot tapping	Impatience
Leaning backward	A relaxed attitude
Leaning forward	Interest
Open palms	Honesty
Rubbing hands together	Excitement

See also COMMUNICATION.

body narcissism Excessive interest in one's body and especially the erotic zones, such as the genitals or breasts. Psychoanalytic theory holds that this interest is particularly noticeable in young children when boys and girls begin to explore their bodies. Signs of narcissism might be evident in preoccupation with elimination activities, sexual response to masturbation and fear of injury to parts of the body. When the excessive interest in one's body continues throughout adulthood, the condition may be reason for psychological counseling.

See also BODY IMAGE; NARCISSISM.

body therapies Body therapies encompass ancient Eastern traditions of spirituality and cosmology along with contemporary Western neuromuscular and myofascial systems of skeletostructural and neuroskeletal reorganization. They postulate that the body holds memory of trauma and that therapy must address body sensations.

Ancient disciplines in the category of body therapies include yoga, t'ai chi, Zen, Taoism, Tantra and Samurai. In the 20th century, Wilhelm Reich observed that clinical patients with emotional disturbances all demonstrated severe postural distortions. This observation helped to uncover more connections between the body-psyche and led to the development of the Reichian school of body therapy.

Another modern pioneer in the field was Moshe Feldenkrais, who postulated that the human organism began its process of growth and learning with one built-in response, the "fear of falling." All other physical and emotional responses were learned as the human organism grew and explored. To attain the full potential of the body-mind-emotions-spirit, there must be, according to Feldenkrais, "reeducation of the kinesthetic sense and resetting of it to the normal course of self-adjusting improvement of all muscular activity." This would "directly improve breathing, digestion, and the sympathetic and parasympathetic balance, as well as the sexual function, all linked together with the emotional experience." Feldenkrais believed that reeducation of the body and its functions was the essence of creating unity of the being. His method has helped many people with problems of back pain, whiplash and lack of coordination. The method is also used to help people who have temporomandibular joint syndrome (TMJ), which is a collection of symptoms, including pain, that affect the jaw, face and head, often brought about by anxieties, stress and tension.

Four Systems of Body Therapies

Although many systems overlap and encompass aspects of the others, body therapies can be divided into four general categories, based on their methods.

Physical manipulation systems include the connective tissue work of the Ida Rolf school (Rolfing) and the deep tissues release systems such as myofascial release used by John Barnes, an American physical therapist.

Energy balancing systems include Chinese acupuncture and acupressure, polarity and Jin Shin Jytsu.

Emotional release systems include bioenergetics, primal therapy and rebirthing.

Movement awareness systems include those of Aston, Feldenkrais, Trager and Aguado.

For information:

Feldenkrais Guild of North America
3611 SW Hood Avenue, Suite 100
Portland, OR 97201
Phone: (800) 775-2118 or (503) 221-6612

North American Society of Teachers of the
    Alexander Technique
P.O. Box 517
Urbana, IL 61801

Phone: (217) 367-6956

Rolf Institute
P.O. Box 1868
Boulder, CO 80306
Phone: (303) 449-5903

See also ACUPUNCTURE; ACUPRESSURE; ALEXANDER TECHNIQUE; AYURVEDA; COMPLEMENTARY THERAPIES; MASSAGE THERAPY; MIND/BODY CONNECTIONS; T'AI CHI; YOGA.

Eisner, Betty. "Body Work and Psychological Healing." *Advances* 13, no. 3 (summer 1997) 64–66.
Feldenkrais, Moshe. *Explorers of Humankind.* San Francisco: Harper & Row, 1979.
———. *Awareness Through Movement.* San Francisco: Harper & Row, 1972.
Feltman, John, ed. *Hands-On Healing.* Emmaus, Pa.: Rodale, 1989.

bondage   A form of sexual activity in which one person pretends to enslave the other to arouse sexual pleasure in one or both partners. Bondage may involve heterosexual or homosexual participants and may include threats or acts of humiliation and danger, with the enslaved person restrained by chains, ropes or other devices. Discipline is a variation of bondage that involves sadomasochistic activities such as whipping. Partners usually have a signal to use when the activity exceeds pleasurable limits.

See also PERVERSION, SEXUAL.

bonding   The psychological process through which a mother forms a loving relationship with her child (also known as maternal bonding and paternal bonding). This may begin when a woman feels her baby move in her uterus for the first time, when she hears the first fetal heartbeat or during or after childbirth. Bonding develops further as she and her husband care for their newborn baby. According to M. H. Klaus and J. H. Kennel, authors of *Maternal-Infant Bonding* (1976), the first hour after birth is an especially critical time for bonding and is the "early sensitive period" when mother and child are particularly receptive to each other. When childbirth occurred mainly at home, mothers and infants were together after childbirth and there was little concern about bonding. Today many hospitals encourage parents to spend the first hours after delivery with their newborn and have arranged rooms so that the baby can remain with the mother after delivery.

Bonding is indicated by behaviors such as smiling, following, clinging, calling or crying when the mother leaves the child. This kind of behavior is the basis for later emotional attachments and is part of a series of normal developmental stages.

borderline personality disorder See PERSONALITY DISORDERS.

boredom A state of mind that is almost always the creation of the person who is bored. As a result, some people seem bored with everything, while others are bored with nothing. For some people, boredom is a self-imposed prison which keeps them from trying new things or having new, life-enriching experiences. Boredom often occurs within individuals who thrive on excessive stimulation and is not a function of environmental or social causes but of the reduction in stimulation.

Some people view things as boring because they are afraid of failure. In his book, *A New Guide To Rational Living*, Dr. Albert Ellis said: "Viewing failure with fear and horror, some people avoid activities that they would really like to engage in." The rationale of such people is: If life is boring, nothing is worth doing. Thus, if nothing is worth doing, a person can hardly fail.

Overcoming Boredom

Overcoming boredom depends on whether people are bored because they cannot live without excitement, or whether they are bored because they have chosen to remain in a shell of inaction. Life is not supposed to be thrilling all the time. If you crave continuous thrills, reduce your expectations for excitement. If you are encased by the stresses of boredom, try to face reality. Get out and do one new thing each day, such as talk to some new people, volunteer somewhere or write letters. Boredom carried to the extreme can be a threat to health in that it can lead to depression and anxiety.

For further information:

The Boring Institute
P.O. Box 40
Maplewood, NJ 07040
Phone: (201) 763-6392

See also DEPRESSION; GENERAL ADAPTATION SYNDROME; SELYE, HANS.

Kahn, Ada P. *Stress A to Z: A Sourcebook for Facing Everyday Challenges.* New York: Facts On File, 2000.

brain The center and largest and most complex portion of the central nervous system. The brain includes all of the higher nervous centers that receive stimuli from the sense organs, interprets and correlates information and is the source of motor impulses. Located within the skull, it is also the best protected part of the central nervous system.

The cerebrum is in the upper portion of the skull. It is the largest part of the brain and consists of the right and left cerebral hemispheres, which handle some of the more advanced processes of the nervous system. Some of these areas have been charted, and it is possible to determine the corresponding changes in certain areas of the body when certain parts of the brain are damaged. Separate parts of the cerebrum have certain functions. For example, sensory portions receive and interpret sensations of vision, hearing, touch, heat, pressure and others. Motor portions control muscles and movement, and association areas handle higher mental processes, such as memory, reasoning and analysis.

Below the cerebrum and toward the back part of the skull is the cerebellum, which controls many activities of the body below conscious level. For example, it automatically deals with reflexes of posture and balance, coordination of muscles and maintenance of muscle tone. Damage to the cerebellum, or inherited defects in it, make it difficult for an individual to move parts of the body properly. When there is a disturbance of a portion of the cerebellum, only the parts of the body on the same side as the disturbance are affected.

The midbrain, in front of the cerebellum, connects various divisions of the brain, including the brain stem and the medulla oblongata (spinal bulb), a control center for functions such as blood circulation and breathing. The spinal cord, which sends nervous system messages to and from the lower portions of the body, merges into the brain stem.

The thalamus is above the midbrain; it is an important center for processing and interpreting various sensations in the body (including pain) and is closely coordinated with the sensory parts of the cerebrum. The thalamus is thought to play a role in one's general mood or affect.

The hypothalamus is in the brain stem and takes on part of the brain's tasks of maintaining fluid balance in the body, sensing hunger, regulating body temperature and signaling a need for sleep or wakefulness. The hypothalamus secretes a hormone and other substances that aid in regulating water in the system and converting food and blood substances to energy (metabolism). Improper functioning of the hypothalamus may contribute to obesity, and when anxiety or excitement makes a person sweat and the heart beat faster, it is the hypothalamus that sends out messages for these reactions throughout the nervous system. Emotional tone may be affected by the chemical functions of neurons in the hypothalamus (depression, mania, anxiety and panic attacks).

Meninges surround the brain structures and extend down to enclose the spinal cord. These are membranes in three layers known as the dura mater (outer layer), arachnoid (middle layer) and the pia mater (inner layer). The meninges form spaces for the cerebro-spinal fluid, which helps to cushion the brain and spinal cord against injury and to keep nerve tissues moist and lubricated. This fluid becomes altered with various diseases; samples of spinal fluid are sometimes taken with a lumbar (lower back) puncture, also known as a spinal tap. This is done by insertion of a needle between the lumbar vertebrae. Examination of the spinal fluid can help diagnose infectious meningitis (inflammation of the meninges), as well as some types of brain hemorrhage or tumors. Spinal fluid defects are sometimes detected at birth. When this occurs, the pressure may enlarge a child's head (hydrocephalus). Treatment for hydrocephalus includes tapping the fluid to reduce the pressure and draining the fluid through a plastic tube inserted in the child's stomach.

Brain Disorders

Some brain disorders are characterized by symptoms rather than causes. These include migraine, narcolepsy (excessive episodic sleepiness) and idiopathic epilepsy (epilepsy of unknown cause), although epileptic seizures can also have specific causes, such as a tumor or infection.

Thought, emotion and behavioral disorders are generally described as emotional, mental or psychiatric illness. In some cases there is no obvious physical brain defect or disorder, although with many illnesses, such as depression and schizophrenia, there is often an underlying disturbance of brain chemistry.

See also ALCOHOLISM; AMYGDALA; BLOOD BRAIN BARRIER; BRAIN CHEMISTRY; BRAIN DEATH; BRAIN ELECTRICAL ACTIVITY MAPPING; BRAIN IMAGING; BRAIN SYNDROME, ORGANIC; BRAIN TUMORS.

brain chemistry   Since the 1950s, researchers have learned an increasing amount of knowledge regarding brain chemistry. At first they noted that certain medications had mood-altering qualities. For example, some patients taking reserpine, a drug used to control blood pressure, became depressed. Some patients taking iproniazid to treat tuberculosis became euphoric. These and other observations led researchers and clinicians to studies indicating that mood disorders can be a function of a biochemical disturbance and can be stabilized with antidepressant drugs.

In animal brain tissue studies, biogenic amines—a group of chemical compounds—have been shown to regulate mood. Two of the amines, serotonin and norepinephrine, seem to be particularly important and are concentrated in areas of the brain that also control drives for hunger, thirst and sex.

Although there has been considerable progress in understanding the role of brain chemistry in depression and other mental health disorders, much is still unknown about the role of brain chemistry and mental health. There is evidence that in some types of depression there are abnormalities in brain function and that some individuals with major depressive disorders have too little or too much of certain neurochemicals the antidepressant drugs relieve. Imbalances in a neurotransmitter set up a chemical imbalance in the hypothalamus, leading to an imbalance of a hormone in the pituitary and causing the adrenal glands to produce too much cortisol, which in turn has widespread physiological effects.

Tricyclic antidepressant drugs seem to enhance certain neurotransmitters. Monoamine oxidase inhibitors (MAOIs) lead to an elevation of the levels of amine messengers in certain regions of the brain; as the brain becomes filled with extra amounts of chemical transmitters, the presumed chemical amine deficiency is corrected.

Effects of lithium are less clearly understood, but some researchers theorize that lithium stabilizes the chemical-messenger levels, so that cycling in amine concentrations is less likely to occur.

See also ANTIDEPRESSANT MEDICATIONS; BRAIN; DEPRESSION; LITHIUM; NEUROTRANSMITTERS.

Roesch, Roberta. *The Encyclopedia of Depression.* New York: Facts On File, 1991.

brain damage   Death or degeneration of nerve cells and areas within the brain. There may be damage to particular areas of the brain, resulting in specific defects of brain function, such as loss of coordination, or more diffuse effects, causing mental retardation or severe physical disabilities.

Hypoxia, not enough oxygen reaching the brain, may occur during birth. A baby's brain cannot tolerate a lack of oxygen for more than about five minutes. At any age, hypoxia may occur as a result of cardiac arrest (stoppage of the heart) or respiratory arrest (cessation of breathing), as well as from other causes such as drowning, electric shock or prolonged convulsions.

Diffuse damage may also result from an accumulation of substances poisonous to nerve cells in the brain, such as phenylketonuria or galactosemia; damage may also result from inhaling or ingesting pollutants such as mercury compounds or lead. Brain damage may also be caused by infections of the brain and, in rare cases, may occur following immunizations.

Localized brain damage sometimes happens following head injury, especially penetrating injuries. In later life, it occurs as a result of stroke, brain abscess or brain tumor. At birth, local brain damage caused by a variety of factors can lead to kernicterus, a condition characterized by disorders of movement and sometimes mental deficiency.

Cerebral palsy may result from brain damage that occurs before, during or after birth. It is characterized by paralysis and abnormal movements; it is often associated with mental retardation and, in some cases, deafness. Disturbances of movement, speech or sensation or epileptic seizures may result from head injury, stroke or other causes of localized or diffuse brain damage.

Treatment to improve some physical and mental functions following brain damage include physical therapy, speech therapy and occupational therapy. Some improvement may be expected in many cases after brain damage, as the individual learns to use other parts of the brain and other muscle groups.

Congenital Defects

Infants are sometimes born with damage due to genetic or chromosomal disorders, such as Down's syndrome and cri du chat syndrome. Structural defects arising during fetal development may be untreatable, such as microcephaly (small head), or fatal, such as anencephaly (congenital absence of the brain). Other defects can be corrected even while the fetus is in the uterus.

See also BRAIN TUMORS; CEREBRAL PALSY; DOWN'S SYNDROME.

brain death   A concept meaning that a person is dead if the brain is dead; this is not a point on which all theologians, doctors and lawyers agree. Although still controversial, a widely accepted definition of the term with four criteria was proposed in 1968 by a Harvard Medical School committee: unresponsiveness to touch, sound and all other external stimuli; no movements and no spontaneous breathing; no reflexes; and a flat EEG, or the absence of all electrical activity in the brain as measured by the electroencephalogram.

There are various attitudes about brain death. One holds that the brain is dead only when the cerebral cortex—or the part of the brain humans use for thinking—stops functioning. Another attitude is that before the brain can be declared dead, the brain stem, which regulates lower processes, must also stop functioning.

The Harvard criteria are used by some, but not all, American states; other countries have differing definitions. Recognition of brain death permits physicians to certify death even when the heart and lungs continue activity with connections to life-sustaining equipment but when there is no brain function.

brain electrical activity mapping (BEAM) A technique using a computer to perform spectral analysis of data from an electroencephalogram (EEG). The BEAM technique calculates the relative quantity of each brain-wave frequency as detected by each recording electrode location, showing patterns that may be too subtle to detect on a routine EEG. BEAM or brain mapping has been used in psychiatric research to study schizophrenia.

See also SCHIZOPHRENIA.

brain imaging Computer-assisted methods to permit physicians and researchers to see detailed anatomical structures, abnormalities and actions within the brain; it is also known as brain scan or scanning. With imaging or scanning techniques, determinations can be made about the neurobiologic bases of mental disorders. For example, the size, shape and position of tumors or a specific area in the brain responsible for epileptic seizures or other conditions can be pinpointed. Images can indicate to physicians brain functions based on differences in metabolism or biochemical differences among different anatomical areas. Brain imaging or scanning techniques use X ray, radioactivity and radio waves to produce detailed visualizations of the brain.

X ray

An X ray produces pictures of the bony structures of the skull but not the brain itself. However, with an X-ray image, a physician can sometimes detect erosion in the inner side of the skull, possibly indicating a brain tumor, as a growth can wear away bone. In some cases, bleeding inside the brain can also be detected with an X ray.

Angiography

This technique involves injecting a dye into an artery leading to the brain and then taking X rays, which show blood vessels in the brain. It is sometimes used to help diagnose some brain hemorrhages, aneurysms, abnormalities of blood vessels and other circulation disorders.

Computerized Axial Tomography (CAT)

Scanners that X-ray the brain in cross section, allowing the computer screens to display views of "slices" of the brain from various angles. In use since the early 1970s, CAT scanning reveals images of the brain substance itself, including pictures of the fluid-filled cavities of the brain (ventricles) that may indicate blood clots, aneurysms, abscesses, tumors or evidence of strokes. To help differentiate normal from abnormal brain tissue, contrast dye is often used.

Magnetic Resonance Imaging (MRI)

A technique that does not involve use of radiation and is particularly useful in showing tumors of the back of the skull. CAT and MRI have replaced previously used techniques of radionuclide scanning, which involved the use of radioactive isotopes to detect abnormalities of the blood vessels, tumors and other lesions.

Positron Emission Tomography (PET)

This technique combines use of radionuclides with CAT scanning and may reveal activities in various parts of the brain. Metabolic activity and the effects of specific drugs can be studied in humans with mental disorders yielding evidence of biochemical changes with this noninvasive procedure.

Ultrasound Scanning

Ultrasound waves cannot penetrate bones of a mature skull but are useful in premature or very young infants. It can be used to detect hydrocephalus and ventricular hemorrhage in premature babies.

With ultrasonography, sound waves above the range of human hearing are sent into the head and bounce back, with echoes varying according to the tissue reached, helping to locate any displacement of the midline of the brain because of the pressure of a tumor. Repeated scans can be performed, as no radiation is involved.

brain scan See BRAIN IMAGING.

brain stem See BRAIN.

brain syndrome, organic Disruptions of mental functioning and consciousness resulting from physical (organic) causes rather than psychological origins. Causes include degenerative diseases, such as Alzheimer's disease, imbalances of metabolism, reactions to medications, infections, vitamin deficiencies and effects of tumors, strokes or trauma.

Symptoms may range from slight confusion to coma or may include memory impairment, hallucinations, delusions and disorientation. A chronic form of organic brain syndrome results in a progressive decline in intellectual functions. Treatment includes dealing with underlying causes wherever possible; treatment is most likely to be helpful in the acute stages of the illness.

See also ALZHEIMER'S DISEASE; BRAIN TUMORS; DEMENTIA.

brain tumors Any growth in the brain, more commonly a term referring to a cancerous growth within the brain substance. Brain tumors can be benign or malignant. Intrinsic tumors are those that arise from brain tissue or grow within the brain. Metastatic tumors are those that grow within the brain after having spread to the brain from another region of the body.

Brain tumors occur at all ages and reach peak incidence in individuals in their fifties and sixties. Classification of brain tumors is based on the cell type from which the tumor originated and can be determined by removing the tumor surgically and analyzing it microscopically.

Diagnosis of brain tumor is often difficult because tumors may cause very generalized symptoms. As tumors grow and occupy more space within the cavity of the skull, pressure on the brain increases. When the tumor presses on specific regions of the brain, there may be more specific complaints, such as headache, nausea, vomiting, partial blindness, double vision, seizures or weakness. There may be changes in personality, changes in speech and impaired memory and judgment. However, individuals with one or more of these symptoms should not rush to the conclusion that they have a brain tumor.

Physicians use brain imaging or brain scanning techniques to help diagnose brain tumors. Forms of treatment include surgery, radiation and chemotherapy.

brainwashing A form of mind control related to propaganda or political indoctrination. In its most extreme form, it was practiced by Communist governments, particularly during warfare. Some American prisoners of war who were incarcerated in China during the Korean War returned with their personalities and attitudes changed. They had been conditioned to the point that they made no attempt to escape their captors. Some came home with feelings that rejected America and accepted Communist propaganda. They also showed no interest in returning to their families. The same techniques—characterized by isolating individuals from friends and families and keeping them socially deprived, exhausted and overworked—are employed by cults professing a wide range of beliefs that promise to "save" the subject. People with low self-esteem and severe identity problems who are socially isolated or reject their own family values are particularly susceptible.

Although situations and techniques of brainwashing vary, there are common elements that are used to change thought patterns and deeply held values. For example, the subject is made to feel totally out of control, that his needs and actions are subject to an authority before which he is powerless. He may be subjected to mental or physical harassment and his deeply held beliefs ridiculed. As much as possible, he is made to feel that his future is uncertain and he must rely on the person who is controlling him. As his body weakens from the treatment, his thought processes become disorganized and he will agree to almost anything. His suggestibility increases as his self-esteem decreases. He begins to feel guilty about past behavior that is at odds with his captors' standards. As he becomes more agreeable to his captors' wishes, he is rewarded and his living conditions improve, only to deteriorate again if he regresses.

While true brainwashing is rare outside the realms of warfare and totalitarian governments, members of religious cults that flourished in the years following the 1960s showed evidence of techniques similar to brainwashing, such as changed speech and behavior patterns, obedience to an authoritarian leader and a rejection of friends and family outside the cult.

Johnson, Joan. *The Cult Movement.* New York: Franklin Watts, 1984.
Somit, Alters. "Brainwashing," In *International Encyclopedia of the Social Sciences,* vol. 1, edited by David Sills. New York: Macmillan, 1968.

brain waves   Electrical currents pulsing through brain cells. Although weaker than those in the heart, they can be detected by an electroencephalograph (EEG), a machine that records changes in electrical pressure and frequency on a moving graph. Physicians use the EEG as well as brain electrical activity mapping (BEAM) to study the brain and diagnose brain disorders. There are differing patterns of brain waves. Alpha waves occur when an individual is in a state of relaxed awareness. In a state of alertness, the brain gives off beta waves. When one is sleeping deeply, lying anesthetized during surgery or is suffering from severe brain damage, delta waves occur. Theta waves are a combination of mixed waves. In 1932, Edgar Adrian (1889–1977), a British electrophysiologist, won a Nobel prize for demonstration of brain waves.

Studies of sleep using EEG have shown specific abnormalities in the delayed onset of rapid-eye-movement (REM) sleep in many depressed patients.

See also BRAIN; BRAIN DAMAGE; BRAIN ELECTRICAL ACTIVITY MAPPING (BEAM); BRAIN IMAGING.

breath-holding spells   See BREATHING.

breathing   Breathing involves respiration and ventilation. Respiration puts oxygen into body cells and ventilation removes the excess carbon dioxide. Poor breathing habits diminish the flow of gasses to and from the body, making it harder for individuals to cope with stressful situations or situations threatening good mental health.

With increased awareness of how one breathes, and by incorporating certain controlled breathing techniques into relaxation practice, a person may be able to quiet thoughts, calm emotions, deepen relaxation and control blood pressure and other physical functions. Although breathing seems very easy and very normal, relearning breathing techniques can help many individuals who suffer from phobias, anxieties and panic attacks. Some performers and athletes learn this technique in order to combat stage fright or performance anxiety.

Breathing is controlled by the autonomic, or involuntary, nervous system. Breathing patterns change during different psychological states. For example, in a state of calm and relaxation, breathing becomes deeper and more rhythmic. Under stress, breathing is shallow and irregular. When frightened, an individual may even hold his or her breath. However, breathing patterns can be consciously controlled in order to influence the autonomic system toward relaxation, thereby interrupting the physiological arousal that can lead to stress-related disorders and high blood pressure.

Styles of Breathing

Most people breathe in one of two patterns: one is chest, or thoracic, breathing, and the other is abdominal or diaphragmatic breathing. Chest breathing, which is usually shallow and often rapid and irregular, is associated with anxiety and other emotional distress. When air is inhaled, the chest expands and the shoulders rise to take in air. Anxious people may experience breath holding, hyperventilation (constricted breathing), shortness of breath or fear of passing out. When an insufficient amount of air reaches the lungs, the blood is not properly oxygenated, the heart rate and muscle tension increases and the stress response is triggered.

Abdominal, or diaphragmatic, breathing is the natural breathing of sleeping adults. The diaphragm contracts and expands as inhaled air is drawn deep into the lungs and exhaled. When breathing is even and unconstricted, the respiratory system performs efficiently in producing energy from oxygen and removing waste products.

What Makes Breathing Inefficient?

Many people who often feel very anxious also often have breathing-related complaints. Some can't seem to catch their breath or get enough air. Others may frequently sigh, yawn or swallow. Some breathe too deeply and hyperventilate. Symptoms associated with hyperventilation resemble those of panic disorder. Researchers have noted the overlap between hyperventilation, anxiety and stress symptoms. It has been found that patients will hyperventilate when asked to think back to unpleasant or anxiety producing events.

Physical conditions associated with breathing difficulties, particularly hyperventilation, include hypertension, allergies, anemia, angina, arthritis, arrhythmias, asthma, colitis, diabetes, gastritis, headaches, heart disease and irritable bowel syndrome.

Deep, diaphragmatic breathing is a cornerstone for many relaxation therapies. Many therapeutic techniques (some known as complementary therapies) and behavior therapies incorporate control of breathing as a basis because the cycle of stress can be altered with breath control. Individuals who have mastered these techniques find that as soon as they are aware of a stressor, they become aware of their breathing and try to control their stress using deep, slow breaths. By contrast, holding the breath, as well as shallow, irregular breathing, can initiate and augment many stressful feelings and physiological responses. Posture can also affect breathing. Keeping the body in alignment allows greater lung capacity.

REDUCING STRESS WITH DIAPHRAGMATIC (ABDOMINAL) BREATHING

- Lie down comfortably on your back on a padded floor or a firm bed with eyes closed, arms at your sides and not touching your body, palms up, legs straight out and slightly apart and toes pointed comfortably outward.
- Focus attention on your breathing. Breathe through your nose. Place your hand on the part of your chest that seems to rise and fall the most as you inhale and exhale.
- Rest your hands lightly on your abdomen and slow your breathing. Become aware of how your abdomen rises with each inhalation and falls with each exhalation.
- If you have difficulty breathing into your abdomen, press your hand down on your abdomen as you exhale and let your abdomen push your hand back up as you inhale.
- Observe how your chest moves; it should be moving in synchronization with your abdomen.

Breathing and Yoga

Yoga is a more than 2,000-year-old method for developing and unifying mind, body and spirit. Yoga practitioners have long recognized the relationship between breathing and health, and they maintain that the life force is carried in the breath. Breathing exercises to control breathing are incorporated into yoga postures (asanas) and practices. Yoga practitioners believe that extending and deepening the breathing process draws breath all the way down to one's heels, and that deep and slow breathing can increase longevity.

Breath-holding Spells

Childhood breath-holding spells, a common and frightening phenomenon that occurs in healthy, otherwise normal children, are a source of stress for parent and child alike. Treatment of children with breath-holding spells has largely focused on providing reassurance to families after a diagnosis has been made.

Some children use breath-holding as an act of rebellion or a demonstration of autonomy. When children know that they can terrify their parents with this behavior, the behavior becomes somewhat reinforced. According to Francis DiMario Jr., M.D., Department of Pediatrics, University of Connecticut Health Center, Farmington, "It is neither feasible nor helpful for parents to attempt to avoid circumstances that may provide emotional upset in their child. Even though pain and fear may serve as provocatives, simple frustration and the expression of autonomy are both normal and expected in young children."

If parental anxiety leads to continuous attempts at appeasement, the child may soon learn to manipulate the parent with the threat of crying. This does not imply a willful attempt at breath-holding, since in some cases these spells are reflexive and unpredictable. There is, nonetheless, the potential for parents to reinforce behavioral outbursts if appropriate calm firmness is not displayed at times of customary disciplining.

Should a breath-holding spell occur, have the child lie on his or her back, face upward, to protect the child's head from inadvertent injury and aspiration.

For information:

American Lung Association
1740 Broadway
New York, NY 10019
Phone: (212) 315-8700

See also AUTONOMY; BEHAVIOR THERAPIES; BIOFEEDBACK; COMPLEMENTARY THERAPIES; GUIDED IMAGERY; HEADACHES; HYPERVENTILATION; IRRITABLE BOWEL SYNDROME; MEDITATION; PANIC ATTACKS AND PANIC DISORDER; PERFORMANCE ANXIETY; PHOBIA; STAGE FRIGHT; YOGA.

Brownstone, David, and Irene Franck. *The Parent's Desk Reference.* New York: Prentice Hall, 1991.
Kahn, Ada P. *Stress A to Z: A Sourcebook for Facing Everyday Challenges.* New York: Facts On File, 2000.
Kerman, D. Ariel. *The H.A.R.T. Program: Lower Your Blood Pressure Without Drugs.* New York: HarperCollins, 1993.
Masaoka, Yuri, and Ikuo Homma. "Anxiety and Respiratory Patterns: Their Relationship During Mental Stress and Physical Load." *International Journal of Psychophysiology* no. 2 (Sept. 1997): 153–59.
"RX: Breathing for Health and Relaxation." *Mental Medicine Update* IV, no. 2 (1995).

brief psychotherapy   A form of therapy, often effective in "crisis management" situations, limited to 10 to 15 sessions. Active and goal directive techniques and procedures are used by the therapist. Brief psychotherapy is useful for some individuals and in some group settings to treat a variety of mild disorders. Recent studies have found brief therapy effective in certain forms of depression and anxiety disorders.

See also ANXIETY DISORDERS; BEHAVIORAL THERAPY; PSYCHOTHERAPY; SEX THERAPY.

bronchial asthma   See ASTHMA, ANXIETY AND DEPRESSION.

bruxism   Grinding or clenching of the teeth. This habit usually occurs during sleep, but some indi-

viduals unconsciously do it during the day. In some cases it is caused by unresolved stress; in other cases, it may be related to the occlusion of the teeth when they are brought together.

Some individuals who seek treatment for bruxism are given low doses of anxiolytic drugs to help them relax, particularly before bedtime. Ongoing bruxism may result in wearing away and loosening of the teeth and jaw stiffness. When causative problems cannot be easily resolved, dentists devise bite plates (similar to those worn by athletes during high-contact sports) to be worn at night.

See also STRESS.

bulimarexia   See EATING DISORDERS.

bulimia   See EATING DISORDERS.

bullies   People who take on a type of intimidating, aggressive behavior that may take place at any time of life but is of great concern among children and teenagers. Research has shown that of a group of 20 school children, one is a bully and one a victim. Male bullies are more likely to use physical size and power to intimidate; female bullies are more likely to use verbal harassment.

Bullies have been thought to be compensating for anxieties or failure, but in actual fact they have been found to be self-confident people who look down on their victims and see violence as a positive way to solve problems. Some bullies tend to have parents who show them little warmth, give them a great deal of freedom but also punish them harshly.

Bullies tend to be drawn to children who are smaller, physically weaker and less secure than the average child. Children who are being bullied may show it by a changed attitude toward going to school, school phobia, lowered performance in school, behavior on weekends that differs from school days, taking detours coming home from school to avoid the bully and odd requests for money that is actually used to satisfy the bully's demands.

Parents may find it difficult to handle a situation that involves their child and a bully, in part because children are frequently ashamed of being bullied. Parents must also tread a fine line between avoiding violence or revenge and teaching their children to stick up for themselves. Parents must also try to determine whether their own intervention will improve or exacerbate the situation.

See also SCHOOL PHOBIA.

Kesler, Jay; Ron Beers; and LaVonne Neff. *Parents and Children.* Wheaton, Ill.: Victor Books, 1987.

bupropion hydrochloride   An antidepressant (trade name: Wellbutrin) that is chemically unrelated to tricyclic or other known antidepressant agents and is not a monoamine oxidase (MAO) inhibitor. Compared with tricyclic antidepressants, it is a weaker block of the neuronal uptake of serotonin and norepinephrine and, to some extent, also inhibits the neuronal reuptake of dopamine.

This drug is contraindicated in individuals who have a seizure disorder, as the incidence of seizures with this drug may exceed that of other marketed antidepressants by as much as fourfold; but this is only an approximation, since no direct comparative studies have been conducted. It is also contraindicated in individuals who have a current or prior diagnosis of bulimia or anorexia nervosa because of higher incidence of seizures noted in such persons treated by the drug. Additionally, taking bupropion hydrochloride and an MAO inhibitor at the same time is contraindicated. At least 14 days should elapse between discontinuing an MAO inhibitor and starting bupropion. Adverse reactions commonly encountered with this drug may include difficulty sleeping, dry mouth, headache, constipation, nausea, vomiting and tremor.

See also ANTIDEPRESSANT MEDICATIONS; DEPRESSION; MONOAMINE OXIDASE INHIBITORS; TRICYCLIC ANTIDEPRESSANT MEDICATIONS.

burnout   The progressive loss of energy, purpose and idealism leading to stagnation, frustration and apathy. It strikes anyone in any job, from top executive to mother with small children to singles "with everything going for them." It has nothing to do with intelligence, money or social position. Victims are usually high achievers, workaholics, idealists, romantics, competent self-sufficients and overly conscientious souls. Their common denominator is the assumption that the real world will be in harmony with their dreams. They hold unrealistic expectations of themselves, their employers and society and often have a vague definition of personal accomplishment. In their attempt to gain some distance from the source of anguish, they contract their world down to the smallest possible dimension and/or take on more and more work.

Physical symptoms of burnout include excessive sleeping, eating or drinking, physical exhaustion, loss of libido, frequent colds, headaches, backaches, neckaches and bowel disorders. The burnout victim desires to be alone, is irritable, impatient and withdrawn and complains of boredom, difficulty concentrating and burdensome work. Fellow workers may notice indecisiveness, indifference, impaired performance and high absenteeism. Intellectual curiosity declines, identity diffuses and interpersonal relationships deteriorate. "Overloaded," "tired of thinking" and "I don't know what I'm doing anymore" express the inner agony.

Burnout begins slowly and progresses gradually over weeks, months and years to become cumulative and pervasive. It runs the gamut from initial enthusiasm to stagnation to frustration to apathy in an ever downward spiral.

Recovery from burnout is possible through rediscovery of self and the formation of new attitudes about living.

The following is a series of guidelines suggested by Dorothy Young Riess, M.D., Pasadena, California:

- Recognize that no one job (or personal relationship) is a total solution for life. Variety is the spice of life.

- Learn how to put priorities where they belong, and stop trying to be "all things to all people."

- Set aside personal time (no phone, no TV, no eating or reading) and answer the vital questions "Where am I going?" "What do I want to achieve?" and "How am I going to do it?"

- Develop competence in simple tasks to enhance optimism and lift depression.

- Learn how to accept reality and assume responsibility for self.

- Differentiate between authentic personal goals and those foisted on you by someone else.

- Create an "outside life" of family, friends, interest and activities unrelated to work.
- Strive for variety in work; avoid routine.
- Develop a support system that emphasizes problem solving, for example, "How can I improve on this situation?"
- Learn how to manage personal time.
- Establish an exercise program at least three times a week.
- Take minivacations.

See also CHRONIC FATIGUE SYNDROME; DEPRESSION.

Reprinted with permission of Dorothy Young Riess, M.D. from *Better Health Newsletter,* Pasadena, Calif., vol. 3, no. 1 (Feb. 1987).

Burton, Robert (1577–1640) See ANATOMY OF MELANCHOLY.

BuSpar Trade name for buspirone hcl.
See also BUSPIRONE HYDROCHLORIDE.

buspirone hydrochloride A drug (trade name: BuSpar) approved for use by the Food and Drug Administration in 1986, used primarily in treating generalized anxiety disorder. Research shows that buspirone's effect on chronic anxiety is equal to that of diazepam, although its effects are not apparent for one or two weeks. In clinical trials, the drug was considered as effective for treating anxiety as benzodiazepines, and some clinicians considered it an advance because it lacked some side effects of other tranquilizers. For example, it may cause less drowsiness than other tranquilizers and does not produce physical dependency in individuals after prolonged use. It is considered safer to take in conjunction with alcohol because it does not exacerbate effects of alcohol as the benzodiazepines do, and it is less likely to be overused because it does not give users a euphoric high. However, side effects include headache, lightheadedness, dizziness and nausea.

See BENZODIAZEPINE MEDICATIONS.

"butterflies" in the stomach The feeling of uneasiness in the stomach is often referred to as "butterflies." Caused by a contraction of the abdominal blood vessels, this is a common experience among those who must make a speech in public, perform before an audience, appear for a job interview or participate in any type of activity that causes feelings of nervousness or apprehension.

See also NERVOUS.

butyrophenones A class of antipsychotic drugs, including haloperidol.

See also ANTIPSYCHOTIC MEDICATIONS; HALOPERIDOL.

cacolalia   An impulse to use obscene words.
See also PERVERSION, SEXUAL.

caffeine   A stimulant of the central nervous system primarily consumed in coffee and tea but also present in cola drinks, cocoa, certain headache pills, diet pills and over-the-counter medications such as Nodoz and Vivarin. Regular use of over 600 mg. a day (approximately eight cups of percolated coffee) may cause chronic insomnia, anxiety, depression and stomach upset.

Caffeine is a naturally occurring alkaloid found in many plants throughout the world. It was first isolated from coffee in 1820 and from tea leaves in 1827. Both "coffee" and "caffeine" are derived from the Arabic word *gahweh* (pronounced "keh-veh" in Turkish).

In beverage form, caffeine begins to reach all body tissues within five minutes; peak blood levels are reached in about 30 minutes. Normally, caffeine is rapidly and completely absorbed from the gastrointestinal tract. Little can be recovered unchanged in urine, and there is no day-to-day accumulation in the body.

Caffeine increases the heart rate and rhythm, affects the circulatory system and acts as a diuretic. It also stimulates gastric acid secretion. There may be an elevation in blood pressure, especially during stress. Caffeine inhibits glucose metabolism and may thereby raise blood sugar levels.

Caffeine is a mild behavioral stimulant. It may interfere with sleep and may postpone fatigue. It appears to interact with stress, improving intellectual performance in extroverts and impairing it in introverts. When taken before bedtime, caffeine may delay the onset of sleep for some individuals, may shorten sleep time and may reduce the average "depth of sleep." It also may increase the amount of dream sleep (REM) early in the night while reducing it overall.

While caffeine in moderate doses may, for some individuals, increase alertness and decrease fatigue, regular use of 350 mg. or more a day may result in a form of physical dependence. (Coffee contains 100 to 150 milligrams of caffeine per cup; tea contains about half, and cola about one-third, that amount.) Interruption of such use can result in withdrawal symptoms, the most prominent of which is sometimes severe headache, which can be relieved by taking caffeine. Irritability and fatigue are other symptoms. Regular use of caffeine produces partial tolerance to some or all of its effects.

Caffeine and Panic Attacks

Individuals who have panic attacks should avoid caffeine, as it has been known to produce panic attacks in susceptible individuals. About half of panic disorder sufferers have panic experiences after consuming caffeine found in four to five cups of coffee. Research may determine whether caffeine has a direct or causative effect on panic or simply alters the body state, which triggers a panic cycle as perceived by the individual. Caffeine may produce its effects by blocking the action of a brain chemical known an adenosine, a naturally occurring sedative.

Caffeine Intoxication (caffeinism)

Caffeine intoxication is an organic disorder caused by recent consumption of over 250 mg. of caffeine and involving at least five of the following symptoms: restlessness, increased anxiety, nervousness, excitement, insomnia, frequent and increased urination, gastrointestinal complaints, rambling thought and speech, cardiac arrhythmia, periods of inexhaustibility, psychomotor agitation and increases in phobic reactions in phobic individuals.

See also CAFFEINE; PANIC ATTACK; PANIC DISORDER; SLEEP.

Doctor, Ronald M., and Ada P. Kahn. *Encyclopedia of Phobias, Fears, and Anxieties.* New York: Facts On File, 1989.

O'Brien, Robert, and Sidney Cohen. *Encyclopedia of Drug Abuse.* New York: Facts On File, 1984.

cannabis   A plant (*Cannabis sativa*) commonly known by many names, including marijuana, maconha and hashish. Cannabis has been known to humans since 2500 B.C., when it was listed in a Chinese book of pharmacology. Cannabis has been used in times past for treatment of headaches, arthritis, malaria, stomach ailments and constipation. Its euphoria-producing properties are well known throughout the world. It is abused because of its effects, and its possession is illegal in the United States and many other countries. It is widely believed that cannabis abuse leads to other, more dangerous forms of substance abuse.

carbamazepine   An anticonvulsant (trade name: Tegretol) used to treat depression, though not approved as of the early 1990s by the U.S. Food and Drug Administration for this use. Some manic-depressives who cannot tolerate lithium do well on carbamazepine. Some individuals who have many cycles (up to four) during a year appear to do less well on lithium and better on carbamazepine. Valproate is another anticonvulsive, marketed under the trade name of Depakote.

See also ANTIDEPRESSANT MEDICATIONS; LITHIUM; MANIC-DEPRESSIVE ILLNESS.

Kravitz, Howard, and Jan Fawcett. "Carbamazepine in the Treatment of Affective Disorders." *Medical Science Research* 15, no. 1 (Jan. 1987).

Zajecka, J. M.; J. Fawcett; and M. S. Easton. "Treatment of Psychotic Affective Disorders." *Current Opinion in Psychiatry* 3 (1990).

carbon dioxide sensitivity   An abnormal sensitivity to inhaling small amounts of carbon dioxide, which causes symptoms of hyperventilation, trem-

bling, facial flushing, blurring of vision and dizziness. Individuals prone to panic attacks have occurrences of their disorder upon inhaling carbon dioxide because of increased activity in the locus coeruleus (a small area of the brain rich in neurotransmitters). Such panic attacks occur in nearly all predisposed individuals but rarely in non–panic attack individuals.

See also ANXIETY DISORDERS; LACTATE-INDUCED ANXIETY; NEUROTRANSMITTERS; PANIC ATTACK.

caregivers   Individuals who are health care professionals, social workers, friends or family members of a child, elderly, ill or disabled person who cannot completely care for himself.

Within families, the responsibility of the caregiver has usually fallen heavily on women. This tendency has not changed even though other institutional options are available; 75 percent of care of the elderly is still provided by a family member. Now other social forces are making the responsibility particularly difficult. Social mobility and shrinking family size may make some women the sole relative responsible for care of both their own and their husbands' aging parents. At the same time, women are moving into highly responsible professional positions at about the time in life that their parents need care. The Older Women's League in Washington, D.C. has determined that at least a third of all women over age 18 can expect to be continuously in the caregiver role from the birth of their first child to the death of their parents. According to the American Association of Retired Persons, some women are pressured to turn down promotions, avoid traveling and even take early retirement to care for aging parents.

The caregiver role can be extremely draining of both physical and mental energy. Caregivers may feel powerless and depressed in the face of the suffering of a loved one and may somehow feel that they should be able to give their own youth and health. Professional caregivers must be on guard against both the tendency to build a wall around themselves or allowing the constant pain and suffering they see to dwarf their own needs.

As caregivers have a considerable amount of power and work in a close, personal relationship with their charges, frequently with little or no supervision, the position is vulnerable to abusive behavior. Recently more attention has been focused on this problem by government and the media. Children are more frequently victims of sexual abuse by their caregivers. The elderly are more often subjected to neglect or emotional and financial abuse.

See also AGING; ALZHEIMER'S DISEASE; ELDERLY PARENTS.

Boyd, Malcolm. "Finding Strength in Peace." *Modern Maturity* 34 (June–July 1991).
"The Daughter Track: Are You Prepared to Be a Lifetime Caregiver?" *Glamour* (May 1990).
Yovanovich, Linda. "A Caregiver's Guide to Self-care." *Nursing* 21 (Oct. 1991).

castration Removal of the ovaries or the male testes by surgery, or inactivation of these glands by radiation, drugs or infections. In males and females, castration changes the hormonal balance of the individual, with the possible result of reducing libido. However, with appropriate counseling, behavioral changes need not result from castration.

Women whose ovaries are removed (oophorectomy) are put into a state of premature menopause and may experience menopausal symptoms, such as hot flashes. Estrogen replacement therapy is helpful for many women.

Removal of the male sex glands has been practiced historically in many cultures and was probably first performed in ancient Egypt and other Near Eastern cultures. Hundred of young boys were castrated in one religious ceremony and their genitals offered sacrificially to the gods. Castrated males were used as eunuchs to guard women in harems. If the operation was performed after puberty, the penis would be of adult size and capable of erection, because the adrenal glands continue to produce androgen even after the testes have been removed.

The term "castrating" is also used to refer to a psychological threat to the masculinity or femininity of an individual. The term "castrating woman" usually refers to a wife or mother who emasculates a man or men in the psychological sense through domination and derogatory remarks and behavior.

The term "castration complex" is used by psychoanalysts to refer to the unconscious feelings and fantasies associated with loss of the sex organs; in males, this relates to loss of the penis, while in females, the belief that the penis has already been removed. In boys, fear of losing the penis is associated with punishment for sexual interest in the mother (the Oedipus complex). It is also associated with threats of castration as punishment for masturbation and the discovery that girls do not have a penis. In girls, the castration complex takes the form of a fantasy that the penis has already been removed as a punishment, for which they blame their mother (Electra complex).

See also ELECTRA COMPLEX; MENOPAUSE; OEDIPUS COMPLEX.

Kahn, Ada P., and Linda Hughey Holt. *The A to Z of Women's Sexuality.* Alameda, Calif: Hunter House, 1992.
Katchadourian, Herant A., and Donald T. Lunde. *Fundamentals of Human Sexuality.* New York: Holt, Rinehart and Winston, 1972.

castration complex See CASTRATION.

Catapres See CLONIDINE.

catastrophize The habit of imagining that the worst case scenario will happen. People who frequently catastrophize have little self-confidence, low self-esteem, difficulties making positive and desirable life changes, and many have social phobias.

An example of catastrophizing is saying to oneself, "If I go to the party no one will know me and I won't have a good time," or "If I take this new job I'll fail because I don't have the right computer skills."

Catastrophizing causes anxieties and is a threat to good mental health because the habit keeps people in situations they might really prefer to change, such as improving their social life, changing jobs, or moving to a new city. With positive self-talk and learned techniques to improve self-esteem, the habit of catastrophizing can be overcome. In severe cases, various psychotherapies may be helpful, particularly cognitive behavioral therapies.

See also BEHAVIORAL THERAPY; COGNITIVE BEHAVIOR THERAPY; PSYCHOTHERAPIES; SELF-ESTEEM; SOCIAL PHOBIA.

Kahn, Ada P. *Stress A to Z: A Sourcebook for Everyday Challenges.* New York: Facts On File, 2000.

Kahn, Ada P. and Sheila Kimmel. *Empower Yourself: Every Woman's Guide to Self-Esteem.* New York: Avon Books, 1997.

catatonia   A physical state marked by an apparent lack of responsiveness to the point of near stupor and either muscular rigidity or the "waxy flexibility" of the muscles in which, if placed in one position, the individual will stay that way until moved to another. Catatonia is a clinical syndrome seen in association with affective disorders, organic mental syndromes, schizophrenia and some neurological diseases. Since the availability of modern antipsychotic medications, catatonia has been diagnosed less frequently, owing to the masking of symptoms or the aborting of a catatonic state by the medications.

The term was first used by Karl Kahlbaum in 1887 to name a state of lowered tension. The term was later absorbed by Emil Kraepelin into his subtypes of dementia praecox and later still became the 20th-century diagnostic category of catatonic schizophrenia.

In catatonic stupor, the individual may be immobile, mute and unresponsive and yet fully conscious. In catatonic excitement, the individual may exhibit uncontrolled and aimless motor activity. Such patients may assume bizarre or uncomfortable postures, such as squatting, and maintain them for long periods. With prolonged catatonic excitement and resultant restraint, hyperthermia that may cause death or residual nervous system damage may result. This condition is called lethal catatonia.

Catatonic schizophrenia is a subtype of schizophrenia dominated by stupor or mutism, negativism, rigidity, purposeless excitement and bizarre posturing. This subtype of schizophrenia is reported to be less common than in the past, possibly because of modern medications.

See also SCHIZOPHRENIA.

catharsis   Therapeutic release of anxiety by talking about disturbing feelings and impulses. It also means bringing to the surface and reliving events and experiences stored in the unconscious mind that produced the anxiety symptoms. Catharsis occurs during psychotherapy and group therapy.

cathexis   An investment of mental energy in an object of any kind, such as a person, a goal or a social group. When one attaches emotional significance to them, such objects are said to be cathected.

CAT scan   See BRAIN IMAGING.

Celexa   Trade name for citalopram, a serotonin specific antidepressant medication.

central nervous system (CNS)   Part of the nervous system consisting of the brain and spinal cord; the CNS is primarily involved in the control of mental activities and in coordinating incoming and outgoing messages. All sensory impulses are transmitted from the CNS, and all motor impulses originate there. The CNS coordinates activities of the entire nervous system; the CNS is affected by many psychotropic drugs, anxiolytic drugs and antidepressant drugs.

See also ANTIDEPRESSANT MEDICATIONS; DEPRESSION.

cerebellum   See BRAIN.

cerebral cortex   See BRAIN.

cerebral palsy   The word "cerebral" refers to the brain; palsy refers to a lack of muscle control. Cerebral palsy involves muscular coordination problems related to the brain. Almost all cerebral palsy cases begin before or during birth. Brain cells may be damaged in various ways. For example, there may be insufficient oxygen reaching the brain during labor if pressure squeezes off the umbilical cord's blood supply. There may be brain damage to a child born of a mother who had rubella during her pregnancy (vaccines now can reduce this cause to a minimum). There may be blood incompatibility between the mother and father; this can be detected before conception to reduce the number of cases of cerebral palsy from this cause.

There is no cure for cerebral palsy, but corrective exercises, braces and surgery help many children born with the disease. The condition can be complicated by parents and friends creating emotional problems for the child as well as the family. As with any other chronic disease, empathy, understanding and moral support from those around the patient will be helpful to all.

See also CHRONIC ILLNESS.

cerebrospinal fluid (CSF)   The fluid within the central canal of the spinal cord, four ventricles of the brain and the subarachnoid space of the brain. The CSF protects vital tissues from damage by shock pressure.

See also BRAIN.

cerebrum   See BRAIN.

certification   The process of preparing the legal documents necessary for the procedure of commitment to a mental institute for detention and treatment. The term is also used to refer to the formal signing of a statement of cause of death issued by a medical practitioner. Additionally, the term is used to indicate that a medical specialty board has approved a physician as a specialist (board certification).

change of life   A term referring to menopause.

See also MENOPAUSE.

checking   A symptom of obsessive-compulsive disorder (OCD). Checking is the repetitious act of looking to see that one's door is locked or one's stove has been turned off. As a common sense precaution, most people do check for these and other important matters. However, when the checking becomes a ritual and takes up most of one's time, it is a symptom of an obsession. About one-third of all sufferers of OCD have checking as a symptom. Checking seems to be more common in men than women.

See also OBSESSIVE-COMPULSIVE DISORDER.

chemical dependencies   See ADDICTIONS.

chemical imbalance   See ANTIDEPRESSANT MEDICATIONS; BRAIN CHEMISTRY.

chest pains   See ANGINA PECTORIS.

child abuse   See FAMILY VIOLENCE.

childbirth   The birth of a child, usually by passage through the birth canal. Many women view childbearing as a transition to adult female sexuality. In many cultures, the figure obtained during pregnancy—wider hips, extra body fat, more rounded contours—is equated with the sexuality of fertility. Other cultures try to separate childbirth from female sexuality and may equate a feminine ideal with slimness and a less rounded image. For most women, childbearing is viewed as an important sexual rite of passage, owing both to the pride of bearing a child and to the often sexually satisfying process of nursing and snuggling an infant. Some male partners find the process of pregnancy and childbirth appealing sexually, and a close bonding of partners occurs; other men have great difficulty in relating to a woman as a mother and a sexual object at the same time.

Natural and Prepared Childbirth

In the latter half of the 20th century, many women became concerned about using pharmacologic methods to relieve pain and render them literally unconscious during the birthing procedure. Indeed, many older mothers believe that they "missed out" on the entire process of giving birth to their children because of pharmacologic interventions. The term "natural childbirth" generally refers to childbirth without drugs or medical intervention. The term is specifically used to refer to a movement toward unmedicated deliveries started by Fernand Lamaze (1891–1957), a French obstetrician.

Interest in natural childbirth began developing during the 1940s and 1950s when the use of drugs for pain relief and medical procedures such as routine episiotomies, shaves, enemas and sterile technique during hospital deliveries removed the woman and her family from a sense of participation in the childbirth process. While the specific methods for childbirth put forward by LaMaze, Dick-Reed and Leboyer vary, they all incorporate nonmedical relaxation techniques as a "natural" method of pain control during labor. In addition, they question the need for routine medical procedures and advocate a more active participation in labor by the woman and lay labor coach, often meaning the father of the baby. The movement has expanded to include the use of birthing rooms (rooms in which labor and delivery take place in a homelike setting) and the inclusion of extended family and friends in the delivery process. Some women choose to have their babies delivered at home to assure being surrounded by their family members. Some women opt for delivery by specially trained nurse-midwives rather than physicians. Nurse-midwives, however, have the backup of physicians in case of medical emergencies.

The term "prepared childbirth" became popular in the early 1990s; it includes prenatal exercise classes and a wide variety of breathing and relaxation techniques.

Special Mental Health Concerns Relating to Childbirth

Some women approach childbirth with many concerns because of reports from friends and relatives. First-time mothers, in particular, are anxious about the unknown aspects related to childbirth. Some first-time fathers who attend the birthing event have anxieties as well. Some men and women have a fear of the entire birthing process, which is known as maieusophobia. While some fear pain, others fear blood, doctors and the uncertainties of facing parenthood. Women often become anxious about many of the practical details surrounding the birthing experience, such as wondering if they will recognize the start of labor and getting to the hospital on time.

Women whose babies are delivered by cesarean section have concerns that the procedure denies them what they believe should be a natural experience. Women who have cesarean sections wonder if they will be able to have subsequent children by vaginal delivery. This depends on whether or not the reason for the cesarean section was a one-time occurrence (such as a breach presentation), if the cesarean scar is strong and if the physician is agreeable to a subsequent normal labor, assuming that the woman's pelvis is wide enough for a baby's head.

See also BONDING; PARENTING; POSTPARTUM DEPRESSION.

Beauvoir, Simone de. *The Second Sex.* New York: Modern Library, 1968.
Eisenberg, Arlene; Heidi Eisenberg Murkoff; and Sandee Eisenberg Hathaway. *What to Expect When You're Expecting.* New York: Workman Publishing, 1984.
Kahn, Ada P., and Linda Hughey Holt. *The A to Z of Women's Sexuality.* Alameda, Calif.: Hunter House, 1992.

chiropractic medicine Chiropractic medicine deals with the relationship between the skeleton and the nervous system and the role of this relationship in restoring and maintaining health. Many people visit chiropractors to relieve stress that interferes with their mental health and causes physical discomforts.

According to chiropractic philosophy, the body is a self-healing organism and all bodily function is controlled by the nervous system. Abnormal bodily function may be caused by interference with nerve transmission and expression. This interference can be caused by pressure, strain or tension on the spinal cord, spinal nerves or peripheral nerves as a result of a displacement of the spinal segments or other skeletal structures.

The art of the chiropractic practitioner involves detecting and correcting problems of the vertebral subluxation complex. Subluxation refers to a slight dislocation or biomechanical malfunctioning of the vertebrae (bones of the spine). According to the International Chiropractors Association, subluxation can irritate nerve roots and blood vessels which branch off from the spinal cord between each vertebrae. The irritation causes pain and dysfunction in muscle, lymphatic and organ tissue, as well as imbalance in normal body processes.

Causes of subluxation include stress, falls, injuries, trauma, inherited spinal weaknesses, improper sleeping habits, poor posture, poor lifting habits, obesity, lack of rest and little or no exercise.

Chiropractors restore misaligned vertebrae to their proper position in the spinal cord through procedures known as "spinal adjustments," or manipulations. The adjustment itself does not directly heal the body. Rather, it is the resulting alignment of misaligned spinal vertebrae that restores balance so that the body can function more optimally.

Although chiropractic medicine is often chosen as therapy for headache, temporomandibular joint syndrome (TMJ), whiplash and bursitis, it may not be the treatment of choice for all medical problems or conditions.

Choosing a Chiropractor

Before choosing a chiropractor, ask him or her to fully explain the benefits, risks and costs of all diagnostic and treatment options. Interview more than one doctor of chiropractic medicine before making a decision on the practitioner.

For information:

American Chiropractic Association
1701 Clarendon Boulevard
Arlington, VA 22209
Phone: (703) 276-8800

American College of Chiropractic Orthopedists
1030 Broadway, Suite 101
El Centro, CA 92243
Phone: (619) 352-1452

See also COMPLEMENTARY THERAPIES; TEMPORO-MANDIBULAR JOINT SYNDROME.

McGill, Leonard. *The Chiropractor's Health Book: Simple, Natural Exercises for Relieving Headaches, Tension and Back Pain.* New York: Crown Trade Paperbacks, 1997.
Rondberg, Terry A. *Chiropractic First: The Fastest Growing Healthcare First . . . Before Drugs or Surgery.* Chandler, Ariz.: The Chiropractic Journal, 1996.

chlamydia   See SEXUALLY TRANSMITTED DISEASES.

chlordiazepoxide   An antianxiety drug (trade name: Librium); one of a group of drugs known as benzodiazepines. It is effective in the management of generalized anxiety disorder and is also used to ameliorate the symptoms of alcohol withdrawal and as a preanesthetic medication. It is considered more useful in relieving anxiety than most non-benzodiazepines.

See also ANXIETY; ANXIOLYTIC MEDICATIONS; BENZODIAZEPINE MEDICATIONS; CENTRAL NERVOUS SYSTEM.

chlorpromazine   A tranquilizer (trade name: Thorazine). The first antipsychotic drug marketed, it is used primarily to treat schizophrenia, other psychoses or mania. It is used less commonly in schizoaffective disorder or major depression with psychotic features, paranoia, intractable hiccups, disturbed behavior associated with mental retardation, nausea and vomiting. The drug has a relatively low potency; it is one of the most sedative antipsychotic drugs, but tolerance to this effect usually develops. It is probably best tolerated by patients under 40 years of age. In older patients, the incidence of dizziness, hypotension, ocular changes and dyskinesia increases, although the latter is more commonly associated with the more potent antipsychotic agents.

See also TRANQUILIZER MEDICATIONS.

cholinergic medications   The word "cholinergic" pertains to nerve cells and organs that are activated by the neurotransmitter acetylcholine. Cholinergic drugs are agents that increase the activity of acetylcholine or have effects similar to those of acetylcholine, such as facilitating the transfer of nerve impulses between cells. These drugs are used as substitutes for acetylcholine in therapy and research, as they resist destruction by enzymes that usually deactivate acetylcholine. Cholinergic drugs are also known as parasympathetic drugs. Cholinergic drugs are frequently used to reverse the anticholinergic effects of many therapeutic agents to promote normal bowel and bladder function (for example, postsurgery).

See also ANTICHOLINERGIC MEDICATIONS.

Chopra, Deepak (1947–)   Indian-born physician whose philosophy of healing, disseminated through books, tapes, lectures and clinics, is based on the Indian holistic system called Ayurveda. He was once a disciple of Maharishi Mahesh Yogi, but he formed his own organization in 1993. Among his books are the best-selling *Ageless Body, Timeless Mind: The Quantum Alternative to Growing Old* (1993) and *The Return of Merlin* (1995), a work of fiction.

He graduated from the All-India Institute of Medical Sciences in New Delhi and moved to the United States in 1970. He completed an internship at Huhlenbert Hospital in Plainfield, New Jersey, moved to Boston in 1971 and taught at several medical schools affiliated with Tufts University, Harvard University and Boston University. He worked for 14 years as an endocrinologist in a Boston-area hospital. Since 1993 Chopra has been executive director of the Sharp Institute for Human Potential and Mind/Body Medicine in southern California.

Chopra claims the mind/body connection can reduce stress, facilitate healing, lead to inner peace and even reverse the aging process. His mind/body programs incorporate massage, yoga, meditation, herbal supplements, nutritional guidelines and exercise regimens. He recommends doing something that brings joy, concentrating fully on that activity, reducing distractions at work, and finding inner satisfaction in daily tasks.

In a chapter on longevity in *Ageless Body,* Chopra outlines some suggestions which may be useful for those wishing to reduce stress in their lives. Techniques include listening to your body's wisdom, living in the present, taking time to be silent and meditating to quiet the internal dialogue.

For information:

Chopra Center for Well Being
7590 Fay Avenue, 403
La Jolla, CA 92037
Phone: (619) 551-7788

Sharp Institute for Human Potential and
　Mind/Body Medicine
3131 Berger Avenue
San Diego, CA 92123
Phone: (619) 541-6737

See also AYURVEDA; COMPLEMENTARY THERAPIES; IMMUNE SYSTEM; MEDITATION; MIND/BODY CONNECTION; RELAXATION.

Chopra, Deepak. *Ageless Body, Timeless Mind: The Quantum Alternative to Growing Old.* New York: Crown, 1993.
———. *Unconditional Life.* New York: Bantam, 1992.
———. *Creating Health.* Boston: Houghton Mifflin, 1991.
———. *Quantum Healing.* New York: Bantam, 1989.

chromosome   All members of a species normally have the same number of chromosomes. The normal number for humans is 46 chromosomes, or 23 pairs, which contain the genes for specific hereditary traits. Chromosomes are usually invisible strands or filaments of DNA, RNA, or other molecules carrying the genetic or hereditary traits of an individual. Chromosomes are located in the cell nucleus and are visible through a microscope only during cell division. Defects in chromosomes can result in birth defects or hereditary disorders. For example, mental retardation is caused by absence of part of a chromosome, a defective chromosome or an extra chromosome. A condition known as trisomy 21 is one that is associated with 85 percent of Down's syndrome cases. There are three number 21 chromosomes in the body cells instead of the normal pair. The extra chromosome may come from either the father or the mother. Some writers use trisomy 21 as a synonym for Down's syndrome.

See DOWN'S SYNDROME; GENETIC COUNSELING; MENTAL RETARDATION.

Chromosome 21   See CHROMOSOME; DOWN'S SYNDROME.

chronic fatigue immune dysfunction syndrome (CFIDS)   Another name for chronic fatigue syndrome. Some physicians and patients prefer this name because it suggests an immunological component to the disorder.

See also CHRONIC FATIGUE SYNDROME.

chronic fatigue syndrome (CFS)   Illness characterized by fatigue that occurs suddenly, improves and relapses, bringing on debilitating tiredness or easy fatigability in an individual who has no apparent reason for feeling this way. It is stressful to the sufferer because the profound weakness caused by CFS does not go away with a few good nights of sleep, but instead steals a person's vigor over months and years. Depression is probably a major part of the syndrome.

While the illness strikes children, teenagers, and people in their fifties, sixties and seventies, it is most likely to strike adults from their mid-twenties to their late forties. Women are afflicted about twice to three times as often as men; the vast majority of those who suffer this illness are white. Because young urban professionals were most afflicted during the 1980s, the name "yuppie flu" was attached to CFS. However, most individuals felt that this name trivialized their illness.

Symptoms of CFS

CFS can affect virtually all of the body's major systems: neurological, immunological, hormonal, gastrointestinal and musculoskeletal. According to the National Institutes of Health, CFS leaves many people bedridden, or with headaches, muscular and joint pain, sore throat, balance disorders, sensitivity to light, an inability to concentrate and inexplicable body aches. Secondary depression, which follows from the disease rather than causing it, is just as disabling. However, knowing that there is a chemical basis for mood swings and that they are directly related to illness can be reassuring.

Symptoms wax and wane in severity and linger for months and sometimes years. Some individuals respond to treatment, while others must function at a reduced level for a long time. However, for all sufferers, the cumulative effect is the same; namely, the illness transforms ordinary activities into tremendously stressful challenges. They cannot tolerate the least bit of exercise, their cognitive functions become impaired, and their memory, verbal fluency, response time and ability to perform calculations and to reason show a marked decrease.

Disruption of sleep patterns cause the CFS sufferer additional stress. Despite constant exhaustion and desire for sleep, they rarely sleep uninterrupted, nor do they awake feeling refreshed. Some have severe insomnia, while others have difficulty maintaining sleep. There is often not enough rapid-eye movement sleep (REM), which is considered necessary for a good night's rest.

Many CFS sufferers experience stressful disorders of balance and of the vestibular system, both of which are modulated by the inner ear. They sometimes feel dizzy, lightheaded or nauseous. Even walking can be difficult, with sufferers tilting off balance or stumbling for no apparent reason. Some individuals with balance disorders develop phobias, such as a fear of falling; sometimes the phobias are so strong that they render the sufferer housebound.

CFS causes stresses on everyone concerned. Those in their support circles can reduce their stress by being helpful, understanding, and available to listen. Sufferers are likely to feel estranged from some of their friends because they believe that no one really understands their feelings of emotional and physical exhaustion. This belief is exacerbated because many sufferers think that others do not take their illness seriously. In addition, some friends and family members may fear that CFS is contagious and try to maintain a distance from the sufferer. (Medical opinion seems to indicate that CFS is not contagious). Friends, family and other members of support circles can reduce a sick individual's stress by being helpful, understanding and available to listen. Spouses face the issue of reduced sexual activity, although both partners can satisfy their needs by engaging in sexual activity during peak periods of energy.

Diagnosing CFS

Diagnosing CFS is stressful for physicians and patients because many of the symptoms are like those of other disorders. Until the mid-1980s, many CFS patients were misdiagnosed as suffering from depression, accused of malingering, encouraged to undergo stressful, costly and inappropriate laboratory tests or simply pushed aside by the medical community because of lack of understanding of the disease. In recent years, however, studies on the immune system, viruses, and the physiological effects of stress have contributed to better understanding of CFS. Individuals with CFS no longer have to feel abandoned by their physicians or fear that they are "going crazy" because no one takes their illness seriously.

Treatment for CFS

Many therapies have been tried on CFS sufferers. Usually a plan is devised for each patient, depending on symptoms. Pharmacological therapies include use of antidepressant drugs, pain relieving drugs and muscle-relaxing drugs.

Other therapies include deep relaxation, yoga, biofeedback and visualization therapy to relieve stress and chronic pain. Nutritional therapies emphasize certain vitamins, such as Vitamins A, B6, B12, C and E, as well as zinc, folic acid, and selenium, all of which are said to have immune-boosting potential.

Oil extract from the seeds of the evening primrose plant is another medicine which some CFS patients have found helpful. The theoretical basis for its use (although not scientifically proven in known double-blind studies) is that evening primrose oil contains gamma-linolenic acid (GLA), which converts in the body to prostaglandin, a vital substance in the regulation of cellular function.

Role of Self-help and Support Groups

Several nationwide organizations encourage research and political advocacy and also provide lists of local support groups. CFS sufferers may find relief from some stressors and help with practical and emotional needs through these organizations. For information:

Chronic Fatigue Immune Dysfunction
   Syndrome Society
P.O. Box 230108
Portland, OR 97223
Phone: (503) 684-5261

Chronic Fatigue and Immune Dysfunction
   Syndrome Association
P.O. Box 220398
Charlotte, NC 28222
Phone: (704) 362-CFID

National Chronic Fatigue Syndrome
   Association
919 Scott Avenue
Kansas City, KS 66105
Phone: (913) 321-2278

See also BIOFEEDBACK; DEPRESSION; INSOMNIA; PHOBIAS; SUPPORT GROUPS; YOGA.

Feiden, Karyn. *Hope and Help for Chronic Fatigue Syndrome.* New York: Prentice Hall, 1990.
McSherry, James. "Chronic Fatigue Syndrome: A Fresh Look at an Old Problem." *Canadian Family Physician* 39 (Feb. 1993).

chronic illness   Chronic illness often brings with it physical symptoms, such as pain, and emotional consequences that can be more far reaching than the disease itself. Emotional consequences affect not only the patient but the immediate caregivers and family as well. Many families let anxieties take over their lives; in other cases, depression arises while coping with illness and the threat of possible loss of physical functioning or life itself.

Many ill persons turn to substance abuse to escape their pain and fears about disability and death. Anger, denial or perceived helplessness leads others to abandon treatment or assume a "why me" attitude that gives them a pessimistic view of their world.

According to Lloyd D. Rudley, M.D., an attending psychiatrist at the Institute of Pennsylvania Hospital, Philadelphia, the crucial issue is "whether you can get past the stage of rage, sadness and overwhelming anxiety. Will you resume the initiative for living or become psychologically paralyzed?" Dr. Rudley says that many people become trapped by emotions that do not serve them well.

Reactions to illness are similar to the stages of grief. First there is shock and a feeling of many losses, including a sense of control, autonomy and the way things used to be. Those who suffer from chronic illness might suffer losses ranging from having to give up a cherished sport or favorite food to impaired speech or the inability to bear children. Stress and symptoms of depression may follow, including hopelessness, self-blame, shattered self-esteem or withdrawal. The ill person may develop many fears, including one of being active again, while others may deny the realities of their condition and overdo activities too soon.

Many chronically ill people do not comply with instructions from their physicians. This may take the form of not showing up for physical therapy, refusing medication or driving a car against the physician's advice. Individuals with emphysema may continue to smoke. According to Dr. Rudley, "People want to think everything will be normal again if they follow the doctor's orders. When things don't work this way and there is no magic formula, a patient may give up on treatment."

Some individuals neglect medical advice as a means of getting more attention. Others who harbor shame or guilt about their condition may punish themselves, in effect, by not complying with prescribed treatment. Forces of denial may be at work, too, in whose who try to "bargain with illness" by following some recommendations but not others.

An individual's prior coping abilities will determine how well he or she responds when illness occurs. However, even when symptoms of illness go into remission or the person adjusts successfully, a whole new set of external problems may discriminate against him or her, or family dynamics can change dramatically.

"Patients need to accept that illness changes them permanently, that a change in lifestyle is necessary," advises Dr. Rudley. Healthy acceptance is achieved when people come to terms with their illness as a part of who they are, "forming a sort of coexistence with it."

Some individuals feel certain "benefits" from being chronically ill. Such motivations are referred to as secondary gains and increase the likelihood of the individual continuing to be ill or to have symptoms. Common benefits of illness include receiving permission to get out of dealing with a troublesome problem, situation or responsibilities of life, getting attention, care or nurturing from people around them and not having to meet their own or others' expectations.

Ill health affects every area of a person's life, including marriage, family, work, financial affairs and future plans. Professional counseling can help individuals and their families adapt to changes brought on by chronic illness. Counseling may help individuals who have insomnia or disrupted sleep, feel a need to hide their illness, observe an increased use of drugs or alcohol, fail to follow treatment recommendations or have prolonged depression, marked negative personality changes, feelings that they are "victims," undue fears about resuming activities, obsessive anxiety or preoccupation with death.

See also ANXIETY; CAREGIVERS; COUNSELING, DENIAL; DISABILITIES; ELDERLY PARENTS.

"Conquering the Psychological Hurdles of Chronic Illness." *The Quill*, Pennsylvania Hospital, Philadelphia (fall 1991).

circadian rhythms   Circadian rhythms are cyclical biological activities that repeat at approximately 24-hour intervals. They are coordinated by an inherent timing mechanism known as a biological clock. Alertness and mental capability seem to be most available to us when we follow our internal clocks. Most people's "clocks" are synchronized to the sun's 24-hour cycle. For example, sunrise means waking and working, and sundown means dinner and sleep. However, individuals who are shift workers find that their "day" is reversed. Most shift workers go home to sleep during the day when their bodies want to be awake and then have to work at night when their bodies want to sleep.

The circadian rhythm of body temperature is a marker for internal clocks. Body temperature rises and falls in cycles parallel to alertness and performance efficiency. When body temperature is high, which it usually is during the day, alertness and performance peak, but sleep is difficult. A lower temperature (generally during the night) promotes sleep but hinders alertness and performance.

See also BIOLOGICAL CLOCK; SHIFT WORK; BIORHYTHMS.

Insights into Clinical and Scientific Progress in Medicine, Rush-Presbyterian–St. Luke's Medical Center, 14, no. 3 (1991).

circumstantiality   See THOUGHT DISORDERS.

civil rights   The concept of civil rights gives legal expression to the desire for equal treatment in regard to participation in government, employment, housing and education. Civil rights were once thought to be only the rights of the individual in relation to government, but through legislation and practice the civil rights concept has now extended to many other social institutions.

Racial discrimination has been the most significant target of civil rights activities and legislation. Following the Civil War, the 13th Amendment to the Constitution abolished slavery, the 14th Amendment made people born or naturalized in the United States citizens and the 15th Amendment gave blacks the right to vote. Discriminatory practices against blacks continued until the 1950s, when a variety of civil rights actions and legislation gave blacks equal access to education and seating on public transportation. The Civil Rights Act of 1964 gave blacks equal access to public accommodations and ended such contradictory and insulting situations as those encountered by black entertainers who could perform—but not be served—in a restaurant or club. Racial discrimination in housing was attacked by the Civil Rights Act of 1968, which prohibited discriminatory practices in financing, advertising, showing, selling and renting property. Affirmative action legislation has also attempted to give blacks equal access to education and employment. The latter movement has given rise to actions based on feelings of reverse discrimination involving white men who feel that hiring quotas give blacks and women an unfair advantage in being accepted for employment or for educational opportunities.

The social changes of the 1960s also made the civil rights of women an important issue. Although some individual states had given women the right to vote, it was not until 1920 that the federal government guaranteed women's suffrage with the 19th Amendment. The Civil Rights Act of 1964 included the prohibition of employment discrimination based on sex as well as race and established the Equal Employment Opportunity Commission to investigate charges of unequal treatment or harassment. Pregnancy or the possibility thereof is no longer an acceptable reason for dismissing or refusing to hire a woman, although her employment may be terminated if pregnancy actually interferes with her work. An important recent issue has been the exposure of women of childbearing age to radiation, which might affect a developing fetus. The unsuccessful attempts to pass the Equal Rights Amendment were the product of feelings that other constitutional amendments and antidiscriminatory legislation were not strong enough to guarantee women equal opportunities.

Other issues that have been considered sources of discrimination and freedom of expression are grooming and appearance codes. For example, young men who prefer long hair have pointed to perfectly acceptable longer hairstyles on women as proof that a school or employer who insists on haircuts for men is being discriminatory. With the aging population, age discrimination has also become an important issue and a target of federal legislation.

On some occasions, one set of civil liberties seems to be in conflict with another. For example, a person's right to choose personal associates or to express himself freely may be in conflict with civil rights principles; such rights are generally upheld if they do not conflict with the interests of society as a whole.

Civil Rights and the Mentally Ill

Rights of hospitalized psychiatric patients are defined by states. The only right an involuntarily committed person loses is the right to liberty.

Some examples of civil rights are guaranteed. These include the right to dispose of property; to execute instruments such as wills and deeds to property; to make purchases; to enter into contracts; to vote; and to retain a driver's license and a professional license. However, under certain circumstances, a license can be revoked if the holder suffers from a mental condition that makes him or her incapable of practicing that profession. In such a situation, due process rights would be afforded the individual before the license would be suspended or revoked. In addition, a court procedure, often depending on expert testimony, can appoint a conservator in the case where a person can no longer manage her money and personal affairs because of illness.

See also AGING; WOMEN'S LIBERATION MOVEMENT.

"Civil Rights," in *The Guide to American Law,* vol. 2. St. Paul: West Publishing, 1983.
McFarland, Gertrude K., and Mary Durand Thomas. *Psychiatric Mental Health Nursing.* Philadelphia: J. B. Lippincott, 1991.

clanging See THOUGHT DISORDERS.

claustrophobia An intense fear of being in closed places, such as elevators, phone booths, small rooms, crowded areas or other confined spaces. The word comes from the Latin word *claustrum,* meaning "lock" or "bolt." Claustrophobia is one of the most common fears. Most people feel slightly uncomfortable in a closed space, but true phobics may have a panic attack and will tend to avoid such places. Some fear they will suffocate, while others have specific fears relating to the enclosure, such as an elevator or airplane that may suddenly fall. For some individuals, claustrophobia begins after a bad experience involving an enclosed space, such as being locked in a closet or room. With behavioral therapy techniques, many people overcome this phobia.

See also AGORAPHOBIA; PANIC DISORDER; PHOBIA.

client-centered therapy A form of therapy developed by Carl Rogers (1902–   ), an American psychologist. Also known as Rogerian therapy, the technique is a nondirective approach that aims to encourage the individual's personal growth. Emphasis is placed on the individual's uniqueness of personality. This type of therapy led to many other developments in the field of psychology during the middle of the 20th century.

See also BEHAVIORAL THERAPY.

climacteric See MENOPAUSE.

climate and mental health Effects of climate on mental health is an ongoing subject for research, even though the subject has been studied and analyzed since Aristotle and Hippocrates wrote on the subject. Climate has an effect on housing, sports and leisure activities, transportation, work and the types of products and businesses that are necessary to satisfy basic human needs.

Cool climates have generally been considered easier to live in than areas that are consistently too hot for human comfort. It has only been recently that air conditioning has been perfected and become widespread in industrialized countries. Greater control over the environment has been thought to give greater impetus to creativity and change. Inhabitants of cool climates have generally been thought to be more industrious and goal-oriented than those who live in warm climates. Cooler climates require that the body burn and produce energy more quickly and therefore stimulate activity. On the other hand, cold weather raises blood pressure, is generally hard on the circulatory system and tends to make even people who spend most of their time in sedentary activi-

ties indoors crave foods high in fat and starch. Warmer climates slow the body's metabolism and, if humidity is added to the heat, produce a more languid lifestyle. Stormy and changeable weather, which is usually accompanied by sudden barometric changes, may produce irritability and mood changes because the rising and falling pressure affects body fluids.

Some authors and researchers have attempted to connect a population's religious and philosophical outlook to its environment. For example, inhabitants of a forest civilization may develop beliefs about spirits or other metaphysical phenomena from their observations of trees and animals. An open desert atmosphere might give a completely different outlook.

Relationship of Weather and Violence
One correlation between weather and human activity that is supported by statistics is the relationship between hot weather and violence. Figures show that crimes and riots are far more likely to occur in hot weather than in cool or rainy weather.

Palmer, Bruce. *Body Weather*. Harrisburg, Pa.: Stackpole Books, 1976.
Sherrets, S. D. "Climate and Personality," In *Encyclopedia of Psychology*. vol. 1, edited by Raymond J. Corsini. New York: Wiley, 1984.

clinical depression See AFFECTIVE DISORDERS.

clinical psychology A branch of psychology specializing in the study, diagnosis and treatment of behavior disorders. Clinical psychology became popular in the United States during the late 1940s and 1950s. Much of the research in clinical methods, diagnosis and therapy has taken place within departments of clinical psychology. In most states, clinical psychologists must be licensed to treat clients and have a Ph.D. degree. Training for a Ph.D. in clinical psychology includes course work, development of research skills and clinical practice.

See also PSYCHOLOGY.

clinical trials See RANDOMIZED CLINICAL TRIALS.

clitoris   An erectile organ of the female external genitalia that is the center of sexual feeling and stimulation. It is located at the top of the folds where the labia majora and labia minora (larger and smaller lips) meet. The term is derived from the Greek word *kleiein,* meaning "to shut or close." Because it contains many nerve endings, the clitoris is sensitive to tactile stimulation during sexual activity. Many women enjoy stimulation of the clitoris as a means of increasing sexual excitement and reaching orgasm.

The clitoris is composed of tissue that becomes engorged with blood during sexual arousal, causing the clitoris to become erect. The clitoris has a sensitive tip called the glans, which has many nerve receptors, making it extremely sensitive to touch. The size of the clitoris and the degree it projects from under the clitoral hood varies from woman to woman.

The clitoris originates from the same embryonic tissue as the penis. The prepuce, or clitoral hood, covers the clitoris from the external folds of the labia minora, and stimulation of the labia minora may have the same effect as direct stimulation of the clitoris.

The term "clitoral orgasm" refers to an orgasm induced by direct stimulation of the clitoris, manually by the woman herself (masturbation), by contact with and motion of the penis, by the partner's mouth or tongue or by a sexual aid such as a vibrator.

Clitorism and Clitoridotomy

Clitorism is prolonged clitoral erection, a painful and dangerous condition similar to priapism in the male. Clitoridotomy is the surgical excision of the prepuce of the clitoris, a procedure somewhat equivalent to circumcision of the male.

Surgical Removal of the Clitoris

Clitoridectomy, the surgical removal of the clitoris, was performed during the 19th century in Europe as a means of controlling masturbation and nymphomania. Clitoridectomy was first performed in the United States in the late 1860s and was practiced until the first two decades of the 20th century. Today, clitoral amputation is rarely performed except in cases of severe enlargement, to relieve a disorder of continuous clitoral erection or as a result of a neoplasm or other serious medical problem. However, among many African societies, Islamic groups and the Pano Indians of Ecuador, removal of the clitoris is practiced ritualistically, in the belief that the absence of the clitoris will prevent a woman from experiencing orgasm and enjoying sexual intercourse.

See also MASTURBATION; ORGASM.

Goldenson, Robert, and Kenneth Anderson. *Sex A-Z.* London: Bloomsbury Publishing Limited, 1987.
Hite, Shere. *The Hite Report.* New York: Macmillan, 1976.
Kahn, Ada P., and Linda Hughey Holt. *The A to Z of Women's Sexuality.* Alameda, Calif.: Hunter House, 1992.

clomipramine   A tricyclic antidepressant drug (trade name: Anafranil). It has been widely used as an antidepressant drug in Europe for many years. In the 1980s, open and controlled studies demonstrated that clomipramine had an antiobsessional action as well. The drug is now used in the treatment of depressive disorders, panic disorder with and without agoraphobia, and phobic disorders and is approved in the United States for obsessive-compulsive disorder (OCD). Research indicates that approximately 50 to 75 percent of patients (children and adults) with OCD respond favorably but seldom completely. Most commonly, six to eight weeks of treatment is required, although patients will occasionally respond in only two weeks. Continued behavioral therapy as well as drug therapy for six months to a year in responsive patients is recommended to minimize relapse.

See also ANTIDEPRESSANT MEDICATIONS; MONOAMINE OXIDASE INHIBITORS; OBSESSIVE-COMPULSIVE DISORDER; PANIC DISORDER.

American Medical Association. *AMA Drug Evaluations Annual, 1991.* Chicago: AMA, 1991.

clonazepam   A drug (trade name: Klonopin) with anticonvulsant effects, which has been demonstrated to have potential benefits in the acute treatment of mania. It is a member of the benzodiazepine class of drugs. For certain individuals, it has been helpful in treating anxiety disorders and tardive dyskinesia (a drug-induced movement disorder). Both psychological and physiological dependence have been reported; withdrawal symptoms similar to those observed with barbiturates have occurred following sudden withdrawal of clonazepam.

See ANTICONVULSANT MEDICATIONS; BENZODIAZEPINE DRUGS; TARDIVE DYSKINESIA.

Fawcett, Jan, and J. M. Zajecka. "Treatment of Psychotic Affective Disorders." *Current Opinion in Psychiatry 3* (1990).

clonidine   A drug used to treat high blood pressure (trade name: Catapres). It is also rarely used as an anxiolytic drug for some individuals. It has antimanic properties, and alone or in combination with lithium it may have advantages over neuroleptics in the acute stages of mania. Side effects include drowsiness, sedation and, in some cases, depression. Clinical studies are under way to determine additional uses and efficacy in a variety of disorders.

Clonidine is considered an adrenergic autoreceptor agonist; it acts on the central nervous system, reducing the action of the sympathetic nervous system by altering the brain-chemical balance. The brain then slows the heart rate and decreases action in some nerves that control blood vessel constriction. It is also prescribed for some symptoms during menopause.

The trend is toward using carbamazepine (an anticonvulsant drug) much more than clonidine, especially in mania.

See ANTICONVULSANT MEDICATIONS; BLOOD PRESSURE; CARBAMAZEPINE; MENOPAUSE.

clozapine   An antipsychotic drug used to treat schizophrenia (trade name: Clozaril). It was approved for use in the United States in 1989 and appears to be an effective treatment for some schizophrenic patients who do not respond to other drugs. It is not a cure but seems to improve symptoms of some schizophrenia patients so that they can function in the community and benefit from rehabilitative services and therapy. One advantage of clozapine over other antipsychotic drugs is that its use does not seem to cause severe movement disorders known as tardive dyskinesia.

Patients taking this drug should be closely monitored by a physician to guard against a fatal decrease in the promotion of white blood cells, a weakening of the immune system in response to the drug.

See also SCHIZOPHRENIA.

Clozaril   See CLOZAPINE.

clorazepate   Generic name of the benzodiazepine medication known as Tranxene.

See also BENZODIAZEPINE DRUGS; PHARMACOLOGICAL APPROACH.

cluster headaches   See HEADACHES.

Clytemnestra complex   A woman's obsessive impulse to kill her husband in order to possess one of his male relatives. The term is derived from the classical myth in which Clytemnestra, wife of Agamemnon, fell in love with her husband's cousin, then killed Agamemnon and was herself later killed by her son, Orestes.

See also OBSESSIVE-COMPULSIVE DISORDER.

cocaine   An addictive drug that stimulates the central nervous system and induces feelings of euphoria. Cocaine is most often found in the form of white powder and is typically ingested by inhaling or "snorting," usually through a straw or other tube, into the nose. It can also be injected into the veins. After conversion back to its base form, cocaine can be smoked, which is known as "freebasing."

Cocaine use can lead to severe psychological and physical dependence. It can increase the pulse, blood pressure, body temperature and respiratory rate. Paranoid psychosis, hallucinations and other mental health problems can result from cocaine use. Cocaine use also causes bleeding and other damage to nasal passages. Cocaine-related heart and respiratory failure can lead to death.

In pregnancy, cocaine use endangers the unborn child, who may be born prematurely, with low birth weight, a variety of serious birth defects and later learning and behavioral problems.

Crack is a form of cocaine base that is smoked and is most highly addictive. Cocaine is sometimes used with other drugs. The cocaine-heroin combination is called a "speedball," and the cocaine-PCP mixture is known as "space base."

Different users react to the drug in different ways. However, many experience an instant feeling of enormous pleasure known as a "rush." Initially it may also make the user feel energetic and self-confident. However, the pleasurable feelings produced by cocaine are followed by depression and fatigue, known as a "crash." To avoid the "crash," users take more cocaine, establishing a cycle of use and dependency that is extremely difficult to end and often requires lengthy treatment.

Cocaine is produced from the coca leaf in two stages to yield coca paste and then cocaine base. The coca leaf is grown primarily in Peru, Bolivia and, to a lesser extent, Colombia. The conversion to the white crystalline powder form, cocaine HCl, is done primarily in Colombia but occurs elsewhere in the Andean region.

See also SUBSTANCE ABUSE.

Media Resource Guide on Common Drugs of Abuse. Public Relations Society of America, National Capital Chapter, Fairfax, Va., September 1990.
O'Brien, Robert, and Sidney Cohen. *Encyclopedia of Drug Abuse.* New York: Facts On File, 1984.

codeine   A drug obtained from the juice of an unripe white poppy. It is chemically similar to morphine, also an opium derivative, but milder. It is commonly used as a painkiller in tablet form and in cough medications. Codeine has a mild sedative reaction. Use of codeine causes the body to build up a tolerance that stimulates the user to need an increasing amount of the drug to achieve a desired result.

See also ADDICTION; SUBSTANCE ABUSE.

codependency   A relationship is which the participants have a strong need to be needed but also continue to create their mutual needs in a detrimental, weakening manner in order to preserve the dependent relationship. One example of a codependent relationship is one in which a husband covers up for his wife's alcoholism. He does the household chores, drives the children to their activities and explains her problem as an "illness." He is an enabler, because he makes it possible for her to continue with her addiction.

Another example of a codependent relationship is one in which a parent continues to compensate for or cover up a child's difficulties in school or with the law, thinking that he is protecting the child. It is often interpreted that this behavior persists because preserving the child's flaws and immature behavior will keep her forever dependent on the parent. Since codependency is viewed as a type of addiction, the advocates of the codependent theory feel that these tendencies can be overcome with a process similar to the recovery process used by Alcoholics Anonymous.

Codependence has been loosely defined and overgeneralized, attempting to include almost every problem as an addiction when other possible causes are not identified.

Codependency has been criticized for promoting tendencies to blame the parent-child or other relationships for individual problems and failures rather than accepting responsibility for one's own actions. The codependent philosophy has also been called yet another symptom of self-absorption and narcissism.

See also AGORAPHOBIA; ALCOHOLISM.

Becnel, Barbara. *The Co-dependent Parent.* San Francisco: Harper, 1991.
Rieff, David. "Victims All?" *Harper's* (Oct. 1991).
Wells, Marolyn, Cheryl Glickauf-Hughes, and Katherine Bruss. "The Relationship of Codependency to Enduring Personality Characteristics." *Journal of College Student Psychotherapy* 12, no. 3 (1998) 1: 25–38.

cofactors   Factors that do not cause a disorder alone but that can intensify effects of other causative factors. For example, stress can be a cofactor in a viral disease, and burnout or grief can be cofactors in depression.

See BURNOUT; DEPRESSION; STRESS.

coffee   Many people rely on coffee to relieve stress. Having a cup of coffee is also considered a social experience, as it is an opportunity for individuals to sit together and relax for a few moments of conversation. Coffee is primarily a stimulant, as it contains caffeine. Some individuals believe that coffee gives them a feeling of instant energy and use coffee to help wake themselves up or recharge themselves throughout the day. This is so because it affects the central nervous system, increasing the heart action in rate and strength. There is also increased activity of the kidneys, and brain centers are aroused. Different individuals can tolerate different levels of caffeine in coffee. Those who have cardiac conditions or hyperthyroidism, in which the heart is already overstimulated, should reduce their coffee intake. Some people are overly sensitive to caffeine, while others overdose themselves, developing anxiety, insomnia and irritability, all symptoms of "caffeinism." Individuals complaining of anxiety symptoms or insomnia should be evaluated for excessive caffeine use or hypersensitivity.

See also CAFFEINE; CENTRAL NERVOUS SYSTEM; STRESS.

cognitive dysfunction Problems with retention or use of information, judgment or the ability to learn and think. For example, in Alzheimer's disease, cognitive dysfunction begins early on in the course of the disorder. There may be elements of cognitive dysfunction in depression as well as many other disorders.

Certain medications may cause dose-related, reversible cognitive dysfunction as side effects. For example, tricyclic antidepressants and antihistamines, because of their anticholinergic side effects, may reduce short-term memory and word-finding ability at high doses; the newer selective serotonin reuptake inhibiting (SSRI) drugs, such as Prozac and Zoloft, do not. Benzodiazepine tranquilizers, such as alprazolam (Xanax), may also reduce short-term memory at higher doses. Reduction of dose will reverse these temporary effects, unless the problem is related to another underlying cause, such as depression.

Cognitive dysfunction is used in another psychotherapeutic context to refer to dysfunctional attitudes (heightened self-criticism, low self-esteem) that lead to depression and anxiety.

See also COGNITIVE THERAPY.

cognitive therapy A therapeutic approach based on the concept that anxiety problems result from patterns of thinking and distorted attitudes toward oneself and others and that changing one's thinking alters one's behavior. Cognitive therapy is used to treat depressed individuals and others who have anxieties and phobias. One innovator during the late 1970s was Aaron Beck (1921–), an American psychiatrist. Earlier forms of cognitive therapy were introduced by Albert Ellis in the last 1960s under the name Rational Emotive Therapy (RET).

Cognitive therapy, like behavior therapy, has the goal of helping the individual change the unwanted behavior. It differs from radical behavior therapy in that it does not focus only on overt behavior for therapy. Instead, cognitive therapy emphasizes the importance of the individual's thoughts, feelings, imagery, attitudes and hopes and their causative relationship to behaviors.

See also BEHAVIORAL THERAPY; DEPRESSION.

Beck, A. T. *Cognitive Therapy and the Emotional Disorders.* New York: International Universities Press, 1976.
Beck, A. T. et al. *Cognitive Therapy of Depression.* New York: Wiley, 1979.

coital death Death resulting from a heart attack or respiratory failure during sexual intercourse, which occurs rarely among coronary patients engaging in prolonged and highly active intercourse and coital positions that excessively raise the heartbeat and blood pressure. This is a common fear of many men after heart surgery or after a heart attack. Women also fear that their mates might die during sexual intercourse as a result of vigorous activity. With appropriate counseling, couples learn to overcome this fear.

coitus Sexual intercourse; also known as copulation or coition. The term is derived from the Latin word *coire*, meaning "to go together." It usually implies insertion and penetration of the penis in the vagina. Coitus can take many different forms regarding positions, duration and speed.

Coital Positions

Couples use many positions, called coital postures or intercourse positions, during coitus to enhance or maintain excitement and pleasure, as well as for comfort, or to improve or reduce the likelihood of conception. Different couples find their own unique advantages in certain positions and also discover what pleases them. The man-above position (commonly known as the "missionary position") is most common. Other erotic postures include face to face; woman above; side by side; sitting; standing; kneeling; and rear entry.

Coital movements by a male and female during intercourse vary, but in general, intercourse begins with slow, gentle penetration by the penis into the vagina; movements of the penis become progressively deeper and faster and may involve temporary withdrawal or interruption. The woman can move her pelvis in the same general pattern until both reach orgasm or the point of satisfaction.

Coitus à la vache, meaning "in cow fashion," is a French term for heterosexual intercourse in which the woman is in the knee-chest position with the man kneeling behind her and entering the vagina from the rear.

Coitus analis is a Latin term for anal intercourse.

Coitus ante portas (Latin for "coitus before the door") is a sexual activity with the penis between the woman's thighs instead of penetrating the vagina. This practice is common among adolescents as a contraceptive technique (not adequate) or as a way to prevent rupturing the hymen. It is also known as interfemoral intercourse, *coitus inter femora,* intracrural intercourse.

Coitus a tergo ("coitus from behind") is heterosexual intercourse with the man's penis entering the woman's vagina from the rear, as in *coitus à la vache.* It is also called *coitus a posteriori.*

Coitus in ano ("coitus in the anus") is anal intercourse between heterosexual or homosexual couples. It is also called *coitus per anum, coitus in anum* and *coitus analis.*

Coitus in axilla ("coitus in the armpit") is intercourse between heterosexual or homosexual couples in which the penis is inserted in the armpit of the partner.

Coitus in os (mouth coitus) is a term for fellatio.

Coitus intra mammas ("coitus between breasts") refers to sexual intercourse in which the penis is inserted between the woman's breasts, which she may press together with her hands. It is also called *coitus intermammarius.*

Coitus more ferarum is an obsolete term for intercourse from the rear; it is derived from the Latin words meaning "coitus in the manner of beasts."

Coital Techniques

Coitus incompletus is an alternative term for coitus interruptus or withdrawal, a contraceptive technique in which the penis is withdrawn from the vagina before ejaculation. Although this may be the oldest form of contraception, mentioned in zthe Book of Genesis, it is an unreliable technique because semen may be emitted before orgasm.

Coitus reservatus is a deliberate suppression of orgasm in the male, as ejaculation approaches. It is also called *coitus prolongatus.*

Kahn, Ada P., and Linda Hughey Holt. *The A to Z of Women's Sexuality.* Alameda, Calif.: Hunter House, 1992.

coitus condomatus   Use of a condom during sexual intercourse.

See also SAFE SEX.

coitus interruptus   A contraceptive technique involving the man's withdrawal of the penis from the vagina before ejaculation; it is also known as the withdrawal method. Its main advantage is that no supplies are needed. The disadvantages are that it requires a high level of motivation, self-control and practice by the male. It also interferes somewhat with the sexual response cycle and satisfaction of both the man and the woman. It is not an effective contraceptive method, since failures can occur due to either failure to withdraw before ejaculation or due to leakage of small amounts of semen prior to ejaculation.

See also SEXUAL RESPONSE CYCLE.

color   Color carries with it psychological associations that are expressed in language. For example, we are "green with envy," "see red" and have the "blues." Many people associate certain musical tones or other sounds with colors. Certain clear shades of red, orange and yellow are associated with food and are very appetizing. Tinting food with blue, violet or other mixtures of colors has been found to make it unappetizing.

Attraction to colors changes somewhat with age. Babies tend to be attracted to yellow, white, pink and red. Older children are less attracted to yellow and tend to like colors in the order of red, blue, green, violet, orange and yellow. As adults mature, blue tends to become a favorite color, possibly because of changes in the eye itself and the way it sees color. Differences in light perception between dark and light eyes may account for the fact that brunettes tend to prefer red and blondes blue.

Studies have determined that colors have certain psychological and physical effects. For example, red is the strongest and most stimulating of colors. It has been shown to increase hormonal activity and to raise blood pressure. Red stimulates creative thought and is a good mood elevator but is not conducive to work. Orange shares many of the qualities of red but, especially in its combined forms, is considered more mellow and easy to live with. Yellow's characteristic of being the most visible color makes it useful for signs or other purposes that promote safety. It also seems to have a good effect on metabolism. Green and blue green have been found to be relaxing colors that promote work requiring concentration and a meditative atmosphere. Blue has the opposite effect of red. It lowers bodily functions and promotes a restful atmosphere; however, it may be depressing if used too extensively. Being surrounded with blue has caused participants in psychological tests to underestimate time periods and the weight of objects. Purple, a combination of red and blue, has a neutral effect. In large amounts, it is disturbing because the eye does not focus on it easily. Monotonous use of the same color has been found to be more disturbing than a variety of colors.

Healing and mystical properties have been ascribed to color throughout history. Ancient peoples associated colors with the houses of the zodiac and with the elements. Color was highly important in the practice of magic. The superstitious feel that blue and green divert the power of the evil eye. Color has been important in religious symbolism and ritual. For example, in Judaism red, blue, purple and white have been considered divine colors.

In Chasidic sects, women are forbidden to wear red or other bright colors that draw attention to themselves. Green, the color of life and rebirth, is important in Christianity. In many cultures even close to modern times, red was considered to have healing properties to the extent that it was thought beneficial to actually surround a patient with red clothing, red furnishing and covers and give him or her red food and red medicine.

Fear of colors is known as chrematophobia, chromophobia and chromatophobia.

See also BLOOD PRESSURE; CREATIVITY.

Birren, Faber. *Color Psychology and Color Therapy.* Secaucus, N.J.: Citadel Press, 1961.

coma   When the cortex of the brain cannot be aroused, an individual is said to be in a coma. Many syndromes can produce coma, including cerebral hemorrhage; large cerebral infarction; blood clots in the brain; tumors; failure of oxygen supply; nutritional deficiency; poisonings; concussion and other trauma; and electrolyte disorder.

Metabolic problems impair function in the brain, and when nerve impulses are abnormal, a state of coma ensues. Diabetic coma is one of the metabolic coma-producing diseases. Treatment of diabetic coma is specific, usually beginning with massive doses of insulin. On the other hand, excessive insulin can cause coma in diabetics from hypoglycemia (low blood sugar), requiring immediate administration of sugar (glucose). In other types of coma, measures are taken to ensure that no further damage will be done to the brain. This means being sure that breathing is normal and that the heart is functioning properly. Glucose is given intravenously to assure sufficient nutrition to the brain. Careful diagnosis and special therapy are essential. Medication may be necessary to combat an infection in another organ that led to the coma.

See also BRAIN; DIABETES.

combat fatigue   See POST-TRAUMATIC STRESS DISORDER.

combat neurosis   See POST-TRAUMATIC STRESS DISORDER.

commitment People requiring psychiatric care are hospitalized through either a voluntary or an involuntary admission. A voluntary admission involves the individual signing into a treatment source of his own free will. An individual who enters a facility voluntarily may reject any type of treatment prescribed and may sign himself out of the facility at any time. Involuntary admission, or involuntary commitment, is the process by which an individual suffering from a severe mental disorder is legally deprived of her freedom. An individual may be committed legally in most states if she is likely to physically harm herself or other people or is unable to physically care for herself. Physicians who have examined the person explain to the court, usually in writing, why they believe the person should be placed in a mental institution.

Commitment is unpopular, as it forces a physician to make a decision that deprives a person of his liberty against his wishes. Yet physicians are held responsible for making the decision to avoid harm (death from suicide) to the patient or others (homicide). Patients may also be so severely ill that they are unable to care for themselves physically (maintain nutrition, protection from the elements) or exhibit lack of judgment that physically endangers the patient. The certified patient is entitled to a defense attorney, and the decision to exact the commitment must be made by a judge based on the evidence. The procedure is set up to protect people who are mentally ill while at the same time protecting individual rights.

See also LEGAL ISSUES.

communication A process through which meanings are exchanged between individuals. When individuals feel understood, they have communicated effectively: They are in control of events, other people trust and respect them, and in work settings, they feel valued. Communicating effectively enhances health and self-esteem, nurtures relationships and helps people maintain good mental health.

Failure to Communicate

When individuals do not communicate well, they feel misunderstood, frustrated, distressed, defensive and often hostile, all of which increase their stress level. Faults and flaws in communication habits, as well as communication gaps, cause stress to many people and those with whom they interact on all levels, from the most intimate to the most distant of acquaintances. People who don't communicate effectively are more vulnerable to disease; they can be hostile and confrontational, and they are at increased risk for heart disease. People who feel misunderstood report more depression and more mood disorders of the kind shown to weaken the immune system. When communication breaks down, heart rate speeds up, cholesterol and blood sugar levels rise, and they become more susceptible and sensitive to headaches, digestive problems and pain. In work settings, communication gaps can reduce productivity, make workers irritable and even increase the risk of accidents.

Differences in Male-Female Communication Styles

According to Bee Reinthaler, a personnel communications specialist, differences between communications styles of male and female managers in business can cause problems in efficiency and in accomplishing goals. Males in the corporate world often use a complex combination of business, sports and military jargon. Their behavior is action-oriented and competitive. On the other hand, women generally are more demonstrative and frame their speech with qualifiers, questions and questioning intonations. They express doubts, uncertainties and feelings more frequently than men.

According to Reinthaler, when women wait for men to speak first, they create an image of incompetence. "Men may then fall into the stereotypical role of treating women as incompetent, and the stereotypical interaction continues in a destructive way. It would be more effective if managers of both genders would 'speak the same' language."

"Many women attempt to crack the male communication code in the workplace until something happens that shows they have underestimated its complexities," says Candiss Rinker, an expert in the science and practice of change management. She explains that women have been socialized from childhood to avoid direct communication about difficult issues, so they often use a sugar-coated approach that other women understand, but men do not.

Deborah Tannen, linguistics professor, says gender differences put women in a double bind at work that is not as evident in personal relationships. "Workplace communication norms were developed by men, for men, at a time when there were very few women present. The situation is aggravated when women hold positions of authority. If they talk in ways expected of women, they may not be respected; if they talk in ways expected of men, they may not be liked," says Tannen, author of *Talking From 9 to 5: How Women's and Men's Conversational Styles Affect Who Gets Heard, Who Gets Credit and What Gets Done at Work.*

Removing the Stress from Your Communication Style

Individuals should apply the old "golden rule" in communicating with others. They should speak the way in which they would like to be spoken to and listen to others the way they hope others will listen to them. It is important that they learn to express their likes and dislikes in a tactful and diplomatic way. They will find that when they are more direct, other people will be more responsive. With slight adaptations, these suggestions may be useful in communicating with children, siblings, parents, coworkers, bosses or acquaintances and should be helpful in most situations.

IMPROVING MENTAL HEALTH BY AVOIDING COMMUNICATION GAPS

- *Learn to cope with criticism.* Receiving criticism causes stress. The impact on our mood and body depends more on how we describe the negative feedback to ourselves. Ask yourself: Does this seem reasonable? Is it fact or opinion? Are there others who might confirm or dispute this view? How would others have behaved?
- *Learn to listen.* Listening is an active process requiring openness and receptivity. Keep your mind free of distracting reactions, responses, judgments, questions and answers.
- *Observe your own body language.* Research shows that more than half of what we communicate is conveyed by body language. Smiling, frowning, sighing, touching or drumming fingers give out strong messages. Women tend to smile more than men, nod their heads and maintain more continuous eye contact while listening and speaking than men. Under stress or in new situations, this tendency becomes even more pronounced.

- *Recognize and respect differences in conversational styles.* Styles of conversing play a major role in triggering misunderstandings. For example, women tend to ask more personal questions than men. Men more often give opinions and make declarations of fact.
- *Become more assertive.* Speak and act from choice, and stand up for your rights without being aggressive.
- *Learn to say no when you want to.* Avoid feeling resentful, frustrated or guilty. Take time before you respond to a request. You need not give lengthy explanations for saying no.
- *Try to resolve conflicts when you recognize them.* Use "I" statements whenever possible, rather than attacking the other person with a "you" statement. Make sure you understand each other's concerns, positions or feelings by summarizing what you have heard.

See also ASSERTIVENESS TRAINING; BODY LANGUAGE; IMMUNE SYSTEM; RELATIONSHIPS; SELF-ESTEEM.

Kahn, Ada P. *Stress A to Z: A Sourcebook for Facing Everyday Challenges.* New York: Facts On File, 2000.

Reardon, Kathleen Kelley. *They Don't Get It, Do They?: Communication in the Workplace—Closing the Gap Between Women and Men.* New York: Little, Brown, 1995.

Reinthaler, Bee. "Verbal Communications." *The Professional Communicator* (Fall 1991).

Sobel, David S. "Rx: Prescriptions for Improving Communication." *Mental Medicine Update* 3, no. 2 (1994).

Tannen, Deborah. *Talking From 9 to 5: How Women's and Men's Conversational Styles Affect Who Gets Heard, Who Gets Credit and What Gets Done at Work.* New York: William Morrow, 1994.

Tingley, Judith C. *Genderflex: Men and Women Speaking Each Other's Language at Work.* New York: Amacom, 1995.

comorbidity　The simultaneous appearance of two or more illnesses, such as the occurrence of alcohol dependence and depression. The association may reflect a causal relationship between one disorder and another, or an underlying vulnerability to both disorders. Also, the appearances of the illnesses may be unrelated to any common etiology or vulnerability.

compensation　A defense mechanism by which one attempts to make up for real or imagined deficiencies. It may be an unconscious or conscious process. Sometimes people strive to make up for these perceived defects of physique, performance skills or psychological attributes in genuine ways.

See also DEFENSE MECHANISMS.

competency (to stand trial) See LEGAL ISSUES.

competition One of many situations present in American life that induces stress and affects mental health. It encourages individual achievement and the need to win. As such, it is the extreme opposite of another American concept—teamwork—which teaches us to respect others, appreciate their strengths and weaknesses, share our skills and knowledge and help others meet their goals.

Early in life, children on the playing field experience the contradiction of competition and teamwork. Thus begins a source of stress we carry through much of our adulthood. Competition encourages comparisons between ourselves and others, both on a social and economic level; this in turn affects our feelings of self-esteem.

See also AUTONOMY; CONTROL; SELF-ESTEEM; TYPE A PERSONALITY.

complementary therapies A set of practices that, depending on the viewpoint, either complement or compete with conventional medicine in the prevention and treatment of concerns related to mental health and other diseases. Complementary therapies are often referred to as "alternative" therapies.

According to David Edelberg, M.D., writing in *The Internist* (September 1994), the terms "complementary" and "alternative" therapies commonly refer to anything that is not conventionally practiced or taught in medical school. In 1994, there were more than 200 fields of alternative medicine. Alternative fields can be divided into four broad categories: traditional medicine, such as Chinese or Native American; hands-on body-work, psychological or psychospiritual medicine and many holdovers from the 19th century, such as chiropractic and homeopathy.

Complementary therapies for dealing with anxieties and healing mind as well as body, include emotional release therapies with or without body manipulation, emotional control or self-regulating therapies, religious or inspirational therapies, cognitive-emotional therapies and emotional expression through creative therapies. Some of these have been known by such names as encounter groups, gestalt therapy, primal therapy, EST, bioenergetic psychotherapy, Rolfing, transcendental meditation and biofeedback.

It is important to note that complementary therapies are not subject to scientific scrutiny through controlled efficacy studies with placebo or comparisons of treatments. They are accepted and promoted as helping on the basis of "anecdotal evidence" stemming from individual reports of success. Some may be truly helpful while others may be useless or ineffectual.

Many individuals find relief for anxiety-induced conditions from one or a combination of complementary therapies either along with or after seeking traditional care. For example, mental imagery is rated one of the six most commonly used alternative treatments among cancer patients and is believed by physicians as well as patients to reduce both the pain and distress of symptoms. However, as with other medical conditions, individuals should not overlook traditional psychiatric or medical treatments in favor of alternative therapies because they may be robbing themselves of valuable time as their condition progresses.

Complementary vs. Conventional Care

Conventional medical practitioners adhere to scientific models and methodologies that many complementary medical practitioners believe focus too exclusively on reductionist and physiochemical explanations of biological phenomena. Proponents of complementary medicine suggest that this approach shows limited understanding of health and disease and, in particular, of interactions between mind/body connections, psychological, social and biological factors that influence coping with stress and disease processes.

Advocates of complementary approaches, in recent decades known also as "holistic" (or "wholistic") medicine, regard the influence of psychological factors and cognitive processes as equal to, if not more powerful than, the insights and methods of conventional medicine in coping with stress and disease and improving clinical outcomes.

For most of the 20th century, the generally accepted model for understanding biological phenomena and intervening therapeutically was the allopathic method. It achieved scientific, economic and political primacy over the competing models such as osteopathic medicine, homeopathy, chiropractic and other alternative approaches. However, the public's interest in complementary therapies has grown tremendously during the last two decades of the 20th century.

In a survey by the Harvard Medical School researchers reported that more than a quarter of the people they interviewed saw a physician regularly but were also employing another treatment, usually with their doctor's knowledge. One in ten respondents were relying on nontraditional treatments exclusively. The study emphasized the widespread acceptance of "alternative medicine," a variety of unrelated practices from acupuncture to yoga, that are promoted as having healing benefits. The common factor between them is that they have not yet been subjected to scientific review, the process most of the Western world uses to determine whether a treatment is safe and effective.

A landmark study published in 1993 in the *New England Journal of Medicine* showed that far more people visited providers of complementary therapies—an estimated 425 million in 1990—than visited primary care physicians (388 million) during the same time period. The study, conducted by David Eisenberg and colleagues, found that one-third of Americans used alternative medical treatments. In addition, most of the expense for these visits, $10.3 billion, was out-of-pocket.

Herbal and "Folk" Therapies

In many cultures, herbs and other natural and botanical products are used to relieve anxiety-induced health conditions instead of modern diagnostic techniques and pharmacological treatments. Herbs are used to cure specific illnesses, improve health, lengthen life and increase sexual vigor and fertility.

Herbal medicine may have begun with the Greeks and spread across Europe with the Roman conquests. However, the development of an organized approach to using herbs took place in central Europe and the British Isles. Practices and beliefs in folk medicine are preserved in isolated, traditional cultures such as settlements in Appalachia and Native American tribes. Folk medical treatments have developed by serendipity, trial and error, without the benefit of the scientific method. Since folk cultures generally mix religious and spiritual beliefs with concepts of health and illness, they attribute disease to causes other than the natural causes recognized by conventional medicine. In folk beliefs, mental or physical illness may be caused by divine retribution for transgression or by the will of spirits and other magical beings. Folk healers pass down techniques from one generation to the next and may jealousy guard their secrets.

Because of immigration to the Western world at the end of the 20th century, many practitioners of Western medicine are learning about folk medicine, so that they may better communicate with patients from other cultures.

Increasing Interest by Insurers

Increasingly, some health insurers are paying for complementary therapies, removing some of the financial stress involved in seeking these treatments. A study reported in the *Journal of Health Care Marketing* (spring 1995) indicated the mechanisms through which each of three complementary therapies (chiropractic, acupuncture and biofeedback) gained some credibility and acceptance by insurers from the government, third-party insurance companies and HMOs. Results indicated that these therapies have each achieved at least moderate success in obtaining third-party reimbursement.

Choosing Alternative Therapies

Individuals who decide to take an unproven therapy should let their physician know what they are doing. He or she will need to take the effects of that treatment into account when evaluating their care. Be wary when encountering claims that a treatment works miracles, such as rejuvenating skin or curing cancer with no pain or side effects. Watch out for contentions from proponents of a treatment that the medical community is trying to keep their "cure" a secret from the public. Also, be wary of any demands by the practitioner that a complementary treatment be substituted for a currently accepted practice. According to *Harvard Women's Health Watch* (June 1994), while there may be little harm in adding an alternative practice such as meditation or massage therapy to a therapeutic regimen, replacing a valid treatment with one that has no proven efficacy may have serious consequences.

Watch out for claims that the treatment is better than approved remedies just because it is "natural." Natural products are not necessarily more benign than agents synthesized in a laboratory. A drug is any substance that alters the structure or function of the body, regardless of its source. It is important to remember that many plants contain toxic substances that can be harmful when taken in uncontrolled doses.

For information:

Ayurvedic Institute
P.O. Box 23445
Albuquerque, NM 97192-1445
Phone: (505) 291-9698

National Center for Complementary and
  Alternative Medicine
National Institutes of Health
6120 Executive Boulevard, Suite 450
Rockville, MD 20892-9904
Phone: (301) 402-4741

Sharp Institute for Human Potential and
  Mind/Body Medicine
8010 Frost Street, Suite 300
San Diego, CA 92123
Phone: (800) 82-SHARP

See also ACUPUNCTURE; AYURVEDA; BIOFEEDBACK; CHIROPRACTIC MEDICINE; CROSS CULTURAL INFLUENCES; GUIDED IMAGERY; HOLISTIC MEDICINE; MEDITATION; MIND/BODY CONNECTIONS; RELAXATION; ROLFING; TRANSCENDENTAL MEDITATION.

* Reprinted with permission from *Encyclopedia of Phobias, Fears, and Anxieties,* Ronald M. Doctor and Ada P. Kahn. (New York: Facts On File, 2000).

Eisenberg, D. et al. "Unconventional Medicine in the United States: Prevalence, Costs, and Patterns of Use." *New England Journal of Medicine* 328 (1993): 246–252.

Facklam, Howard. *Alternative Medicine: Cures or Myths?* New York: Twenty-First Century Books, 1996.

Gellert, George. "Global Explanations and the Credibility Problem of Alternative Medicine." *ADVANCES: The Journal of Mind-Body Health* 10, no. 4 (Fall, 1994).

Goldberg Group, The Burton, compilers. *Alternative Medicine: The Definitive Guide.* Puyallup, Wash.: Future Medicine Publishing, 1993.

Goldfinger, Stephen E. "Alternative Medicine: Insurers Cover New Ground." *Harvard Health Letter* 22, no. 2 (Dec. 1996).

Goleman, Daniel, and Joel Gurin, eds. *Mind/Body Medicine: How To Use Your Mind For Better Health.* Yonkers, New York: Consumer Reports Books, 1993.

Gordon, James S. *Manifesto For a New Medicine: Your Guide to Healing Partnerships and Wise Use of Alternative Therapies.* Reading, Mass.: Addison-Wesley, 1996.

Morton, Mary, and Michael Morton. *5 Steps to Selecting the Best Alternative Medicine.* Novato, Calif.: New World Library, 1996.

Roach, Mary. "My Quest for Qi." *Health* (March 1997).

Weil, Andrew. *Eight Weeks to Optimum Health: Proven Program for Taking Full Advantage of Your Body's Healing Power.* New York: Alfred A. Knopf, 1997.

complex Ideas that are linked together and related to feelings that affect an individual's behavior and personality. For example, a person may have suffered an early experience that made him feel inferior; he may have an inferiority complex as an adult. He may react by being timid or do just the opposite and act aggressively to compensate for his true feelings. Individuals who act like bullies often have superiority complexes and believe (or at least act as though they do) that they are superior to those around them.

Well-known complexes are the Oedipus complex and Electra complex, in which, according to Freudian thought, the individual is attracted to the parent of the opposite sex.

See also ELECTRA COMPLEX; OEDIPUS COMPLEX.

compliance The agreement by an individual in following treatment outlined by a physician or therapist. In some cases, compliance may mean changing lifestyle habits, such as stopping smoking or eating less. Compliance also refers to following a prescribed drug regimen, taking pills on time as prescribed or omitting certain foods because they cause adverse drug reactions. An example of the last is omitting foods that contain tyramine if one is taking a monoamine oxidase inhibitor (MAOI) for depression. Various studies show a strong relationship between recovery, health and compliance with treatment recommendations.

According to Jan Fawcett, M.D., Department of Psychiatry, Rush-Presbyterian-St. Luke's Medical Center, Chicago, the term "adherence" might be used instead of compliance, because it puts more of a burden on the clinician to form a therapeutic alliance with the patient, which increases behavioral compliance and possibly enhances the therapeutic effect of the medication administered.

Many variables may affect antidepressant treatment compliance, according to Dr. Fawcett. Patient characteristics, including their social matrix, are important and must be addressed. The treatment setting (study or office) and differences, such as acute or maintenance treatment, require attention to different strategies for obtaining compliance. Appropriate education must be provided to the patient regarding side effects. Clinical features of the illness, including severity, duration and comorbid conditions are important to assess for planning a treatment and compliance strategy.

See also ANTIDEPRESSANT MEDICATIONS, NON-COMPLIANCE.

Fawcett, Jan. "Compliance: Definitions and Key Issues." *Journal of Clinical Psychiatry* (1995): 4–8.

compulsion   See OBSESSIVE-COMPULSIVE DISORDER.

compulsive disorder   See OBSESSIVE-COMPULSIVE DISORDER.

computerized axial tomography (CAT)   See BRAIN IMAGING.

computers   Machines promoted as tools to simplify tasks, and thus save time and effort. The computer is designed to serve as an extension of employees' skills and capabilities. Implied is that the user is in control and the computer maintains the burden of adaptation. In fact, in many cases, the opposite is true.

For lower-level employees, use of computers may diminish skill levels and autonomy, decrease morale and increase mental health problems. While these workers report that the computer makes their work more enjoyable, they also report job changes associated with computers that involve stressors, including increased time pressures and reduced possibilities for control of the task. Added to that is the stress of having their work on the computer monitored by the computer itself, which collects all aspects of employees' activities and centralizes the information for management review.

For higher-level employees, computers seem to have increased the work done and set new standards of higher quality. With the advent of desktop and laptop computers, professionals in all fields are expected to do their own word processing, spread sheets, electronic mail and presentation preparation. This has allowed management to cut back on staff. Although computers are a powerful technology, they are continuously changing the way we do business and, thus, have become a major stressor for employees at all levels.

See also AUTONOMY; CONTROL.

concurrent therapy   Simultaneous treatment of husband and wife and possibly other family members in marital therapy or psychotherapy, either by the same or different therapists.

See also SEX THERAPY.

conditioning   Procedures to change behavior patterns. Conditioning techniques are used in therapy for several mental health conditions, including anxieties and phobias. There are three main types of conditioning: classical, operant, and modeling.

In classical (Pavlovian) conditioning, two stimuli are combined: one adequate, such as offering food to a dog to produce salivation (an unconditioned response), and the other inadequate, such as ringing a bell, which by itself does not have an effect on salivation. After the two stimuli have been paired several times, the inadequate or conditioned stimulus comes to elicit salivation (now a conditioned response) by itself.

Operant conditioning is also considered a method of learning. Operant conditioning involves the strengthening or weakening of some aspect of a response (for example, its form, frequency or intensity) based on the presentation of consequences. Two basic forms of operant learning are contingency management and operant shaping. Contingency management involves the manipulation of existing stimuli that precede or signal the behavior (such as taking cookies out of the cupboard to stop a child from climbing and opening the cupboard) or manipulation of stimuli that follow it as consequences (reinforcement or punishment).

Operant shaping involves gradually and systematically reinforcing responses until a long-range desired new behavior is achieved. Shaping is also known as behavior shaping, approximation conditioning or reinforcement of successive approximations.

The term "operant conditioning" was coined by Burrhus Frederic Skinner, (1904–90) an American psychologist who applied an understanding of operant conditioning to psychotherapy, language, learning, educational methods and cultural analysis.

The principles of operant conditioning have been the basis for programs that successfully treat a wide range of human behavior problems, habit problems and behavioral deficiencies, as well as elicit and maintain new behavior development.

Unlike classical and operant conditioning that require repeated trials for new learning or behavior, modeling results in behavior acquisition by observation. Subsequent performance of the new behavior may rely on operant reinforcement and past history of the observer.

See also BEHAVIOR THERAPY.

Doctor, Ronald M., and Ada P. Kahn. *Encyclopedia of Phobias, Fears and Anxieties,* 2nd ed. New York: Facts On File, 2000.

condom   A cylindrical sheath of rubber placed on the penis prior to coitus (sexual intercourse) that catches seminal fluid and prevents sperm from entering the vagina and impregnating the woman. Condoms are also known commonly as "rubbers" or "sheaths."

Condoms also act as barriers to bacteria, helping to prevent sexually transmitted diseases (STDs) from passing between partners. The condom should be put on the penis before any contact and should be properly removed after ejaculation, so that no sperm makes contact with the vagina. However, condoms are not 100 percent effective in preventing the spread of certain sexually transmitted diseases, because the male scrotum, if infected, may spread the infection to a partner.

In the 1980s, during the escalation of the AIDS (acquired immunodeficiency syndrome) epidemic, the use of condoms was promoted as a safe sex measure and means of reducing the risk of the spread of AIDS and STDs.

Advantages of using a condom as a contraceptive include relatively low cost, availability without a physical examination or prescription and protection against STDs. Disadvantages include the care in user behavior required to make it effective and its reputation for dulling sensation in the penis.

The condom may have been invented by Dr. Condom, a physician in the court of Charles II (1650–1685). However, the first published report of condom use to prevent venereal disease was in the work of the Italian anatomist Fallopius in 1564.

Historically, the French have referred to the condom as the "English cape," and the English have referred to it as the "French letter."

See also ACQUIRED IMMUNODEFICIENCY SYNDROME; COITUS; SAFE SEX; SEXUALLY TRANSMITTED DISEASES.

conduct disorder   Also known as juvenile delinquency; the largest single group of mental health disorders during adolescence. The rate is approximately 20 percent in adolescent boys and 2 percent in adolescent girls. Adolescents are responsible for a substantial proportion of violent crimes, accounting for over 18 percent of all arrests for violence. The escalation of such deviant behavior in adolescents is twice that of the adult rate.

The adolescent prone to violence often has low self-esteem, is easily frustrated, has difficulty controlling impulses and has repressed rage. About 50 percent of adolescent delinquents progress to serious antisocial behavior as adults. Adolescent delinquency also predicts a high rate of alcohol abuse in adulthood.

Factors that lead to conduct disorder seem to be both social and biologic. Social factors include poverty, overcrowding, parental unemployment, broken homes and parental rejection. The youth may have had poor parenting techniques and received harsh, punitive discipline. Many boys with conduct disorders had fathers who also engaged in delinquent behavior as adolescents. Some adolescent delinquents have a history of serious medical and neurological illness. Many are more accident-prone than their peers and have been victims of birth injury and physical abuse as young children. Another factor is the presence of a depressive disorder; aggressiveness and antisocial behaviors are the externalized expression of the disorder. Research studies are beginning to show that treatment of underlying depression may reduce aggressive and antisocial behaviors.

In younger children as well as adolescents, conduct disorder may include some of the following behaviors:

Steals without confrontation of a victim on more than one occasion (including forgery); steals with confrontation of a victim (e.g., mugging, purse snatching, extortion, armed robbery)
Runs away from home overnight at least twice while living in parental or parental surrogate home (or once without returning)
Often lies (other than to avoid physical or sexual abuse)
Deliberately engages in arson
Often truant from school (for older person, absent from work)
Breaks into someone else's house, building or car
Deliberately destroys others' property (other than by fire setting)
Is physically cruel to animals or people
Forces someone into sexual activity
Uses a weapon in more than one fight

See AGGRESSION; PERSONALITY DISORDERS; ADOLESCENCE, AGGRESSIVE BEHAVIOR in Bibliography.

Davis, Kenneth; Howard Klar; and Joseph T. Coyle. *Foundations of Psychiatry.* Philadelphia: W. B. Saunders, 1991.

confabulation   See KORSAKOFF'S SYNDROME.

confidentiality   See LEGAL ISSUES.

conflict resolution   The ability of people to come out of an encounter respecting and liking each other. This is a win-win situation in which the stress of anger and confrontation are minimized, and those involved are able to be heard, to express their position and articulate their needs.

AVOID THREATS TO GOOD MENTAL HEALTH WITH CONFLICT RESOLUTION

- Think before speaking.
- Say what you mean and mean what you say.
- Listen carefully to the other person.
- Do not put words in the other person's mouth.
- Stick to the problem at hand.
- Refrain from faultfinding.
- Apply the same rules to handling personal and business conflicts.

See also COMMUNICATION.

congenital defects   Malformations or other bodily disorders that are present at birth; also known as birth defects. Some birth defects manifest themselves years later. Some birth defects can be prevented with genetic counseling before pregnancy.

See also CHROMOSOME; DOWN'S SYNDROME; GENETIC COUNSELING; GENETIC DISORDERS.

conscience   The part of the mind that provides judgment of one's own values and actions. Conscience plays an important role in developing a positive self-image and avoiding feelings of guilt and shame.

See also BODY IMAGE; SELF-ESTEEM.

consent, informed   Agreement to a plan for medical care, surgery or other type of therapy. In some cases, informed consent must be obtained from the individual to prescribe certain drugs that are used for research purposes only. In all cases, individuals who enter therapy for a mental health condition should be informed about choices of therapy, possible side effects of medications if a medication is prescribed for them and desired outcome, before going ahead with the therapy plan. In a legal sense, informed consent also refers to the right of a health professional such as a therapist to release information learned in therapy sessions only upon the consent of the patient involved.

See also LEGAL ISSUES.

constipation   Inability to have a bowel movement. Many people cause themselves stress and worry because they do not have a bowel movement every day. However, many healthy people may not have a movement for several days and suffer no ill effects. Advertising for laxatives seems to have created an "illness" called "irregularity," which laxatives are said to cure. A better approach to solving the problem is through diet and exercise. A diet rich in fiber, including fresh fruits and vegetables as well as whole grains, will help establish patterns of regularity.

Emotional factors, such as tension, frustration and resentment, may result in constipation. Tensions may cause the muscles of the intestines to tighten, or contract, in what is called spastic constipation. This is often a part of the syndrome known as irritable bowel syndrome.

Elderly people often suffer from constipation, in some cases because of diminishing tone of intestinal and other muscles, as well as the slowing down of body signals from reduced efficiency of the nervous system.

See also IRRITABLE BOWEL SYNDROME.

content, latent   See DREAMING.

contract (therapeutic contract)   A mutually agreed upon statement of the changes an individual desires to accomplish through psychotherapy; it is also known as a therapeutic contract. Some therapists ask the individuals to put their goals in writing. In many cases, the contract is revised several times as therapy progresses.

See also PSYCHOTHERAPIES.

contraindication   Circumstances in which a drug should not be prescribed for a particular person. For example, the stimulant dextroamphetamine would not ordinarily be prescribed for an individual who has high blood pressure.

Contraindications may be considered absolute, that is, never considered justified, or relative, implying that a procedure may entail significant risk or adverse effects. Use of a treatment in the face of the relative contraindications should be weighed against the risks of not giving treatment.

control   Having a feeling of control over one's life—including everyday events and their outcomes—is a factor in maintaining good mental health. Although people do not always consciously think about their level of control while things are going well for them, they are aware of losing control when their sense of control is threatened. For example, agoraphobics fear having a panic attack while they are away from a safe place because they fear losing control of themselves in ways such as fainting or becoming ill. Individuals who are fearful of flying remain that way because they feel totally out of control while in the hands of the pilot. While individuals cannot always control the event, such as fly the airplane, they can learn to control their own responses to stressful situations. For example, a phobic person can learn relaxation techniques to control the rapid breathing that occurs when he faces a feared situation. In that sense, he then takes control of the situation.

control group   This group is involved during many drug tests and other experiments in which one factor is being tested. In the control group, the specific factor is deliberately left out. An example is a drug test for a new high blood pressure drug, in which the control group may be given a placebo instead of the new drug.

conversion reaction   An emotional conflict transformed into a physical symptom. Often the emotional problem is too painful for the person to face consciously, so the conflict is converted into a sensory or motor disability. For example, a person may have what appears to be a real paralysis of an arm or leg when there is no organic cause for the disability.

convulsions   Involuntary spasmodic contractions of muscles. This can be accompanied by loss of consciousness that occurs with certain neurological disorders as well as during withdrawal of central nervous system depressants or following an overdose of a stimulant.

See also EPILEPSY; SEIZURES.

coping The psychological and practical solutions that people must find for extremely distressing situations, as well as everyday challenges. Examples of these situations are dealing with cancer, caring for an aging relative, readjusting after the death of a loved one, facing unemployment and dealing with random nuisances.

Arthur A. Stone and Laura S. Porter, writing in *Mind/Body Medicine* (March 1995), defined coping as "constantly changing cognitive and behavioral efforts to manage specific external and/or internal demands that are appraised as taxing or exceeding the resources of the person." Different individuals develop different ways of coping, through which they learn to adapt their responses and reduce their stress and anxieties.

To some, "coping" means getting on with life and letting things happen as they may. To others, it is consciously using the skills they have learned in the past when facing problem situations. Coping can mean anticipating situations, or it can mean meeting problem situations head-on. For example, managers who are able to handle employees in everyday situations become nervous and jittery when anticipating giving a public speech. In a serious medical crisis, some people cannot cope with their own illness, but they manage to muster strength to care for a loved one.

Individuals can learn new coping skills from mental health professionals as well as those who practice alternative or complementary therapies, such as meditation and relaxation training. Relaxation and deep breathing techniques can help overcome the stress involved in a difficult situation.

Better Coping for Better Mental Health

When Hans Selye (1907–82), an Austrian-born Canadian endocrinologist and psychologist, wrote his landmark book *The Stress of Life,* he described the general adaptation syndrome. The secret of health, he said, was in successful adjustment to ever-changing conditions.

Research studies have shown that people who cope well with life's stresses are healthier than those who have maladaptive coping mechanisms. In his book, *Adaptation to Life,* George Valliant, a Harvard psychologist, summarized some insights about relationships between good coping skills and health. He found that individuals who typically handle the trials and pressures of life in an immature way also tend to become ill four times as often as those who cope well.

Stone and Porter reported that coping efforts may have direct effects upon symptom perception, as well as indirect effects on physiological changes, disease processes, mood changes, compliance with physician's instructions and physician-patient communication.

See also BEHAVIOR THERAPY; BREATHING; COMMUNICATION; GENERAL ADAPTATION SYNDROME; HARDINESS; MEDITATION; RELAXATION.

Locke, Steven, and Douglas Colligan. *The Healer Within.* New York: Mentor, 1986.
Selye, Hans. *The Stress of Life.* New York: McGraw-Hill, 1956.
———. *Stress Without Distress.* Philadelphia: J. B. Lippincott Company, 1974.
Stone, Arthur A., and Laura S. Porter. "Psychological Coping: Its Importance for Treating Medical Problems." *Mind/Body Medicine* 1, no. 1 (March 1995).

copulation See COITUS.

cortisol A hormone secreted by the adrenal cortex, also known as hydrocortisone. Cortisol is released in response to stress. Depressed individuals show consistently increased concentrations of plasma cortisol. In contrast to normal patients, depressed patients also do not consistently suppress their plasma cortisol levels in response to dexamethasone. Dexamethasone suppresses cortisol secretion by acting on receptors at the hypothalamopituitary level to "turn off" adrenocorticotropic hormone (ACTH) and, in turn, cortisol; in depressed individuals this feedback mechanism is deficient.

See also AUTONOMIC NERVOUS SYSTEM; BIOLOGICAL MARKERS.

cotherapy   A form of psychotherapy in which more than one therapist works with an individual or group. Cotherapy is also known as combined therapy, cooperative therapy, dual leadership, multiple therapy and three-cornered therapy. Cotherapists work in various areas. For example, in sex therapy, one therapist is a male and the other is female, which encourages both viewpoints in sexuality problems affecting a married couple.

See also MARRIAGE; SEX THERAPY.

counseling   A term used to cover a variety of professional services available to an individual with a mental health concern. Such services may range from a trained social worker to a psychiatrist. Services may be provided in a school or employment setting or in a health center.

Counseling may be available for an individual, a couple or a family. When one is seeking counseling, help can be obtained by calling a local hospital or looking in the yellow pages of the telephone directory under psychologists or psychiatrists. Some listings have the heading "counselors." There are also many self-help and support groups in which members who have similar situations share experiences. A sense of improvement takes place for many participants in the group because they realize that they are not alone with their problems and concerns.

As anyone can claim to be a "professional counselor," it is wise to learn what training the counselor has had and whether he or she is certified by any state agency or professional board.

See also PSYCHOTHERAPIES; SUPPORT GROUPS.

countertransference   A term first identified in the psychiatrist-patient relationship. Countertransference in a general sense is any strong emotional reaction by a therapist to a patient. As the converse of transference, it is the displacement onto the client of the helping person's feelings that arise from the helping person's early childhood experiences with significant persons. Such distortions can interfere with the therapist-patient relationship. Indications of this process at work may be the therapist having sexual or aggressive fantasies toward the patient, dreaming about the patient, having extreme feelings of liking or disliking the patient, preoccupation with the patient in nonclinical situations and defensiveness with others about interventions with the patient.

Therapists in training who experience these feelings discuss them with their supervisors, who help them decrease these distortions.

While it is not uncommon for expert therapists to encounter countertransference feelings, they are by virtue of their training and self-understanding expected to be able to identify these feelings and use them to enhance therapy rather than distort and block therapeutic progress.

See also PSYCHOANALYSIS; PSYCHOTHERAPY; TRANSFERENCE.

Cousins, Norman (1915–1990)   American author, professor of medical humanities and leader in biobehavioral healing. Cousins managed to heal himself of a life-threatening disease and a massive coronary attack. Both times he used his own regimen of nutritional and emotional support systems as opposed to traditional methods of treatment. The experiences are detailed in his books, including *Anatomy of an Illness as Perceived by the Patient* (Bantam, 1981), a worldwide best-seller, and *The Healing Heart: Antidotes to Panic and Helplessness* (Norton, 1983).

Cousins is sometimes described as the man who laughed his way to health, a simplified explanation of the controversial healing method he employed when he was diagnosed in the mid-1960s as having ankylosing spondylitis, a degenerative disease that causes breakdown of collagen, the fibrous tissue that binds together the cells of the body. Almost completely paralyzed and given only a few months to live, Cousins checked himself out of the hospital and moved into a hotel room. While maintaining a positive mental outlook, he took massive doses of vitamin C and exposed himself to high doses of humor, including old movies and books by James Thurber, P.G. Wodehouse and Robert Benchley. In his book *Anatomy of an Illness,* Cousins wrote: "I made the joyous discovery that ten minutes of genuine belly laughter had an anesthetic effect and would give me at least two hours of pain-free sleep."

In 1980, about 15 years after his major illness, Cousins suffered a near-fatal heart attack in California. According to an article in the *Saturday Review,* Cousins told his physicians at the UCLA Intensive Care Unit that they were "looking at what is probably the darndest healing machine that has even been wheeled into the hospital." The article said that "Cousins makes his body a personal laboratory and befriends the society within his skin. He refused morphine; he asked for a change in the visiting routine to ensure rest. Gradually he improved."

When facing the treadmill stress test with fear, Cousins realized that his fear was a factor in slowing his progress, so he adopted a more relaxed lifestyle, changed his diet and specifically avoided stress-producing situations. When he did the treadmill test again, he approached it in a relaxed manner, listened to classical music and comedy tapes and had a better result.

A *Saturday Review* article commenting on *The Healing Heart* said that "It was not a medical textbook, but a study of awareness, listening, trust, choice, and intention about the intelligent use of a benevolent, centering will. It is about communication and partnership between the healer and the healed. It addresses as complementary the art of medicine and the science of medicine, the person and the institution, and freedom of choice and professional responsibility. The book affirms hope and belief as biologically constructive forces, with belief guided by knowledge and tempered by reason."

At one point, Cousins interviewed 600 people with malignancies and found that in many cases their disease took a sharp turn for the worse when they received their diagnosis. He determined that a physician can activate the healing process by building up both his or her and the patient's confidence and creating a partnership for healing.

See also COMPLEMENTARY THERAPIES; HUMOR; IMMUNE SYSTEM; LAUGHTER; RELAXATION.

Cousins, Norman. *The Healing Heart: Antidotes to Panic and Helplessness.* New York: Norton, 1983.

———. *Anatomy of an Illness as Perceived By the Patient.* New York: Bantam, 1981.

Kahn, Ada P. *Stress A to Z: The Sourcebook for Facing Everyday Challenges.* New York: Facts On File, 2000.

couvade A custom followed in some non-Western societies in which the father feels ill and stays in bed before and during delivery of the child. He may even show some symptoms of pregnancy and pangs of childbirth. The custom may be a sympathetic reaction or a means of drawing evil influence away from the wife and baby.

There are references in medical literature to severe behavioral or mental problems associated with paternity: episodes of delirium; psychotic decompensation generally of a paranoid nature; panic attacks; and even cases of false pregnancy. Expectant fathers may become hyperactive, sometimes resulting in increased incidence of sports injuries. There may also be an increase in aggressive behavior leading to fights and alcohol abuse. Fathers have been known to engage in avoidance behavior, disappearing during the delivery. There is also a significant increase in the number of divorces and suicides during the postpartum period and a decrease in libido and frequency of sexual relations.

Today psychosomatic symptoms are the main characteristic of the couvade syndrome. Some men have reported digestive problems, nausea, vomiting, abdominal pain or bloating or a change in appetite or weight. Toothache is reported with surprising frequency.

In contemporary American society, pregnancy has an impact on the expectant father, frequently in the form of physical symptoms, as well as in the form of anxiety, difficulty sleeping and changes in family and professional relationships. Pregnancy can also affect sexual activity, as well as the use of alcohol and tobacco. An increasing number of fathers-to-be are reducing their intake of alcohol and tobacco prior to conception because research has suggested that alcohol and nicotine in sperm may influence fetal development.

Since the 1960s in the United States an increasing number of young fathers have attended prepared childbirth classes with their wives, in which they learn and practice breathing techniques during pregnancy so that they can be birthing "coaches" later on. Doing so gives them a sense of participating in the event and probably contributes to a reduction of their own psychosomatic symptoms.

See also CHILDBIRTH; PREGNANCY.

* Adapted from LaPlante, Patrice. "The Couvade Syndrome." *Canadian Family Physician* 37 (July 1991).

covert modeling Imagining or actually observing another person performing a behavior or action, and then imagining the particular consequences. For example, a person who feels extremely anxious about speaking in public can imagine another person getting up on the stage, delivering a talk, answering questions and feeling successful about the situation. The next step in the concept is for the individual to picture himself or herself doing the same thing at a reduced level of anxiety.

See also BEHAVIOR THERAPY; COVERT REHEARSAL; PSYCHOTHERAPIES.

covert rehearsal An imagery technique in which an individual in therapy is asked to imagine himself or herself effectively doing an anxiety-producing task. The individual may repeat the visualization many times, considering different alternatives and outcomes. This procedure often follows covert modeling. The goal of the technique is to motivate the individual to believe that he or she can face the situation or do the task at a reduced level of anxiety.

See also BEHAVIOR THERAPY; COVERT MODELING; COVERT REINFORCEMENT; PSYCHOTHERAPIES.

covert reinforcement A technique used in psychotherapy in which the individual imagines two responses to an action or situation, one which produces much anxiety and one which produces little. For example, the person first imagines seeing another give a public speech (covert modeling), then practices covert rehearsal (imagining giving the speech), finally imagines that the speech has been given, and that there was a favorable audience response without an undue level of anxiety.

See also BEHAVIOR THERAPY; COVERT MODELING; COVERT REHEARSAL; PSYCHOTHERAPIES.

crack The street name given to tiny chunks or "rocks" of freebase cocaine, a smokable form of the drug extracted from cocaine hydrochloride powder in a simple chemical procedure using baking soda, heat and water. Crack is even more rapidly physically and psychologically addictive than powdered cocaine. Cocaine powder breaks down with heat and so cannot be effectively self-administered by smoking. In contrast, base cocaine or "freebase," which has been chemically "freed" from its hydrochloride salt, readily vaporizes into smoke by heat. Inhalation of the smoke gets the cocaine rapidly into the bloodstream through the lungs, faster than if powder cocaine is snorted. Extremely high blood levels of cocaine produced and delivered to the brain by smoking crack increase the likelihood of serious toxic reactions, including potentially fatal brain seizures, irregular heartbeat and high blood pressure. Congestion in the chest, wheezing, black phlegm and hoarseness may also result from smoking crack.

Use of crack by pregnant women can cause fetal loss or damage and babies with low birth weights, who are extremely sensitive to noise, touch and other stimuli and cry frequently. Anyone who uses it is vulnerable to developing an addiction.

See also COCAINE; SUBSTANCE ABUSE.

Media Resource Guide on Common Drugs of Abuse. Public Relations Society of America, National Capital Chapter, Fairfax, Va., September 1990.

cranial nerves Twelve pairs of nerves that emerge directly from the brain and mediate several of our senses. All but two of the nerve pairs connect with the brain stem, the lowest section of the brain. The other two, the olfactory and optic nerves, link directly with parts of the cerebrum, the main mass of the brain. Studies suggest that visual and olfactory stimuli may affect mood and motivation in significant ways without the awareness of the person affected.

All the nerves emerge through various openings in the skull, and many then divide into major branches.

See also BRAIN.

crank The name for illegal methamphetamine, a potent stimulant that attracted attention during the 1960s and early 1970s when it was popularly known as speed, meth and crystal. At low doses, crank effects include insomnia, dizziness, confusion, a sense of increased energy and alertness, suppressed appetite and feelings of well-being followed by depression. At higher doses, crank may produce severe anxiety, hallucinations, paranoid thinking and extremely aggressive behavior. Very high doses may result in convulsions, coma, cerebral hemorrhage and death.

Crank is easily manufactured in illicit "basement" laboratories and is sold as yellow or off-white powder, chunks or crystals wrapped in foil or plastic bags or in capsule form. When first used, crank is frequently inhaled. Users learn to inject the drug, to obtain a brief but powerful euphoria or "rush," similar to that produced by crack cocaine. Crank users describe the feeling as an intense pleasure jolt or shock that pushes them to use the drug repeatedly.

See also COCAINE; SUBSTANCE ABUSE.

Media Resource Guide on Common Drugs of Abuse. Public
   Relations Society of America, National Capital Chapter, Fairfax, Va., September 1990.

creativity   An unusual association of words or ideas and ingenious methods of problem solving, which may involve using everyday objects or processes in original ways. A free and voluminous flow of ideas is also part of the creative process even though most of the ideas may not be truly creative. The technique of brainstorming is related to this aspect of creativity.

Although some aspects of the creative process have been defined and identified, creativity is a difficult mental activity to study or even to define because of its inherent subjectivity and various forms of manifesting itself in different areas of life. Behaviorists even adopt the position that there is no such thing as a creative act; what appears to be new is, in fact, "old wine in new bottles" or arrived at by luck and random experimentation. However, most discussions of creativity contain the concepts of the new, novel or unique or whether an idea is actually a combination of existing and known elements and ideas in a new way. For example, Shakespeare created dramatic masterpieces without using original plots. Another element of creativity is its relation to reality, to something others can relate to or use. A unique solution to a problem is not, in the end, creative if it does not work. A work of art may be original but not truly creative unless it relates somehow to experiences, feelings or thoughts—even though previously undefined—of the observer. Some creative ideas, however, are ahead of their time and may not be understood or appreciated until after the creator's lifetime.

The Creative Process

Researchers and biographers of creative individuals have identified certain stages in the creative process. Often the scientist or artist will identify an area of work that he wishes to attack, but after approaching it in a rational manner, he leaves it feeling dissatisfied and returns to less creative endeavors for a period that has been called incubation. A frequent experience is that after this period a solution or artistic concept may come rather suddenly, which then must be fleshed out, elaborated or tested. The ability to let go of proven reasonable concepts, to reach out beyond ordinary thought and then to return to test and rework the fruits of these irrational explorations is thought by many experts to be central to the creative process.

Certain personality and intellectual characteristics have been found to correlate with creativity. Although intelligence and creativity are thought to be separate mental gifts, and not all intelligent people are creative, intelligence does seem to be necessary to creativity. Creative people have been found to be leaders and independent thinkers. They are self-assured and unconventional and have a wide range of interests. Since they are frequently involved in their own thoughts and inner life, they tend to be introverted and uninterested in social life or group activities. Passion for their field of work and a sense that what they do will eventually be recognized and make a difference are also qualities that support creativity.

There is a somewhat prevalent attitude that creative people have a reputation of being mentally unstable. Some experts say that creativity is actually limited or impossible in the presence of severe neurosis. Both tests and observations indicate that while creative individuals may have unusual personality structures and the potential for extreme behavior, they also possess extremely strong mechanisms for keeping these tendencies under control. On the other hand, studies of creative individuals have shown that a common element is a severe childhood trauma or loss, such as the death of a parent, and that many have a period of mental disturbance. Depression seems to be common among the creative. A common pattern is a period of depression followed by an explosion of creative thought and work.

Measuring creativity has challenged mental health professionals. For example, J. P. Guilford (1897–1987), who explored this area in the 1960s, described two areas of thinking: convergent or narrow, focused thinking and divergent thinking, which allows the individual to let her mind roam and explore a broad spectrum of ideas. Guilford felt that the latter type of thinking was most creatively productive. Under Guilford's direction, the Torrance Tests of Creative Thinking were developed at the University of Southern California.

Researchers have also taken an interest in stimulating and increasing creativity. It has been found that an individual's creativity may increase or decrease according to her environment and work habits. For example, changing the atmosphere, time of day and even clothing for work may make certain people more or less productive. Techniques, such as brainstorming and other group techniques, encourage the flow of ideas. Certain techniques of thought may allow the distancing that gives a fresh view of the project or problem.

Although creativity is strongly associated with the arts, it is equally important to fields such as science, business and manufacturing.

See also BRAINSTORMING.

Benson, P. G. "Creativity Measures," in Corsini, Raymond J., ed., *Encyclopedia of Psychology,* vol. 1. New York: Wiley, 1984.

Levy, Norman, and Harold Kelman. "Creativity: Horney's View," In *International Encyclopedia of Psychiatry, Psychoanalysis and Neurology,* vol. 3, edited by Benjamin Wolman. New York: Van Nostrand, 1977.

Weisberg, Robert. *Creativity, Genius and Other Myths.* New York: W. H. Freeman and Company, 1986.

Creutzfeldt-Jakob disease (CJD)   A rare fatal brain disease caused by a transmissible infectious agent, possibly a virus. Failing memory, changes in behavior and a lack of coordination are some of the symptoms observed in the early stages of the disease. The disease progresses rapidly, usually causing death within one year of diagnosis. According to the Alzheimer's Disease and Related Diseases Association, examination of brain tissue reveals distinct changes unlike those seen in Alzheimer's disease. No treatment is available to stop the progression of the disease.

See also ALZHEIMER'S DISEASE.

crime, witnessing   See POST-TRAUMATIC STRESS DISORDER.

crisis   A turning point, for better or worse, in an acute disease, an emotionally significant event or radical change in status in a person's life. The anxiety involved in a crisis situation may result from a combination of the individual's perception of an event and his or her ability or inability to cope with it. Some people cope better with a crisis situation than others.

Crisis intervention is often necessary to provide immediate help, advice or therapy to individuals with acute stress or psychological or medical problems. Many crisis intervention centers utilize telephone counseling. For example, in cities throughout the United States, there is a suicide hotline for those contemplating ending their lives. In some cases, a rape victim's first step toward seeking professional assistance is to call a rape crisis hotline. When a bombing or shooting occurs in a public place, crisis intervention services are provided for survivors who witnessed the event in an effort to prevent the onset of or ameliorate post-traumatic stress disorder (PTSD).

Crisis Intervention

The goal of crisis intervention is to restore or improve the individual's equilibrium to the same level of functioning as before the crisis. Many different types of therapists and self-help groups provide crisis intervention. Therapy may include talking to the stressed individual and appropriate family members or short-term use of appropriate prescription medications. However, crisis intervention is not a substitute for longer term care. Through therapy, the individual may learn to immediately modify certain environmental factors as well as interpersonal aspects of the situation causing the crisis. Emphasis should be on reducing stress and anxiety, promoting self-reliance and learning to focus on the present. Longer term therapy is helpful after the individual has regained some degree of composure and coping skills.

See also COPING; GENERAL ADAPTATION SYNDROME; POST-TRAUMATIC STRESS DISORDER; SELF-HELP; SUICIDE; SUPPORT GROUPS.

Kahn, Ada P. *Stress A to Z: A Sourcebook for Facing Everyday Challenges.* New York: Facts On File, 2000.

criticism   Comments directed to another regarding behavior, appearance, performance, quality of work or other personal characteristics. Criticism may be favorable but is usually regarded as the opposite of praise.

Receiving criticism may lower one's self-esteem and even make one reluctant to do or try certain activities. For example, when a child receives negative criticism regarding his singing ability from a teacher, the child may become reluctant to sing out loud again. Some individuals who have social phobias have them because of a fear of criticism. Examples are fears of public speaking, eating in public or writing in public.

Normal self-esteem is required to self-correct ineffective behavior that is continued. The capacity to accept criticism that is appropriate and modify behavior is often associated with self-improvement and success. Narcissistic individuals or others with very low self-esteem cannot accept even appropriate criticism.

Some depressed people take criticism very harshly and sink even deeper into their feelings of worthlessness and helplessness.

Children as well as others who are in the position of being students or followers thrive on encouragement rather than criticism, since they are actually in an inferior position to a parent, teacher or supervisor. Parents may be tempted to coax children out from bad to good behavior with rewards, but the end result is really rewarding objectionable behavior, rather than providing constructive solutions. Criticism should genuinely define what is desirable and undesirable. Directions that are positive, clear and specific are more likely to produce results than short, general commands, such as "behave yourself." When criticism is essential, the child's attempt should be viewed as important. It is more productive to focus criticism on the task or skill than on the person and to avoid comparison with other students or siblings.

Criticism is usually not pleasant for the one being criticized and is often also unpleasant for the critic. In work situations, some supervisors find it difficult to offer criticism to employees. In some situations, supervisors avoid direct criticism, which may actually make problems worse. Putting criticism in writing is a way to avoid direct confrontation but may seem harsher than intended and gives the employee no immediate opportunity to respond. Writing a memo to a group criticizing acts that only a few have committed is another way of avoiding confrontation, but this usually offends the innocent and makes the guilty feel that what they are doing is a common practice. Employers may also have a tendency to mix praise and blame in such a way that the employee takes neither seriously.

Some supervisors may have a tendency to scrutinize the employee too closely and make general comments about his behavior in addition to what is needed to resolve the situation. Any criticism of an employee that fails to get to the heart of the problem and to deal with elements of the problem that may recur is counterproductive. A supervisor should expect that her criticism of an employee should be a learning experience for him as well.

See also ANXIETY DISORDERS; INFERIORITY COMPLEX; PHOBIA.

Leach, Penelope. *The Child Care Encyclopedia.* New York: Knopf, 1984.
Platt, J. M. "Encouragement." In *Encyclopedia of Psychology,* vol. 1, edited by Raymond J. Corsini. New York: Wiley, 1984.
Quick, Thomas. *Person to Person Management; An Executive's Guide to Working Effectively with People.* New York: St. Martin's, 1977.

cross-cultural influences   Beliefs and behaviors that may not be concordant with those of currently practiced, Western-style biomedicine. This is an area of concern to therapists who treat mental health concerns as the influx of immigrants into

American society adds new dimensions to skills needed to treat these individuals.

Therapists and patients often hold different models of health and illness that may influence the effectiveness of communication during a clinical visit as well as the outcome of treatment. For example, there may be significant differences in the ways anxiety is described and experienced. Lee Pachter, writing in the *Journal of the American Medical Association*, March 2, 1994, defines a "cultural group" as a group of people who share common beliefs, ideas, experiences, knowledge, attitudes and behaviors. Most clinical encounters can be regarded as an interaction between two cultures— the culture of medicine and the culture of the patients. Therapists and patients may have different explanatory models for sickness. An explanatory model is the way an individual conceptualizes a sickness episode, including beliefs and behaviors concerning etiology, course and timing of symptoms, reasons for becoming sick, diagnosis, treatment and roles and expectations of the sick individual.

Perceptions of Depression and Anxieties

Depression and anxiety disorders are viewed in different ways in different cultures. For example, studies indicate that agitation is a more common symptom among Japanese, South Indian and North Indian depressives than among Western depressives. Feelings or delusions of guilt are somewhat less common among Indians than Westerners.

Indian studies during the 1970s indicated a fairly high degree of hypochondriasis, which is noticeable as bowel consciousness and concern about sexual potency and the genital organs. Chinese studies during the 1940s described the *shook yang,* in which an individual fears retraction of the genitals and death because of this process.

In comparison studies of Indian and British depressed persons (1970s), certain differences were noted that may reflect cultural influences. For example, the Indians complained more about physical symptoms than the British. Physical symptoms have also been observed in studies of African depressives. Individuals emphasize their symptoms based on what local medical people consider illness. Purely psychological symptoms are often dismissed as not of much consequence in less sophisticated groups. Rural Indians may use the body to express inner tensions and anxieties. Differences in such symptoms were noted among British and Indian soldiers under extreme stress during World War II.

Interpretation of guilt among depressives varies between cultures. For example, some Indians attribute their present suffering to possible bad deeds in a previous life. In the Indian social system, conformity is highly valued and the assumption of responsibility for one's actions is less well developed. Thus the individual fears failure rather than a loss of self-esteem because he is concerned about what others will say.

Symptoms of obsession and paranoia appear more frequently in Western studies than among Indian depressives. This may be because rituals are accepted daily practices in some Indian socioreligious systems, and thus such systems are not considered irregular by the individual or his relatives. Also, Westerners tend to be more competitive than Indians, and this tendency may explain a higher degree of suspicious paranoid attitude.

Some specific differences between cultures include mourning practices, feelings of shame, guilt and projection, the interoperation of the sick role and methods of child training.

Mourning practices differ among cultures, and the process of grief influences the occurrence of depression. For example, in some societies, religion promises continued interaction with the deceased and the possibility of reparation for whatever wrongs may have been done. However, acceptance of loss may be inhibited if customary rites and beliefs lose significance in rapidly acculturating groups. Whether mourning leads to depression depends on the degree of ambivalence in the individual's relationship to the lost person or object. Such relationships are affected by the interaction between parent and child, and particularly the relationship of father to child in patriarchal, traditional societies, which differs from that in most Western cultures.

Shame and guilt influence depression and anxieties. Depression may be rare among illiterate

Africans because of the lack of self-reproach, self-responsibility and a lack of individual competition, as well as a fatalistic attitude. Researchers during the 1950s and 1960s agreed that in Africa, depression is relatively light and short, without feelings of sin and guilt. There is a relative infrequency of manic symptoms and a very low suicide rate.

Early missionary reports indicated that Japanese guilt feelings were not related to sexual and sensual bodily expressions but instead connected with family obligations. The Japanese (according to a 1960 study by P. M. Yap) have a term that literally means repaying one's parents; infractions of this obligation cause feelings that Westerners call "guilt." Different individuals feel guilty about different things, depending on their culture. In Japanese literature, more first-born than last-born males are among those who become depressed. This may occur because in the Confucian system, the eldest son has a heavy responsibility, especially when the father dies.

Projection (a defense mechanism by which unacceptable impulses are attributed to others or personal failures are blamed on others) is used in many cultures. In some societies in which religion teaches that the individual is evil because of a supernatural cause, there is also a mechanism for absolution, atonement and relief of guilt in the individual. In many Asian societies, rites of worship or reverence serve a similar function. Some individuals will project guilt and depression to some evil "personality" that possesses and inhabits one's being. These are alternative reactions to depression and are influenced by differences in education and social class.

How people experience the sick role differs among cultures. For example, the "lost soul" belief (when it seems that they have no spirit and are depressed) in South America may also give cultural support to the depressed person in the condition called *susto*, which does not call for medical attention. Illiterate groups, including the lower classes in advanced cultures, tend to define the sick role in physical terms and visit doctors with physical problems instead of psychological ones.

Child training influences how depression, anxieties and fears are expressed in later life. Guilt feelings may be influenced by parental severity in child training. Withholding of love and affection may increase self-aggression, and aggression seems to turn inward more readily when the mother, rather than the father, gives punishment. Variables in societies include types of parental dominance, use of verbal, love-oriented technique as opposed to physical punishment, the size of the family, the number of siblings, the presence of mother surrogates and social class or culture pattern.

There is a high prevalence of post-traumatic stress disorder (PTSD) among refugee groups from Southeast Asia and Central America who fled violence and state terror. Researchers studying these groups have found a high co-occurrence of depressive disorder and dissociative experiences. The term "cultural bereavement" has been proposed as a diagnosis that more fully captures the nature of the syndrome of traumatic losses experienced by refugees.

In Japan, a type of social phobia (*taijin kyofusho*) has been identified in which the primary symptom is the fear of embarrassing others, rather than oneself. In New Guinea and Melanesia, "cargo anxiety" occurs out of a belief that ancestral spirits will arrive, bringing valuable cargo. Locals destroy existing food supplies in expectation of better items to come. Insecurity and dissatisfaction with the existing way of life are thought to lead to such delusions.

Anxiety Disorders in India vs. the United Kingdom

One study comparing phobic individuals in India and those in the United Kingdom indicated several differences. The British sample contained more individuals with agoraphobia and social phobias. The Indian sample contained more individuals who had phobias of illness and sudden death. The lower incidence of agoraphobia among the Indians may be explained by the fact that while agoraphobia generally occurs more among females than males, Indian women are traditionally housebound, and an inability to venture out by themselves may not be considered unusual behavior. More important, this difference may be explained by the differences in social structure between India and the United Kingdom. In India, for example, social life is defined by one's roles, such as son, husband, father, grandson or neighbor, whereas in Western

POSSIBLE RELATIONSHIPS OF SOCIOCULTURAL VARIABLES TO DEPRESSION

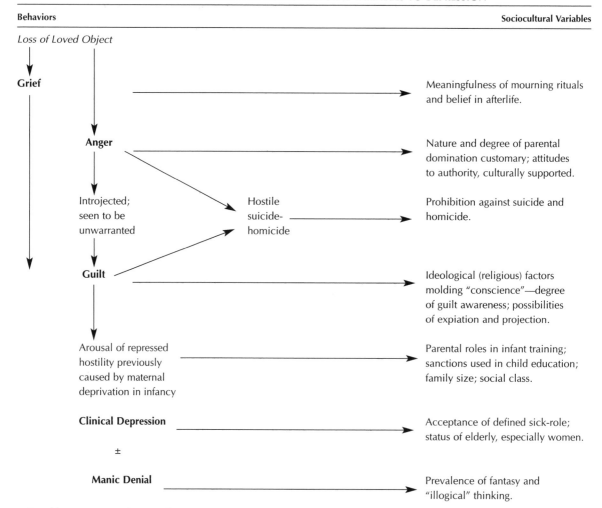

Behaviors   **Sociocultural Variables**

Loss of Loved Object

Grief → Meaningfulness of mourning rituals and belief in afterlife.

Anger → Nature and degree of parental domination customary; attitudes to authority, culturally supported.

Introjected; seen to be unwarranted → Hostile suicide-homicide → Prohibition against suicide and homicide.

Guilt → Ideological (religious) factors molding "conscience"—degree of guilt awareness; possibilities of expiation and projection.

Arousal of repressed hostility previously caused by maternal deprivation in infancy → Parental roles in infant training; sanctions used in child education; family size; social class.

Clinical Depression → Acceptance of defined sick-role; status of elderly, especially women.

±

Manic Denial → Prevalence of fantasy and "illogical" thinking.

Adapted from P. M. Yap, "Phenomenology of Affective Disorder in Chinese and Other Cultures," CIA Foundation Symposium/Transcultural Psychiatry (London, 1965), p. 98.

cultures the focus is on individuality and independence. Thus the Indian may feel less social pressure than Westerners, and this lack of social pressure may play a role in the incidence of agoraphobia and social phobias. It may also be that fear of social situations is not recognized as a condition requiring medical help. Also, poor health education and less-than-adequate health services in general may heighten anxieties about illness and death.

Culturally Sensitive Care Is Necessary

Pachter encourages "culturally sensitive" health care. This means a system that respects the beliefs, attitudes and cultural lifestyles of its patients. It is a system that acknowledges that culturally constructed meanings of illness are valid concerns of clinical care.

See also ACCULTURATION; ANXIETY; COMMUNICATION; DEPRESSION; GUILT; HYPOCHONDRIASIS; MIGRA-

PATTERNS OF DEPRESSION IN THREE CULTURES

	West	Nigeria	India
Incidence	Common	Rare (artifact?)	Common
Sick role	Acknowledged	Not acknowledged (no word for depression)	Acknowledged
Hypochondriasis	Less common	Common	Common
Paranoid symptoms	Uncommon	Most frequent	Rare
Guilt feelings	Frequent	Almost absent	Rare
Retarded/agitated	R > A	A > R	A > R (artifact?)
Fugitive impulse	Not described	Common (wander into jungle)	Frequent (renunciation)
Suicide	Common	Rare	Less common

Adapted from J. S. Neki, "Psychiatry in South-East Asia," *British Journal of Psychiatry,* 123 (1973): 257–269.

TION; PARANOIA; POST-TRAUMATIC STRESS DISORDER; SELF-ESTEEM; SICK ROLE.

* *Adapted from:* Doctor, Ronald M. and Ada P. Kahn. *Encyclopedia of Phobias, Fears, and Anxieties* (New York: Facts On File, 2000).

Chambers, J. et al. "Phobias in India and the United Kingdom." *Acta Psychiatrica Scandinavia* 74 (1986): 388–391.

Friedman, Steven. *Cultural Issues in the Treatment of Anxiety.* New York: The Guilford Press, 1997.

Howells, J.G. and M.L. Osborn. *A Reference Companion to the History of Abnormal Psychology.* Westport, Conn.: Greenwood Press, 1984.

Neki, J.S. "Psychiatry in South-East Asia." *British Journal of Psychiatry* 123 (1973): 257–269.

Pachter, Lee M. "Culture and Clinical Care." *Journal of the American Medical Association* 271, no. 9 (March 2, 1994).

Tan, Ai Girl. "Implicit Theories of Stress: A Cross-Cultural Comparison between Japanese and Malaysians." *Japanese Journal of Social Psychology* no. 1 (Sept. 1995): 11–10.

Teja, J.S. et al. "Depression Across Cultures." *British Journal of Psychiatry* 119 (1970): 253–260.

Yap, P.M. "Phenomenology of Affective Disorders in Chinese and Other Cultures." London: CIA Foundation Symposium/Transcultural Psychiatry, 1965.

crowding A large mass of people or animals. In Hans Selye's landmark book, *The Stress of Life* (1976), he suggested that in humans, crowding may make men more competitive, somewhat more severe and like each other less, whereas women tend to be more cooperative and lenient and to like each other more.

Selye speculated that residential crowding in itself does not produce psychological or physical symptoms of stress and anxiety. In fact, under certain conditions, interpersonal contact is supportive, as long as the people know that they have the space to get away from each other when they want to. His studies, however, did not reflect later 20th century anxieties from heavy traffic, high-rise living, air pollution, noise and other features associated with contemporary urban life.

See also AUTONOMY; CONTROL; GENERAL ADAPTATION SYNDROME; PERSONAL SPACE; SELYE, HANS; STRESS.

Kahn, Ada P. *Stress A to Z: The Sourcebook for Facing Everyday Challenges.* New York: Facts On File, 2000.

crying A vocal expression of emotion, accompanied by tears. It is both a cause of stress and a stress reliever, depending on the situation. For example, at funerals, it is a normal response to grief; at weddings, it is a response to happiness. As a natural reaction based in social custom and personal experience, people cry when they are very sad or very glad. Movies are known as "tear-jerkers"; and no sight rouses more tears than soldiers returning home. Sometimes, people cry because they cannot cope any longer with stressful situations. There may be stress from pain, or real or anticipated losses of status, security or friendship.

According to William Frey, a biochemist, giving in to a good cry is cathartic. "Emotional tears contain a higher protein concentration than tears that are shed when the eye is irritated by onion vapor. We are quite literally crying it out, removing chemicals that have built up in the body due to stress."

Certain emotional disorders include crying as a symptom. In a depressive state, an individual may cry easily and without cause. In severe depression, an individual may lose the capacity to cry or weep, despite a feeling of profound sadness. In a newborn baby, crying clears the eyes and both inflates the lungs and removes secretions from the lungs; they also cry to indicate hunger and pain.

See also DEPRESSION; GRIEF.

Kahn, Ada P. *Stress A to Z: The Sourcebook for Facing Everyday Challenges*. New York: Facts On File, 2000.

cults   The original concept of the cult was religious. Groups known as cults, which grew out of the thoughts and attitudes of the 1960s, frequently had a religious philosophy and were often started by religious leaders. These groups may also have social or political reform as their goal, possibly even including terrorism.

The cult experience varies. One new recruit to the "Moonies," or members of the Reverend Sun Myung Moon's Unification Church, recalled being awakened on his first morning in the cult by a guitarist singing "You Are My Sunshine." Jim Jones, a former Disciples of Christ minister, led his followers, members of the People's Temple, into isolation and mass suicide in Guyana.

Despite their differences, cults do share certain similarities. They seem to have arisen from a time period when social values were questioned and thought to be inadequate. New recruits are frequently young people who, although they may be emotionally stable, lack family and close friends and are searching for relief from confusion or emotional distress. Cults welcome new members with an attitude of caring and acceptance that creates a strong emotional experience for the new member. Once in the cult, the new members behavior and attitudes are dictated by strong pressure in a very close-knit atmosphere. Members are made to feel that there are continually higher levels of commitment or sanctity that they can attain in relationship to the group often involving considerable psychological or physical stress. Questioning the values of the group is looked upon as evil or sinful. Members who were experiencing problems before their entrance into the group are reminded that to return to the outside would be to return to those difficulties. Cult leaders tend to be charismatic individuals who may be considered to be divine by group members. Their whims, desires and opinions are obeyed without question.

Family and friends of recruits are usually distressed by their affiliation, which sometimes seems to occur with no warning. They observe strange speech and behavior patterns if the recruit maintains contact at all. Some new cult members sever all close ties and disappear. In response to cult movements, certain groups and individuals have undertaken deprogramming efforts that attempt to extricate group members, usually at the request of their families. Deprogrammers may use force or coercion to remove members and have been accused of using brainwashing techniques similar to those used by the cults to hold their members.

See also BRAINWASHING.

Galanter, Marc. *Cults, Faith, Healing and Coercion*. New York: Oxford University Press, 1989.
Johnson, Joan. *The Cult Movement*. New York: Franklin Watts, 1984.

culture shock   See ACCULTURATION; MIGRATION.

Cushing's syndrome   Excessive production of glucocorticoids (cortisol) by the adrenal cortex. The term is also applied to a benign tumor of the pituitary gland. There is a continuous loss of protein from the body, indicated by skin changes and weakened bones. Blood glucose is increased, and there may be glucose in the urine despite increased insulin secretion. In women there may be loss of menses. Diagnosis is made on the basis of puffiness of skin, masculinizing effects, increased blood pressure, higher-than-normal glucose levels in the blood and high amounts of excreted corticoid steroids in the urine. The disease is treated by partial removal of the cortex portion of the adrenal glands.

Patients with Cushing's syndrome may suffer from depression, confusion, organic psychosis and suicidal tendencies. Cushing-like syndrome can be induced by taking corticoid-like steroids (for example, prednisolone, cortisone) for various medical conditions such as lupus erythematosus, Crohn's disease and severe asthma.

See also ADRENAL CORTEX; ADRENAL GLAND; COR-TISOL.

cyclothymia A mood disturbance in which one has moods of elation and depression. Cyclothymia is now categorized as a mild type of bipolar (manic-depressive) disorder. To be diagnosed as having cyclothymia, a person must have at least two years of this disorder (one year for children and adolescents) and many periods of depressed mood or loss of interest or pleasure usually unrelated to external sources. With cyclothymia, the person is not as socially or occupationally impaired as with severe depression or manic episodes, but anxieties develop because of rapid mood changes. Cyclothymia usually begins in adolescence or early adult life. It is equally common in males and females.

See also AFFECTIVE DISORDERS; BIPOLAR DISORDER; DEPRESSION; MANIC-DEPRESSIVE ILLNESS; DEPRESSION AND AFFECTIVE DISORDERS in BIBLIOGRAPHY.

American Psychiatric Association. *Diagnostic and Statistical Manual of Mental Disorders,* 4th ed., rev. Washington, D.C., 1994.

cyproterone acetate An antiandrogenic drug (trade name: Cyproteron/Androcure) used in some women to counteract effects of excess male hormones. Some women develop facial hair and other masculine features as a result of a disorder of the adrenal gland or after use of hormonal therapy for cancer. Cyproterone acetate also has been used to control precocious puberty in boys and in sexual offenders to reduce sex drive.

dance therapy A form of creative therapy that permits expression of emotion through movement. It can be used with a wide variety of patients, from those who have no serious disorders to those who do. Many individuals who will not speak about their mental health concerns will indicate something about them with movement. Therapists who use this technique are usually trained in dance and body movement as well as psychology. Dance therapy alone does not relieve symptoms of ill mental health but may be used in conjunction with other therapies.

See also COMPLEMENTARY THERAPIES.

Darvon Trade name for dextropropoxyphene hydrochloride, a synthetic derivative of opium. This drug is a moderately strong painkiller and has sedative effects. It also has the potential for the development of tolerance as well as psychological and physiological dependence.

See also SUBSTANCE ABUSE.

date rape See RAPE, RAPE PREVENTION AND RAPE TRAUMA SYNDROME.

dating A social process by which individuals become acquainted with each other and develop a relationship which may lead to friendship, romance, a sexual relationship and/or marriage. It is stressful for participants of all ages.

For young people, dating is a rite of passage from childhood to adulthood. Some young people begin dating during their teen years, while others wait until their college years. There are often issues of self-esteem, and many are held back from dating because of negative feelings about themselves. Others may have the additional anxieties of criti-

cism of their dates by their parents. Additionally, peer pressure can make young people drink, smoke or enter sexual relationships before they are ready, and they may suffer the stresses of pain and guilt because of their actions.

Individuals who are divorced or widowed find themselves back in the dating scene. Many concerns felt by young people hold true for older people, too. For single parents, dating presents particular stresses as young children often "screen" their parents' dates. Some children ask embarrassing questions, such as "Are you going to marry my daddy?"

Despite the anxieties inherent in dating, the process allows people a socially acceptable way of getting acquainted with others.

TIPS TO REDUCE ANXIETIES IN DATING

- Know something about the person's background before the date.
- Accept "blind" dates only arranged by people you know and trust.
- Seek out people who treat others with respect.
- Date people who share your values.
- Avoid people who are overly critical or abusive.

See also CRITICISM; DIVORCE; INTIMACY; PUBERTY; RELATIONSHIPS; REMARRIAGE; SELF-ESTEEM.

Vedral, Joyce L. *Boyfriends: Getting Them, Keeping Them, Living Without Them.* New York: Ballantine, 1990.

day care Although certain types of day care have been available for many years, recent changes in the economy, employment and family patterns have made day care an important and emotionally charged issue. The women (and men) who want a family and career ("having it all") are faced with the dilemma of day care versus staying at home with the child. Many parents feel some degree of guilt about seeking day care for their children. However, as a practical matter, it has become economically more difficult to support a family on one income. Additionally, wives and mothers who are not forced to work for financial reasons are encouraged by modern thinking to feel that the position of being a housewife and mother is not rewarding. Still, others faced with the specter of a high divorce rate may want to keep up their skills and have their own employment benefits "just in case." For the single-parent family with small children, some type of child care is a necessity. Social mobility has also increased the need for some type of daytime child care. At one time, mothers could frequently depend on grandmothers for daytime child care. Now a grandmother may be hundreds of miles away and working herself.

Many children today are still taken care of by a sitter in either their own or the sitter's home. However, the day-care situation does offer certain benefits. Children learn to socialize with their peers before entering school. Day-care centers are licensed and run by professionals. They may offer educational programs, toys and equipment that would not be available through a sitter. On the other hand, children sometimes object to being in a situation that is not homelike. Lack of concentration of children in a given geographic area may mean that day care is distant or unavailable. Day care may be more costly than care at home. However, credentials of day-care operators must be carefully checked. During the 1980s, several cases of child abuse were alleged.

Today some day-care centers have a separate area for sick children. Day-care centers specifically for sick children have been set up either independently or in pediatric wards of hospitals. Studies of the effects of day care on children have not shown that children suffer any real difficulties from participation in day care. However, a recently released study found that children who spend 30 or more hours a week in day care are markedly more aggressive (than those who are cared for by a parent) by the time they reach kindergarten. In some cases, children from deprived backgrounds benefit from day care; however, putting children in the hands of caregivers may lessen the extent to which mothers

can influence their child with their own values and standards.

A more recent trend in day care is the establishment of facilities for daytime care of elderly persons, whose condition does not necessitate institutional care but who have difficulty performing certain daytime activities alone. A recent study by Northwestern University showed that while this service is used, there is not the potential demand that was anticipated.

With the increasing number of women in the workforce and their advance to positions of increasing responsibility, day care has, to a certain extent, become a corporate responsibility. A day-care center in the mother's place of employment solves transportation problems and allows the parent to visit with the child during the daytime. The Stride Rite Corporation in Cambridge, Massachusetts, is an example of a company that has started a program combining care of both small children and elderly dependents of employees in the same facility.

See also CAREGIVERS; WOMEN.

Edmundson, Brad. "Where's the Day Care?" *American Demographics* 12 (July 1990).
Gallo, Nick. "Too Sick for School?" *Better Homes and Gardens* (Sept. 1990).
Kantrowitz, Barbara. "Day Care: Bridging the Generation Gap." *Newsweek* (July 16, 1990).
Maynard, Firedelle. *The Child Care Crisis.* New York: Viking, 1985.

daydreaming Letting one's thoughts wander with specific direction. People of all ages daydream. Office workers may be seen staring out the window, seemingly at nothing. Children may be seen watching birds or flowers, sometimes in a trance-like state. For many people daydreaming may be the forerunner for creativity and developing great ideas or inventions or for taking new directions in life. In daydreaming, one's mind is free to roam without inhibition and self-censorship or criticism from others. Different ways of looking at work, play and family situations are often developed during moments of daydreaming. When workers or children are looking out the window instead of doing homework, they may be daydreaming; to an observer, however, it is difficult to tell if the child is developing an idea for the future or is simply bored.

When daydreaming is filled with impossible fantasies and one lives in the daydreams instead of reality, one's mental health may be considered impaired.

deadlines Most people experience anxiety or stress in meeting or failing to meet a date or time by which something must be done. Once they have fallen behind, it is difficult to catch up. They find that rushing adds to their anxiety and decreases effectiveness. Ineffectiveness leads to frustration. Some people become moody or emotional, and they blame themselves or others for the deadline failure.

The key to avoiding the anxiety produced by deadlines is to set realistic time schedules, enlist help needed when deadlines go awry and negotiate new deadlines when it appears that for one reason or another, deadlines are going to be missed. For individuals to keep a positive outlook, they should break deadlines down to a series of small steps; as each step is completed, they will feel some success, and that success, in turn, will keep them motivated toward their final goal.

See also AUTONOMY; CONTROL.

Kahn, Ada P. *Stress A to Z: The Sourcebook for Facing Everyday Challenges.* New York: Facts On File, 2000.

deafness and hearing loss Loss of hearing, either complete or partial. Hearing is related to many things, including problems within the ears themselves, overall body health, the emotions and the external environment. Estimates are that about a quarter of a million people in the United States are completely deaf, and about 3 million have major hearing problems. Many individuals who begin to lose their hearing try to draw attention away from their loss or cover up for it. Hearing aids help many individuals, but some are embarrassed to wear one or fear that others will think less of them if they do. Some people associate loss of hearing with aging and hence postpone getting a hearing aid to preserve their image of youthfulness.

A number of factors can contribute to deafness, including heredity, subjection to noise exposure,

damage to the eardrum (by insertion of a foreign object into the ear canal) and certain illnesses (encephalitis). Often hearing loss is rooted to a buildup of cerumen (ear wax) in the ear canal. This can be removed through a simple procedure by an audiologist or ENT (ear, nose, throat) specialist. (Patients should never do this themselves.)

People tend to shut off certain sounds at certain times and admit only what is interesting and significant. For example, in some nursing homes, it has been observed that individuals say they cannot hear but suddenly perk up when ice cream or something they like is mentioned.

The term "psychogenic deafness" pertains to such mental shutting off of hearing carried to an extreme. Some patients with mental illnesses may have such a strong subconscious desire not to hear that they become completely deaf even though they have physically normal ears.

The term "psychosomatic deafness" pertains to a situation in which actual physical deterioration occurs in the ear in response to a mental or emotional problem. There also may be combinations of both physical and mental hearing difficulties.

One who suspects he has a hearing loss should consult an audiologist to undergo a hearing test.

See also PSYCHOSOMATIC (PSYCHOSOMATIC ILLNESS).

death Death and dying are major emotionally charged issues. Many people fear death as well as the process of dying. Although death is something everyone will eventually face, it is one of the least talked about topics in Western society. However, as medical science has created ways to prolong life even in those with terminal illness, an increasing number of people are beginning to "take charge" of their own deaths by preparing legal documents such as living wills and giving others durable power of attorney so that they will not be kept artificially alive on respirators or other machines. On these legal documents, people can specify the types of life support systems they do and do not want. For example, one person may say that he will not tolerate being tube-fed when he can no longer keep food down in the normal way; another might want nutrition provided but not assistance in breathing. This permits a physician to omit more heroic treatment efforts without civil or criminal liability.

Legal definitions of death vary. At one time it was simply when the heartbeat and breathing stopped. Now it is recognized that the brain is the basis for life, and "brain death" has supplanted the breath and heart tests for death. People whose hearts and lungs have stopped working can be maintained for years on machines, but no one is really "alive" when they are brain dead. Brain death means an unconscious state in which the person has no reflexes, cannot breathe or maintain a heartbeat. The electroencephalogram (EEG) of the person would be flat, without any regular oscillations indicating function of the brain. Brain death occurs naturally within a few minutes after the heart stops, because oxygen necessary for life would not be carried through the blood to the brain.

In most states a physician must certify death and indicate the time, place and cause. In some cases, circumstances of death play a major role in insurance payments. When there are suppositions of homicide or suicide, the situation takes on additional dimensions.

Death is an ethical issue for physicians and health care professionals. Some patients who are near death ask for a death-inducing potion or instrument. Physicians are faced with the ethical and legal dilemma of providing assistance in such cases. There have been instances in which loved ones provide such assistance, sometimes incriminating themselves in subsequent unpleasant legal situations. The question of assisted suicide is both a moral and legal issue. It is also a mental health issue, since severely depressed individuals may feel hopeless as a symptom of the depression. It is possible for them to develop the conviction that they have a terminal illness and ask for assistance in committing suicide, when successful antidepressant treatment would change their outlook.

In the latter part of the 20th century, many people choose the place for their death. Some who have terminal illnesses opt to go home rather than stay in the hospital with its impersonal surroundings, despite its high-technology equipment. Others opt for hospice care, where all of the patients are facing death very soon.

Religious beliefs console many people as their own death approaches or after the death of a loved one.

"Advance Directives" and Dying with Dignity

While medical science has created ways to prolong life even in terminal cases, an increasing number of people are beginning to "take charge" of their own deaths using advance directives—legal documents that allow individuals to specify the types of life support systems they do and do not want. For example, one man may say he will not tolerate being tube-fed when he can no longer keep food down in the normal way, while another will want nutrition provided but not assistance in breathing or respirators. This permits a physician to omit heroic treatment efforts without civil or criminal liability.

"Dying with dignity" is a term that gained popularity during the 1980s and 1990s when high technology enabled health care practitioners to maintain terminally ill people on life support systems. Wanting to "die with dignity," individuals can plan ahead by executing a document known as an advance directive, in which they make treatment wishes known while still healthy. In 1991, the federal Patient Self-Determination Act was enacted; it states that health care providers must give patients information about advance directives, including living wills and durable power of attorney for health care.

Living will. A living will allows people to specify when and under what conditions they want treatment to be withheld, should they suffer a terminal illness. They can spell out, for example, that if an irreversible coma occurs, they do not want lifesaving measures to be taken. In some states, the living will must be signed by the person executing it, as well as two witnesses who are at least 18 years old.

When the physician determines and notes in the medical record that the patient has met four specific conditions, a living will goes into effect. The four criteria are that the patient has a condition which is terminal, incurable and irreversible, and death is imminent. Additionally, some state laws regarding living wills do not recognize the withdrawal of hydration and nutrition. Individuals who do not wish fluids and nutrition to be administered when they meet the four conditions required for a living will either cross those items off from the living will document, or execute a durable power of attorney for health care spelling out this wish.

Durable power of attorney for health care. This document allows people, as principals, to appoint another person, known as the agent, to make medical care decisions in case they become mentally or physically incompetent. The document permits one to determine at what point the power of attorney becomes effective and the scope of the agent's decision-making powers. Durable powers of attorney enable people to give very specific directions about what treatment they do and do not want.

Advance directives may be revoked at any time while one is still competent. If it is necessary to revoke a durable power of attorney after individuals become incapacitated, legal action may be necessary. Advance directives become part of the permanent medical record. However, health care providers are not bound to carry out an advance directive that conflicts with state legislation, and it is important for concerned individuals to check the laws of each state involved for optimal peace of mind.

See also BRAIN DEATH; CAREGIVERS; END OF LIFE ISSUES; GRIEF; LEGAL ISSUES; NEAR-DEATH EXPERIENCES; STRESS; SUICIDE; TERMINAL ILLNESS.

Circirelli, Victor G. "Personal Meanings of Death in Relation to Fear of Death." *Death Studies* 22, no. 8 (Dec. 1998): 713–733.
Galt, Cynthia P., and Bert Hayslip Jr. "Age Differences in Levels of Overt and Covert Death Anxiety." *Omega: Journal of Death and Dying* 37, no. 3 (1998): 187–202.
Logue, Barbara. *Last Right: Death Control and the Elderly in America*. New York: Lexington Books, 1993.

decision making   The mental process of making choices and choosing options. Some decisions are made easily, while others are arrived at after considerable struggle. Decision making produces anxiety because it involves addressing alternatives, options and possibilities for reassessment at a later time.

The most important decisions people make usually focus on their health and well-being, affect other people, involve large amounts of money and require risk taking. Because many people are uncomfortable taking risks, doing so may generate anxiety and, in turn, that anxiety can interfere with making the best decisions.

Information used in making decisions is extremely important. How people perceive a situation and past experiences with similar situations, as well as their own background and culture, play a large part in the decision-making process. Problems may occur when complete information is not gathered or not carefully analyzed in terms of where it has come from.

See also COPING; GENERAL ADAPTATION SYNDROME.

decompensation   A breakdown in the psychological defense mechanisms that help individuals maintain good mental functioning. Decompensation may occur under stress or in mental disorders such as anxiety, depression or psychoses with hallucinations or delusions.

See also ANXIETY; DEFENSE MECHANISMS; DELUSION; DEPRESSION; HALLUCINATION.

deconditioning   A technique used in behavioral therapy; also known as desensitization. Under a therapist's guidance, individuals are gradually exposed to the situation or event that causes them anxiety responses. In time, they are exposed to the situation at its maximum. Instead of responding with their former, unwanted response, to which they had become conditioned, they are desensitized to the event and no longer respond with their unwanted behavior, which might have been extreme anxiety or a panic attack.

See also BEHAVIORAL THERAPY.

defense mechanisms   Techniques that individuals use to preserve and protect their self-esteem as well as to control their reactions to situations and life circumstances. Individuals may or may not be aware that they are putting their own defense mechanisms into play. Defensive behaviors are a way in which people cope with daily life, including ordinary as well as extraordinary circumstances. People have a wide variety of defense mechanisms, ranging from projection (blaming someone else for one's situation), rationalization (justifying questionable behavior by defending its propriety) and sublimation (rechanneling sexual energy into creative projects). Denial is another defense mechanism. The presence of pathological denial (of a drinking problem) is often seen in people with alcoholism or substance abuse problems. In cases of extreme child abuse, dissociation—a splitting of one's mind from the physical circumstance—becomes a defense mechanism. While defense mechanisms can be helpful in coping with daily life, excessive use of such devices and dependence on them can be a threat to good mental health.

In follow-up studies of the Harvard University class of 1934, Dr. George Vaillant found that though virtually all of his subjects had significant life crises, those who overcame them tended to have "mature" defenses such as suppression (the capacity to focus on only the most important issue at the time) and a good sense of humor. Those who were overwhelmed by life crises tended to employ "less mature/more primitive" defenses (blaming others) and denial (not admitting the presence of a problem to oneself).

See also DISSOCIATION; DISSOCIATIVE DISORDERS; MULTIPLE PERSONALITY DISORDER.

déjà vu   The French term for "already seen," this refers to a sensation that an event seemingly happening for the first time has been experienced before. The feeling is sometimes accompanied by a sense of what is going to happen next. The sensation may cause a sense of disorientation because of the gap between rational, objective knowledge and feelings.

Déjà vu experiences may be profound and may last several days in epileptic patients. In normal individuals the experience is usually brief.

The déjà vu experience has been explained by the possibility that there may be a link between the current situation and a past situation that cannot be remembered. Another possibility is that the feelings experienced in the new situation may be so similar to a previous situation or experience that there is a sense of repetition. Still, another explanation of déjà vu is that the situation was experienced before in a dream or imagined situation.

See also EPILEPSY; MEMORY.

Harre, Ron, and Roger Lamb, eds. *The Encyclopedic Dictionary of Psychology.* Cambridge: MIT Press, 1983.
Nicholi, Armand M. Jr., ed. *The New Harvard Guide to Psychiatry.* Cambridge: Belknap Press of Harvard University, 1988.

delibidinization   A term used in psychoanalysis to refer to elimination or neutralization of a sexual aim, also known as desexualization. An example is diverting an impulse toward voyeurism (scopophilia) to curiosity about an intellectual matter.

delinquency   See ANTISOCIAL PERSONALITY DISORDER; CONDUCT DISORDER.

delirium   A deranged state of mind characterized by a clouding of consciousness, disorientation regarding time and place, memory disturbances, severely impaired concentration and slowing of the EEG (brain waves). There may be hallucinations, and delirious people may believe that they see and hear things that are not there. Delirium may be associated with high fevers in diseases such as pneumonia, meningitis and encephalitis. Alcohol and morphine or a head injury can induce delirium. Treatment requires constant medical and nutritional supervision.

See also DELIRIUM TREMENS.

delirium tremens   An acute mental disturbance characterized by delirium, trembling and excitement (abbreviated as "DTs") that occurs after periods of chronic alcoholism. It can also occur during withdrawal from alcohol. It is rare in individuals under age 30 or after less than three or four years of chronic alcoholism. A person with the DTs has rapid pulse and often a high temperature, perspires copiously, has terrifying visual hallucinations (dogs, rats) and paranoid delusions and may have convulsions similar to those in epilepsy. Often a patient will not remember anything that occurred during her bout with DTs. If not treated, DTs may be fatal.

See also ALCOHOLISM; DELIRIUM.

delusion   A strong but false mental conception of an event or image. Delusions are classified as nonbizarre (events that could happen but did not, such as being followed) and bizarre (totally impossible, such as visits from Martians). Most people at some time think small lies to themselves or indulge in a moment of wishful thinking to protect themselves against anxiety. However, when a person can no longer distinguish between fact and fiction, he is having a delusion. To the delusion sufferer, his fantasy is real, and no amount of information will change his attitude.

One common delusion seen by mental health professionals is the delusion of grandeur, which arises from feelings of insecurity or inferiority. A person who believes that he is Elvis Presley or Winston Churchill is escaping from negative feelings he has about himself. Another common delusion is that of persecution. A person who is hostile to others may not admit to this feeling but instead believes that other people (such as the FBI) are harassing her, bugging her telephone or following her. A delusion of illness (often terminal cancer) is fairly common in persons suffering from severe psychotic depression.

Delusions are one of the characteristics of delusional disorder (nonbizarre delusions) or schizophrenia, especially paranoid schizophrenia.

See also DELUSIONAL JEALOUSY; SCHIZOPHRENIA.

delusional jealousy   A term for a paranoid jealousy reaction marked by a delusion that one's spouse or lover is unfaithful; an obsolete term for this habit is amorous paranoia. Such individuals constantly watch for indications of infidelity and justification of their suspicion and may make up evidence if no evidence is available. In males, this type of behavior is known as the Othello syndrome.

Case reports suggest successful treatments with newer medications such as fluoxetine (Prozac).

dementia   A loss of functions such as thinking, remembering and reasoning severe enough to interfere with one's daily functioning. Symptoms may also include personality changes and changes in behavior and mood. While not a disease, dementia is a group of symptoms that may accompany certain conditions or diseases.

The most common cause of dementia is Alzheimer's disease. Other diseases that produce dementia include Parkinson's disease, Pick's disease, Creutzfeldt-Jakob disease, amyotrophic lateral sclerosis (Lou Gehrig's disease) and multiple sclerosis. Other conditions that can cause or mimic dementia include hydrocephalus, depression, brain tumors, thyroid disorders, nutritional deficiencies, alcoholism, infections (for example, meningitis, syphilis, AIDS), head injuries and drug reactions. Some of these conditions may be treatable and reversible.

Individuals suspected of having dementia should be examined by a physician experienced in the diagnosis of such disorders, as well as evaluated by a psychologist, and have a thorough laboratory testing. A competent diagnosis will help the individual obtain treatment for reversible conditions and help both the individual and the family plan future care.

Persons with dementia have symptoms that require specialized care. Individualized planning is necessary, based on the symptoms and degree of impairment. Treatment should be aimed at helping patients make the most of their remaining abilities and helping family members cope with the burden of the patient's increasing care needs.

Multi-infarct dementia (MID)

Multi-infarct dementia, also known as vascular dementia, is mental deterioration caused by multiple strokes (infarcts) in the brain. MID may appear suddenly, as many strokes can occur before symptoms are apparent. Such strokes may damage areas of the brain responsible for specific functions, such as calculating or remembering. There may also be generalized symptoms, such as confusion, disorientation and changes in behavior. MID may appear similar to Alzheimer's disease. According to the Alzheimer's Disease and Related Disorders Association, Inc., MID and Alzheimer's disease coexist in 15 to 20 percent of dementia patients.

Risk factors for MID include a history of high blood pressure, vascular disease, diabetes or previous stroke. While MID is not reversible or curable, recognition of an underlying condition, such as high blood pressure, may help lead to a specific treatment that may slow the progression of the disorder.

To help identify strokes in the brain, brain scanning techniques such as computerized axial tomography (CAT) and magnetic resonance imaging (MRI) are used.

For information on dementia and related disorders, contact:

Alzheimer's Disease and Related Disorders
    Association, Inc.
70 East Lake Street
Chicago, IL 60601-5997
Phone: (800) 621-0379
in Illinois, (800) 572-6037
or (312) 853-3060

See also ALZHEIMER'S DISEASE; BRAIN IMAGING; CREUTZFELDT-JAKOB DISEASE (CJD); DEPRESSION; HUNTINGTON'S DISEASE (HUNTINGTON'S CHOREA).

Demerol   The trade name for the drug meperidine hydrochloride. Many of its pharmacologic properties and indications are similar to those of morphine. The drug is considered a synthetic derivative of opium; it is useful in medical situations but also subject to abuse.

As a pain reliever, Demerol is widely used in anesthetic premedication, in balanced anesthesia and in obstetric analgesia (pain relief). It is preferred to morphine for obstetric use because its rapid onset of action and shorter duration usually permit greater flexibility, possibly with less effect on neonatal respiration. However, it can produce significant respiratory depression in the newborn infant proportional to the fetal blood concentration. This can be minimized by giving small incremental doses intravenously during labor.

In individuals who are taking antipsychotic drugs, sedative drugs or other drugs that depress the central nervous system, the dose of Demerol should be carefully adjusted and reduced. Severe toxic reactions and even death have followed the use of Demerol in patients receiving monoamine oxidase inhibitors (MAOIs).

See also OPIOID SUBSTANCE ABUSE; PAIN; SUBSTANCE ABUSE.

American Medical Association. *AMA Drug Evaluations Annual, 1991.* Chicago: AMA, 1991.

denial   A mechanism for coping with everyday life as well as crises; also known as a defense mechanism. Using denial, an individual can filter out anxiety-producing thoughts and ideas. Denial is largely an unconscious mechanism, although at times it seems to be at a conscious level. For example, individuals who are terminally ill and fear death will deny the severity of their illness. Children who are abused by their parents will deny the abuse, yet some—because of the severity of their abuse—develop a dissociative disorder, such as multiple personality disorder. The antidote for extreme denial is facing reality and coping with it in the present.

Denial should be distinguished from the defense of suppression, a diverting of attention from minor threats or problems in order to focus all attention on dealing with a major current threat or problem. Suppression is a mature defense that allows individuals to cope with stressful events by focusing attention.

See also DEFENSE MECHANISMS.

deoxyribonucleic acid (DNA)   The primary determinant of hereditary traits passed on from generation to generation through the genes and chromosomes. This substance is the most important part of the nucleus of the cell.

See also CHROMOSOME; HEREDITY.

dependency   Psychological or physical reliance on other people or on drugs. In the case of dependence on people, it is a feeling that assistance from others is necessary for emotional or financial security or other reasons and is expected and actively sought. The person who is dependent looks to others for nurturance, guidance and decision making. It is not uncommon for a highly dependent person to feel resentment toward the depended-upon person or feel "controlled by him." This can be illustrated by the observation that in a relationship "anger equals dependency," a problem seen between adolescents and their parents, sometimes in marriages or in elderly people who have become dependent on their children. The solution, when possible, is to attain emotional and economic independence.

A dependency on drugs (or alcohol) means that one uses the drugs as a means of coping with everyday life and cannot get along without them. A codependent person is one who enables another to be dependent on a drug habit or to continue with a mental disorder such as agoraphobia.

See also AGORAPHOBIA; ALCOHOLISM; CODEPENDENCY; SUBSTANCE ABUSE.

dependent personality disorder A personality disorder characterized by a pattern of dependent and submissive behavior. Such individuals usually lack self-esteem and frequently belittle their capabilities; they fear criticism and are easily hurt by others' comments. At times they actually bring about dominance by others through a quest for overprotection.

Dependent personality disorder usually begins in early adulthood. Individuals who have this disorder may be unable to make everyday decisions without advice or reassurance from others, may allow others to make most of their important decisions (such as where to live), tend to agree with people even when they believe they are wrong, have difficulty starting projects or doing things on their own, volunteer to do things that are demeaning in order to get approval from other people, feel uncomfortable or helpless when alone and are often preoccupied with fears of being abandoned.

See also DEPENDENCY; PERSONALITY DISORDERS; SELF-ESTEEM.

American Psychiatric Association, *Diagnostic and Statistical Manual of Mental Disorders,* 4th ed., rev. Washington, D.C., 1994.

depersonalization A state of feeling unreal. The sensation usually comes on suddenly and may be momentary or last for hours. People in this state may feel that they are elsewhere looking down on themselves, watching themselves. Depersonalization is sometimes accompanied by derealization, a feeling that the world is unreal. An otherwise healthy person may experience depersonalization, especially during a time of extreme fatigue or sorrow. It is a frightening experience because it makes the individual feel out of control during the episode. People who have agoraphobia and panic attacks sometimes experience depersonalization, particularly if they hyperventilate (rapid, shallow breathing). Depersonalization also occurs in some drug users, as an adverse effect to some antidepressant drugs, during a migraine headache attack and in some forms of epilepsy.

When episodes of depersonalization that are severe enough to impair an individual's social and occupational functioning occur frequently, the disorder is known as depersonalization disorder.

See also DISSOCIATIVE DISORDERS; SCHIZOPHRENIA; SCHIZOTYPAL PERSONALITY DISORDER.

American Psychiatric Association. *Diagnostic and Statistical Manual of Mental Disorders,* 4th ed., rev. Washington, D.C., 1994.

Deprenyl Trade name for selegiline, a drug that in some research projects has been shown to slow the progress of Parkinson's disease. It was approved for use in the United States in 1989. Additional research is under way concerning the drug and its use in neurological disorders.

See also PARKINSON'S DISEASE.

depressants Agents, such as drugs, that reduce or slow down functions (metabolism) or activities of the central nervous system or brain. Examples of depressants are alcohol, barbiturates and tranquilizers. These agents must be differentiated from drugs that may cause depression.

See also ALCOHOLISM; BARBITURATE DRUGS; TRANQUILIZER DRUGS.

depression A mood or affective disorder characterized by sadness, dysphoria, hopelessness, despair, personal devaluation and helplessness. (An affective disorder refers to a condition involving the external expression of an internal state [mood or emotion]). Some depressions are marked by anxiety, withdrawal from others, loss of sleep or excessive need for sleep, constant fatigue, loss of appetite or compulsive eating, loss of sexual desire, lethargy or agitation, an inability to concentrate and make decisions and possibly exaggerated guilt feelings or thoughts.

The term "depression" applies to a condition on a continuum of severity. It can be a temporary mood fluctuation, a symptom associated with a number of mental and physical disorders, and a clinical syndrome encompassing many symptoms, such as major depression or dysthymic disorder. When psychological, physical or interpersonal functioning is affected for over two weeks because of depression, it can be considered a mental health problem. Depression is the most common and most treatable of all mental health problems. On the other hand, it has been shown to be second only to severe heart disease in days of work lost, and in its more severe forms carries a 15 percent lifetime risk of suicide.

Depression can appear at any age, although major depressive episodes peak at age 55 to 70 in men and 20 to 45 in women. Recent studies have shown a trend for earlier onset of depression, especially in females. About 20 percent of major depressions last two years or more, with an average duration of eight months. About half of those experiencing a major depression will have a recurrence within two years.

Some victims of depression have episodes that are separated by several years, and others suffer clusters of episodes over a short time span. Between episodes, such individuals function normally. However, 20 to 35 percent of sufferers have chronic depression that prevents them from functioning totally normally.

Estimates are that 2 to 3 percent of men and 4 to 9 percent of women suffer a major depression at any given time in the United States. The lifetime risk may be as high as 10 percent for men and 25 percent for women. About 66 percent of those who suffer from depression fail to recognize the illness and do not get treatment for it.

Symptoms

Depressed individuals usually have pervasive feelings of sadness, hopelessness, helplessness and irritability. Often they withdraw from human contact but do not admit to symptoms. They may also experience noticeable change of appetite, either significant weight loss when not dieting or weight gain; change in sleeping patterns, such as fitful sleep, inability to fall asleep or sleeping too much; loss of interest in activities formerly enjoyed; feelings of worthlessness; fatigue; an inability to concentrate; feelings of inappropriate guilt; indecisiveness; re-

curring thoughts of death or suicide or even attempting suicide.

Many depressed individuals have chronic mental and physical feelings that appear to have no end in sight and cannot be alleviated by happy events or good news. Some depressed people are so disabled by their condition that they cannot build up enough energy to call a friend or relative or seek medical help. If another person calls for them, these people may refuse to go because of hopelessness that they can be helped. Many depressed persons will not follow advice and may refuse help and comfort. Persistence on the part of family and friends is essential because in many cases depression is the illness that underlies suicides. On the other hand, it is common for those patients to see general physicians with "medical" complaints.

Causes

There is no single cause for depression. It is related to many factors, including a family history of depression, psychosocial stressors, diseases, alcohol, drugs, gender and age. Depression occurs in mood disorders, anxiety disorders, psychotic disorders, adjustment disorders and psychoactive substance use disorders, including alcoholism. Individuals who have personality disorders, especially obsessive-compulsive, dependent, avoidant and borderline personality disorders, are susceptible to depression.

Psychosocial Factors

An individual's lack of confidence in her interpersonal skills and personality traits such as overdependency on others as a source of support and self-esteem, perfectionism and unrealistic expectations work together with psychosocial stressors to cause depression. Such psychosocial events include death of a spouse, loss of a job and, for some, urban living.

Social Learning Theory

Some psychologists say that stress disrupts involvement with others, resulting in a reduction in degree and quality of positive reinforcement. This leads to more negative self-evaluation and a poor outlook of the future. Depressed people view themselves and the world negatively, which leads to a further sense of low self-worth, feelings of rejection, alienation, dependency, helplessness and hopelessness.

Cognitive Theory

Often unrecognized negative attitudes toward the self, the future and the world result in feelings of failure, helplessness and depression. These distorted attitudes may activate a prolonged and deepening depressive state, especially under stress. Learning what they are, understanding their negative distortions and challenging those hopeless and negative thoughts in real life can reverse both depression and a tendency for future depression.

Psychoanalytic Theory

A psychoanalytic position regarding depression is that a loss, or a real or perceived withdrawal of affection, in childhood may be a predeterminant of depression in later life. Sigmund Freud and Karl Abraham mentioned the role of ambivalence toward the lost love object, identification with the lost object and subsequent anger turned inward.

Later theories suggested an unrealistic expectation of self and others and loss of self-esteem as essential components leading to depression. Depression arising after a saddened reaction in experiencing loss may result from a failure to work through the loss.

Interpersonal Theory

This theory emphasizes the importance of social connections for effective functioning. An individual develops adaptive responses to the psychosocial environment during early developmental experiences. When early attachment bonds are disrupted or impaired, the individual may be vulnerable later on to more interpersonal and social problems that lead to depression.

Genetic Factors

Some individuals may be biologically predisposed to develop depression, based on genetic factors that researchers do not yet fully understand. There are genetic markers that indicate susceptibility to manic-depressive illness, and considerable research has been under way in the last 25 years toward understanding the biochemical reactions controlled by these genes.

There is considerable evidence that depression runs in families. For example, if one identical twin suffers from depression or manic-depression, the other twin has a 70 percent chance of also having the illness. Research studies looking at the rate of depression among adopted children have supported this finding. Depressive illnesses among children's adoptive family had little effect on their risk for the disorder; however, among adopted children whose biologic relatives suffered depression, the disorder was three times more common than the norm. Among more severe depressives, family history is more often a significant factor.

Neurotransmitter Theory

Recent research indicates that people suffering from depression have imbalances of neurotransmitters, natural biochemicals that enable brain cells to communicate with each another. Three biochemicals that are often out of balance in depressed people are serotonin, norepinephrine and dopamine. An imbalance of serotonin may cause the anxiety, sleep problems and irritability that many depressed people experience. An inadequate supply of norepinephrine, which regulates alertness and arousal, may contribute to the fatigue, depressed mood and lack of motivation. Dopamine imbalances may relate to a loss of sexual interest and an inability to experience pleasure. Several neurotransmitter imbalances may be involved, and research is finding other neurotransmitters that may be important in clinical depression.

Cortisol

Another body chemical that may be out of balance in depressed people is cortisol, a hormone produced by the body in response to extreme cold, fear or anger. In normal people, cortisol levels in the blood peak in the morning and decrease later in the day. In depressed people, however, cortisol peaks early in the morning and does not level off or decrease in the afternoon or evening. Recent research in animals suggests that abnormal elevations of cortisol sustained over three months may cause changes in brain structure.

Environmental Influences

Environment plays an important role, although researchers view depression as the result of interaction of environmental as well as biologic factors. Historically, depression has been viewed as either internally caused (endogenous depression) or externally related to environmental events (exogenous or reactive depression). Major changes in one's environment (such as a move or job change) or any major loss (such as a divorce or death of a loved one) can bring on depression. Feeling depressed in response to these changes is normal, but when it becomes a severe long-term condition (over one month) and interferes with effective functioning, it requires treatment.

Some environmental factors related to depression include being unemployed, elderly and alone, poor, single and a working mother of young children. However, depression changes an individual's way of looking at ordinary life stresses so as to exaggerate the negative aspects, leading to feelings of being hopeless, helpless and overwhelmed.

Illness

Psychological stressors caused by physiological dysfunctions can lead to depression. For example, a debilitating disease can severely restrict usual lifestyle, resulting in depression. Any illness that impinges on cerebral functioning and impairs blood flow to the brain can produce depression. Such illnesses may include adrenal cortex, thyroid, and parathyroid dysfunctions and many neurological, metabolic and nutritional disorders, as well as infectious diseases.

Medications as a Cause

Some medications have been known to cause depression. For example, during the 1950s, doctors learned that some people taking reserpine, a medication for high blood pressure, suffered from depression. Since then, depression has been noted as a side effect of some tranquilizers, hormones and a number of medications. However, alcohol is more likely to cause depression than any medication.

Adolescent Depression

Recognizing depression in oneself or in one's children or students is important. Depression is an illness and should be treated as such with available help. Adolescence is a period of demanding and complicated conflicts that lead many young people to develop anxieties, negative self-esteem and fears about their future. Some develop depression when overwhelmed by peer pressure, feelings of loneliness, powerlessness and isolation. Low performance in school can also lead to a feeling of rejection.

The lack of ability to embrace what life has to offer often results in boredom, which may be an indicator of vulnerability to depression.

Contributing factors to adolescent depression may include exaggerated concerns, misperceptions and continual self-criticism. Cognitive behavior therapies focus on these processes.

Symptoms related to adolescent depression include:

Sadness; feelings of helplessness or hopelessness
Poor self-esteem and loss of confidence
Overreaction to criticism
Extreme fluctuations between boredom and talkativeness
Sleep disturbances
Anger, rage and verbal sarcasm; guilt
Intensive ambivalence between dependence and independence
Feelings of emptiness in life
Restlessness and agitation
Pessimism about the future
Refusal to work in school or cooperate in general
Increased or decreased appetite; severe weight gain or loss
Death wishes, suicidal thoughts, suicide attempts

Depression in a young person may be somewhat different from that in an adult because adolescents do not always understand or express feelings well. Some of their symptoms may be overlooked as part of growing up. There is a strong cycle of "getting into trouble" and feeling depressed. A teenager may be depressed because of being in trouble, or in trouble because of being depressed. Depression in adolescents is sometimes linked to poor school performance, truancy, delinquency, alcohol and drug abuse, disobedience, self-destructive behavior, sexual promiscuity, rebelliousness, grief and running away. The young person may have felt a lack of support from family and other significant people and a decrease in the ability to cope effectively. In many instances where depression is attributed to adolescent conflicts, it turns out that depressive episodes are the beginning of mood cycles related to recurrent major depression, bipolar disorders or dysthymia, which require expert diagnosis and psychiatric treatment.

Melancholia

Melancholia is a severe form of depression that may originate without any precipitating factors, such as stress. This is in contrast to a reactive depression, which occurs after some stressful life event such as loss of a job or divorce.

Seasonal Mood Disorder (Seasonal Affective Disorder)

Some individuals have mood symptoms related to changes of season, with depression often occurring most frequently during winter months and improvement in the spring. Many of these individuals experience periods of increased energy, productivity and even euphoria in the spring and summer months. Also called seasonal affective disorder, this type of depression has often been found responsive to light therapy.

Treatments

A variety of therapies and medications help people of all ages who have depression. Estimates are that between 80 and 90 percent of all depressed people can be effectively treated. Many types of therapists provide help. In general, therapists use "talk" treatment to try to understand the individual's disturbed personal and social relationships that may have caused or contributed to the depression. Depression, in turn, may make these relationships more difficult. A therapist can help an individual understand his or her illness and the relationship of depression and particular interpersonal conflicts. If psychotherapy is not helpful or the depression is of such a severe level that there is a loss of work, function or persistent and increasing suicidal ideation over one to three months, medications may be needed to lift the depression in conjunction with therapy.

Psychoanalysis. Treatment of depression with psychoanalysis is based on the theory that depression results from past conflicts pushed into the unconscious. Psychoanalysts work to identify and resolve the individual's past conflicts that have led to depression in later years.

Short-Term Psychotherapy. In the mid-1980s, researchers reported effective results of short-term psychotherapy in treating depression. They noted that cognitive/behavioral therapy and interpersonal therapy were as effective as medications for some depressed patients. Medications relieved patients' symptoms more quickly, but patients who received psychotherapy instead of medication had as much relief from symptoms after 16 weeks and their gains may last longer. Data from this and other studies may help researchers better identify which depressed patients will do best with psychotherapy alone and which may require medications.

Cognitive/Behavioral Therapy. This therapy is based on the understanding that people's emotions are controlled by their views and opinions of the themselves and their world. Depression results when individuals constantly berate themselves, expect to fail, make inaccurate assessments of what others think of them, overvalue situations, catastrophize and have negative attitudes toward the world and their futures. Therapists use techniques of talk therapy to help the individual replace negative beliefs and thought patterns.

Electroconvulsive Therapy (ECT). Use of ECT to treat depression has declined in the last two decades as more effective medications have been developed. However, ECT is still used for some individuals who cannot take medications because of their physical conditions or who do not respond to anti-depressant medication. ECT is considered as a treatment when all other therapies have failed or when a person is suicidal.

SIGNS AND SYMPTOMS OF DEPRESSION

Psychological

- Loss of interest
- Unexplained anxiety
- Inappropriate feelings of guilt
- Loss of self-esteem
- Worthlessness
- Hopelessness
- Thoughts of death and suicide
- Tearfulness, irritability, brooding

Physical

- Headache, vague aches and pains
- Changes in appetite and changes in weight
- Sleep disturbances
- Loss of energy
- Psychomotor agitation or retardation
- Loss of libido
- Gastrointestinal disturbances

Intellectual

- Slowed thinking
- Indecisiveness
- Poor concentration
- Impaired memory

Self-help

Many depressed individuals in self-help groups share ideas for effective coping and self-care for depression. These include regular exercise, more contact with other people (for example, in special interest groups) and coping with exaggerated thoughts (such as self-deprecation) and catastrophizing by introducing more realistic thoughts and supporting them.

The National Depressive and Manic-Depressive Association is a national self-help organization, formed in the early 1980s. Chapters throughout the country meet locally to help members cope effectively with depression. For more information, contact:

Depression and Related Affective Disorders Association (DRADA)
Johns Hopkins Hospital, Meyer 3-181
600 N. Wolfe Street
Baltimore, MD 21287
Phone: (410) 955-4647
Fax: (410) 614-3214
Web site: www.med.jhu.edu/drada

National Alliance for the Mentally Ill
2101 Wilson Boulevard, Suite 302
Arlington, VA 22201
Phone: (703) 524-7600 or (800) 950-6264
Fax: (703) 524-9094
Web site: www.nami.org

National Depressive and Manic-Depressive Association
730 North Franklin Street, Suite 501
Chicago, IL 60610

Phone: (800) 826-3632
Fax: (312) 642-7273
Web site: www.ndmda.org

National Institute of Mental Health
6001 Executive Boulevard
Bethesda, MD 20892
Phone: (800) 421-4211
Web site: www.nimh.nih.gov

National Mental Health Association
1020 Prince Street
Alexandria, VA 22314
Phone: (703) 684-7722

See also AFFECTIVE DISORDERS; AGORAPHOBIA; ANTIDEPRESSANT MEDICATIONS; ANXIETY; MOOD DISORDERS; PSYCHOTHERAPIES; SUICIDE.

Fawcett, Jan. "The Detection and Consequences of Anxiety in Clinical Depression." *Journal of Clinical Psychiatry* 58 (Dec. 1997): 35–40.
Garland, E. Jane. "Adolescent Depression." *Canadian Family Physician* 40 (Sept. 1994).
Greist, John H., and James W. Jefferson. *Depression and Its Treatment: Help for the Nation's #1 Mental Problem.* Washington, D.C.: American Psychiatric Press, 1984.
———. *Depression and Its Treatment.* New York: Warner Books, 1994.
Karp, David Allen. *Speaking of Sadness: Depression, Disconnection, and the Meanings of Illness.* New York: Oxford University Press, 1996.
Klerman, Gerald. *Suicide and Depression among Adolescents and Young Adults.* Washington, D.C.: American Psychiatric Press, 1986.
Warneke, Lorne. "Management of Resistant Depression." *Canadian Family Physician* 42 (Oct. 1996): 1,973.

Depression and Related Affective Disorders Association (DRADA)   DRADA is a nonprofit organization focusing on manic-depressive illness and depression. DRADA distributes information, conducts educational meetings and runs an outreach program for high school counselors and nurses. DRADA helps organize support groups and provides leadership training programs and consultation for those groups.

depth psychology   An approach to therapy that emphasizes unconscious mental processes as the source of emotional symptoms such as depression, anxieties and personality disorders. An example of depth psychology is Freudian psychoanalysis. Historically, other noted therapists have also used a depth approach, including Karen Horney, Carl Jung and Harry Stack Sullivan. Included in the category of depth psychology are other techniques that investigate the unconscious, such as hypnoanalysis, narcosynthesis and psychodrama.

desensitization   A behavioral therapy procedure sometimes used in treating anxiety disorders; it is also known as systematic desensitization. In this procedure, individuals learn relaxation techniques, to imagine their responses in difficult situations, ultimately face their feared or highly emotionally charged situations and practice new, more acceptable responses. An example is learning to travel by airplane and not experience a panic attack.

See also BEHAVIORAL THERAPY.

"designer drugs"   A term applied to synthetically manufactured drugs that mimic the appearance and/or effects of other drugs. Many have been falsely depicted as synthetic heroin. One such drug is China White, also known as fentanyl. Hundreds of times more powerful than heroin, fentanyl has been responsible for deaths and overdoses. Ecstasy (XTC, or more properly named 3,4-methylene-dioxyamphetamine) is also considered a designer drug. Several "designer drug" users have developed symptoms similar to those produced by Parkinson's disease, characterized by uncontrollable tremors, drooling, impaired speech and muscular paralysis. Designer drugs are sometimes chemically synthesized to utilize novel chemical structures to produce enhanced effects and to avoid the structure of outlawed drugs of abuse.

Designer drugs are usually taken orally. Although tolerance levels are unknown, this class of drugs has a stormy history of compulsive use. The long-term effects are also unknown. They may be particularly dangerous when used in combination with alcohol and other drugs.

Designer drugs affect developing fetuses in ways similar to those of the drugs they mimic. For exam-

ple, fentanyl acts like heroin, Ecstasy like amphetamines.

See also AMPHETAMINE DRUGS; HALLUCINOGENS; HEROIN; METHAMPHETAMINES; SUBSTANCE ABUSE.

Media Resource Guide on Common Drugs of Abuse. Public Relations Society of America, National Capital Chapter, Fairfax, Va., September 1990.

desipramine   A tricyclic antidepressant (trade names: Norpramin and Pertofrane) that is as effective as imipramine in the treatment of depression. Side effects are similar to those produced by imipramine, but anticholinergic and sedative actions are less pronounced. Thus desipramine may be especially useful in patients who are particularly sensitive to these effects, such as the elderly. These drugs are also sometimes used to treat headaches due to nonorganic causes and to treat attention-deficit hyperactivity disorder in some selected cases.

See also ANTIDEPRESSANT MEDICATIONS; HEADACHES; TRICYCLIC ANTIDEPRESSANT MEDICATIONS.

Desyrel   Trade name for trazodone hydrochloride, an antidepressant drug that is not related to the tricyclic antidepressant drugs or the monoamine oxidase inhibitors (MAOIs). Controlled studies have demonstrated that trazodone is as effective as amitriptyline and imipramine in patients with major depressive disorders and other types of depressive disorders. Because of its sedative effect, trazodone is generally more useful in depressive disorders associated with anxiety. It does not aggravate psychotic symptoms in patients with schizophrenia or schizoaffective disorders.

In therapeutic doses, trazodone inhibits the neuronal uptake of serotonin. Experimentally, prolonged administration decreases the number of serotonin receptors.

See also ANTIDEPRESSANT MEDICATIONS; DEPRESSION; SEROTONIN.

detoxification   The removal of poisons from the body, either by the body itself or with medical treatment. In current usage, the term usually applies to the process by which a person overcomes alcoholism or other addictive drugs. During the

1970s, hemodialysis was used in the United States to remove a polypeptide believed to cause schizophrenia. Initial research findings were not replicated, and dialysis units in the United States are no longer used to treat mental illness. However, dialysis is used in the detoxification of patients after potentially lethal overdose ingestions.

See also ALCOHOLISM.

dexamethasone suppression test (DST) See BIOLOGICAL MARKERS.

dextroamphetamine A drug that is a stimulant for the central nervous system. It is prescribed for narcolepsy (a rare condition characterized by excessive sleepiness) and also in some cases to treat children with hyperactivity. It is no longer recommended as an appetite suppressant for people who want to lose weight.

Dextroamphetamine is one of a group of drugs commonly known on the street as "uppers." However, some individuals may actually feel sedated when taking a test dose of dextroamphetamine. When the drug is used on a prolonged basis, its stimulant effects lessen and a higher dose must be taken to produce the desired effect. Seizures and high blood pressure may result from overdoses.

See also SUBSTANCE ABUSE.

Diagnostic and Statistical Manual of Mental Disorders, Fourth Edition A categorical guide for classification of mental disorders published by the American Psychiatric Association in 1994. Mental disorders are grouped into 16 major diagnostic classes, such as, anxiety disorders and mood disorders. The book is used for clinical, research and educational purposes. It is used by psychiatrists, other physicians, psychologists, social workers, nurses, occupational and rehabilitation therapists, counselors and other health and mental health professionals who wish to base a diagnosis of mental disorders, including anxieties and phobias, on standardized criteria. It was planned to be usable across settings, including inpatient, outpatient, partial hospital, consultation-liaison, clinic, private practice, primary care and with community populations.

Efforts were made in the preparation of *DSM-IV* to incorporate material that may be useful in culturally diverse populations in the United States and internationally. Thus *DSM-IV* includes three types of data specifically related to cultural considerations. First, there is a discussion of cultural variations in the clinical presentations of certain disorders not included in the *DSM-IV* classification. Next, there is a description of culture-bound syndromes that have not been included in the *DSM-IV* classification. Finally, there is an outline to assist the clinician in systematically evaluating and reporting influences of culture on a patient.

The first edition of the book appeared in 1952. The early categories were voted on by members of the American Psychiatric Association. The recent edition was revised over a period of nearly seven years and prepared by teams of physicians and researchers, including those from The National Institute of Mental Health (NIMH), National Institute on Drug Abuse (NIDA) and the National Institute on Alcohol Abuse and Alcoholism (NIAAA). Categories were formed by empirical studies. Field trials helped bridge the boundary between clinical research and clinical practice by determining how well suggestions for change that are derived from clinical research findings apply in clinical practice.

The editors of *DSM-IV* acknowledge that the title *Diagnostic and Statistical Manual of Mental Disorders*, unfortunately, implies a distinction between "mental" disorders and "physical" disorders. Literature documents that there is much physical in mental disorders and much mental in physical disorders.

American Psychiatric Association. *Diagnostic and Statistical Manual of Mental Disorders*, 4th ed., rev. Washington, D.C., 1994.

Diana complex A psychiatric term for a woman's repressed desire to be a man. The name comes from the Roman deity Diana, who filled a masculine role as goddess of hunting and protectress of women.

See also COMPLEX.

diazepam An antianxiety drug (trade name: Valium), effective in the management of generalized anxiety disorder and panic disorder in appropriately selected patients. It is also used for skeletal muscle relaxation, for seizure disorders, for pre-anesthetic medication or intravenous anesthetic induction and for alleviating abstinence symptoms during alcohol withdrawal. Diazepam is one of a group of benzodiazepine drugs.

Psychological and/or physical dependence can result from overuse or inappropriate use.

See also ANTIANXIETY MEDICATIONS; ANTIDEPRESSANT MEDICATIONS; BENZODIAZEPINE MEDICATIONS.

dieting   Following a special or modified diet for the purpose of losing weight. Motivation to be as thin as fashion models unrealistically causes many people, particularly women, to begin dieting. Dieting produces anxieties because losing weight is not easy. It means setting realistic goals. It requires time—often a year for positive results—for some people; it means hard work, both in losing the weight and keeping it off. It is also stressful because many people perceive themselves as overweight, whether this is the case or not.

Some dieting approaches involve extensive behavior modification. These programs offer support groups and education about good nutrition and exercise. Most importantly, they offer help in altering the individual's behavior in order to limit food intake, increase physical activity and reduce the stress of the current social pressures to be thin.

There are dangers involved in dieting. Donna Ciliska, in *Canadian Family Physician* (January 1993), said: "The drive for thinness in women as they strive to be what our culture demands has contributed to poor nutrition, an increase in eating disorders, a decrease in self-esteem, discrimination against overweight people, and a diminished bank account. Paradoxically, being overweight is more common in men and poses more of a health risk; the social pressure for them to be thin is less severe than for women. Fewer men seek weight loss programs."

Individuals who believe that they are overweight should have a physical examination from their family physician to determine whether they are actually overweight or are weight-, shape- or food-obsessed. If overweight, further assessment is necessary; if not overweight, they need supportive strategies to help them feel better about themselves

and referral to community resources to help them with their concern.

For information:

American Dietetic Association
216 W. Jackson Boulevard, Suite 800
Chicago, IL 60606
Phone: (312) 899-0040

Food and Nutrition Information Center
National Agricultural Library Building,
    Room 304
Beltsville, MD 20705
Phone: (301) 504-5414

See also BODY IMAGE; EATING DISORDERS; OBESITY; SELF-ESTEEM; SUPPORT GROUPS.

Ciliska, Donna. "Women and Obesity." *Canadian Family Physician* (Jan. 1993).
Hamilton, Michael et al. *The Duke University Medical Center Book of Diet and Fitness*. New York: Fawcett Columbine, 1991.
Kahn, Ada P. *Stress A to Z: A Sourcebook for Facing Everyday Challenges*. New York: Facts On File, 2000.
Thomas, Patricia, ed. "Dieting May Be a Losing Proposition." *Harvard Health Letter* 19, no. 10 (Aug. 1994).

disabilities   A temporary or permanent loss of a faculty. It may refer to physical disabilities, such as the loss of a leg or of hearing, or mental capabilities, such as retardation or autism. Coping with a disability causes anxiety for the one who has the disability and also for parents, siblings, children and other loved ones who face caring for the disabled person.

Persons who become disabled often struggle with the anxiety of trying to be like everyone else. Because of their disability they may feel a loss of self-esteem, compounded, in many cases, by limitations in their living situations. According to Reverend John A. Carr of the Yale-New Haven Medical Center, who was born with the congenital absence of both hands and one foot, "Coping with a handicap will depend on how human interactions occur, to allow more or less progress toward meaningful life." In his book, *Coping with Crisis and Handicap*, Reverend Carr recommends open dialogue between those who are disabled and those who are not; it is essential because "in denying our efforts to fight for a world more open to the handicapped, whether we refer to architectural or attitudinal barriers, we may be denying ourselves accessible avenues we will need later."

Coping with a Disability in the Family

Mary S. Challela, Director of Nursing and Training at the Eunice Kennedy Shriver Center for the Mentally Retarded at the University of Massachusetts Medical School, Waltham, Massachusetts, defines "parental coping" as "managing the day-to-day activities of meeting the disabled child's needs, the parents' needs, and those of other children in the family, in a realistic manner. Before parents can be expected to assume any of these tasks effectively, they must be allowed and encouraged to respond emotionally to the crisis of disability." How parents react, she explains, is influenced by how and when they are told of the abnormality, their degree of social isolation, the type and severity of the disability, social class and education, attitudes of families and friends and information received from and attitudes of professionals. Parents need emotional support and counseling in dealing with the initial and subsequent crises, education in learning how to care for the child's special needs, guidance in dealing with other family members and continued interest and encouragement.

According to Allen C. Crocker, Children's Hospital Medical Center, Boston, there are many emotions generated in the sister or brother of a disabled child, including "concern, curiosity, protectiveness, frustration, sorrow, grief, anxiety, longing, unhappiness, jealousy and resentment. The elements of stress assuredly exist and are troubling to consider."

Many professionals urge special support for siblings, and they value the role of self-help groups for parents, siblings and other family members. Such groups can help resolve problems and feelings, serve as a socializing agency for all concerned and provide a way to reach out to others in similar situations. Also, these support groups provide an important exchange of resources and often become an important force for obtaining services through legislation and social pressure.

In some cases, it may be an elderly parent who becomes disabled. Coping mechanisms for relieving the stresses of the situation include obtaining professional guidance and social support.

For information:

Architectural and Transportation Barriers
 Compliance Board
1331 F Street NW, Suite 1000
Washington, D.C. 20530
Phone: (202) 272-5434, (800) 8972-2253 or (800) USA-ABLE

Mobility International, U.S.A.
P.O. Box 3551
Eugene, OR 97403
Phone: (503) 343-1284

National Information Center for Children and
 Youth with Disabilities
P.O. Box 1492
Washington, D.C. 20013
Phone: (202) 884-8200

See also COPING; GENERAL ADAPTATION SYNDROME; SELF-ESTEEM; SUPPORT GROUPS.

Milunsky, Aubrey, ed. *Coping with Crisis and Handicap.* New York: Plenum Press, 1981.

disorientation Confusion about time, place and personal identity. Disorientation on a very temporary and sometimes fleeting basis occurs in many mental health disorders, including psychoses, schizophrenia, dissociative disorders, panic attacks and agoraphobia. Disorientation can also result from head injuries or intoxication. A disoriented person's speech may be unclear and behavior confused, and the person may be unable to answer clear questions about name, address and present whereabouts. Disorientation is most common in organic mental disorders causing dementia or stroke or after epileptic seizures.

See also AGORAPHOBIA; PANIC ATTACK.

disruptive behavior disorders See ANTISOCIAL PERSONALITY DISORDER; CONDUCT DISORDER.

dissociative disorders Disruptions of the usually integrated functions of consciousness, memory, identity or perception of the environment. According to the *Diagnostic and Statistical Manual of*

Mental Disorders, 4th ed. the disturbances may be sudden or gradual, transient or chronic. There are several major disorders included in this classification:

Dissociative amnesia: Characterized by an inability to recall important personal information, usually of a traumatic or stressful nature, that is too extensive to be explained by ordinary forgetfulness.
Dissociative Fugue (formerly psychogenic fugue): Characterized by sudden, unexpected travel away from home or one's customary place of work, accompanied by an inability to recall one's past and confusion about personal identity or the assumption of a new identity.
Dissociative Identity Disorder (formerly multiple personality disorder): Characterized by the presence of two or more distinct identities or personality states that recurrently take control of the individual's behavior, accompanied by an inability to recall important personal information that is too extensive to be explained by ordinary forgetfulness.
Depersonalization disorder: Characterized by a persistent or recurrent feeling of being detached from one's mental processes or body that is accompanied by intact reality testing.
Dissociative Disorder Not Otherwise Specified: For insurance coding purposes, this category includes disorders in which the predominant feature is a dissociative symptom but that do not meet the criteria for any specific dissociative disorder.

In evaluating dissociative disorders, a cross-cultural perspective is important because some dissociative states are a common and accepted expression of cultural activities or religious experience in many societies. Also, it is essential to rule out any physiological causes that may contribute to depersonalization and dissociation.

See also CROSS-CULTURAL INFLUENCES; DEPERSONALIZATION.

American Psychological Association. *Diagnostic and Statistical Manual of Mental Disorders,* 4th ed., rev. Washington, D.C., 1994.

dis-stress   Hans Selye (1907–1982), an Austrian-born Canadian endocrinologist, differentiated between the unpleasant or harmful variety of stress called *dis-tress* (from the Latin *dis* = bad, as in dissonance, disagreement) and *eustress* (from the Greek *eu* = good, as in euphonia, euphoria). During both distress and eustress, the body undergoes virtually the same nonspecific responses to various stimuli acting upon it. However, certain emotional factors, such as frustration and hostility, are particularly likely to turn stress into distress.

See also COPING; EUSTRESS; FRUSTRATION; GENERAL ADAPTATION SYNDROME; HOSTILITY; SELYE, HANS; STRESS.

Selye, Hans. *Stress Without Distress.* New York: J. B. Lipincott, 1974.
———. *The Stress of Life,* rev. ed., New York: McGraw-Hill, 1978.

disulfiram   A drug used in overcoming alcoholism (trade name: Antabuse). When taken with alcohol, this drug interacts with body chemistry to produce uncomfortable and sometimes dangerous or fatal reactions. The unpleasantness of this interaction is the basis for its adjunctive use to help a motivated individual to stop the consumption of alcohol. The drug should be used with supportive counseling or psychotherapy.

See also ALCOHOLISM; ALCOHOLISM in BIBLIOGRAPHY.

diversity   A word that relates to any group of people that is mixed in terms of race, religion, ethnicity and gender. Because diversity may be perceived as an approach to quotas in schools or in the workplace, the concept can be a source of anxiety for those involved. Stress also arises between individuals from diverse backgrounds because of cultural differences. Respect for, and understanding of, these differences can make diversity a successful concept in business, religious and community activities.

It is effective for businesses to have diversity in their workforces because no business can afford to ignore any population segment. Companies dependent on direct sales to customers must pay attention to the differing cultures in their marketplace.

Additionally, the business management process can benefit from the imagination and creativity generated from diverse viewpoints.

Conducting diversity awareness workshops is one way companies have introduced the idea of valuing personal differences. However, these workshops are only the first step in creating an environment in which previous prejudices are erased and a true sensitivity to diverse employee needs prevails.

See also ACCULTURATION; COMMUNICATION.

divorce The legal ending of a marriage. During the 1980s, about half of all marriages ended in divorce. Women and men who seek divorce do so because they have any one of a wide range of problems in their marriage, which may include a poor sexual relationship, differences in goals or financial problems. Divorce differs from annulment, in which a court declares that a marriage has been invalid from its beginning; reasons for annulment vary among states and countries.

Many divorced individuals marry again. According to researcher Judith Wallerstein, Center for the Family in Transition, Corte Madera, California, 60 percent of second marriages fail, particularly if one or more of the mates bring children into the marriage.

Meeting new people and dating after divorce brings anxieties and concerns about acquiring a sexually transmitted disease, such as AIDS (acquired immunodeficiency syndrome).

Many divorced people remember being treated poorly, perhaps exploited, suspecting infidelities and feeling angry. Depending on what triggered the anger, it may not be easy to forget. However, if appropriately contained, one's anger will not interfere with adjusting to a new life.

Feelings of failure are common when a marriage breaks up. Usually what individuals do is what they thought best under the circumstances; lack of success in the marriage should not reflect on their sense of self-worth in other areas. Most divorced individuals learn from their experiences and bring new insights to new relationships.

According to Ada P. Kahn, in "Divorce: For Better Not For Worse," a brochure published by the Mental Health Association of Greater Chicago, recent studies show that when parents are wretched, children do not feel that keeping the marriage together on their behalf is a gift. There is no advantage for children when parents stay in a marriage in which they cannot resolve basic issues.

Kahn advised that parents should explain divorce to their children, that it was a rational decision, deliberately and carefully undertaken with full recognition of how difficult it would be. Children have the right to know why, with the explanation given in language suited to their age and understanding. Parents should try to communicate what divorce will mean for them, very specifically how it will affect their visiting and living arrangements. Children should be assured that they will not be forced to take sides, they have permission to love both parents and both will continue to love them. More complex explanations are in order in the case of desertion or abuse. In every instance children must be assured that they are not responsible for the rupture and that they are not responsible for healing it.

As a consequence of divorce, many children feel a diminished sense of being parented, because their parents are less available, emotionally, physically or both. The child feels that he or she is losing both parents. This is a common but usually temporary part of the divorce experience.

The most serious long-range effect is that children feel less protected in their growing-up years and, having seen a failed man-woman relationship, become concerned that they will repeat their parents' mistakes. Parents should address this issue by talking about it or being ready to talk when children ask questions. Parents should not continue to fight the battles that persisted during the marriage. Parents should not criticize their former mate in front of the children. Doing so will encourage the child to grow into adulthood with fears about man-woman relationships. Divorced parents must realize that they are role models in the divorce just as they were in the marriage.

Rebuilding life after divorce may be complicated and difficult. Most experts offer the following advice; take one step at a time; start by choosing one step you really need or would like to take; seek out resources for your particular needs in the community; churches, synagogues and community mental health agencies may be able to help.

See also MARRIAGE; SEXUALLY TRANSMITTED DISEASES.

Kahn, Ada P., and Linda Hughey Holt. *The A to Z of Women's Sexuality.* Alameda, Calif.: Hunter House Publications, 1992.

Wallerstein, Judith S. *Second Chances: Men, Women, and Children a Decade after Divorce.* New York: Ticknor & Fields, 1989.

dizziness A feeling of being unsteady, lightheaded or faint. Most people describe dizziness as a feeling of spinning, turning or falling in space or of standing still while the objects around them are moving. (Medically, this is termed vertigo.) Dizziness is often a symptom of a phobic reaction. People who come into contact with their feared object may react with weak knees, sweaty palms and dizziness, which may intensify their physical sensations, making them fear that they will faint, have a heart attack on the spot or die.

During a phobic reaction or a panic attack, an individual may hyperventilate (breathe more than they need to). This results in a drop in the carbon dioxide in the blood, which causes constriction of blood vessels in the brain. Dizziness as a result of an emotional feeling usually disappears when the phobic object is removed or when the person gets to a place of safety.

For many people, dizziness also accompanies seasickness. Some sailors advise keeping one's eyes on the horizon to give one a steady spot to watch. In most cases, dizziness disappears when the individual sets foot on land. Dizziness as a result of intoxication with alcohol usually subsides after a period of sleep.

See also AGORAPHOBIA; PANIC ATTACK.

DNA See DEOXYRIBONUCLEIC ACID.

domestic violence Abuse of spouses, children or parents in the home. This may take the form of spouse-battering, child abuse, incest or abusing elders. All of these situations are extremely stressful to the victims, as well as to others in the family.

The abuser may behave violently as a response to particular stressors in his or her life. Various mental health issues may be involved.

Domestic violence happens in all strata of society, and there are many more cases than official records indicate because it is often covered up out of fear and shame. Characteristics of victims of family violence include anxiety, powerlessness, guilt and lack of self-esteem.

Professionals who treat victims of family violence are concerned with getting the victims, usually women or children, away from the abuser and into therapy before the abuse becomes too severe and additional stressors arise. Some perpetrators, as well as victims, of family violence compound their difficulties with the use of alcohol or drugs.

Battered Women

Battered women are victims of physical assault by husbands, boyfriends or lovers. Battering may include physical abuse sometimes for the purposes of sexual gratification, such as breaking bones, burning, whipping, mutilation and other sadistic acts. Generally, however, battering is considered part of a syndrome of abusive behavior that has very little to do with sexual issues. Drug and alcohol-related problems are more common among families with battering behaviors. Women who select and choose to remain in abusive relationships were also often abused as children. Many women stay in such relationships without reporting the abuse and without seeking counseling. Batterers often were abused themselves as children.

Women who are abused by their husbands or boyfriends not only sustain injuries from physical beatings but also suffer many mental and emotional scars, including post-traumatic stress disorder (PTSD), depression and anxiety.

Help for battered wives is available. First, physical protection, often provided by women's shelters within the community, must be assured for the woman and her children. Second, social support services must provide economic protection, since women often stay in abusive relationships due to a lack of practical economic alternatives. Finally, psychotherapeutic intervention should be aimed at both batterer and victim to trace antecedents of the violent behavior, correct substance abuse problems and substitute positive coping mechanisms for violent behavior patterns.

Most abused women do not seek help until beatings become severe and have occurred over a period of time, often two to three years. Some women are too embarrassed to ask for help or believe that if they report the beating to police they will not be taken seriously. The majority of women who seek help because of family violence are between age 20 and 60. In 75 percent of households in which abuse takes place, the husband or boyfriend is an alcoholic or on drugs.

A study at the University of California San Franciso during 1992 indicated many details about the living conditions and circumstances surrounding battered women. According to the study, the battered women who were interviewed did not depend on their violent partner for most of their financial support; almost 30 percent had jobs, and many had income from families, welfare, social security and other sources.

Among other findings, 40 percent of the women had to be hospitalized for injuries. One in three of the women had been attacked with a weapon, most often a knife or a club; four had been shot. One in 10 was pregnant when beaten; 30 percent of the group said they had been abused before they were pregnant. In about half the cases, the husbands or boyfriends drank heavily or abused drugs: Eighty-six percent of the women had been beaten at least once before in a previous relationship.

According to Kevin J. Fullin, M.D., St. Catherine's Hospital, Kenosha, Wisconsin, as many as one in two women has suffered from an episode of domestic violence sometime in her life. Due to such a high rate, physicians and healthcare workers are developing new approaches to domestic violence in order to increase its detection. They are attempting to properly identify anyone who comes to a hospital with a domestic abuse situation. The child or adult suspected of being abused is questioned in a non-threatening, non-judgmental manner without any other family members present. The goals of this confidential questioning are to find the real cause of the problem and to do something to stop the abuse.

WHAT BATTERED WOMEN CAN DO

- Leave the scene of the abuse; stay with a friend or family member who will be supportive emotionally and provide a safe haven.
- Leave the home when the abuser is absent to eliminate confrontation.
- Take bank records, children's birth certificates, cash and other important documents along with clothing and personal items.
- If possible, photograph or videotape any consequences of abuse, such as injuries to yourself or damage to the home. These could be important for possible later court proceedings.
- Call the police and file a police report. Obtain an order of protection as soon as possible.
- Seek counseling for yourself and your children; join a support group along with others who have been victims of family violence.

Battered Child Syndrome

Battered child syndrome includes rough physical handling by caregivers, which results in injuries to the baby or child. This can cause a failure to grow, a disability and sometimes death. Studies have shown that parents who repeatedly injure or beat their babies and children have poor control of their own feelings of aggression, or may have been abused or psychologically rejected as children.

The syndrome is found among people with stable social and financial backgrounds, as well as in parents who are mentally unstable, alcoholic or drug-dependent. In most states, laws require physicians to report instances of suspected willfully inflicted injury among young patients. When it appears that the children will continue to be battered, steps are taken to remove the children from the home.

Legal Rights of Domestic Violence Victims

Until the latter years of the 20th century, police and the legal system often viewed domestic violence as a private matter—not a crime. Now, in many states, the police may arrest a batterer if there is evidence of abuse. Civil actions might include legal separation, child custody, child support and divorce. One common civil action in cases of domestic violence is a temporary restraining order, which involves making a complaint and going to a hearing to obtain a legal document that limits how close a person may come to a woman and her children.

A criminal complaint can be filed in addition to or instead of civil actions. A criminal complaint involves a police investigation, and if enough evidence is found, may lead to an arrest and involvement of the judicial system.

For information:

National Coalition Against Domestic Violence
P.O. Box 34103
Washington, D.C. 20043-4103
Phone: (212) 638-6388

National Council on Child Abuse and
 Family Violence
1155 Connecticut Avenue NW
Washington, D.C. 20036
Phone: (202) 429-6695
E-mail: nccafv@aol.com

See also ADDICTION; AGGRESSION; ALCOHOLISM; ANXIETY; CODEPENDENCY; CONTROL; COPING; DEPRESSION; GUILT; INCEST; POST-TRAUMATIC STRESS DISORDER; SELF-ESTEEM; SUPPORT GROUPS.

Doctor, Ronald M., and Ada P. Kahn. *Encyclopedia of Phobias, Fears, and Anxieties. New York: Facts On File, 2000.*
Shannon, Kari. "Domestic Violence Detection at St. Catherine's." *Chicago HealthCare (Dec. 1991).*

dopamine   A precursor of the neurotransmitter norepinephrine. A deficiency of dopamine in the brain is a diagnostic sign of Parkinson's disease. The dopamine hypothesis is a concept holding that schizophrenia is caused by an excess of dopamine in the brain, owing either to an overproduction of dopamine or a deficiency of the enzyme necessary to convert dopamine to norepinephrine. Neurons that release dopamine also control the so-called pleasure system in humans and animals. The addicting effects of cocaine and amphetamine stimulants have been attributed to their effect on hyperstimulation of the dopamine-pleasure system, thus producing feelings of artificially induced euphoria, excitement and pleasure beyond that of everyday life. It also causes changes in brain chemistry to promote a need for the substance in order to achieve a state of well-being, thus producing addiction. Recent research has suggested that other addictions such as alcoholism and narcotic addiction may also be based on the function of the dopamine-pleasure system. Dopamine also controls the release of certain hormones from the anterior pituitary gland (for example, prolactin).

Dopaminergic drugs are those that affect the production or utilization of dopamine. Drugs that enhance the maintenance of adequate levels of dopamine have therapeutic value in the treatment of Parkinson's disease. A commonly used dopaminergic drug is levodopa (L-dopa).

See also BRAIN; NEUROTRANSMITTERS; NOREPINEPHRINE; PARKINSON'S DISEASE; SCHIZOPHRENIA.

Doral   Trade name for the benzodiazepine medication quazepam.

See also BENZODIAZEPINE DRUGS; PHARMACOLOGICAL APPROACH.

Dossey, Larry (1940–)   A Dallas, Texas physician, lecturer and author of *Healing Words: The Power of Prayer and the Practice of Medicine* and *Meaning and Medicine: Lessons from a Doctor's Tales of Breakthrough and Healing.* Much of his writing is directed toward helping readers relieve stress in their lives.

He believes that American society is in the grips of a "time sickness" epidemic. He defines this as a disorder in which we feel so overloaded and stressed by schedules that our bodies rebel and we respond to all ringing bells—alarm clocks, telephones—as signals to get ready for action. Our bodies pump stress hormones, which in turn suppress immune response. Cholesterol and stomach acidity is increased. "The end result" he says, "is frequently some form of 'hurry' sickness, expressed as heart disease, high blood pressure, insomnia, irritable bowel syndrome."

About Dossey's best-selling books, a reviewer in *Whole Earth Review* (fall 1993), said: "Modern medicine is based on standardization, the assumption that the criteria for symptoms, prognoses and curative practices can be measured and objectified. Individuals with a set of symptoms are expected to be helped by the same course of treatment, and the percentage who will recover can be predicted. Dossey brings us quite a different perspective, one which taken to its extreme would create a totally different and ultimately individualized medicine."

Dossey emphasizes that meaning, or the significance one attaches to an interpretation of an event, has been overlooked in modern medical practice. Significant life events which are highly stressful, such as death of a spouse or loss of a job, can have a very different subjective meaning. Each unique interpretation of a similar event will bring about stress in different ways. Dossey also writes about the placebo effect, miracles and the power of prayer.

Dossey divides the history of medical practice into several eras: Era I was and remains based on the materialist theory of disease and its treatment. Era II discovered the mind/body link; it conceives of the mind as implicated in healing, although it understands the mind as local, existing within the body and limited by the body's position in time and space. Era III medicine, he continues, expands this understanding by focusing on how the powers of the mind work between people.

See also COMPLEMENTARY THERAPIES; FAITH HEALING; PLACEBO EFFECT; PRAYER.

Kahn, Ada P. *Stress A to Z: The Sourcebook for Facing Everyday Challenges.* New York: Facts On File, 2000.
Dossey, Larry. *Healing Words: The Power of Prayer and the Practice of Medicine.* San Francisco: Harper, 1993.
———. *Meaning and Medicine: Lessons from a Doctor's Tales of Breakthrough and Healing.* New York: Bantam, Doubleday, 1991.

downers A popular street term for a class of drugs that subjectively cause sedation or relaxation, including barbiturates and synthetic derivatives, other non-barbiturate sleeping pills, benzodiazepine drugs and even dextromethorphan, a synthetic narcotic in cough syrup and antihistamine drugs that cause sedation as a side effect. They are prescription drugs (and sometimes over-the-counter medications used legitimately as tranquilizers and sleeping pills. The most common depressant, usually classified by itself, is alcohol. Barbiturates have very similar effects, while tranquilizers are less sedating. These are highly addictive, both psychologically and physically, and are associated with intense withdrawal problems. The state of intoxication associated with true depressants is similar to that of alcohol: a weak and rapid pulse, slow or rapid shallow breathing, cold and clammy skin, drowsiness and impaired motor function.

These drugs are usually in tablet or capsule forms, which are swallowed. Some abused barbiturates include Amytal, Fiorinal, Seconal and Phenobarbital. Other well-known depressants that are abused include tranquilizers such as Equanil and Miltown and sleeping pills such as Doriden and Placidyl. The use of sedative hypnotics with alcohol is particularly dangerous and can lead to death.

The terms "downer" and "upper" are frequently used incorrectly. Alcohol, sometimes considered an "upper" or euphoriant for the first hour or two after ingestion (depending on amount ingested), later becomes a "downer" as it produces intoxication and central nervous system depression. Even small doses of barbiturates will make some individuals "high" or "up" depending on environmental stimulation. The terms "downer" and "upper" therefore have misleading meanings that ignore dosage and time-related drug effects.

See also BARBITURATE DRUGS; BENZODIAZEPINE MEDICATIONS; SUBSTANCE ABUSE.

Down's syndrome A chromosomal abnormality that results in mental handicap and a characteristic physical appearance. People with Down's syndrome have 47 instead of the normal 46 chromosomes. In most cases the extra chromosone is number 21; the disorder is also called trisomy 21.

About one in 650 babies born is affected with Down's syndrome. The incidence of affected fetuses rises with increased maternal age to about one in 40 among mothers over age 40. Pregnant women over age 35 and those with a family history of Down's syndrome are usually offered chromosome analysis of the fetus's cells after they have been obtained by amniocentesis or chorionic villus sampling. If the fetus is found to be affected, termination of the pregnancy may be one of the options.

While there is no cure for Down's syndrome, such children can make the most of their capabilities through appropriate educational opportunities. In some cases, institutional care is necessary. For some children, improvement of facial appearance can be made with plastic surgery.

Until the second half of the 20th century, many Down's syndrome children did not live beyond their teen years because of birth defects and their susceptibility to infection. Now advances in medical and surgery techniques and improved long-term care facilities have extended their life expectancy; however, most do not live beyond early middle age.

Caring for a child with Down's syndrome presents particular parenting problems and an exceptional degree of patience. The degree of mental handicap varies; the child's IQ may be anywhere from 30 to 80. Almost all affected children are capable of a limited amount of learning and, in some cases, reading. Usually affected children are cheerful and affectionate and get along well with people.

See also MENTAL RETARDATION.

doxepin hydrochloride A tricyclic antidepressant medication also used as an antianxiety medication; sold under the trade names of Adapin and Sinequan. When prescribed for adult patients of all ages, it is safe and well tolerated, even in elderly patients. For many individuals, doxepin helps relieve symptoms of depression, insomnia, anxiety, fear and worry.

See also ANTIANXIETY MEDICATIONS; ANTIDEPRESSANT MEDICATIONS; TRICYCLIC ANTIDEPRESSANT MEDICATIONS.

dream analysis Interpretation of a person's dreams as part of psychotherapy or psychoanalysis. However, many people try to self-analyze their dreams or talk to their families about their dreams. Dream analysis is based on the concept developed by Sigmund Freud that an individual's repressed feelings and thoughts are revealed in a disguised way in dreams. The therapist analyzes the dreams, based on an understanding of the individual's personality, character traits, family ties and background. Patient and therapist make associations and try to determine the meaning of the dream.

See also DREAMING; SLEEP.

dreaming Mental activity that occurs when one is asleep. Dreaming usually involves many vivid sensory images, such as sights, sounds, motion, touch and even smell or taste. For many people, dreaming is a continuation of activities and thoughts from the previous day, and there are no deeply hidden meanings. They may be sorting out events from the day in a distorted way because of the lack of the conscious, awake mind. For others, images in dreams may be symbols of unconscious thoughts. Symbols in dreams may mean nothing or may refer to death, family members and sexual functions.

Dreaming occurs during periods of rapid eye movement (REM) sleep, which last about 20 minutes and occur four or five times a night. Disruptions of schedule or sleep deprivation, depression, stress and drug use often interfere with REM time. Necessary biochemical changes occur at REM and non-REM times that are essential for normal daytime functioning. People who are awakened during periods of REM sleep usually can report their dreams clearly. Those who awaken normally may not remember dreams at all or only in a fragmentary way. Fear of dreams is known as oneirophobia.

More recently, dreaming has been thought to be a form of unconscious problem solving during sleep. Attempts have been made to help people use dreams positively to solve problems that emerge in dreaming.

According to Larry Dossey, M.D., executive editor, *Alternative Therapies*, there is a trend in medicine toward honoring dreaming experience of patients and looking at the role of dreaming for the patient. Dossey differentiates between healing, wisdom, danger, death, disasters, good fortune and prodromal dreams.

For information:

Association for the Study of Dreams
P.O. Box 1600
Vienna, VA 22183
Phone: (703) 242-8888

Community Dream Sharing Network
P.O. Box 8032
Hicksville, NY 11802
Phone: (516) 735-1969 or (516) 796-9455

See also DREAM ANALYSIS; SLEEP.

Dossey, Larry. "Dreams and Healing: Reclaiming a Lost Tradition." *Alternative Therapies* 5, no. 6 (Nov. 1999): 12–117.

drug abuse See ADDICTIONS; ALCOHOLISM; SUBSTANCE ABUSE.

drug addiction See ADDICTIONS; SUBSTANCE ABUSE.

dual sex therapy The team approach to sex therapy developed by William H. Masters (1915–), an American physician, and Virginia Johnson (1925–), an American psychologist. Dual sex therapy is based on the theory that two therapists are needed—one male and one female—because male therapists acting alone cannot be expected to fully understand the feelings and reactions of a woman, and a female therapist acting alone cannot be expected to fully understand male sexuality. However, when they collaborate in the process, therapy will be more effective.

See also SEX THERAPY.

durable power of attorney See DEATH; END OF LIFE ISSUES.

dying with dignity See DEATH.

dysfunctional family A term indicating that the developmental needs of one or more members of a family are not being met. Often, the basic problem is poor communication between family members, even though they live in the same household. An example of a dysfunctional family is one in which there is marital conflict and a young child who is showing signs of aggressive behavior in school. The parents may be unaware that their behavior is causing a great deal of stress for the child, which he expresses in aggressive behavior instead of talking about it with his parents.

In a dysfunctional family, there is little emphasis on encouraging each child to develop autonomy. An example is a family that expects its adolescent child to obey curfew rules appropriate for a younger child.

Dysfunctional families do not deal constructively with difficult times. For example, when a child becomes seriously ill, there may be little communication about the illness between family members, or there may be unexpressed feelings of guilt. Alcoholism and substance abuse tends to lead to dysfunctional families, as the substance abuser cannot be depended on or to fulfill expectations. Families in which there is domestic violence, child abuse or spouse abuse are dysfunctional.

Family therapy is helpful in improving life situations for members of dysfunctional families. In therapy, family members learn to improve their communication skills and learn new coping skills to deal with everyday problems as well as major life stressors.

See also COPING; STRESS.

dyskinesia Abnormal muscular movements usually caused by a brain disorder. These may include uncontrolled twitching, jerking or writhing movements that interfere with the individual's willful movements. Such movements may involve the whole body or only a group of muscles, such as those around the eye. Dyskinesias may be caused by brain damage at birth or may be side effects of certain drugs, such as some drugs used to treat psychiatric illnesses. When dyskinesias are caused by drugs, the problem often ceases when use of the drug is stopped. However, prolonged use of some antipsychotic drugs can result in a permanent or chronic condition known as tardive dyskinesia.

See also TARDIVE DYSKINESIA.

dyslexia A reading disability characterized by difficulty in recognizing written symbols. Those with the disorder tend to reverse letters and words. Writing from dictation is difficult for such children. Those with the disability feel frustrated and often develop reduced self-esteem because they feel different from their peers. Specific remedial teaching can help such children learn to overcome their deficit. It is important that parents avoid pressuring the child and offer praise for the child's accomplishments. Many individuals who were dyslexic as children are successful at completing educational programs and entering highly professional and public careers.

dysmenorrhea Painful menstruation. Many women experience pain and cramps in their back and lower abdomen during menstruation. Dysmenorrhea may occur for many reasons and can cause stress, frustration, absenteeism from work, withdrawal from social and family obligations and a sense of "missing out" on several days a month. An understanding of the physiology involved as well as medical intervention can help women cope with this aspect of life.

Primary dysmenorrhea is menstrual pain that occurs in the absence of any observable pelvic lesion. Mechanical dysmenorrhea is a form of the disorder resulting from an obstruction, such as narrowing of the cervix (stenosis), that prevents the normal flow of menstruation from the uterus. Primary dysmenorrhea is often associated with the beginning of menstrual flow and may occur in the presence of an underdeveloped uterus or the presence of clots in the cervix or both. Spasmodic dysmenorrhea pain usually increases over a period of several hours and then subsides. Some women experience a diminution of dysmenorrhea after their first pregnancy.

Functional or congestive dysmenorrhea, also known as psychogenic dysmenorrhea, may increase during periods of anxiety or stress. However, most dysmenorrhea is due to the production of chemicals, called prostaglandins, in the uterine lining that cause powerful contractions. These cramps are effectively treated with drugs (such as ibuprofen) that inhibit prostaglandin formation. When these agents do not work, other disorders such as endometriosis may be found.

See also MENSTRUATION.

dysmorphic disorder   A disorder in which a normal-appearing individual is preoccupied with some imagined defect in appearance. If there is a slight anomaly, the individual's concern is grossly excessive. This is associated with anorexia nervosa and other eating disorders in which the person perceives herself as obese.

This disorder has been related to a number of single-symptom disorders and severe obsessional disorders. The delusional disorders, which include morbid jealousy, have been reported to respond to treatment with selective serotonin-uptake inhibiting medications such as fluoxetine (Prozac) and Pimozide.

See also EATING DISORDERS.

dyspareunia   Sexual intercourse that is painful for the woman. Pain may occur for many reasons, including dryness of the vagina, tightness of the vaginal muscles, a vaginal infection, an infection of the urethra or urinary tract or a local irritation, such as from a spermicide or the material of a condom or diaphragm. The first step in reducing discomfort during sexual intercourse is a discussion with one's partner.

For some women, psychological factors play a part. If they have experienced pain in the past, they may fear its recurrence. This happens to some women who have been abused as children or raped. Some women may fear pregnancy or acquiring a sexually transmitted disease and are not able to relax during intercourse. Tension and anxiety or a lack of adequate stimulation before actual penetration may contribute to pain during intercourse. During foreplay (stimulation before intercourse), the vaginal walls secrete lubricating fluid that makes intercourse more comfortable. However, after menopause and during breast feeding, many women find that secretions are not sufficient; a water-soluble jelly may be helpful as a lubricant. Hormone replacement therapy postmenopausally also helps to increase lubrication and thicken the skin of the vaginal wall.

A change in position during intercourse can help relieve pain for some women. They may feel a discomfort when the penis contacts their cervix (the neck of the uterus) and can avoid discomfort by less deep penetration. A pain felt deep in the pelvis may be caused by endometriosis, ovarian tumors or cysts or some other condition that should be investigated and treated by a physician as soon as possible.

Medical treatments, psychological counseling and sex therapy are available to help these conditions.

See also COITUS.

Kahn, Ada P., and Linda Hughey Holt. *The A to Z of Women's Sexuality.* Alameda, Calif.: Hunter House, 1992.

dysphoric mood   A mood in which one feels sad, despondent and discouraged with anxiety and tension. A dysphoric mood may be a symptom of depression.

See also AFFECTIVE DISORDERS; DEPRESSION.

dyssomnia A category of sleep disorders. Dyssomnias include disorders of initiating or maintaining sleep, such as insomnia or hypersomnia. These differ from other sleep disorders, such as nightmares and sleep-walking.

See also SLEEP.

dysthymic disorder A chronically depressed mood that occurs for most of the day, more days than not, for at least two years. According to the *Diagnostic and Statistical Manual of Mental Disorders,* 4th ed., individuals with this disorder describe themselves as feeling sad or "down in the dumps." Children may show signs of irritability.

During period of depressed mood, individuals may experience poor appetite or overeating, insomnia or hypersomnia, low energy or fatigue, low self-esteem, poor concentration or difficulty making decisions and feelings of hopelessness.

See also AFFECTIVE DISORDERS; DEPRESSION.

American Psychiatric Association. *Diagnostic and Statistical Manual of Mental Disorders,* 4th ed., rev. Washington, D.C.: 1994.

dystonic reaction A state of abnormal muscle tension that sometimes occurs as a side effect of neuroleptic medications. There may be spasms of the eyes, eyelids, face, neck and back muscles. In rare instances, spasms of the larynx and pharynx can cause asphyxia. The side effect is alleviated by changing to a lower dose of medication or to another, less potent antipsychotic or by using anti-Parkinsonian medications prophylactically in conjunction with the antipsychotic.

eating disorders Compulsive misuse of food to achieve some desired physical and/or mental state. They can cause severe weight loss, ill health and psychological impairments. Eating disorders share common addictive features with alcohol and drug abuse, but unlike alcohol and drugs, food is essential to human life, and proper use of food is a central element of recovery.

People with eating disorders may be experiencing anxiety in some aspect of their lives which they think will be improved by dieting in excess. There is low self-esteem and a mortal fear of fatness. When sufferers acknowledge their compulsive behavior, their stress is often expressed in feelings of depression and a wish to commit suicide. Sufferers typically hide their illness; typically, people with eating disorders feel they don't deserve to be helped, although when family, friends, or coworkers discover their illness, they try to help, and this creates a great deal of stress for all concerned.

Estimates indicate that there are 8 million reported victims of eating disorders in the United States—7 million are women (although the number of males is increasing) between the ages of 15 and 30. Eating disorders can be cured when the sufferer accepts treatment; an estimated 6 percent, however, of all reported cases die.

Anorexia Nervosa

Anorexia nervosa is a syndrome of self-starvation in which people willfully restrict their intake of food out of fear of becoming fat; this withholding results in life-threatening weight loss. Anorexics (people who suffer from anorexia nervosa) "feel fat" even when they are at normal weight or dangerously thin. When emaciated, anorexics often deny their illness and develop an active disgust for food. Deaths from anorexia nervosa are higher than from any other psychiatric illness.

Causes of anorexia vary widely. Many anorexics are part of a close family and have special relationships with their parents. They are highly conforming, anxious to please and may be obsessional in their habits. There is speculation that girls who refrain from eating wish to remain "thin as a boy" in an effort to escape the burdens of growing up and assuming a female sexual and marital role. Another contribution to the increase in anorexia is contemporary society's emphasis on slimness as it relates to beauty. This is particularly prevalent in the fashion and advertising industries, with their images of overly thin models. Most women diet at some time, particularly athletes and dancers who seem more prone to the disorder than other women.

Symptoms include severe weight loss, wasting (cachexia), food preoccupation and rituals, amenorrhea (cessation of the menstrual period) and hyperactivity (constant exercising to lose weight). The anorexic may suffer from tiredness and fatigue, sensitivity to cold and loss of hair.

Eating disorders sometimes result in other mental health disorders, including depression personality disorder and schizophrenia. Individuals may suffer from withdrawal, mood swings and feelings of shame and guilt. Both anorexics and bulimics develop rituals regarding eating and exercise. They often are perfectionists in habits, such as clothes and personal appearance, and have an "all or nothing" attitude about life.

Bulimia

Bulimia is characterized by recurrent episodes of binge eating followed by self-induced vomiting, vigorous exercise and/or laxative and diuretic abuse to prevent weight gain. Most people view vomiting as a disagreeable experience, but to a bulimic, it is a means toward a desired goal.

Another eating disorder is bulimarexia, which is characterized by features of both anorexia nervosa and bulimia. Some individuals vacillate between anorexic and bulimic behaviors. After months and perhaps years of eating sparsely, the anorexic may crave food and begin to binge, but the fear of becoming overly fat leads her or him to vomit.

Bulimics may be of normal weight, slightly underweight or extremely thin. Bingeing and vomiting may occur as much as several times a day. In severe cases, it may lead to dehydration and loss of potassium, causing weakness and cramps.

A Cycle of Addiction

Behaviors of anorexics and bulimics are driven by the cycle of addiction. There is an emotional emptiness, which in turn leads to the psychological pain of low self-esteem. The individual looks for a way to dull the pain using addictive agents (starvation or bingeing), which usually results in the need to purge or in medical problems. Finally, suffering from guilt, shame and self-hate, the individual goes back to a routine of starvation and/or bingeing and purging.

Treatment

Medical problems caused by the disorder should be diagnosed and managed first. When the medical complications are severe, an individual may be hospitalized to stabilize physical functions and monitor nutritional intake. Often small feedings are carefully spaced because the patient cannot handle very much food at one time. In some cases, antidepressant medications are begun during the hospital stay.

In the late 1990s, treatment of eating disorders cost an excess of $30,000 a month. Many patients need repeated hospitalizations and can require treatment extending two years or more. Some therapists believe that anorexia/bulimia is never cured but merely arrested. However, some behaviorists believe that weight gain indicates a cure. There are several therapies used in treating with eating disorders; these different options should be discussed with the individual's therapist. A major part of therapy for eating disorders involves help-ing the individual rethink her or his perception of body image, because often it is the perceived flaws that led to the eating disorder in the first place.

Many people with eating disorders are treated on an outpatient basis. There may be weekly counseling that include individual and group sessions for outpatients and family, marital therapy and specialized support for eating disorders.

For information:

National Association of Anorexia Nervosa and
  Associated Disorders (ANAD)
Box 7
Highland Park, IL 60035
Phone: (847) 831-3438

Anorexia Nervosa and Related Eating Disorders
P.O. Box 5102
Eugene, OR 97405
Phone: (503) 344-1144

BASH (Bulimia Anorexia Self Help)
c/o Deaconess Hospital
6150 Oakland Avenue
St. Louis, MO 63139
Phone: (800) 762-3334

See also BODY IMAGE; DEPRESSION; SELF-ESTEEM.

Fowler, Sandra J., and Cynthia M. Bulik. "Family Environment and Psychiatric History in Women with Binge-Eating Disorder and Obese Controls." *Behaviour Change* 14, no. 2 (1997): 106–112.
Kasvikis, Y.G. et al, "Past History of Anorexia Nervosa in Women with Obsessive-Compulsive Disorder." *International Journal of Eating Disorders* 5, no. 6 (1985).

ECG   See ELECTROCARDIOGRAM.

echolalia   Compulsive repetition of what is said by another person. The accent, tone and words of the speaker are mimicked. This occurs in some people with autism and some forms of mental retardation; it is an unusual symptom of catatonic schizophrenia.

echopraxia   Compulsive imitation of the movements and gestures of another person. Echopraxia often accompanies echolalia.

See also ECHOLALIA.

ECT   See ELECTROCONVULSIVE THERAPY.

EEG   See ELECTROENCEPHALOGRAM.

Effexor   Trade name for venlafaxine, a newer antidepressant medication with dual reuptake blocking capacity for serotonin and norepinephrine.

ego   A region of the mind believed to contain both conscious and unconscious parts, which serves a mediating role between bodily needs, (id) and the external world. People acquire certain moral and ethical demands as they mature, and these are taken into account by the ego in this mediating function. The ego is also responsible for planning and thinking.

Most ego functions are automatic. A basic ego function is adaptation to reality, which is accomplished by delaying drives and calling up defense mechanisms as safeguards against unacceptable impulses.

Individuals use defense mechanisms to protect the ego from conflicts; such defense mechanisms include projection, repression and sublimation.

Sigmund Freud said the ego was one of three aspects of mental functioning, along with the id and superego. The ego lets one reason, test reality and solve problems, while the id modifies instinctual impulses following wishes of the person's conscience (superego).

See also DEFENSE MECHANISMS; FREUD, SIGMUND; ID; SUPEREGO.

ejaculation   The emission of semen from the penis at orgasm, usually during intercourse or masturbation. Ejaculation disorders are conditions in which ejaculation occurs before or very soon after penetration, does not occur at all or in which the ejaculate is forced back into the bladder. Because ejaculation disorders interfere with the completion and enjoyment of sexual intercourse, they are very stressful for men, as well as for their partners who do not always know how to help and may feel some blame.

Early ejaculation is ejaculation occurring within 10–60 seconds after penile penetration; it is also known as premature ejaculation. It is the most common sexual problem in men, often because of overstimulation, anxiety or stress about sexual performance.

Inhibited ejaculation is a rare condition in which erection is normal but ejaculation does not occur. It may be psychological, or it may be a result of a complication of other disorders or drug use.

Retrograde ejaculation occurs when the valve at the base of the bladder fails to close during an ejaculation. This forces the ejaculate backward into the bladder. Retrograde ejaculation may be the result of a neurological disease, or it can occur from pelvic surgery, surgery on the neck of the bladder or after a prostatectomy.

Treatment for ejaculation difficulties may begin with a visit to a physician, a urologist or a sex therapist.

See also SEX THERAPY; SEXUAL RESPONSE.

Elavil   Trade name for amitriptyline hydrochloride, a tricyclic antidepressant drug. It is as effective as imipramine in the treatment of depressive episodes of major depression, bipolar disorder, dysthymic disorder and atypical depression. Concomitant administration of amitriptyline with an antipsychotic drug can be beneficial in schizoaffective disorder and depression with psychotic features. It is used to help control abnormal eating behavior in bulimic patients and may also be useful in the prevention of migraine headaches and in some patients with chronic pain, including tension-type headache that is unresponsive to analgesic therapy.

Though effective, amitriptyline has a high rate of such side effects as sedation, dry mouth, constipation and weight gain associated with its use. It is highly toxic in overdose.

See also ANTIDEPRESSANT MEDICATIONS; HEADACHES.

Eldepryl   Trade name for the monoamine oxidase inhibitor antidepressant medication selegiline.

See also ANTIDEPRESSANT MEDICATIONS; PHARMACOLOGICAL APPROACH.

elderly parents   Caring for elderly parents is an increasingly common and complicated issue in today's society. There are many emotional and practical challenges involved when middle-aged adults begin to assume a bigger role in their parents' affairs and cope with their own feelings about this "role reversal."

Knowing when to take a more active role in parents' lives as they get older is a question many middle-aged adults face. They should be attentive for changes in the parents' judgment and ability to take care of themselves and their affairs. Elderly parents may present a variety of needs. Some may need physical assistance and others emotional assistance. Some may need financial help. As their behaviors change, one should try to determine to what extent those changes are part of a lifelong personality style. The adult child should also ask others who know the parent if they see changes, too. One may want to seek professional help in making this evaluation.

Many middle-aged children feel awkward about being responsive to their parents' needs without being overprotective. To overcome this awkwardness, children should talk to their parents, find out how they perceive their circumstances and discuss mutual concerns. They can agree to explore the situation further and work together toward a mutually agreeable approach. If the parent does not acknowledge problems, one can keep the dialogue going by asking how they would advise a friend in similar circumstances. This technique may help everyone focus more clearly on immediate needs and solutions.

Most older people want to live independently as long as possible. There are many noninstitutional arrangements for those who become increasingly dependent. Many participate in adult day-care programs, some have meals delivered to their homes, others live semi-independently with daily outside help and some live in "retirement projects" with a nurse on duty. One should encourage one's parents to stay involved with friends and to enjoy as many activities as they can.

As parents age, they may decide that it is in their own best interests to discuss and review their options. Some, despite increased physical or mental frailty, may want to keep things as they are.

Social workers usually advise not rushing things, unless needs are immediate and obvious. When difficult questions arise, all people—the elderly included—may not be ready to make decisions. They may want more time before talking about the problem again. One should consider involving others, such as grandchildren, trusted friends or a family doctor, in discussions. Everyone responds in different ways to different individuals. It may be useful to determine which individuals one's parents are most likely to listen to and involve those people in discussions.

As elderly parents become more dependent, interpersonal role relationships change. The adult child may experience a range of emotions and possibly the reappearance of long-forgotten feelings. For example, in some families, adult children may have always felt grateful to their parents and now feel able to finally repay their parents in financial, emotional and physical ways. In other families, however, adult children who already have other heavy responsibilities may find additional dependency too much to accept and feel overburdened, resentful or guilty about their inability to help.

Parents may feel resentful about losing their independence and direct their hostility toward the grown-up child. In such cases, one must keep in mind that their hostility is really directed at the situation and not necessarily at the child.

Taking on more responsibility for one's parents is an evolving process. At first one may feel uneasy and uncertain in taking control from parents. There are likely to be conflicts as different people perceive problems in different ways. Some people resist recognizing problems. Sometimes one sibling does not want to accept the fact that the parent is becoming dependent. In time, children and parents become more comfortable with the role reversal and move toward new patterns of meeting everyday situations.

As parents age, many begin thinking more about death and will offer their wishes regarding life-prolonging interventions. Increasingly common living will arrangements help ease the ethical dilemma of decision making when facing a parent's major illness or prolonged disability. A living will is a legal document that can allow a child to do what the parent desires when the time comes.

Recognizing signs of mental health problems in the elderly is important. In general, the elderly as a group are as mentally healthy as the general population. Nevertheless, there are some illnesses specific to this age group that can affect their behavior, judgment and memory. For example, elderly parents may be overly fearful of losing control of what is going on around them. Symptoms may be mild, such as sadness, loneliness, irritability or confusion, or they may be severe, such as depression, agitation or delusions. One should watch for such symptoms and get appropriate help. There are specialists in geriatric mental health who can be consulted.

Many adult children find that they cannot cope alone with elderly parents. In many cases it is too much for one individual, or one couple, to care for aging parents. There may be reasons why others cannot be involved in the responsibility; one may have few or no other family members, or they may live far away or already have heavy demands on themselves.

The idea of sharing responsibilities is important for the major caregiver and also to increase the number of people to whom parents continue to relate. One can consult the local Office on Aging to get some ideas about available services in the community, such as day care, meals, recreation, living arrangements and respite help. Many such programs feature sliding-scale fees. Additionally, community mental health programs have specialists in the care of older adults who can provide counsel and suggest support groups to help share concerns and practical approaches.

For adult children whose parents live in distant places, local social workers are affiliated with networks that can help arrange for long-distance care of elderly parents.

TIPS FOR TALKING WITH AN ELDERLY PARENT

- Be patient in starting your discussion.
- Set goals for each discussion. Be realistic.
- Discuss his/her wishes; permit parents to maintain their dignity and keep a sense of control.
- Use specific examples: "I've been concerned about your safety at home since your neighbor, Maggie, broke her hip."
- Suggest some options; explain advantages and disadvantages.

- Make some specific short-term and long-term plans to give both of you peace of mind.

See also DEATH; SUPPORT GROUPS.

Kahn, Ada P. *Stress A to Z: The Sourcebook for Facing Everyday Challenges.* New York: Facts On File, 2000.
Kahn, Ada P. *Becoming a Parent to Your Parents.* Mental Health Association of Greater Chicago, 1988.

Electra complex   According to Sigmund Freud, a term relating to a relationship of a daughter to her father during an early stage of psychosocial development. The presumed desire of a young girl to sexually possess her father is a parallel to the Oedipus complex boys presumably develop toward mothers. In mentally healthy individuals, these unconscious feelings are resolved as the individual moves into a more mature stage of development.

The name of this complex comes from Electra, a mythical figure, daughter of Agamemnon, king of Mycenae. While Agamemnon was at war, his wife Clytemnestra, and her lover conspired to kill her husband upon his return to usurp his kingdom. To avenge her father's death, Electra planned to murder her mother and the lover.

See also COMPLEX; MYTH; OEDIPUS COMPLEX.

electrocardiogram (ECG, EKG)   A record of the electrical impulses that precede contraction of the heart muscle. Wave patterns are known as P, Q, R, S and T. The ECG is a useful means of diagnosing disorders of the heart, many of which produce deviations from normal electrical patterns, Individuals who have anxieties and panic disorder may suffer from heart palpitations or a very fast heartbeat; a physician may request an ECG for them to rule out heart problems. In the ECG, electrodes are placed on the individual's chest and amplified by the electronic machine that creates the electrocardiogram, or the printed tracing of the patterns of the heartbeat.

An abnormal ECG may help to diagnose a myocardial infarction (heart attack), tissue damage, arrhythmia (abnormal heart rhythm), coronary insufficiency (coronary artery sclerosis) or other cardiac condition. The ECG is often used along with increasingly vigorous levels of exercise on a treadmill or in a battery-operated recorder

(Holter monitor) worn for 24 hours to diagnose heart disease more accurately.

electroconvulsive therapy (ECT)   A treatment involving the use of anesthesia and administration of muscle relaxants and oxygen that produces a convulsion by passing an electrical current through the brain; it is also known as electroshock therapy. Historically, this treatment was used for a variety of serious symptoms of mental illness. Under close medical monitoring, it is given to carefully selected patients with psychosis or severe depression who are unresponsive to treatment, especially patients with high levels of suicide risk. ECT has been shown to affect a variety of neurotransmitters in the brain, including GABA, norepinephrine, serotonin and dopamine. It is also sometimes used to treat acute mania and acute schizophrenia when other treatments have failed. The number of ECT treatment needed for each person is determined according to the therapeutic response. Individuals with depression usually require an average of six to 12 treatments; commonly, treatments are given three or four times a week, usually every other day. After a course of ECT treatments, such patients are usually maintained on an antidepressant drug or lithium to reduce the risk of relapse of the condition. ECT has a high rate of therapeutic response (80 to 90 percent) but may have a relapse rate of 50 percent in one year, which can be reduced to 20 percent with maintenance medication.

The treatment can be lifesaving in people who are too medically ill to tolerate medication or who are not eating or drinking (catatonic). Side effects, including memory loss, are not uncommon. Patients must give informed consent to ECT, similar to any operative procedure.

See also DEPRESSION; SCHIZOPHRENIA.

electroencephalogram (EEG)   An instrument that measures small electrical discharges from cortical areas of the brain through electrodes placed at standardized locations on the scalp. Irregularities are identified by examining patterns produced on a graph. EEG is used to study sleep and dreaming and in diagnosing brain tumors and epilepsy. It is also often one of many tests a physician will recommend for an individual who suffers from severe headaches, chronic insomnia and other disorders.

See also HEADACHES; INSOMNIA.

electroshock treatments   See ELECTROCONVULSIVE THERAPY.

ELISA test   (enzyme-linked immunosorbent assay) A laboratory test commonly used in the diagnosis of infectious diseases, and a highly sensitive screening test for evidence of the presence of HIV antibodies, considered a causative agent of AIDS (acquired immunodeficiency syndrome).

Tests found positive by this procedure are usually followed with another confirmatory assay (in the late 1980s, the Western blot confirmatory assay). Learning about a positive test result causes considerable stress and increasing dilemmas for many individuals. Therefore, appropriate counseling and expert interpretation should be done before and after test results are known.

See also ACQUIRED IMMUNODEFICIENCY SYNDROME.

emotional charge   The buildup of anger, rage and hurt feelings, stored in the body and mind. An emotionally charged discussion is one in which one or more of the participants have built up a store of emotions and often "let loose," sometimes speaking without thinking first. An example of emotional charge is often shown at a support group for individuals who care for aging parents and feel overwhelmed by their circumstances. When they finally talk about their feelings to others with many of the same concerns, they "let loose."

Emotional Health Anonymous   A national self-help program to offer support to men and women who have experienced emotional problems and illnesses. The self-help groups of this program use a modified version of the 12 steps to recovery of Alcoholics Anonymous to help participants during and after their crisis periods. Founded in 1970, the program has support groups throughout the United States as well as in other countries.

For information, contact:

Emotional Health Anonymous
General Service Office

2430 San Gabriel Boulevard
San Gabriel, CA 91779
Phone: (818) 573-5482

See also SUPPORT GROUPS.

emotions   A range of feelings humans experience. These may include anger, joy, happiness, sadness, gladness, despair, love, disgust, fear or surprise. How an individual feels is unique to that individual, and it is impossible to describe feelings, although people try through psychotherapy and creative release (song, poetry, etc.).

Emotions are also expressed at times with sweaty palms, weak knees or rapid heartbeat, such as when the individual is feeling fear or anxiety.

Researchers say that experiencing emotional feelings begins before the age of two months when a baby first smiles, and emotions continue to develop as the infant realizes how separation from the mother feels. As we grow older, our emotional reactions are influenced by experiences. For example, before a job interview we may feel nervous; before a happy occasion we will probably feel joy or gladness.

Emotion is important to an infant's development of good mental health in later life. Researchers have found that lack of loving attention and a trusting relationship during infancy may result in later difficulty with normal emotional development. A child may be emotionally deprived if there is frequent separation from parents during the first few years of life and bonding does not occur. Children who are emotionally deprived often crave attention and have difficulty coping with frustration.

The term "emotional problems" or "emotional disorders" is used to apply to many mental health difficulties. How people express their emotions is an important aspect of mental health. Many emotional responses are considered within the range of normal. When responses are out of the range of normal, such as pervasive sadness in depression, mental health is threatened.

empathy   An ability to mentally feel and understand what someone else is feeling. People who have been in the same situation as another can empathize. For example, a widow can have empathy with another individual who recently lost a spouse.

employee assistance programs (EAPs)   Programs that identify employees whose personal problems adversely affect their job performance, they provide the employee and their immediate families with confidential, professional assistance. From the employer's point of view, whatever EAPs can do to improve the mental health of employees helps make the business run more efficiently.

Employee assistance programs (EAPs) have been in existence for more than 50 years. Most authors trace their origin to the founding of Alcoholics Anonymous in 1935. In the 1960s and 1970s, the scope of EAPs began to include help for employee problems such as depression and other mental health concerns, drug abuse, divorce and other family difficulties. In the 1980s and 1990s, these programs have been expanded to include issues such as environmental stress, corporate culture, managing rapid technological change and retraining.

According to the Employee Assistance Professional Association (Arlington, Virginia), in the early 1990s, about one-third of the nation's workers were covered by some form of an EAP and about 75 percent of the "Fortune 500" companies had EAPs.

How EAPs Work

There are two types of EAPs: internal and external. The majority of EAPs use independent companies that provide EAP services under a contract with the employer.

While the programs are geared to identifying employees whose personal problems may adversely affect their job performance, they also take a proactive stance in helping employees avoid problems before they occur. For example, companies offer their employees seminars on stress reduction, parenting, adolescents and drugs, exercise, health and diet.

EAPs provide referrals to appropriate professional services for employees and their immediate families. Confidentiality is assured; most employees would not use an EAP if they thought their problems would be revealed.

Employers implement EAPs for a variety of reasons. One is the skyrocketing costs related to providing a medical benefits program; another is the huge cost attributed to down time due to employee alcohol addiction and mental health concerns. A four year study of mental health care received by employees of the McDonnell Douglas Corporation estimated that the company could have saved $5.1 million over three years if those employees who did not seek treatment had done so. Employees who used the EAP for chemical dependency also lost 44 percent fewer work days and filed fewer medical claims than those who did not.

Through its EAPs, Hewlett-Packard offers stress management courses to its 56,000 United States employees. Programs range from learning coping skills to dealing with teenage drug abuse. Additionally, Hewlett Packard offers its employees physical activities—membership in health clubs and on-site weight rooms, basketball courts, jogging tracks and nautilus equipment—as a means of stress reduction and an avenue toward healthier lives. Saturn Corporation, an automobile manufacturer headquartered in Tennessee, provides one-on-one counseling much of which is stress-related, by specially trained health care specialists. E.I. Dupont, the Delaware chemical manufacturer, also takes an individualized approach to helping its employees deal with stress.

For information:

Employee Assistance Professionals Association
  Inc.
2101 Wilson Boulevard, Suite 500
Arlington, VA 22201-3062
Phone: (703) 387-1000
Fax: (703) 522-4585
Web site: www.eap-association.com

See also ALCOHOLISM; DEPRESSION.

Kahn, Ada P. *Stress A to Z: The Sourcebook for Facing Everyday Challenges.* New York: Facts On File, 2000.

empty nest syndrome   A mild form of depression that occurs in middle-aged people when their children grow up and leave home. Typically, the syndrome seems to affect women more than men, and particularly women whose lives have focused on their children at the expense of engaging in activities for their own fulfillment. Such individuals no longer feel needed and feel a void in their life. However, many middle-aged people view children leaving home with a sense of relief and of accomplishing a major life task.

McQuaide, Sharon. "Women at Midlife." *Social Work* 43, no. 1 (Jan. 1998): 21–31.

enabler   A participant in a codependent relationship. The enabler promotes the codependent relationship by compensating for or covering difficulties or flaws in the behavior of the other out of an addictive need to be needed and to keep the relationship going. For example, a parent who continues to support an adult child who should be responsible for herself because the parent enjoys the feeling of the child's dependence would be considered an enabler. Another example is a husband who does all the household chores—shopping, driving children to activities, etc.—and explains that his wife is not feeling well in order to cover for an agoraphobic wife. It is difficult for an individual to live with agoraphobia without an enabler. Many alcoholics and drug addicts also have enablers.

See also AGORAPHOBIA; ALCOHOLISM; CODEPENDENCY; COURTSHIP, LOVE, ROMANCE, RELATIONSHIPS in BIBLIOGRAPHY.

Becnel, Barbara. *The Co-Dependent Parent.* San Francisco: Harper, 1991.

encephalitis   An inflammation of the brain that may result from many causes, including viruses, bacterial infection or lead poisoning. Symptoms may be mild or serious, with fever, convulsions, delirium and coma.

See also BRAIN.

encounter group   A form of small-group therapy in which personal growth is encouraged through sensitivity to others and interactions on an emotional level. A leader functions as a facilitator rather than a therapist and encourages participants to focus on "here and now" feelings and interactions. The term was coined by J. L. Moreno in

1914. In the 1990s, such groups are often referred to as "rap" groups, and individuals with similar concerns come together to discuss mutual concerns, such as depressions, parenting children who abuse drugs, or women who are abused by their husbands.

See also SUPPORT GROUPS.

Endep Trade name for amitriptyline, a tricyclic antidepressant medication.

See also ANTIDEPRESSANT MEDICATIONS; PHARMACOLOGICAL APPROACH; TRICYCLIC ANTIDEPRESSANTS.

endocrine disorders In disorders of the endocrine system, there is either not enough or too much production of a hormone by a gland. Endocrine disorders may cause many symptoms in body functions and behavior related to mental health, such as growth, metabolism, response to stress and sexual activity. Too much hormone production may be a result of a tumor, an autoimmune disease affecting a gland or a disorder of the pituitary or the hypothalamus, which control many other glands. When there is unusual hormone production, there may be a feedback effect on the secretion of hormones by the pituitary and the hypothalamus. To diagnose endocrine disorders, many laboratory and diagnostic tests are used, including tests that measure levels of hormones in the blood and urine.

Examples of endocrine disorders include Addison's disease, thyrotoxicosis and Cushing's syndrome. In Addison's disease, a defective adrenal cortex results in reduced hormone production. In thyrotoxicosis, there is an excess of hormone production. In Cushing's syndrome, there is an excess of adrenocorticotropic hormone (ACTH) secretion by a pituitary tumor.

The most common endocrine disease is hypothyroidism, in which the thyroid gland, for a number of possible reasons, fails to produce enough thyroid hormone to convert food (glucose) into energy. Hypothyroidism may cause fatigue, apathy, a tendency toward weight gain and mental dullness. Decreases in thyroid function can cause depression. Some medications such as lithium can bring out a tendency toward hypothyroidism.

Endocrine disorders can rarely cause mental disorders such as depression or even psychosis.

See also ENDOCRINE SYSTEM; ENDOCRINOLOGY.

endocrine system A series of ductless glands that secrete hormones directly into the bloodstream. Examples include the thyroid gland, which secretes thyroxine; ovaries (in females), which secrete estrogen; testes (in males), which secrete testosterone; and the adrenals, which secrete hydrocortisone. These glands and their secretions regulate the body's rate of metabolism, growth, sexual development and functioning. Some endocrine glands increase their activity during stress and emotional arousal. In research, these hormones appear to have very significant affects on fetal development and even on the central nervous system (brain) in adults.

Recent research is showing that even the supportive cells (glial cells) of the brain may produce hormones, though their function beyond this is not yet known.

See also ADRENAL GLAND; HORMONES.

endocrinology The study of the body's endocrine system and the hormones they secrete. A physician who specializes in diseases of the endocrine system is known as an endocrinologist.

end of life issues Issues that affect the mental health of family members, as well as the person near death. Extreme stress may result because of use or nonuse of medical procedures and lack of communication with health care practitioners.

In 1995, the American Medical Association established the Task Force on Quality of Care at the End of Life "to aid physicians in identifying when in the care-giving process, a transition in care needs may occur, and to identify actions that can be taken to improve the quality of life for those facing the end of life."

Ethical Considerations

In a background paper (dated November 21, 1995), the American Medical Association's Task Force reported that end of life issues have always been fraught with problems that society as a whole has not yet addressed. Through their close relationships with their patients, physicians continue to hold a significant role in how people address these issues. Assuming that patients do not misunderstand the prognosis and treatment options and that they are not suffering from a treatable form of depression, physicians in virtually all cases are morally obligated to abide by the competent patient's directions in the provision or stoppage of life-sustaining treatment. Physicians have an obligation to relieve pain and suffering and to promote dignity and autonomy of dying patients in their care. This includes providing effective and palliative treatment even though it may foreseeably hasten death.

The AMA is also developing a working definition of "futile treatment" that physicians will be able to use in consultation with patients and their families when intensive care is requested and the physician does not believe such treatment has a reasonable chance of benefiting the patient.

Euthanasia and Physician-Assisted Suicide

While competent patients generally retain autonomy in end of life decisions, this does not extend to requests for euthanasia or physician-assisted suicide. Dire social implications are inherent in these issues, and they pose a serious risk of abuse that is virtually uncontrollable, according to the AMA background paper. Such practices are ethically prohibited. They are fundamentally inconsistent with the physician's role as healer, and they could contribute to erosion of the patient/physician relationship.

Importance of End of Life Issues

Patients deserve full information about their clinical status, honest assessment of prognosis and education about potential treatment options, including palliative and hospice care. Physicians should encourage patients to consider their attitudes and beliefs about health care and quality of life prior to a crisis. They should advocate completion of advance directives, a signed paper that states the patient's wishes as to the prolonging of life. At the same time, the medical profession recognizes its responsibility to take actions to enhance the decision-making ability of the ethically, morally and professionally trained medical/health care team, so that this group can be entrusted to provide care for patients at the end of life.

To increase understanding and use of advance directives, in late 1995, the AMA took actions to familiarize physicians with the patient guide, jointly released in October 1995 by the AMA, the American Association of Retired Persons (AARP) and the American Bar Association (ABA), called *Shape Your Health Care Future and Health Care Advance Directives.*

See also DEATH; ELDERLY PARENTS; SUICIDE.

* Adapted from background paper, "Task Force Addresses End of Life Care," American Medical Association, November 21, 1995.

endogenous Arising from causes within the body. The term is often linked with depression (endogenous depression), which refers to a type of depression not due to an identifiable external cause as opposed to an exogenous depression, which may be linked to a death in the family, job loss or other identifiable causes. Such depression may be treated with psychotherapy and/or antidepressant drugs.

See also ANTIDEPRESSANT MEDICATIONS; DEPRESSION.

endogenous depression A type of depression that originates from within the body, as when there is a chemical imbalance, contrasted with a type of depression known as exogenous depression, which is not physiological in origin.

See also ANTIDEPRESSANT MEDICATIONS; DEPRESSION; ENDOGENOUS.

endorphins A group of substances formed within the body that relieve pain and may improve mood. Endorphins have a chemical structure similar to that of morphine. Since the early 1970s, researchers have understood that morphine acts at specific sites called opiate receptors in the brain, spinal cord and at other nerve endings. From this knowledge, they identified small peptide molecules produced by cells in the body that also act at opiate receptors. These morphinelike substances were named endorphins, short for endogenous morphines. Effects of endorphins are noted, for example, in accident victims, who feel no initial pain after a traumatic injury, or in marathon runners, who do not feel muscle soreness until they complete their race.

In addition to their effect on pain, endorphins are considered to be involved in controlling the body's response to stress, regulating contractions of the intestinal wall and determining mood. Addiction and tolerance to narcotic analgesics, such as morphine, are thought to be due or to cause suppression of the body's production of endorphins; withdrawal symptoms that occur when effects of morphine wear off may be due to a lack of these natural analgesics. Conversely, acupuncture is thought to produce pain relief partly by stimulating release of endorphins.

See also MEDITATION; RUNNER'S HIGH.

enkephalins A small group of peptide molecules that are secreted within the brain and by nerve endings such as in the digestive system and adrenal glands. Enkephalins have an analgesic (pain relieving) effect and are thought to affect mood and produce sedation.

See also ENDORPHINS.

enuresis See BEDWETTING.

environment Chemical, physical and biological components that compose the natural world. Stresses caused by the environment can interfere with good mental health. In cities throughout the United States, the number of days when the Pollution Standard Index (PSI), which is a combined reading of five major pollutants—particulate matter, sulfur dioxide, carbon monoxide, ozone and nitrogen dioxide—frequently goes beyond acceptable standards; in fact, PSI can fluctuate from as few as three to well over 200 in any given year. Difficulties in breathing, runny eyes and light-headedness, all sources of stress for the sufferer, are just some of the symptoms caused by bad air.

Inside the home or workplace, environmental hazards continue to prevail. It is estimated that up to 15 percent of the population is sensitive to indoor pollutants, which may be 10 times more concentrated than in nearby outdoor air. Some chemicals found in and around the household and workplace are pesticides, permanent press fabrics, gas-stove fumes, car exhaust and particleboard. Even water causes environmental illnesses; symptoms range from mild to disabling and are often non-specific. Every part of the body can be affected by flulike headaches, muscle aches and fatigue, or more debilitating food intolerance and central nervous system problems such as memory loss, confusion and depression.

For information:

National Coalition Against the Misuse of Pesticides
530 Seventh Street SE
Washington, D.C. 20003
Phone: (202) 543-5450

National Pesticide Telecommunication Network
Texas Tech University Health Sciences Center
School of Medicine Thompson Hall, Room S-129
Texas Tech University
Lubbock, TX 79409
Phone: (800) 858-7378

National Safety Council
1121 Spring Lake Drive
Itasca, IL 60143-3201
Phone: (708) 285-1121

National Safe Workplace Institute
1121 Spring Lake Drive
Itasca, IL 60143-3201
Phone: (708) 285-1121

See also CLIMATE AND MENTAL HEALTH; SICK BUILDING SYNDROME.

Altman, Roberta. *The Complete Book of Home Environmental Hazards.* New York: Facts On File, 1990.

envy An emotional feeling that most people experience at one time or another in which they have a sense that something is lacking in their lives that others may have. For example, they may desire the status or possessions of another person. Usually envious people are unwilling to admit to these feelings. Envy can spring from many types of relationships, but the situations close at hand involving friends, relatives, neighbors or colleagues are generally most intense. It is easier to compare ourselves with people close at hand and to think that their good fortune might have been ours. Because feelings of envy imply that someone is in a superior position and is often considered to be a sinful feeling, people develop various ways of masking or suppressing it. To avoid expressing envy, some people develop snobbish attitudes, gossip, criticize or imply that the person envied is the envious one.

This ability to imagine or mentally project into or identify with an admired person's strengths is an intellectual asset that may enable people to progress and better themselves. However, it becomes negative when it becomes fixated on another person's life without spurring the envious person to better his or her through effort in a constructive way.

Modern American life is full of elements that create envy. For example, the mobile quality of society deemphasizes social class and creates feelings that all things are possible for all people. This can also create feelings of frustration, failure and envy when expectations are thwarted. Mass media, especially television, allows us to view "lifestyles of the rich and famous." Advertising plays on feelings of envy. The "Me Decade" of the 1980s, with its narcissism and the "yuppie" lifestyle, created a climate in which it has been easy for envy to flourish. As one is faced with a wide array of consumer products made available by high technology, it is always possible to feel that someone else has more.

Low self-esteem produces envy that often does not improve by the attainment of material things, status symbols or fame. Normal self-esteem makes envy unlikely but allows creative identification with admired traits in others.

The reverse side of feelings of envy is the fear of being envied. This may be the reason that many people are less willing to talk about their salaries or general financial situation than other topics that might seem far more personal. Members of other societies carry this fear even further by sharing food and other possessions or by avoiding direct compliments, which are seen as a sign of envy and which may bring the power of the "evil eye" to bear on the fortunate person. Even people who find compliments pleasant still quite frequently experience an awkward feeling in accepting them.

See also FRUSTRATION; SELF-ESTEEM.

enzyme-linked immunosorbent assay (ELISA) See ELISA TEST.

enzymes Proteins that regulate rates of chemical reactions in the body. Thousands of enzymes in the human body are produced by cells and tissues. Activities of enzymes are influenced by factors including certain drugs, such as barbiturates, that affect the rate at which others drugs are metabolized. This effect (enzyme induction) causes some drug interactions. Other drugs block action of enzymes. An example is antibiotics, which destroy bacteria by blocking bacterial enzymes.

Enzymes that break down medications in the body are sometimes induced (or increased) by concomitant use of other drugs such as nicotine (as in smoking) or large amounts of alcohol or sedatives. People with induced enzymes may break down and excrete antidepressants or anxiolytic drugs more rapidly, requiring higher than usual doses to achieve effects. If a smoker ceases smoking while taking other medications, the enzymes may no longer be induced and the usual dose may now be too high, causing side effects.

epidemic The sudden and rapidly spreading outbreak of a disease that affects a significant number of people in one location at the same time. An example is influenza, which seems to recur every year. Another is food poisoning, which might affect many individuals who eat the same food at a picnic and become ill. There have been and still are, in parts of the world, epidemics of some diseases, such as measles and chicken pox.

Epidemics cause mental health consequences because the ill people temporarily cannot function with their normal capacity, and the well people become worried about others who are ill and concerned that they will also contract the disorder. There are usually many anxieties and stresses associated with any epidemic.

The increase in the number of AIDS (acquired immunodeficiency syndrome) patients has been referred to an epidemic by the public and has aroused many fears in the general population, including fears of any kind of casual contact with homosexuals and fears among health practitioners of caring for AIDS patients.

See also EPIDEMIOLOGY.

epidemic anxiety Acute anxiety among many members of a given community at the same time. Epidemic anxiety is also known as mass hysteria. Usually a common factor for the anxiety can be identified, and individuals usually recover without long-lasting effects.

Epidemic anxiety has occurred following chemical explosions and similar crises of public safety. In such cases, people commonly report nausea, vomiting and headaches and attribute all such symptoms (whether correctly or not) to the recent event.

See also MASS HYSTERIA.

epidemiology The science that studies prevalence in the distribution of diseases in populations. Unlike clinicians who deal with one patient at a time, epidemiologists study large numbers of people in a community, country or area of the world. Although epidemiology originally dealt mainly with infectious diseases such as plague and cholera, epidemiologists now study many mental health disorders as well as contemporary physical problems such as AIDS.

See also EPIDEMIC.

epilepsy A disorder in which there is a tendency to have recurrent seizures or temporary alterations in one more brain functions. Seizures are neurological abnormalities that come and go that are caused by unusual electrical activity in the brain. Seizures usually happen spontaneously, with no apparent cause, but are a symptom of brain dysfunction; they can result from a variety of diseases or injuries. For example, head injuries, brain infection (encephalitis or meningitis), drug intoxication and alcohol withdrawal states may at times be causes of seizures.

Many epileptics lead normal lives and are healthy between seizures. However, some may be limited in their choice of jobs because of their disorder. Many epileptics wear a tag bracelet or carry a special card indicating that they are epileptic; they should advise people with whom they work about what to do if a seizure occurs.

Historically, epileptic people have often been the subject of fear, avoidance and lack of understanding. Although epilepsy is considered a brain disorder, these people are not "crazy" and should be helped, not shunned, as has happened to some epileptic individuals. Family members, friends and bystanders need to be educated to show understanding and compassion rather than criticism and ridicule. Epileptics remain mentally healthier individuals with a supportive system around them.

Epilepsy occurs in about one in 200 persons, with about 1 million epileptics in the United States. Epilepsy usually begins in childhood or adolescence; when epilepsy develops during childhood and there is a family history of the disease, there is a strong likelihood that symptoms will decrease after adolescence. Many people outgrow it and recover without medication, while others control their disease with anticonvulsant drugs.

In some epileptics, seizures occur at times of extreme stress or fatigue or during an infectious illness. Epileptics can reduce the frequency of seizures by taking appropriate medication and avoiding certain situations known to bring on their seizures. Some epileptics can anticipate an attack when they experience an aura, which is a vaguely uncomfortable feeling of restlessness and irritability.

Symptoms and Types

The occurrence and progression of a seizure depends on the part of the brain in which it arises and how it fans out. For example, generalized seizures may arise over a wide area of the brain and cause loss of consciousness, while partial seizures are usually caused by damage to a more limited area of the brain (temporary lobe epilepsy). Generalized seizures are divided into two main types, grand mal and petit mal (absence) seizures. During a grand mal seizure, the individual becomes unconscious and falls down, and the entire body stiffens, jerks and twitches uncontrollably; breathing is irregular or absent. After the seizure, bladder and bowel control may be lost; the person may feel disoriented and confused and may feel a need to sleep. When the effects are over, in several hours, the individual may have no recollection of the seizure.

During a petit mal, or "absence" seizure, there is a momentary loss of consciousness, without abnormal movements. The individual may lose memory for only a few seconds or up to half a minute. As the attack happens, the individual may appear to be inattentive or daydreaming. In children, these seizures may occur hundreds of times a day and can hinder school achievements.

During simple partial seizures there will be an abnormal twitching movement, tingling sensation or even visual or other hallucinations without warning that last several minutes. With this type of seizure, the individual recalls details of the occurrence. When seizures cause twitching movements on the same side of the body, the term applied is Jacksonian epilepsy.

During complex partial seizures the individual may not respond if spoken to and looks dazed. There may be involuntary actions, such as lip smacking, that usually are not remembered by the sufferer.

Diagnosis

The physician will take a complete history from the individual as well as other family members and do a complete neurological examination and a sleep electroencephalogram (EEG); however, even the sleep EEG cannot always confirm or refute the diagnosis of seizure. Tests of heart function (such as an ECG or Holter monitor) are also used to test for cardiac irregularities as a cause of loss of consciousness. Additionally, CAT scanning of the brain and MRI scanning can give additional information, as can specific blood tests.

Treatment

In most cases, anticonvulsant drugs lessen the frequency of seizures. However, these drugs may have side effects such as drowsiness and impaired concentration. Medications are tailored to the needs of each individual patient and the severity of the disease. In rare cases, brain surgery is recommended when seizure disorders are severe, do not respond to medication and emanate from a single operable area or "focus" in the brain.

Helping During an Epileptic Seizure

Those standing by and witnessing an epileptic attack should watch to see that the individual can breathe while unconscious and is not in any physical danger from the surroundings. The person should not be restrained or held down but permitted to move freely; something soft should be placed beneath the head. Tight clothing, particularly around the neck, should be loosened. The mouth should not be forced open. Reasons to call an ambulance include consciousness not being regained after the seizure, a seizure lasting for five minutes or longer or a second seizure occurring immediately after the first one. Bystanders can be most helpful by remaining calm and reassuring to the sufferer.

See also ANTICONVULSANT MEDICATIONS.

epinephrine A hormone secreted by the adrenal gland; also called adrenaline. Epinephrine (or adrenaline) is sometimes referred to as the "emergency" hormone, as it affects the entire body and is responsible for reactions to fear and anger, such as rapid heartbeat and feelings of nervousness and agitation. Release of epinephrine throughout the body is part of the human body's "fight or flight" readiness response to danger or a threat of danger. Epinephrine is a powerful stimulant; in cases of cardiac arrest, it is injected as a last resort into the heart to start it beating again.

See also ADRENALINE; NEUROTRANSMITTERS.

Equanil Trade name for the antianxiety drug meprobamate.

See also ANXIETY; MEPROBAMATE.

ethical drug A drug that requires a physician's prescription. (An "over-the-counter drug" does not require a prescription.) Psychotropic medications, including antidepressant drugs, are examples of ethical drugs.

ethics There are many aspects to defining ethics; one that fits most circumstances is the biblical one: "Do unto others as you would have others do unto you." Ethics is involved in everyday behavior.

People learn to "do the right thing" according to the unstated or stated rules of each culture.

In health and medicine, many ethical issues are involved. Usually, four basic principles are considered: (1) autonomy: respecting the wishes of the patient; (2) independence: maintaining independence from overbearing technology; (3) beneficence: doing what is best for the patient; and (4) justice: balancing individual needs with the social good. At times these values may conflict, causing additional dilemmas.

Medical science has developed to the point at which it can prolong physiological life. Aspects of ethics are involved, because technologically people can be kept alive after they are physiologically dead. During the mid-1990s, bioethicists, scientists concerned with ethics, still struggle with decisions regarding artificial life-support machines as well as other issues. Bioethicists have techniques for looking at questions about life-prolonging technology, genetic research and testing, organ transplantation, reproduction, AIDS and rationing medical care.

Legal issues as well as ethical issues arise when wishes of the family differ from the scientific pursuit of knowledge possibly derived from watching the progress of a terminally ill patient on life support. Many hospitals now have ethics committees that help make difficult decisions.

In December 1991, a federal Patient Self-Determination Act was enacted, which requires hospitals to tell all patients they have the right to refuse treatment. Some states also have laws. One example is Illinois, which has a Health Care Surrogate Act (September 1991) allowing people to decline such treatment as intravenous feeding or respirators for terminally ill relatives.

Physicians are faced with ethical decisions when terminally ill patients ask for assisted suicide. In most states, a physician cannot legally assist in inducing death.

Another dimension of ethics in medicine involves drug testing. For example, when a promising new drug is tested, some people are involved in trials. An ethical dilemma arises in random tests in which new drugs are compared with inactive placebos to determine the safety and effectiveness of the new drugs.

At one time mentally retarded persons and prisoners were used in medical and psychological tests. This is no longer the case, because they are not in a position to give informed consent.

Many U.S. medical schools are including courses in ethics for physicians. Lawyers take written examinations regarding ethics as part of their licensure procedure.

See also DEATH; LEGAL ISSUES; SUICIDE.

euphoria A state of mind in which one feels extremely exalted, elated and jubilant (euphoric mood). Such a reaction is appropriate after hearing extremely good news, such as passing a major examination, or after a long climb to the top of a mountain. However, when this state occurs inappropriately or is too intense, the individual might be in a manic or hypomanic state or may have manic-depressive illness or bipolar disorder.

See BIPOLAR DISORDER; MANIC-DEPRESSIVE ILLNESS.

eustress A term coined by Hans Selye (1907–1982), pioneer researcher in the field of stress, to refer to "good stress." During eustress and dis-stress (bad stress), the body undergoes virtually the same nonspecific responses to the various positive or negative stimuli acting upon it. However, he explained, the fact that eustress causes much less damage than distress demonstrates that "how you take it" determines whether one can adapt successfully to change.

Examples of "good stress" include starting a new romance, getting married, having a baby, buying a house, getting a new job or getting a raise at work. All these situations, as well as others, demand adaptations on the part of the individual. Both eustress and dis-stress are part of the general adaptation syndrome (GAS), which Selye described as being the controlling factor in how people cope with stresses in their lives.

Later researchers (Thomas Holmes and Richard Rahe) included several "good stress" situations in their social readjustment rating scale, which was designed to be a predictor of ill health. Sources of good stress included marital reconciliation, retirement, and outstanding personal achievement in addition to those named above.

See also COPING; DIS-STRESS; GENERAL ADAPTATION SYNDROME; HOMEOSTASIS; LIFE CHANGE SELF-RATING SCALE; SELYE, HANS; STRESS.

Selye, Hans. *Stress Without Distress*. New York: J. B. Lippincott, 1974.
———. *The Stress of Life*, rev. ed. New York: McGraw-Hill, 1978.

euthanasia   A term relating to inducing the death of another person as a "mercy killing." Some spouses of terminally ill persons wish to help their loved one out of misery by giving them death-inducing potions. Some individuals ask physicians for such drugs, and there have been instances in which physicians have cooperated. However, euthanasia is an illegal procedure in nearly all states, and offenders can be prosecuted. Euthanasia has been referred to as "assisted suicide." The question of whether or not euthanasia should be considered legal is a matter of ethics.

See also ETHICS; SUICIDE.

Eutonyl   Trade name for the monoamine oxidase inhibitor antidepressant medication partyline.

See also ANTIDEPRESSANT MEDICATIONS; MONOAMINE OXIDASE INHIBITORS; PHARMACOLOGICAL APPROACH.

exercise   Exercise can have positive mental health benefits and serve as a way to raise self-image and increase creativity. According to Jeff Zwiefel, M.S., Director, The National Exercise for Life Institute, physical strength and stamina and a confident attitude are the main by-products of exercise. A study at Baruch College, New York, found that people who are stronger and more muscularly fit have a significantly better self-image than their peers. Psychological tests have discovered that those who exercise are more confident, emotionally stable and outgoing than those who are sedentary.

Joan C. Gondola, associate professor of physical education at Baruch College, found the same positive results of exercise on creativity levels when she administered a test on female college students. One group had exercised 20 minutes before the tests and the other group had not; the exercise group had more imaginative responses than those that had not.

The boost in creativity may be attributed to the release of adrenaline and endorphins during exercise. The right side of the brain is stimulated by these chemicals, which control creative and intuitive processes.

Exercise is an excellent way to relieve stress, whether caused by pressures at work, family tensions or grief. However, exercise may also become a compulsion, when the individual drops other responsibilities in favor of improving body image or losing weight. Because of our society's emphasis on a thin, slender body shape, many individuals have become exercise addicts. For some individuals, such addiction interferes with their mental well-being. An example is compulsive exercise that accompanies eating disorders.

For information:

Aerobics and Fitness Association of America
15250 Ventura Boulevard, Suite 310
Sherman Oaks, CA 91403
Phone: (800) 445-5950

National Fitness Foundation
2250 E. Imperial Highway, Suite 412
El Segundo, CA 90245
Phone (213) 640-0145

See BODY IMAGE.

experiential family therapy   A type of family therapy emphasizing experiences between family members and between family members and therapist during therapy. The therapy is based on humanistic approaches that focus on helping family members learn to use symptoms and anxieties constructively. It is also known as symbolic-experiential family therapy.

See also PSYCHOTHERAPIES.

exposure therapy   Behavioral therapies that emphasize changing an individual's responses to phobic situations while gradually increasing exposure to the feared situation. Exposure therapy may be effective for some phobias and for agoraphobia; to be effective, appropriate drug therapy is also used in many cases.

See also AGORAPHOBIA; BEHAVIORAL THERAPY; PHOBIA; PSYCHOTHERAPIES.

Isaac M. Marks. *Living with Fear.* New York: McGraw-Hill, 1978.

extrapyramidal system   A system that influences and modifies electrical impulses sent from the brain to the skeletal muscles. The system consists of nerve pathways linking nerve nuclei in the surface of the cerebrum (the main mass of the brain), the basal ganglia deep within the brain and parts of the brain stem. Degeneration of or damage to parts of the system can cause disturbances in execution of voluntary (willful) movements and in muscle tone and can cause the appearance of involuntary (unwanted) movements such as tremors or writhing motions. Disturbances of this type occur in Huntington's disease, Parkinson's disease and some types of cerebral palsy.

Extrapyramidal side effects can also occur as a result of taking some phenothiazine drugs, used for treating some mental disorders.

See also PHENOTHIAZINE DRUGS.

extroversion   A personality trait that involves characteristics of outgoingness, friendliness, openness and general optimism. Extroverts like to be with people, work well in groups and are often leaders. How and why personality traits develop is unknown. Some say that family background may influence personality traits, but others believe that the basis for the difference between the extroverted and introverted personality lie in the cerebral cortex, the part of the brain involved in learning, reasoning and planning. In brain scans, activity of this area can be visualized. In the extrovert, the cortex is quiet and seems to welcome noisy, exciting situations that arouse it. The introvert's level of cortical arousal is already high, and the introverted personality does not need much outside stimulation and seems to prefer quiet and peace.

Extroverts seem to fall asleep faster than introverts, and extroverts may be less sensitive to pain. The theory about the cerebral cortex was suggested by British psychologist Hans Eysenck. The concept of extroversion was first proposed by C. G. Jung.

See also INTROVERSION.

eye movement desensitization and reprocessing (EMDR)   A technique for treating traumatic experience locked in the nervous system by skillfully combining a representation of the trauma, self-evaluation, emotions and body sensations while experiencing bilateral stimulation (eye movement or tapping sounds, for example). This procedure has empirical support as a trauma treatment. EMDR was developed in the early 1990s by Francine Shapiro, Ph.D., a Northern California psychologist.

Doctor, Ronald M. and Ada P. Kahn. *Encyclopedia of Phobias, Fears and Anxieties.* New York: Facts On File, 2000.

factitious disorder   See MUNCHAUSEN'S SYNDROME.

faith healing   The essence of faith healing, for those who believe in it, is the strong conviction of "mind over matter." For some people, belief in faith healing contributes to better mental health.

Historically, some faith healing takes place with the assistance of a "healer" who places his or her hands on an individual; through the healer's touch, a person is then healed. Faith healing was and still is an accepted phenomenon of Roman Catholicism because certain saints have been thought to have healing powers. The Catholic shrine at Lourdes has gained the reputation for causing miraculous recoveries. Native American religious practice includes rituals intended to promote healing of mental and physical ills. Faith healing is a central doctrine of Christian Scientists who actively discourage reliance on doctors and conventional medicine. Today, there is a renewed interest in faith healing brought about by the resurgence of the fundamental and Pentecostal religious movements. Some of the movements' ministers seem able to cure their congregants' afflictions by arousing in them a religious fervor or hysterical response.

Psychosomatic illnesses are thought to lend themselves best to the faith healing process. To counter the claim that faith healing has succeeded where conventional medical treatments have failed, some skeptics take the position that patients resort to faith healing only when desperate. Feeling that something must work, a person gets into a state of mind in which psychosomatic symptoms disappear, or if the problem is genuinely physical, at least feels better.

Research methods are difficult to apply to faith healing in part because of the questionable psycho-somatic aspects of many diseases. Also, many spontaneous remissions or recoveries from serious or hopeless conditions without the benefit of the faith healing process have been recorded. A psychological study of individuals who had a physical stress condition relieved by faith healing showed that, while there was little indication of mental illness, they had strong denial mechanisms. These denial mechanisms could keep them from recognizing continuing symptoms of their stress.

See also COMPLEMENTARY THERAPIES; DENIAL; IMMUNE SYSTEM; MIND/BODY CONNECTIONS; PLACEBO EFFECT; PRAYER; RELIGION.

Doctor, Ronald M., and Ada P. Kahn. *Encyclopedia of Phobias, Fears, and Anxieties.* New York: Facts On File, 2000.
Galanter, Marc. *Cults, Faith, Healing and Coercion.* New York: Oxford University Press, 1989.
Oxman, T.E. et al. "Lack of Social Participation or Religious Strength and Comfort as Risk Factors for Death After Cardiac Surgery in the Elderly." *Psychosomatic Medicine* 57 (1995): 681–689.
Rose, Louis. "Faith Health." In *Man, Myth and Magic,* edited by Richard J. Cavendish. New York: Marshall Cavendish, 1983.
Sobel, David, and Robert Ornstein, eds. "Faith Heals." *Mental Medicine Update* IV, No. 2 (1995).

familial   A characteristic or disorder that runs in families. Depression seems to run in families, as does panic disorder.

See also DEPRESSION; PANIC DISORDER.

family   Families and other relationships sometimes buffer the mental health challenges faced by individuals during their lifetime. However, for many people, families can also be a source of anxiety and stress. As an example, men and women going through marital problems are especially vulnerable to the effects of relationship conflict. They may suffer from emotional consequences such as depression and can have a compromised immune function leading to an increased rate of physical illness. Caregivers who provide support for family members who are ill are another example of a highly stressed group. A decreased immune function has been observed in spouses caring for mates with Alzheimer's disease.

George R. Parkerson, M.D., and colleagues at Duke University Medical Center reported in the *Archives of Family Medicine* (March 1995) that individuals who see themselves as enduring high family stress are likely to have greater health problems than those reporting low family stress. Patients completed several different surveys that looked at self-esteem, life events and changes, depression and family-induced stress. In addition, information on the number of physician visits, referrals to other physicians, hospitalizations, severity of illness and cost of treatment incurred by these patients was tabulated. Results showed that family stress often had a stronger impact on health outcomes than other types of stress, such as social or financial stress. Those with high family stress scores had more frequent follow-up visits to the clinic, more referrals to specialists, more hospitalizations, a higher severity of illness and incurred higher charges for clinical health care than those with low family stress. They also had fewer social support systems.

In evaluating family stress, researchers used the Duke social support and stress scale (DUSOCS), a 24-item questionnaire; patients indicated personal stress and/or support from each of six different types of family members and four different types of non-family members. In their report, researchers note that "it is important to remember that the study examines only the effect of family stress as perceived by the patient and does not measure family stress in terms of the family as a total system, nor does it measure perceptions of other members of the patient's family."

The Duke University researchers recommended that family physicians identify patients with high family stress and give them the special care they may require to prevent unfavorable outcomes. They suggested that questionnaires such as those used in the study can help identify patients who are at high risk of adverse health-related outcomes and who may not be recognized as such through standard medical history reports, physical exams and medical tests.

Having patients talk about family stress issues with their physicians can be useful. The researchers said that one randomized, controlled trial showed that when family physicians discussed details about stressful and supportive family members with their patients after reviewing questionnaire results, patients said they generally felt better and the process helped them to improve relationships with their families.

See also ALZHEIMER'S DISEASE; COMMUNICATION; DEPRESSION; DYSFUNCTIONAL FAMILY; INTIMACY; RELATIONSHIPS; SELF-ESTEEM.

Burg, M.M., and T.E. Seeman. "Families and Health: The Negative Side of Social Ties." *Annals of Behavioral Medicine* 16 (1994): 109–115.

Parkerson, George R. et al. "Perceived Family Stress as a Predictor of Health-Related Outcomes." *Archives of Family Medicine* 4 (March 1995).

family history When a mental health professional begins treating a new client, the individual will be asked many questions about the physical as well as mental health of parents and siblings. If any first-degree relatives had a history of any mental illness, it is important that the specific illness be discussed, along with information about treatment and long-term course and outcome. The mental health professional may run through a series of specific disorders, because many individuals will not recognize alcoholism or shoplifting in their parents or siblings as emotional problems. Any relevant information about the family background may be included in the family history part of the interview because it will help the mental health professional diagnose and treat the individual.

Honesty and forthrightness on the part of the individual can help in her own diagnosis and treatment.

See also FAMILY THERAPY; PSYCHOTHERAPIES.

family therapy A form of psychotherapy that tends to focus on the family unit or at least the parent and child (in single-parent families). Family therapy, begun in the 1950s, is geared to help individual family members become aware of their reactions and defensive habits and encourages them to communicate more openly with one another.

Typically, the therapy group will consist of both parents, or a parent and stepparent, two separated parents or other parental pairings depending on the environment in which the child lives.

In many cases, the child is brought to a mental health professional because of difficulties in school, such as aggressive behavior, or school phobia. When it becomes clear to the therapist that the child's problems appear to arise from the home situation, the family will be invited to join one or more sessions. Often such families are not dysfunctional families but, because of changing circumstances and demands, may not be providing the understanding and open communication that the child needs at the time.

Family therapy usually focuses on present problems and their practical solutions. Family therapy can be helpful when at least one member has a relatively serious mental illness, such as recurrent depression or schizophrenia. In these situations, family members need reassurance that neither the individual nor members of the family are responsible for the illness. The approach minimizes guilt and permits the patient and family members to find coping methods that may be more consoling and constructive to the patient. For example, a young schizophrenic individual who lives with his parents may need ongoing assistance in developing social skills, while the parents need ongoing assistance in coping with outbursts or anger and emotional withdrawal.

See also PSYCHOTHERAPIES; SEX THERAPY.

family violence Violence against first-degree relatives or those living in the home. In American society, family violence involves acts of incest, physical child abuse, neglect, sexual child abuse, battered women, spouse abuse and marital rape. Family violence happens in all strata of society, and there are many more cases than official records indicate because it is a subject often covered up out of fear and shame.

Characteristics of persons who are victims of family violence include anxiety, powerlessness, guilt and lack of self-esteem.

According to Paulette Trumm, M.D., Director, Women's Program, Forest Hospital, Des Plaines, Illinois, women who are abused by their husbands or boyfriends not only sustain injuries from physical beatings, but they also suffer from many mental and emotional scars, including post-traumatic stress disorder, depression and anxiety. In most cases, the women suffer from low self-esteem; the healing process takes a long time.

Mental health professionals who treat victims of family violence are concerned with getting the women or children away from the abuser and into therapy before the beatings become too severe or other problems arise. Some victims of family violence compound their difficulties with use of alcohol or drugs.

Most abused women do not seek help until beatings become severe and have occurred over a period of time, often two to three years. Some women are too embarrassed or believe that if they report the beating to police, they will not be taken seriously. The majority of women who seek help from family violence are between age 20 and 60. In 75 percent of households in which abuse takes place, the husband or boyfriend is an alcoholic or on drugs.

Many women do not report family violence because they do not have the courage or financial resources to report the attacks and leave. For women who want to break the cycle of violence and abuse, Suzette Rush at Forest Hospital, Des Plaines, Illinois, suggests:

- Leave the abuser; stay with a friend or family member who will be supportive emotionally and provide a safe haven.

- Leave the home when the abuser is absent to eliminate any confrontations.

- Take bank records, children's birth certificates, cash and other important documents along with clothing and personal items.

- If possible, photograph or videotape any consequences of abuse, such as injuries or damage to the home. These could be important for possible later court proceedings.

- Call the police and file a police report. Obtain an order of protection as soon as possible.

- Seek counseling for yourself and your children; join a support group along with others who have been victims of family violence.

Family violence also includes acts of violence against a defenseless, elderly person in the home.

See also ABUSE; DOMESTIC VIOLENCE; DYSFUNCTIONAL FAMILY; INCEST; SUPPORT GROUPS.

McFarland, Gertrude K., and Mary Durand Thomas. *Psychiatric Mental Health Nursing*. Philadelphia: J. B. Lippincott, 1992.
"Women Can Get Help, Support and Healing for Physical and Mental Abuse." *Branching Out*, Forest Health System, Inc., Des Plaines, Illinois (fall/winter 1991).

fantasy Imagining events or objects that are not present. Many people indulge in fantasy, and, in fact, fantasy may lead to creativity. However, when fantasy takes the place of realistic thinking, the individual may have a thought disorder. Fantasies give one the temporary illusion that wishes are being met or desires satisfied.

Many people have fleeting sexual fantasies, sometimes involving people other than their mates or involving acts with their mates. Individuals may fantasize about sexual acts that they have heard about, read about or have seen in pictures. Having sexual fantasies is a normal habit for most individuals, but if carried to an extreme, and if the individual finds satisfaction and fulfillment from a fantasy life, the habit may be considered out of bounds of normalcy and require psychotherapy.

See also PRIMAL FANTASIES; PROCREATION FANTASY.

fatigue See CHRONIC FATIGUE SYNDROME; DEPRESSION.

fear An emotion resulting in intense and unpleasant tension that comes about because of a real threat or the imagination of a threatening situation, as in a phobia. There may be an intense feeling of wanting to escape, together with physiological reactions, which might include weakness, dizziness, rapid breathing, rapid heartbeat, nausea, muscle tension or weakness in the knees. Different individuals have different physiological responses to fear.

The general public often misuses the term "fear" for phobia, and vice versa. Fear is a real and knowable danger and can usually be recognized by others. On the other hand, phobia is an inappropriately fearful response to a situation and out of proportion to the real danger; the danger in a situation perceived by one as phobic cannot be seen or realized by another. Real fear is normal. Chronic phobias that cause avoidance behavior are considered anxiety disorders.

Fear can be a helpful emotion. For example, the fear reaction enables people to get out of the way when they hear the whistle of a train. The fear reaction sets off a signal in the hypothalamus that triggers a release of adrenaline into the body. Adrenaline acts immediately to prepare the body for fight or flight. The heart beats more strongly, breathing deepens, perspiration increases to cool the body, pupils dilate to sharpen vision and the face may turn pale.

See also ANXIETY DISORDERS; FIGHT OR FLIGHT RESPONSE; PHOBIA.

Rosen, Jeffrey B., and Jay Schulkin. "From Normal Fear to Pathological Anxiety." *Psychological Review* 105, no. 2 (April 1998): 325–350.

feedback The sharing of feelings or thoughts without evaluating them or demanding changes. Feedback involves objective information given by a therapist, teacher or parent or by others in a support group. Feedback may help an individual make changes or reinforce certain behaviors. For example, the individual who is fearful of public speaking may develop confidence when he gets very favorable feedback after his first public speech.

See also BEHAVIORAL THERAPY; PSYCHOTHERAPIES.

fertility See INFERTILITY.

fetal alcohol syndrome A condition in which the growth of the fetus is retarded, resulting in possible cranial, facial and limb anomalies as well as mental retardation. This is caused by a woman's heavy alcohol consumption during pregnancy. Even moderate drinking can produce less severe but undesirable effects on the fetus. The National Institute on Alcohol Abuse and Alcoholism advises total abstention from alcohol during pregnancy. It was only in the latter half of the 20th century that the effects of alcohol on a fetus have become better understood. Many deformities and problems in newborns have been eliminated because of this knowledge.

See also ALCOHOLISM.

fibromyalgia   A form of "soft-tissue" or muscular rheumatism that causes pain in the muscles and fibrous connective tissues (ligaments and tendons). It is an accepted clinical syndrome that causes anguish for the sufferer, not only because of the pain and discomfort, but because of the difficulty in having it diagnosed properly.

According to Barry M. Schimmer, M.D., chief, Rheumatology, Pennsylvania Hospital, "For a long time we thought that their problems were psychosomatic and these patients were referred for psychiatric help. Today we know that this condition is very real and needs to be dealt with and treated like any other chronic illness."

The exact cause of fibromyalgia is unknown and there is no known cure. Many different factors trigger the pain including an illness, such as the flu, hormonal changes, or physical or emotional trauma.

Symptoms

The ailment, which affects 3 to 6 million Americans, primarily Caucasian, middle-class women between the ages of 35 to 55, results in muscles becoming tight and tense, and the person feels emotionally drained. Other symptoms of the disease, in addition to pain and constant fatigue, are feeling "down" and anxious; numbness and tingling in the hands, arms, feet and legs; sleep disturbance; tension headaches; subjective swelling; bladder spasms and irritable bowel. Cold weather, extremes of activity, fluctuation of barometric pressure and stress often aggravate the symptoms of fibromyalgia.

Diagnosis and Treatment

Since diagnosis of fibromyalgia is so difficult, a rheumatologist does extensive detective work sorting out the patient's medical history and performing a thorough examination. Said Dr. Schimmer, "When we examine the patient we will find tender 'trigger points' in certain patterns over the neck, shoulders, chest, lower back and hips, and this helps to separate fibromyalgia from other conditions."

Non-steroidal anti-inflammatory agents are used, as are corticosteroids, but they often do not help. Efforts are made to improve sleep. Non-pharmacologic treatment emphasizes aerobic exercise, particularly water aerobics. Light sports, such as swimming, bicycling and walking, are also encouraged. Some people find biofeedback, hypnotherapy, massage and support groups helpful. Many patients, in an acute stage of their disease, worry about having bone cancer or other ominous disorders; some become very anxious. Psychotherapy can help certain individuals overcome the attendant stresses of this disorder.

See also BIOFEEDBACK; MASSAGE THERAPY; PAIN; PSYCHOTHERAPIES; SUPPORT GROUPS.

Epstein, Steven A., Gary Kay, Daniel Clauw et al. "Psychiatric Disorders in Patients with Fibromyalgia: A Multicenter Investigation." *Psychosomatics* 40, no. 1 (Jan./Feb. 1999): 57–63.

McIlwain, Harris H., and Debra Fulghum. *The Fibromyalgia Handbook.* New York: Henry Holt, 1996.

Starlanyl, Devin. *Fibromyalgia and Chronic Myofascial Pain Syndrome: A Survival Manual.* Oakland, Calif.: New Harbinger Publications, 1996.

Williamson, Miryam Ehrlich. *Fibromyalgia: A Comprehensive Approach: What You Can Do about Chronic Pain and Fatigue.* New York: Walker and Company, 1996.

fight or flight response   A reaction to a threatening or stressful situation in which the sympathetic nervous system (SNS) mobilizes the body for maximum use of energy. When a person faces a threatening situation, the SNS causes many physiological reactions, including faster heartbeat, deeper breathing, slower digestion and rising blood pressure.

See also AGORAPHOBIA; ANXIETY DISORDERS; FEAR; PHOBIA.

5-Hydroxytroptophan   See NEUROTRANSMITTERS; SEROTONIN.

flashbacks Images of events that occurred in the past that recur in the mind. This happens to people who have post-traumatic stress disorder (PTSD) as well as victims of violent crimes or witnesses to violent crimes. Flashbacks can be distressing, make individuals fearful, cause insomnia or seriously disrupt sleep. Flashbacks of psychedelic experiences induced in the past by psychedelic drugs such as LSD have been reported.

See also POST-TRAUMATIC STRESS DISORDER.

flat affect An affect or mood that indicates the absence of signs of affective expression. This is often a common symptom of depression.

See also AFFECT; AFFECTIVE DISORDERS; BLUNTED AFFECT; DEPRESSION.

flight of ideas See THOUGHT DISORDERS.

flooding A behavioral therapy technique in which the individual is repeatedly exposed to the precipitating factor for a phobia, panic attack or ritualistic behavior, in combination with a relaxation technique until the individual no longer responds to the situation with anxiety or subsequent ritualistic behavior.

See also BEHAVIORAL THERAPY; DESENSITIZATION.

fluoxetine hydrochloride An antidepressant drug (trade name: Prozac). It is not in the categories of tricyclic antidepressants or monoamine oxidase inhibitors. The efficacy of fluoxetine in treatment of major depression is comparable to that of the tricyclic antidepressant drugs. Most studies have been of moderately depressed outpatients; its efficacy in severely depressed hospitalized patients has not been established. In limited studies in those with bipolar disorder, fluoxetine was useful in treating the depressed component of this illness. The selection of fluoxetine appears to be most appropriate for patients who are at special risk for sedative, hypotensive and anticholinergic side effects caused by other antidepressants. Fluoxetine has a much lower overdose toxicity than other antidepressant medications.

See also ANTIDEPRESSANT MEDICATIONS; DEPRESSION; PHARMACOLOGICAL APPROACH.

flurazepam Generic name for the benzodiazepine medication known as Dalmane.

See also BENZODIAZEPINE DRUGS; PHARMACOLOGICAL APPROACH.

folie a deux A rare psychotic disorder, also known as "shared paranoid disorder." It occurs when the delusions of one individual develop in another person who is in a close relationship with the first individual. In such a situation, the second person did not have a delusional disorder before the onset of the disorder in the other person. Once this disorder was known as paranoid disorder; when it was originally described in the late 19th century, it was given the French name *folie a deux*, or folly between two.

Specifically how this disorder develops is not clearly understood. However, it seems to involve the presence of a dominant person with an established delusional system and a more submissive person who develops the induced disorder, thereby gaining acceptance of the more dominant individual.

See also DELUSION.

folk medicine See COMPLEMENTARY THERAPIES; CROSS-CULTURAL INFLUENCES; FAITH HEALING.

forgetting An inability to retrieve stored memories. This is a common occurrence; mentally healthy people forget short-term as well as long-term memories. They may forget recently made appointments, forget what their boss told them earlier in the day or forget occurrences that happened in childhood. Forgetting is a common experience, just as is the experience of suddenly remembering something that was previously forgotten.

How memory changes over time has been the subject for many scientific studies and has concentrated primarily on two factors, inhibition and loss of retrieval clues. Inhibition refers to how similar kinds of learning, either before or after the event to be remembered, interferes with later recall of that event. Theories about retrieval cues involve the knowledge that recall is easier regarding familiar people, things and situations.

Other theories hold that individuals have "selective" memories and may forget events or situations previously encountered that were unpleasant or even traumatic. This concept is related to repression, which suggests forgetting as a coping mechanism.

Forgetting may be a symptoms of some disorders, such as Parkinson's disease, multiple-infarct dementia, or Alzheimer's disease.

See also MEMORY; PARKINSON'S DISEASE; REPRESSION.

formication   A sensation that ants or other insects are crawling on the skin, sometimes resulting from abuse of cocaine or other drugs. This unpleasant sensation should be distinguished from a delusion in which the individual may believe they have ants, insects or worms on or in them. Scratching of the skin may result in redness or rash and a misdiagnosis of a skin disease.

See also COCAINE; DELUSION.

foster homes   Homes in which children are placed on a temporary or permanent basis. The concept of removing children from abusive or absent parents developed during the latter half of the 20th century. Usually such children are placed by court order or at least at the recommendation of a social service agency. Children of criminals or of known drug abusers or child abusers are sometimes placed in foster homes. Foster homes are usually those of "intact" families, and new residents are incorporated into the family structure as "members." Psychiatric mental health support is provided for the residents as well as for members of the foster family. Usually a formal arrangement with a court or community mental health center is mandatory. Foster homes are regularly monitored by a placement agency.

Children who have grown up in orphanages or mentally retarded children are sometimes placed in foster homes. In some cases, children return to their original families; in other cases, they may continue to live in the same or other foster homes or return to an institution.

fragile X syndrome   A cause of mental retardation resulting from an inherited defect of the X chromosome. After Down's syndrome it is the most common cause of mental retardation in males. Approximately one in 1,500 men is affected; one in 1,000 women is a carrier. The disorder happens in families, and while males are mainly affected, women may carry the genetic defect responsible for the disorder and pass it on to some of their sons or their daughters, who may become carriers of the defect. About one-third of female carriers have some degree of mental impairment.

When a young couple knows that there is a history of the syndrome on either side of the family, genetic counseling should be sought before planning a family.

See also DOWN'S SYNDROME; GENETIC COUNSELING; MENTAL RETARDATION; MENTAL RETARDATION in BIBLIOGRAPHY.

free association   See ASSOCIATION, FREE.

free love   A term meaning sexual permissiveness as advocated by such individuals as George Bernard Shaw, Bertrand Russell, H.G. Wells and, at one time, by the Oneida, New York, community. The permissiveness includes making love with anyone without any restrictions. During the 1950s and 1960s, in the era of "hippies," many young people believed in and engaged in free love as a protest against established values and institutions in the United States. At that time free love was also one of the characteristics of communal living.

Disillusionment on the part of many women and disappointment with the lack of long-term committed relationships have since put limitations on the movement's popularity. The increase of sexually transmitted diseases such as herpes simplex, papilloma virus and AIDS virus infections have severely limited the free love movement in most Western cultures. However, much freer sexual mores exist in certain subcultures, such as central Africa.

See also MARRIAGE.

Freud, Sigmund (1856–1939)   Austrian neurologist and psychiatrist and the originator of psychoanalysis (the "talking cure") as a therapeutic process. Freud's contributions to the study of mental health influenced later thoughts on psychology, child development and personal interactions. His writings provided possibilities for major advances in the scientific understanding of human behavior, particularly in bringing the topic of sex to the attention of the general public and as an appropriate topic for scientific research. Although controversial during his time and continuing to be so, Freud's theories affected subsequent approaches to psychology and psychiatry.

His many writings have influenced literature, history and social sciences. Among his books are *The Interpretation of Dreams* (1900), *Three Essays on the Theory of Sexuality* (1905), *Totem and Taboo* (1913), *Beyond the Pleasure Principle* (1920) and *The Ego and the Id* (1923).

Freud based his treatment on helping the patient bring back to consciousness repressed emotions, reviving and reliving painful experiences buried in the unconscious, thereby releasing painful emotions. Freud replaced the early use of hypnosis with interpretation of dreams, free association and analysis of behavioral and speech lapses now known as "Freudian slips."

The "Freudian view" (Freudianism) holds that people are driven by unconscious and particularly psychosexual impulses. In his method of free association, unconscious sexual conflicts and their repression are viewed as factors in neuroses. These concepts became the keystones of the new discipline he called psychoanalysis, which focused on procedures including interpretation of dreams, analysis of resistance, the transference relationship between the therapist and the patient and a study of the patient's current symptoms in terms of his psychosexual development and early experiences. Freud's theory of personality holds that personality and character traits come from experiences based on early stages of psychosexual development. In psychoanalysis over a period of years, he sought to reconstruct the patient's psychic life from early childhood to the present.

According to Freud's writings, personality has three parts, or forces: the id, representing the instincts one is born with and still harbors in the unconscious, the superego, the voice of civilization and restraint, and the ego, which tries to reconcile the two with each other and with the outside world. There are, of course, inevitable conflicts among these forces.

According to Freud, once the needs of hunger and thirst are met, the id is driven by sexual desire and aggression. In his view, a young child has sexual feelings toward the opposite-sex parent and hates and fears the same-sex parent. Thus a boy who does not rechannel such urges may develop an Oedipus complex and girls may develop an Electra complex.

Freud termed the sex drive or sex energy "libido." He viewed libido as one of two major human instincts, the other being thanatos, or the death instinct. Freud believed that much nonsexual behavior is actually motivated by a redirection of the libido in a process called sublimation, through which sexual motivations are expressed in other ways, such as painting or other creative forms of expression.

Psychosocial Development

Freud believed that psychosocial development included a series of phases. The oral stage comes first, lasting from birth to about one year of age, in which the child derives pleasure from sucking and stimulating the lips and mouth. The second, or anal stage, occurs during the child's second year, during which interest is focused on elimination. The third stage, lasting from about age three to about five or six, is the phallic stage, in which a boy focuses his interest on his penis and derives pleasure from masturbation. During this stage, a girl realizes that she has no penis, envies boys and feels cheated or believes that she once had a penis and that it was cut off. She may even hate her mother for this defect. The latency stage comes next and lasts into adolescence. During this stage, sexual impulses are repressed, but in the genital stage, which begins with adolescence, young women's and young men's interests become more specifically genital. This stage is less self-directed and increasingly directed toward other people as appropriate sexual objects.

According to Freud, people do not always mature from one stage to the next and might remain fixated at one or more stages, so that most adults have some traces of earlier stages in their adult personalities.

Attitudes About Women

Freud believed that "anatomy is destiny" and that women's lack of a penis was a major factor in personality development, leading to lifelong feelings of imperfection, inferiority and jealousy. He believed that women were inherently passive and had masochistic feelings about sexual intercourse.

Freud suggested that women experienced two kinds of orgasm, a clitoral orgasm and a vaginal orgasm (dual-orgasm theory). He believed that the vaginal orgasm was better and more mature than the clitoral orgasm. Later researchers, including Masters and Johnson, disagreed with any distinction between clitoral and vaginal orgasms, as their research indicated that physiologically, female orgasms are the same, regardless of the source of stimulation. Additionally, they found that some clitoral stimulation is almost always involved in reaching orgasm.

In his psychiatric practice, Freud heard reports from women of sexual abuse from their fathers and regarded this as fantasy and an innate need to compensate for their lack of a penis. Followers of Freud, such as Helene Deutsch, accepted Freud's view and argued that a degree of paternal seductiveness was essential to normal feminine development.

Some of Freud's contemporaries as well as later psychiatrists differed with Freudian views, many of which were offensive to the patriarchal Victorian culture that found shocking the notion that innocent children and well-bred women had sexual desires. The first expressions of controversy, in about 1911–1912, by Carl Jung and Alfred Adler, included views that Freud overestimated the role of sexual conflict in developing neuroses. Later, in the early 1920s, Karen Horney initiated and led an effort to indicate flaws in Freud's viewpoints centered around penis envy; her work influenced many subsequent practitioners and writers.

Feminists have objected to much of Freud's theory, including the notion that women are inferior to men and that they are sexually masochistic and passive. Feminists argue that psychoanalytic theory is a male-centered theory. Regarding the dual-orgasm theory, feminists state that Freud's notion includes the necessity of the presence of a penis for sexual satisfaction. Contemporary feminists have denounced Freud as a male chauvinist.

See also ELECTRA COMPLEX; OEDIPUS COMPLEX; PSYCHOANALYSIS; PSYCHOTHERAPIES.

Appignanesi, Lisa, and John Forrester. *Freud's Women.* New York: Basic Books, 1992.

Krull, Marianne. *Freud and His Father.* New York: W.W. Norton, 1986.

Kahn, Ada P., and Linda Hughey Holt. *The A to Z of Women's Sexuality.* Alameda, Calif.: Hunter House, 1992.

Lerman, Hannah. *A Note in Freud's Eye: From Psychoanalysis to the Psychology of Women.* New York: Springer Publishing, 1986.

Mahony, Patrick J. *On Defining Freud's Discourse.* New Haven: Yale University Press, 1989.

Mahoney, E. R. *Human Sexuality.* New York: McGraw-Hill, 1983.

Wallace, Edwin R. *Freud and Anthropology: A History and Reappraisal.* New York: International Universities Press, 1983.

Westerlund, Elaine. "Freud on Sexual Trauma: An Historical Review of Seduction and Betrayal." *Psychology of Women Quarterly* 10 (1986).

Freudian slips   See FREUD, SIGMUND; SLIPS OF THE TONGUE.

friends (friendship)   Friendship is unique among human relationships in the degree of freedom it allows. Individuals have little or no choice in blood relations or neighbors; marriage and employment ties are made cautiously and severed with difficulty. Friendships flow along more easily and casually, developing, changing and dissolving sometimes with little effort or even awareness. Friendships are more flexible and variable than other relationships. Some friendships evolve from shared interests, some simply from a shared history and compatible personalities. Qualities most appreciated in friends include loyalty, trust and an ability to keep a confidence. People want to feel that they can rely on their friends and that their friends will be open and honest with them.

Friendships are involved in maintaining good mental health. Friendships can be supportive in our daily lives as well as during periods of turmoil or crisis. Individuals who experience depression often report a lack of friends, although having a wide circle of friends is not a preventive factor for depression. Some reports have indicated that individuals who have many social contacts may be healthier and actually live longer than those who do not.

Friendships also affect mental health because they may challenge or be challenged by other relationships in contemporary life. For example, an employer, supervisor or teacher, particularly one with an authoritarian personality, may feel that friendships among students or employees give them too much power as a group. In the workplace, a friendship may dissolve when one is promoted and the other stays behind. A friendship may be broken or changed when one friend marries, and disruptive friendships can weaken a marriage. A friend of the opposite sex is frequently unsettling to a spouse or lover. Friends who do not meet with parents' approval can also be a source of family conflict. Friends who decide to share housing or enter into a business partnership sometimes learn about undesirable qualities of the other that could be ignored when the relationship was less formal.

The freedom inherent in friendship has its negative as well as positive aspects. There are fewer social rules about friendship than other relationships, and two people may have entirely different expectations from each other until those expectations clash. The lack of structure for friendships may also allow one friend to take the other for granted until the friendship disintegrates.

Among early humans, friendship was a banding together to avoid danger. In contemporary life, friendship may again play a role in combating the physical and psychological dangers of high crime and anonymity of modern urban life.

The nuclear family of modern life puts increasing pressures on family members to be one another's friends. Parents and children, husbands and wives who, in the past, may have had a network of relatives and longtime friends now turn to their immediate family for friendship, not always with satisfactory results.

A Gallup poll reported in 1990 showed that the typical American places much importance on friendship and indicates some frustrations that people have in forming friendships. Friendship re-

quires time and a certain degree of flexibility. Twenty-five percent of the total surveyed said that they did not have enough time to spend with friends, and 46 percent of those who said they would like to have more friends indicated, almost in contradiction, that they did not have enough time to spend with the friends they had. Working women and couples with children at home were most likely to feel that they had insufficient time to spend with friends.

The survey showed that women and men approach friendship quite differently. Women tended to form more intimate relationships with other women than men with men. One to one activities that promote conversation are more popular with women, whereas men are more likely to get together in groups for activities such as sports or cards. Men rely on their wives for emotional support rather than other men; but many women, even those who are married, often rely on other women. Women are more likely than men to have a best friend of the same sex. Almost a third of the men surveyed said a woman was their best friend.

When participants were asked about arguments with friends, those under age 30 reported more disagreements. Friendship evidently becomes more tranquil with age, possibly because friends settle their differences and learn to recognize sore spots and perhaps because age enables people to recognize and discard difficult relationships.

The survey also measured longevity of friendship. Half of those surveyed keep in touch with a friend they made when they were younger than age 17, and half also keep in touch with friends who live miles away.

People make friends in many ways. In the Gallup report, 51 percent of the 18- to 29-year-olds made most of their friends at school. Of the 30- to 49–year-olds, 51 percent said they made most of their friends through work. From the age of 50 and up, friends came from a greater variety of sources, including church, work, clubs or other organizations.

Despite the emphasis that the participants in the Gallup survey placed on friendship, 71 percent said they did not try particularly hard to make new friends. This may be a reflection of the fact that 75 percent of those surveyed were satisfied with their current friendships; but this may also be a product of conventional wisdom that to give the appearance of eagerly and actively searching for friends in a programmed manner is usually counterproductive.

DeStefano, Linda. "Pressures of Modern Life Bring Increased Importance to Friendship." *Gallup Poll Monthly* (Mar. 1990).

Marty, Martin. *Friendship.* Allen, Tex.: Argus Communications, 1980.

frigidity An obsolete term for the inability of a woman to obtain satisfaction (usually orgasm) during sexual intercourse. Sex researchers Masters and Johnson coined the term "female orgasmic dysfunction" to replace this term. A woman's lack of satisfaction during sexual intercourse may result from a combination of many factors, including a lack of desirability of the partner, lack of adequate stimulation, lack of communication between the partners concerning sexual behaviors and desires and cultural rejection of certain practices. In addition, the fear of desertion or pregnancy may interfere with satisfaction. The amount of time necessary for a woman's arousal and satisfaction varies widely between individuals.

In some cases lack of interest in sexual activity and lack of satisfaction may result from depression, stress, fatigue or alcohol. Narcotics and some tranquilizers may also reduce interest in sexual activity.

Counseling, therapy and prescribed sexual exercises help many women who have orgasmic dysfunction to become more physically responsive and emotionally free to enjoy sexual pleasures.

See also DUAL-ORGASM THEORY; FREUD, SIGMUND; ORGASM; SEXUAL DYSFUNCTION.

frontal lobe Part of the cerebral hemispheres at the frontal or anterior side of the brain, associated with personality factors in humans. Ability for foresight, initiative, judgment (especially regarding consequences of behavior) and tact is affected by frontal lobe defects; but intelligence is apparently not affected.

Frontal Lobe Syndrome

A mental disorder due to lesions in the frontal lobe; it is also known as organic personality syndrome.

Symptoms may include impaired social judgment and impulse control, marked apathy and impairment of purposeful behavior.

Frontal Perceptual Disorders

Difficulties in performing certain problem-solving tasks, such as matching numbers, letters or other symbols, seen in individuals with tumors or other lesions of the frontal lobes.

Leukotomy

A surgical procedure, also called frontal lobotomy, involving severing certain nerve fibers connecting the frontal lobes with the rest of the brain. It was performed as therapy for individuals suffering from certain forms of chronic psychosis resulting in undesirable behaviors or for certain forms of pain. This procedure is no longer used. Cingulotomy is used in certain cases of severe, treatment-resistant depression and obsessive-compulsive disorder.

See also BRAIN.

frottage A form of sexual disorder in which the individual persistently seeks sexual excitement and enjoyment by rubbing against other people. The term is derived from the French, meaning "rubbing," and the individual who displays this type of behavior is known as a *frotteur.* Such an individual may be fearful of engaging in a mature sexual relationship.

See also SEXUAL DYSFUNCTION.

frustration Interference with impulses or desired actions by internal or external forces. For example, internal forces are inhibitions and mental conflicts, and external forces may be from parents, teachers and friends, as well as the rules of society. A mentally healthy person is usually able to cope with a good degree of frustration despite obstacles.

People who are repeatedly and constantly frustrated respond in many ways, some with anger, hostility, aggression or depression; others become withdrawn and passive. Some children and adults who are constantly frustrated show regressive behavior and may become unable to cope with problems on their own.

Modern life is filled with frustrations, from childhood through old age. Some children are frustrated by their parents' high expectations, and many parents are frustrated by their inability to provide material goods for their children. Many individuals are frustrated by lack of job opportunities, layoffs and lack of advancement on their jobs. Other individuals are frustrated in their marriages, while some single individuals feel frustrated by their lack of a partner. Many who are not satisfied in sexual relationships experience ongoing frustration. As people age, many become frustrated by their increasing inability to do things they did at earlier ages. Frustration sets in when retired individuals cannot function independently and must live with their children or in nursing homes.

fugue A psychiatric term for a state of altered consciousness that causes individuals to suddenly flee from home or work, forget their entire past and start a new life with a new name. After recovery, such individuals will recall their earlier lives but not events that occurred during the fugue. This state is also referred to as amnesia and may last hours or days. During a fugue of a few hours, individuals may show symptoms of agitation and confusion. During dissociative or fugue states, people "allow" themselves to behave in a manner that their normal consciousness and good judgment would not permit.

Among many possible causes of fugues are head injuries, epilepsy and dementia. In other cases, fugue states that become extended may be due to an unconscious wish to avoid unpleasant or threatening situations.

Treatment for fugue episodes (when the individuals are brought to treatment) may include hypnotic suggestions or use of amobarbital sodium. Such episodes have been the focus of plots for movies and novels, because the public seems fascinated by others' experiences of amnesia, perhaps out of a secret wish to escape from their own life situations.

See also AMNESIA; DISSOCIATIVE DISORDERS.

GABA   See GAMMA-AMINOBUTYRIC ACID.

GAD (generalized anxiety disorders)   See ANXIETY DISORDERS.

galvanic skin response (GSR)   Measurement of changes in resistance in the skin to emotional or psychological stimulation as measured by an electronic device. Electrical resistance is reduced by sweating activity induced by emotional arousal. As sweat glands are activated by activity, the GSR measures reflect changes in the sympathetic nervous system.

Skin responses are measured by pairing an imperceptibly small electrical current between two electrodes on the skin. Increases in conductance (lowered resistance) are considered reflective of increased autonomic (emotional) activity.

See also SYMPATHETIC NERVOUS SYSTEM.

gambling   Gambling is considered to be a compulsion or addiction when it becomes the only important thing in one's life and all of one's efforts are aimed toward obtaining money to gamble. Although gambling does not involve ingesting a substance, many of the characteristics of compulsive gambling are similar to alcoholism. The National Council on Compulsive Gambling and Gamblers Anonymous have estimated that there are 6 million compulsive gamblers in the United States. The typical compulsive gambler is a married man in his early to mid-thirties who is employed in a field that involves money and possibly high risk such as investment, business or law. Compulsive gamblers are usually outgoing, generous and gregarious but are prone to sudden negative mood swings. Even in serious stages of compulsive gambling, the addict will express concern about his health but not about his addiction. Gamblers Anonymous offers a recovery program similar to Alcoholics Anonymous. The Council on Compulsive Gambling offers a crisis intervention hot line for compulsive gamblers and their families.

People gamble for many reasons. Some simply enjoy the sociability and atmosphere of events surrounding the activity. Some people begin gambling because it helps to relieve a stressful situation. The fascination with the game and the prospect of winning make certain individuals forget their problems. Others find the risk and unpredictability of the game exciting and stimulating. In addition to wanting the actual winnings, some derive a sense of power and importance from winning. They have a sense that when they win, people are watching and admiring them. Some may gamble out of rebellion, since gambling is thought to be sinful by some religious groups. Despite its sometimes seedy, underworld aspects, gambling may also appear to be glamorous to some people. Films frequently depict expensively dressed, sophisticated characters gambling in casinos in exotic locations.

Teenage Gambling

In 1998, the American Academy of Pediatrics reported results of a study indicating that between 76 percent and 91 percent of all teens will have gambled by the time they are seniors in high school. Researchers from Children's Hospital, Harvard Medical School, Boston, discovered that adolescents who gambled reported participating in an increased number of at-risk behaviors in other areas of their lives. Overall, illegal drug use was nearly doubled by teens who had gambled in the past year compared with teens who had not. In addition, gambling teens were approximately twice as likely as non-gambling teens to have been in a fight or to have carried a weapon in the last 30 days. Because research has shown most adult pathologic gamblers start gambling in adolescence and develop their addiction over 10 or more years, the researchers emphasized the need for early intervention programs for teens who gamble.

For information, contact:

Gamblers Anonymous
3255 Wilshire Boulevard, Suite 610
Los Angeles, CA 90010
Phone: (211) 386-8789

National Council on Problem Gambling
John Jay College of Criminal Justice
445 W. 59th Street
New York, NY 10019
Phone: (212) 765-3833

Black, Donald W., and Trent Moyer. "Clinical Features and Psychiatric Comorbidity of Subjects with Pathological Gambling Behavior." *Psychiatric Services* 49, no. 11 (Nov. 1998): 1434–1439.

gamma-aminobutyric acid (GABA) A neurotransmitter in the brain that tends to result in an inhibition of the release of activating neurotransmitters, such as norepinephrine. Some medications bind to the GABA receptors; these include alprazolam, a benzodiazepine (popularly known as Xanax). (A drug "binds" to chemical receptors that are shaped to receive and use it rather than other chemicals.) When taken in therapeutic doses, both diazepam and alprazolam change the shape of the receptor molecule (GABA) they share. Chemical interactions between alprazolam and the diazepam receptor alter metabolism of GABA, which in turn produces a change in cell biochemistry. As this occurs, anxiety is reduced.

See also ALPRAZOLAM; ANXIETY; BENZODIAZEPINE MEDICATIONS; NEUROTRANSMITTERS; PANIC DISORDER; PHARMACOLOGIC THERAPY in BIBLIOGRAPHY.

Ganser's syndrome See DISSOCIATIVE DISORDERS.

gay A word that in the latter part of the 20th century refers to male or female homosexuals, but more often to males. Female homosexuals are known as lesbians.

See also GAY LIBERATION; HOMOSEXUALITY; LESBIANISM; SEXUALITY.

gay liberation A social movement during the mid-20th century in which homosexuals asserted their rights to their individual sexual orientations, sought recognition of their behavior as normal and encouraged reduction of societal prejudices. Many gay organizations were formed to promote homosexual causes and interests.

See also HOMOSEXUALITY; LESBIANISM.

gender identity disorder Gender identity disorder is a type of psychosexual disorder in which an individual's gender identity is incongruent with his or her anatomical sex. Many individuals who believe that they are men or women in the body of the other sex experience anxieties, and some individuals have surgical sex change operations.

According to the *Diagnostic and Statistical Manual of Mental Disorders,* 4th ed. (American Psychiatric Association, 1994), there are two major components of gender identity disorder, both of which must be present to make the diagnosis: (1) a strong and persistent cross-gender identification, which is the desire to be, or the insistence that one is, of the other sex and (2) persistent discomfort about one's assigned sex, or a sense of inappropriateness in the gender role of that sex. Additionally, to make the diagnosis there must be clinically significant distress or impairment in social, occupational or other important areas of functioning.

See also GENDER ROLE; SEXUAL FEARS.

gender role Attitudes and behaviors that are culturally and socially associated with maleness or femaleness, which are expressed to varying degrees by individuals. For example, in Western cultures, the gender role for many women was historically passive and submissive, until the "women's liberation" movement and "sexual revolution" during the latter half of the 20th century. Along with many societal changes, gender roles have also changed significantly. An example is child care, which is no longer exclusively the woman's role, and earning the larger part of the family income is no longer exclusively the man's role. However, changes in gender roles have led to many contemporary mental health problems, such as women's conflicts between motherhood and career and men's fears of inferiority when wives advance more rapidly in their career than they do in theirs.

gene The part of the chromosome containing a code for a specific functional molecule of an organism.

general adaptation syndrome A feeling we now refer to as stress; it was coined by Hans Selye (1907–1982), an Austrian-born Canadian endocrinologist and psychologist in his landmark book, *The Stress of Life* (1956). The GAS is the manifestation of stress in the whole body as it develops over time. It is through the GAS that various internal organs, especially the endocrine glands and the nervous system, help individuals adjust to constant changes occurring in and around them and to "navigate a steady course toward whatever they consider a worthwhile goal."

Dr. Selye was a pioneer in an area that has continued to look at stress as a threat to wellness. The secret of health, he contended, was in successful adjustment to ever-changing conditions. Life, he said, is largely a process of adaptation to the circumstances in which we exist. He viewed many nervous and emotional disturbances, such as high blood pressure and some cardiovascular problems, gastric and duodenal ulcers and certain types of allergic problems as essentially diseases of adaptation.

Selye called his concept the general adaptation syndrome because it is produced only by agents which have a "general" effect on large portions of the body. He called it "adaptive" because it stimulates defense mechanisms. He used the term "syndrome" because individual manifestations are coordinated with and interdependent on each other.

There are three stages in the GAS. Individuals go through the stages many times each day, as well as throughout life. Whatever demands are made on us, we progress through the sequence. The first is an alarm reaction, or the bodily expression of a generalized call for our defensive forces. We experience surprise and anxiety because of our inexperience in dealing with a new situation. The second stage is resistance, when we have learned to cope with the new situation efficiently. The third stage is exhaustion, or a depletion of our energy reserves, which leads to fatigue. Adaptability, Selye continued, was a finite amount of vitality (thought of as capital) with which we are born. We can withdraw from it throughout life, but we cannot add to it.

See also COPING; DEFENSE MECHANISMS; DISSTRESS; EUSTRESS; HARDINESS; HOMEOSTASIS; PSYCHONEUROIMMUNOLOGY; SELYE, HANS; STRESS.

Kahn, Ada P. *Stress A to Z: The Sourcebook for Facing Everyday Challenges.* Facts On File, 2000.
Selye, Hans. *The Stress of Life.* New York: McGraw-Hill, 1956.
———. *Stress without Distress.* Philadelphia: J. B. Lippincott Company, 1974.

generalized anxiety disorders (GAD) See ANXIETY DISORDERS.

generic drug A prescription drug sold under its chemical (generic) name rather than under a patented trade name. Names for generic drugs are chosen and approved by government agencies.

See also ETHICAL DRUGS.

genetic counseling Advising a family about the risk of occurrence of mental retardation or other inherited conditions and the problems that may arise from their occurrence. Genetic counseling requires considerable training and sensitivity. It is often preferable for a mental health professional to refer appropriate couples to specialized centers for this purpose.

In many cases, the need for counseling is recognized by a pediatrician, an obstetrician or another primary care physician after the delivery of a defective child. Such an urgent and unexpected situation may arouse feelings of guilt, anxiety or anger in both parents and physician. While counseling before pregnancy is preferred, and many advances in antenatal diagnosis are aimed at early detection, occasional unanticipated genetic defects appear after delivery. Unfortunately, some of these (e.g.,

Huntington's disease) cannot be recognized until middle age.

Identification of high-risk couples is one method of prevention of birth defects and mental retardation. Concerned potential parents can be advised of the medical facts regarding the severity and prognosis of the genetic disorder, the risk of its recurrence if they already have a retarded child and options available for managing the affected child and for avoiding recurrence.

Individuals interested in receiving professional advice now have numerous resources. The number of genetic counseling centers has increased rapidly in recent years; there are now more than 200 major university-based centers with many satellites.

The March of Dimes Foundation directs its efforts toward prevention of birth defects and improving the outcome of pregnancies. This organization also publishes an international directory of resources relevant to genetic disorders and can refer parents to appropriate genetic clinics.

See also MENTAL RETARDATION; GENETICS in BIBLIOGRAPHY.

Grossman, Herbert J., ed. *AMA Handbook on Mental Retardation.* Chicago: American Medical Association, 1987.

genetic disorders Disorders caused totally or partially by faults in inherited genes and chromosomes of an individual's cells. Some genetic disorders, known as congenital, are present at birth. However, many genetic defects do not become apparent until many years later, and many congenital abnormalities are not genetically caused. Most genetic disorders are familial, which means that one has one or more relatives affected by the same disorder. However, there are times when a child is born with a genetic disorder and no family history of a disorder.

INDICATIONS FOR GENETIC COUNSELING

- Family history of an inherited disorder
- Genetic or congenital anomaly in a family member
- Parent who is a known carrier of a chromosomal translocation
- Woman who has previously given birth to a child (children) with chromosomal aberrations
- Parent who is a known carrier of an autosomal recessive disorder in which in utero diagnosis is possible
- Abnormal somatic or behavioral development in a previous child
- Mental retardation of unknown etiology in a previous child
- Pregnancy in a woman over age 35
- Specific ethnic background that may suggest a high rate of genetic abnormality (e.g., Tay-Sachs disease)
- Three or more spontaneous abortions and/or early infant deaths
- Infertility

There are three general categories of genetic disorders: chromosome abnormalities, unifactorial defects and multifactorial disorders.

Chromosome Abnormalities

When a child is born with an abnormal number of whole chromosomes, or extra or missing bits of chromosomes in the cells, this can lead to multiple disturbances and disorders. Down's syndrome and Klinefelter syndrome, forms of mental retardation, are in this category.

Unifactorial Defects

Unifactorial defects are caused by a single defective gene or pair of genes. These disorders are distributed among members of an affected family according to simple laws of inheritance.

Multifactorial Disorders

These are caused by the additive effects of several genes, along with environmental factors. The pattern of inheritance is less straightforward. Many disorders fall into this category, including asthma, insulin-dependent diabetes and some conditions present at birth, such as cleft lip and palate, schizophrenia and manic-depressive (bipolar) disorder. According to a study reported in the early 1980s, the risk for full siblings of a schizophrenic person to develop schizophrenia is 7 to 8 percent, the children of one schizophrenic parent have a 9 to 12 percent risk and the children of two schizophrenic parents have a 35 to 45 percent risk.

In recent years, studies have revealed a possible link between genetic makeup and alcoholism. Scientists also suspect that genetic factors may underlie personality types and particularly disorders such as manic-depression. Genetic disorders are only a partial explanation, however; as with other mental health disorders, environment may also influence the expression of these conditions. Genetic defects in hearing and vision may lead to a misdiagnosis of mental retardation, and children born with Marfan's syndrome (a genetic disorder with symptoms including a gangly, uncoordinated look) may develop depression because they feel "different" from their peers.

See also ALCOHOLISM; DEPRESSION.

genital stage In Freudian theory, the final or mature stage of psychosexual development. The genital stage or phase follows the oral and anal stages and occurs during adolescence, when sexual interest focuses on a relationship with another. When appropriate transitions from other developmental stages did not occur, once may have difficulty adjusting to sexual relationships and/or marriage.

See also FREUD, SIGMUND.

Geodon Trade name for ziprasidone, an "atypical" antipsychotic medication for the treatment of schizophrenia and other psychoses.

geriatric depression The most common mental health disorder among the elderly. According to the National Institute of Mental Health (NIMH), estimates of depression among elderly people ranges from 10 to 65 percent. Other estimates and epidemiologic studies report that 20 percent of geriatric outpatients are clinically depressed and that up to 75 percent of nursing home patients have some type of mental health disorder. Depression in the elderly takes on much the same form as it does in younger people. For example, the depressed person will have a pervasive feeling of hopelessness and helplessness with regard to improving his or her outlook, not show interest in previously enjoyed activities, may experience insomnia and may become easily distracted and bored.

See also AGING; DEPRESSION; ELDERLY PARENTS.

geriatric depression rating scale (GDRS) A specific screening device to measure depression in the elderly. The GDRS is a 30-item tool with a simple yes/no format that takes only about five to 10 minutes. It has well-established reliability and validity when used with the elderly. The GDRS differs from the Hamilton depression inventory (Ham-D) in that it does not have physical symptoms included on the Ham-D.

See also AGING; DEPRESSION; ELDERLY PARENTS.

Yesavage, J. A. et al. "The Geriatric Depression Rating Scale: Comparison with Other Self-Report and Psychiatric Rating Scales." In *Assessment in Geriatric Psychopharmacology,* edited by T. Crook, S. Ferris, and R. Bartus. New Canaan, Conn.: Mark Powley and Associates, 1983.

geropsychiatry A specialized form of mental health care that addresses the complexities involved between mental and physical illness in the elderly. For example, an elderly patient who might appear to have psychotic symptoms may be experiencing symptoms of toxicity resulting from taking two or more incompatible drugs. Many psychosomatic disorders and chronic conditions manifest themselves with symptoms of depression.

Many physicians specializing in geropsychiatry are located in community hospitals where they can provide a safe and secure environment and offer psychological evaluation in conjunction with medical testing and liaison services for elderly patients being treated for medical or surgical conditions.

An increasing number of hospitals are adding this component to their mental health programs. Some hospitals contract with various organizations who provide these services on a contract basis.

See also AGING; DEPRESSION; ELDERLY PARENTS; GERIATRIC DEPRESSION.

gestalt psychology A type of therapy based on the concept that the whole is more important than the sum of its parts, or that "wholeness" is more important than individual components of behavior and perception. It aims to increase self-awareness by looking at all aspects of an individual within his or her environment. It achieved a good degree of popularity as a means of coping with personal problems and is still practiced by some therapists.

The movement toward this type of psychology was founded in Germany in the early 1900s by a group that adopted the name *gestalt,* meaning "form, pattern, or configuration."

See also PSYCHOTHERAPIES.

Gilles de la Tourette syndrome   See TOURETTE SYNDROME.

glass ceiling   An impenetrable but almost invisible barrier perceived by working women that they believe keeps many of them from rising to the top of their field despite their good qualifications, experience and hard work. This frustration leads to anxiety, depression and less than optimal mental health.

The glass ceiling may take many forms. Qualified women already in the organization may be passed over as men are brought into high-level positions in the organization from the outside for the sake of providing a fresh outlook and new blood. In organizations involving teamwork and negotiations, discussions may be held in such a way that women are kept on the periphery. Teasing and harassment of women may discourage them and make it difficult for some of them to perform. Women who have a "mannish" style may be hired over women who are more feminine and then thought to be strange and unacceptable because they have masculine characteristics. Women in lower-level positions are sometimes given responsible, demanding work that is reflected in neither their title nor salary. As women attempt to progress in an organization, they may be frustrated by performance standards that are higher for them than for men. Women may also be limited by assumptions that there is a feminine management style that is more passive and nurturing toward fellow workers and less goal-oriented and driven than the masculine style.

Women who do make it past the glass ceiling frequently credit the influence of a mentor, spouse or parent. Some women have decided to avoid the glass ceiling by striking out on their own.

See also MENTOR; WOMEN'S LIBERATION MOVEMENT.

Mills, D. Quinn. *Not Like Our Parents: How the Baby Boom Generation Is Changing America.* New York: William Morrow, 1987.

global warming   The idea that human activities can rapidly change the earth's climate; it is a cause for concern and anxiety for people all over the world.

Jean Fourier, a French physicist, was the first to understand the "greenhouse" effect. In 1824 he suggested that the earth stays warm at night because its atmosphere traps sun-warmed gases in the same way a greenhouse holds heated hair. In 1892 Svante Arrhenius, a Swedish physical chemist, predicted that if levels of carbon dioxide in the atmosphere doubled, the average temperature of the earth would rise between 1.5 and 4 degrees Celsius, close to the prediction most climatologists share today.

Activists continue to debate and protest threats to the ecology of the world, such as cutting down rain forests and depleting water supplies.

globus hystericus   See LUMP IN THE THROAT.

gonorrhea   See SEXUALLY TRANSMITTED DISEASES.

"granny dumping"   The term applied to the elderly and often confused Americans who are being abandoned on hospital emergency room doorsteps. According to a report in the *Bulletin* of the American Association of Retired Persons (AARP) (Sept. 1991), anecdotal reports indicate that the number of abandoned elderly is increasing. As of the end of 1991, congressional committees were looking into the problem. Many caregivers feel overwhelmed and unable to continue. According to AARP legislative director John Rother, this is a symptom of the inadequacies of the long-term care policies in the United States. Emergency room physicians say families are so stressed in part because Medicare does not pay for custodial nursing home care or at-home long-term care, because little respite care is available and because families in crisis are often unaware of community resources.

See also AGING; RETIREMENT; AGING in BIBLIOGRAPHY.

"'Granny Dumping': New Pain for U.S. Elders." *Bulletin,* American Association of Retired Persons, vol. 32, no. 8 (Sept. 1991).

grief   An intensely painful emotional reaction caused by the loss of a loved one. Although the expression of grief is unique to each individual, there are recognized stages of grief (bereavement) that have some common characteristics for most people.

At first there may be numbness and an unwillingness to recognize the death (denial). These are defense mechanisms that help the individual cope with the pain of the loss. Numbness is a pervasive feeling that enables the mourner to get through the experience of the funeral and the first few days following the death of the loved one; this may last from a few days to a few months. Hallucinations are also common among the recently bereaved; in some cases, they believe they see the deceased person walk into the room. In the case of a deceased infant or child, the parent may think they see the child in their crib or bed or hear his or her cry or voice.

When the initial feeling of numbness wears off, the individual may feel anger, despair and overwhelmed by the circumstances; these feelings can lead to depression. Many people feel angry that the deceased person deserted them; these are natural feelings that will pass in time. Other physical symptoms are fairly common; some have headaches, and others have insomnia or gastrointestinal complaints. Attempted suicide is an abnormal expression of grief but is not uncommon. There may be an increase in alcohol intake at this time.

The individual may experience intense feelings of helplessness. One may think, "Could I have prevented this from happening? Why wasn't I powerful enough to do something more?" Such thoughts are part of the human condition. People like to feel that they are in control at all times. Death often leaves those behind feeling helpless.

Many people who have experienced loss say that within two years a bereaved person adjusts to the loss and gets on with his or her life. However, overwhelming feelings of loss do recur, and such moods continue to alternate with those of enthusiasm. In the long run, a positive attitude should overcome the depressed feelings.

How well an individual adjusts after a period of grief depends to some degree on his or her immediate support system. If friends and family are nearby, it may accelerate the recovery process. Widowed persons with no relatives and few friends seem to have the most difficult time adjusting to

their losses. Some parents who have lost an infant try to have another baby within a few years; however, the feeling of loss of the first one never really goes away.

Anniversaries of birthdays, weddings and other events come up every year. Individuals who have suffered a loss should recognize and accept that they will feel sad at certain times. What one does to observe treasured memories is a very individual matter, depending on one's tradition. With time, each person learns to do what feels right. Remembering a loved one with joy, instead of sorrow, is an honor to his or her life.

For individuals who continue to suffer in their grief reaction without relief or help from other sources of support, mental health counseling may help. Getting help when one needs it is sign of strength and wisdom. Appropriate referrals for mental health care can be made by a social worker or physician. Support groups for widows and widowers help many people. Knowing that others had the same emotional reactions may help one cope better with getting on with one's life. Those grieving for the loss of a child may also find help in appropriate support groups.

Many organizations offer telephone information and referral services that also suggest sources of help. Crisis telephone lines and centers and hospital emergency rooms are sometimes a fast way of getting help; these numbers should be listed in a special section of local telephone books.

For information on obtaining brochures on grief, contact:

Mental Health Association of Greater Chicago
104 South Michigan Avenue
Chicago, IL 60603-5901
Phone: (312) 781-7780

Other resources:

Afterloss (monthly newsletter)
P.O. Box 2545
Rancho Mirage, CA 92270
Phone: (800) 423-8811

Pregnancy and Infant Loss Center
1415 Wayzata Boulevard, Suite 105
Wayzata, MN 55391
Phone: (612) 473-9372

Parents of Murdered Children
100 E. Eighth Street, Suite B41
Cincinnati, OH 45202
Phone: (513) 721-LOVE

Elisabeth Kubler-Ross Center (workshops,
    regional groups)
So. Route 616
Head Waters, VA 24442
Phone: (703) 396-3441

Theos (groups in the United States and Canada
    for widowed people)
1301 Clark Building
717 Liberty Avenue
Pittsburgh, PA 15222
Phone: (412) 471-7779

See also BEREAVEMENT; DEATH; DEPRESSION;
INSOMNIA; STILLBIRTH; STRESS; SUDDEN INFANT DEATH
SYNDROME.

Kahn, Ada P. "Living with the Death of a Loved One"
    (brochure). Mental Health Association of Greater
    Chicago, Chicago, 1989.
Kubler-Ross, E. *On Death and Dying.* New York: Macmillan, 1971.
Ramsay, R. W., and R. Noorbergen. *Living with Loss.* New
    York: William Morrow, 1981.

group therapy   A term applying to a wide range
of types of therapies and groups. They may be self-
help support groups, without a trained professional
leader, or they may be led by a mental health professional.

A group organized for group therapy attracts
individuals with similar concerns. For example,
such groups may be for recently widowed persons
(grief), for parents who have lost a child to sudden
infant death syndrome, for individuals who are
suffering from depression or for those wishing to
lose weight. Within the group, individuals find that
others share their feelings and experiences; this
helps them feel less alone and less helpless. Problems in interpersonal relationships are sometimes
benefited by a group therapy experience. Individuals may re-create typical problems in their relationships in the therapy group.

See also PSYCHOTHERAPIES; SUPPORT GROUPS.

GSR   See GALVANIC SKIN RESPONSE.

guardianship   Legal appointment of another person to make decisions for one who is not able or
not legally competent to do so. An individual is
considered legally competent if he or she possesses
the requisite natural or legal qualifications, is capable and is legally fit according to appropriate
statutes. However, a mentally ill individual may
not necessarily need a guardian, as not all mental
illnesses interfere with an individual's decision-
making ability.

For all medical and psychiatric procedures,
informed consent must be given. If the individual
cannot be educated appropriately to give informed
consent, a court will appoint a guardian. Substituted consent is the authorization that is given by a
court-appointed guardian on behalf of the incompetent individual.

See also INFORMED CONSENT; LEGAL ISSUES.

McFarland, Gertrude K., and Mary Durand Thomas. *Psy-
    chiatric Mental Health Nursing.* Philadelphia: J. B. Lip-
    pincott, 1991.

guided imagery   A technique to help the individual generate vivid mental images that help reduce
anxieties. It creates positive mental pictures and
promotes the relaxation necessary for a healing
process. The individual pictures an image, such as a
calm, serene lake with sailboats slowing moving
along, breathes in a relaxed manner and becomes
more relaxed. The individual gradually learns to
notice every detail of the imagined scene and how
the sense of relaxation deepens with this self-talk.
He or she learns too that this sense of calm can be
created at any time by breathing and imagining the
positive vision.

Some case studies and clinical reports suggest
that the guided imagery technique may be helpful
in the treatment of chronic pain, allergies, hypertension, autoimmune diseases and stress-related
gastrointestinal, reproductive and urinary symptoms. In addition to direct effects, imagery may
augment the effectiveness of medical treatments, as
well as help people tolerate the discomforts and
side effects of some medications or invasive procedures.

Imagery has qualities that make it valuable in
mind/body medicine and healing; it can bring

about physiological changes, provide psychological insights and enhance emotional awareness. Use of imagery, in some cases, changes the need for medication. Depending on an individual's medical condition, imagery is best used under the supervision of a physician in conjunction with holistic medicine.

Guided imagery can be used alone or together with other relaxation techniques. It is often used in conjunction with hypnosis, although the two techniques are distinct. While hypnosis serves to induce a special state of mind, imagery consists of a focused, intentional mental activity.

For information:

The Academy for Guided Imagery
P.O. Box 2070
Mill Valley, CA 94942
Phone: (800) 726-2070

See also BREATHING; COMPLEMENTARY THERAPIES; HYPNOSIS; IMMUNE SYSTEM; IRRITABLE BOWEL SYNDROME; RELAXATION; STRESS.

Kwekkeboom, Kristine, Karen Huseby Moor, and Sandra Ward. "Imaging Ability and Effective Use of Guided Imagery." *Research in Nursing and Health* 21, no. 3 (June 1998): 189–198.

guilt An emotional response to a perceived or actual failure to meet expectations of self or others. Guilt feelings can be destructive if carried to an extreme. They can be devastating to one's self-esteem and feeling of capability. However, they can also be constructive when the individual begins to understand his or her sources of guilt and learns to cope with this aspect of the human condition.

People experience feelings of guilt throughout life. For example, a young child may be aware of not pleasing his parents with certain behaviors. Later, the individual may experience guilt feelings for not remembering the birthday of a parent or spouse. Depending on differences in conscience, some individuals can steal or commit crimes against others and society and not feel any guilt, while others will suffer from guilt feelings over minor matters. Middle-aged adults experience guilt feeling when dealing with aging parents. Those who find it necessary to admit a parent to a nursing home for care often suffer guilt feelings; in these cases, guilt feelings are often related to previous relationships. Individuals who are in bereavement over a loved one often feel some guilt about not having done enough for the person when he or she was alive. Some parents of infants who die of sudden infant death syndrome have feelings of guilt over not having been able to prevent the death of their child. Such feelings are unfounded but can be troublesome to the sufferer. Mental health counseling can help relieve many of these uncomfortable feelings of guilt.

Some people feel a sense of guilt over certain circumstances because of their religious upbringing. Talking with a member of the clergy or mental health professional may be helpful. Otherwise, parents or spouses of a person who commits suicide, for example, may struggle with guilt feelings for many years, wondering if they could have prevented the death.

There are also legal implications to the concept of guilt, according to cultural mores and statutes.

See also DEPRESSION; GUILTY BUT MENTALLY ILL VERDICT.

guilty but mentally ill verdict Some states have a plea "guilty but mentally ill"; it is recognized in about one-third of the states and is still the subject of constitutional controversy. The disposition of a case in which there is a "guilty but mentally ill verdict" usually results in treatment of mentally ill individuals in a correctional setting instead of putting them in prison.

See also LEGAL ISSUES.

habits Learned responses that one performs automatically and frequently. They may include useful procedures, such as knowing how to use a computer keyboard, taking a shower in the morning or always leaving a key in a certain place. Habits can also be responses to stressful situations, such as scratching the head, nail biting, hair pulling or reaching for a cigarette. These unwanted or undesirable habits, if continued, can contribute to people's stress levels.

Habits can include certain repetitive and ritual behaviors such as those practiced by sufferers of obsessive-compulsive disorder. Stressful habits can be changed by behavior therapy, psychotherapy and the substitution of more constructive habits. Relaxation therapy, guided imagery, hypnosis and biofeedback may also be helpful techniques to overcome these habits.

See also ANXIETY DISORDERS; BEHAVIOR THERAPY; BIOFEEDBACK; GUIDED IMAGERY; HAIR PULLING; HYPNOSIS; NAIL BITING; OBSESSIVE-COMPULSIVE DISORDER; RELAXATION.

Quellette, Judith A., and Wendy Wood. "Habit and Intention in Everyday Life: The Multiple Processes by which Past Behavior Predicts Future Behavior." *Psychological Bulletin* 124, no. 1 (July 1998): 54–74.

hair pulling A habit that involves pulling out scalp hair and sometimes hair on eyebrows, eyelashes and other areas of the body; men may pull out beard and mustache hairs. For many people, hair pulling is a mechanism for coping with stressful situations. They do it when they are feeling nervous or tense, or it is a compulsion, known as trichotillomania.

Some individuals pull hair in front of others, but most often the activity is pursued in secret. The hairs are carefully hidden or disposed of. The hairless areas have distinctive features, which help distinguish trichotillomania from other forms of hair losses and disease; the patches are irregular in outline, not sharply defined, and the hair loss is never complete. Many of the hairs will break off rather than be completely pulled out, so that various amounts of stubble remain. There are usually no signs of inflammation, and the scalp is normal elsewhere.

The habit can be treated with behavior therapy or other forms of psychotherapies.

For information:

The Obsessive-Compulsive Disorder (OCD)
   Foundation
P.O. Box 9573
New Haven, CT 06535
Phone: (203) 772-0565

See also ANXIETY DISORDERS; BEHAVIOR THERAPY; HYPNOSIS; OBSESSIVE-COMPULSIVE DISORDER; PSYCHOTHERAPIES.

Scahill, Lawrence A. et al. "Childhood Trichotillomania: A Clinical Phenomenology, Comorbidy, and Family Genetics." *Journal of the American Academy of Child and Adolescent Psychiatry* 34, no. 11 (Nov. 1995): 1451–1459.

hakomi A form of body-centered psychotherapy based on principles that show individuals ways to live in harmony with themselves and others. It teaches individuals to enter a stage of awareness in which spontaneous and often nonverbal information becomes available and from which basic and unconscious beliefs stem and direct their lives. Many people use hakomi as a way of preventing the harmful effects of stress.

The body stores and expresses what the mind and heart believes. Trained to look at nuances of voice and body language, posture and gesture, hakomi therapists help individuals study these avenues to unexpressed feelings and past trauma and to gain release from the past. Hakomi teaches people how to observe themselves from a step away (witnessing), as well as from inside their present experience. Individuals learn to have a choice in responses. Through the use of witnessing, unwanted defenses can be studied and willingly yielded.

Hakomi is a blend of many philosophies and ideologies, including Eastern philosophy, Western psychology, Taoism, Feldenkrais, Reichian, Rolfing and other structural bodywork therapies, Ericksonian hypnosis, focusing and neurolinguistic programming.

See also BODY THERAPIES; COMPLEMENTARY THERAPIES.

halazepam Generic name for the benzodiazepine medication Paxipam.

See also BENZODIAZEPINE DRUGS; PHARMACOLOGICAL APPROACH.

Halcion Trade name for the benzodiazepine drug triazolam.

See also BENZODIAZEPINE DRUGS; PHARMACOLOGICAL APPROACH.

Haldol See HALOPERIDOL.

half-life See SYNERGY.

hallucinations and hallucinogens Seeing, hearing, smelling, tasting or feeling something that is not there. They are sources of anxiety and stress because these perceptions cannot be reinforced by anyone else. Hallucinations may be disturbing to sufferers, as well as to those who are trying to understand what they are feeling. Hallucinations sometimes occur as a reaction to certain medications, to high fevers and serious illnesses. They also occur in some severe mental disorders, such as schizophrenia.

Reactions to Hallucinogens

Hallucinogens are drugs and agents that produce profound distortions to one's senses of sight, sound, smell and touch, as well as to the senses of direction, time and distance; in other words, hallucinogens produce hallucinations. Although some individuals may resort to hallucinogens for relief from stress, there are no acceptable medical uses for hallucinogens.

People may experience a "high" associated with use of hallucinogens, which may last as long as eight hours. However, there are aftereffects, including acute anxiety, restlessness and sleeplessness. Long after the hallucinogen is eliminated from the body, the user may experience "flashbacks," which are fragmentary reoccurrences of hallucinogenic effects.

Hallucinogens occur naturally but are primarily created synthetically. The most common hallucinogens are LSD (also known as d-lysergic acid diethylamide, lysergic and LSD-25), mescaline, peyote, psilocybin mushrooms, ecstasy (MDMA 3,4-methylenedioxymethamphetamine), and PCP (phencyclidine).

For information:

American Society on Addiction Medicine
5225 Wisconsin Avenue NW, Suite 409
Washington, D.C. 20015
Phone: (202) 244-8948

See also ADDICTIONS; ANXIETY; SUBSTANCE ABUSE.

haloperidol A drug (trade name: Haldol) used primarily to treat schizophrenia and other psychoses. It is also used in schizoaffective disorder and Tourette syndrome and occasionally as adjunctive therapy in mental retardation and the chorea of Huntington's disease. It is a potent antiemetic and is effective in the treatment of intractable hiccups.

Haloperidol can cause significant side effects and toxic effects such as neuroleptic malignant syndrome and tardive dyskinesia.

See also SCHIZOPHRENIA.

hangover A disagreeable physical effect that occurs after consuming too much alcohol, or the disagreeable aftereffects from the use of drugs. Sometimes sleeping medications cause hangover-like symptoms. A hangover is a source of anxiety because it produces physical as well as emotional symptoms that differ among individuals.

Some may experience nausea, vomiting or dizziness, while others may have headaches, sleepiness, unsteadiness, blurred vision, depression or self-pity. For many individuals, symptoms do not occur until several hours after drinking the alcohol, usually when they awaken from sleep. They may blame mixing of drinks, but drinking even one alcoholic beverage alone can cause a hangover.

The distinctive headache experienced as part of a hangover may be due to toxic substances that are released into the bloodstream and cause irritation of the brain membranes. Headaches may also come from the pressure of swollen blood vessels, which is an effect of alcohol. When alcohol promotes excessive urination, the resulting loss of fluid may reduce spinal fluid pressure, which has been known to bring on a headache.

Usually individuals recover from hangovers without medical assistance. Recommendations from physicians generally include aspirin, bed rest and solid food as soon as possible. A cup of coffee and a meal helps most people feel better.

See also ALCOHOLISM AND ALCOHOL DEPENDENCE; DIZZINESS; HEADACHES.

hardiness A term coined by Salvatore Maddi, Ph.D., a University of Chicago psychologist, relating to the stress-buffering characteristics of people who stay healthy. People with hardiness are able to withstand significant levels of stress without becoming ill; those who are more helpless than hardy develop more illnesses, both mental and physical.

In working with executives at a major American employer, Dr. Maddi and colleagues determined three techniques that can augment hardiness, as well as happiness and health: focusing, reconstructing stressful situations and self-improvement.

Focusing is a technique developed by Eugene Gendlin, an American psychologist, and is a way of recognizing signals from one's body that something is wrong, such as tension in the neck or a mild headache. With stress, these conditions worsen. Maddi suggests mentally reviewing where things

are not feeling just right physically and reviewing situations that might be stressful. Focusing increasing one's sense of control over stress enables one to make changes.

Reconstructing stressful situations is a technique in which you think about a recent stressful episode and write down three ways it might have gone better and three ways it might have gone worse. If you can't think of what you could have done differently, focus on a person you know who deals with stress well and think about what he or she would have done. Realize that things did not go as badly as they could have. Also, realize that you can think of ways to cope better with the same situation.

In the self-improvement technique, you accept that there are some situations you cannot control and that you cannot avoid these situations, such as a serious illness or illness of a member of your family, but to regain your sense of control and achieve more effective coping, you choose a new task to master, such as learning how to swim, or develop a new hobby, while dealing with the stressful situation.

Suzanne Kobasa, a psychologist at the City University of New York, also used the term hardiness to identify and measure a style of psychological coping. Some of the characteristics exhibited by people with hardiness included viewing life's demands as challenges rather than threats, responding with excitement and energy to change and having a commitment to something they felt was meaningful, such as their work, community or family. A third trait was a sense of being in control. Having the right information and being able to make decisions can make an important difference in coping with stress.

Issue of Control in Hardiness

A study reported in the *Journal of Personal and Social Psychology* (April 1995) detailed how 276 Israeli recruits completed questionnaires on hardiness, mental health and ways of coping at the beginning and end of a demanding, four-month combat training period. Two components of hardiness, commitment and control, measured at the beginning of the training, predicted mental health at the end of the training. Commitment improved mental health by reducing the appraisal of threat. Control improved mental health by reducing appraisal of threat and by increasing the use of problem-solving and support-seeking strategies.

See also CONTROL; COPING; GENERAL ADAPTATION SYNDROME; LEARNED HELPLESSNESS; STRESS.

Floria, V. et al. "Does Hardiness Contribute to Mental Health During a Stressful Real-Life Situation? The Roles of Appraisal and Coping." *Journal of Personal and Social Psychology* 68 (April 1995) 1: 687–695.

Goleman, Daniel, and Joel Gurin, eds. *Mind Body Medicine: How To Use Your Mind for Better Health.* Yonkers, N.Y.: Consumer Reports Books, 1993.

Kahn, Ada P. *Stress A to Z: The Sourcebook for Facing Everyday Challenges.* New York: Facts On File, 2000.

Padus, Emrika, ed. *The Complete Guide to Your Emotions and Your Health.* Emmaus, Pa.: Rodale, 1992.

hashish A refined form of cannabis (marijuana) that is found in brown or black sheets, "cakes" or "balls." Hashish (or "hash") generally comes from the Middle East, is more potent than marijuana and is smoked in a pipe. The active ingredient is delta-9-tetrahydrocannabinol, which is metabolized in the liver to a related substance that produces intoxicating effects. Hashish oil is extracted from cannabis plant materials to produce a dark, viscous liquid that averages around 20 percent THC.

See also SUBSTANCE ABUSE; MARIJUANA.

Media Resource Guide on Common Drugs of Abuse. Public Relations Society of America, National Capital Chapter, Fairfax, Va., September 1990.

"having it all" An expression that became popular during the 1980s when career women discovered that they could follow their chosen business or profession, get married and raise a family. For many this has become a satisfying way of life, but for others it has involved many frustrations, anxieties and, in some cases, feelings of guilt. Some women feel that they are not giving adequate attention to the marriage and children, are constantly tired and feel some guilt over having their children in day-care centers. Nevertheless, an increasing number of women opt to enter business and professions. Those who are most successful say it is because of the helpfulness and understanding of their spouse.

See also MARRIAGE; WOMEN'S LIBERATION MOVEMENT.

headaches Pains in the head from the outer linings of the brain, as well as from the scalp and its blood vessels and muscles; headaches occur due to tension in or stretching of these structures. They are a source of stress because of their discomfort and unpredictability. They may be caused by a reaction to stressful situations, overindulgence in alcohol, extreme fatigue and certain infections. Headaches are fairly common in depression, sleep disorders and in individuals who have many anxieties, as well as those suffering from boredom. The National Headache Foundation estimates that more than 80 million Americans develop headaches each year that are serious enough to warrant treatment by a physician. They are the most frequent complaint that physicians treat and may indicate a more serious condition.

Types of Headaches

Tension or muscle contraction headaches. This type is caused by a tightening in the muscles of the face, neck or scalp, as a possible result of stress or poor posture; they may last for days or weeks and can cause variable degrees of discomfort. About 90 percent of all headaches are classified as tension headaches.

Cluster headaches. The term refers to the characteristic grouping in a series of attacks; the pain is generally very intense, severe and almost always one-sided; during a series, the pain remains on the same side. In a new series, it can occur on the opposite side. Cluster headaches are not associated with gastrointestinal disturbances or sensitivity to light that typically accompany other vascular headaches, such as migraine.

Temporomandibular joint (TMJ) headaches. These cause a dull ache in and around the ear that gets worse when one chews, talks or yawns. Sufferers may hear a clicking sound on opening the mouth and feel soreness in the jaw muscles. Stress, a poor bite or grinding the teeth may bring on the headache.

Caffeine headaches. These occur in some individuals who drink too much caffeine in coffee, tea and soft drinks. Some people can relieve their symptoms by eliminating drinks containing caffeine from their diet. Others, however, who drink large quantities of the liquids and then stop abruptly, may suffer caffeine withdrawal symptoms, including headaches, irritability, depression and sometimes nausea; relief may occur with ingestion of a caffeinated beverage.

Migraine Headaches

Migraine, or vascular, headaches are characterized by the throbbing sensation that occurs when blood vessels in the head dilate or swell. Migraine is an often debilitating disease that occurs in periodic attacks, with each attack lasting from four to 72 hours. Symptoms may include intense pain, often associated with nausea, vomiting, appetite loss and an unusual sensitivity to light and/or sound. Migraines generally start on either side of the head and usually remain one-sided. Of the 23 million American migraine sufferers, 60 percent are women. Men and women between the ages of 35 and 45 years of age suffer most from migraine headaches, according to a study reported in the *Journal of the American Medical Association* (December 31, 1991). More than three-fourths of migraine sufferers come from families in which other members have the same disorder. The *JAMA* researchers reported that 8.7 million females and 2.6 million males suffer from migraine headache with moderate to severe disability. Of these, 3.4 million females and 1.1 million males experience one or more attacks per month.

"Common" migraine headaches start unexpectedly, while "classic" migraines are usually preceded by a warning symptom known as an aura, which occurs five to 30 minutes prior to the headache. Typically, the aura includes hallucinations of jagged light or color, speech impairment, perception of strange odors, confusion and tingling or numbness in the face or limbs.

Why Migraine Headaches Are so Stressful

Because migraine headaches usually recur, sufferers become concerned that an attack will happen at an unfortuitous time, such as on the day of a graduation, a wedding or an important appointment. Migraine headaches often begin during a period of time filled with anxieties, such as during adolescence or menopause, or around the time of divorce or death of a mate. When a physician diagnoses headaches, the individual's anxieties and coping styles will be considered.

Migraine headaches, which often occur in members of the same family, may result from a predisposing genetic biochemical abnormality. Also, personality traits may play a role in determining who gets migraines. Although there is no typical personality associated with these headaches, some migraine sufferers have characteristics of compulsivity and perfection.

Emotional tension and stress may lead to migraine attacks, because under extreme stress, the arteries of the head and those reaching the brain draw tightly together and restrict the flow of blood. This in turn may result in a shortage of oxygen to the brain. When blood vessels dilate or stretch, a greater amount of blood passes through, putting more pressure on the pain-sensitive nerves in and close to the walls of the arteries.

Common Migraine Triggers

In a susceptible person, the migraine trigger might be something seen, smelled, heard, eaten or experienced; it may be one particular trigger or a combination of factors.

Approximately 20 percent of all migraine sufferers have sensitivity to a specific food or foods. Knowing that certain foods may trigger migraines is an additional source of stress. Many individuals find that certain foods, such as cheese, chocolate, and red wine, containing a substance known as tyramine trigger migraine attacks. Sodium nitrite, a preservative used in ham, hot dogs and many sausages, is a trigger for some people. Although some migraine researchers have recommended that all migraine sufferers avoid these foods, only about 30 percent of people who have migraine headaches experience this reaction to those foods. Not eating or missing meals can cause low blood sugar levels, which also trigger migraine.

Identifying and avoiding the triggers that cause headaches is the one of the most significant management techniques for controlling headache frequency and stress.

COMMON MIGRAINE TRIGGERS

- Dietary habits (see detailed listing following)
- Environmental factors, such as weather, bright lights, glare or noise
- Emotional factors, such as depression, anxiety, resentment or fatigue
- Activity, such as motion from riding in a car or airplane, lack of sleep, too much sleep, eyestrain and a fall or head injury
- Hormones, such as menstrual cycle, oral contraceptives or estrogen supplements
- Medications, such as overuse of over-the-counter pain relievers and some prescription medications

DIETARY FACTORS: POSSIBLE MIGRAINE ATTACK TRIGGERS

- Caffeinated foods and drinks: coffee, tea, chocolate, cocoa, colas/soft drinks
- Alcohol: especially red wine, vermouth, champagne, beer
- Dairy products: aged cheeses, sour cream, whole milk, buttermilk, yogurt, ice cream
- Breads: sourdough, fresh yeast, some types of cereals
- Vegetables: some types of beans (broad, Italian, lima, lentil, fava, soy), sauerkraut, onions, peas
- Snacks: nuts, peanuts, peanut butter, pickles, seeds, sesame
- Meats: organ meats, salted meats, dried meats, cured meats, smoked fish, meats with nitrates (such as hot dogs, sausages, lunch meat)
- Fruits: most citrus fruits, bananas, avocados, figs, raisins, papaya, passion fruit, red plums, raspberries, plantains, pineapples
- Monosodium glutamate (MSG): a flavor enhancer often used in restaurants and in seasoned salt, instant foods, canned soup, frozen dinners, pizza, potato chips
- Soups: particularly those containing MSG, soups made from bouillon cubes
- Desserts: chocolate, licorice, molasses, cakes and cookies made with yeast
- Seasonings and flavorings: soy sauce, some spices, garlic powder, onion powder, salt, meat tenderizers, marinades
- Hunger: missing meals, fasting, dieting

Migraine Headaches, Hormones and Pregnancy

Although migraine headaches are more common in young boys than in young girls, the number of women affected increases sharply after the onset of menstruation. Certain hormonal changes that occur during puberty in girls and remain throughout adulthood may be implicated in the triggering and frequency of migraine attacks in women.

The link between female endocrine changes and migraine headaches is reinforced by the finding that 60 percent of women sufferers involved in a clinical study related attacks to their menstrual cycle. Individual differences exist: attacks may occur several days before, during or immediately after the woman's menses.

In females with migraine, about 77 percent find their attacks disappear completely, occur less often or are milder during pregnancy. In others, attacks either worsen or remain unchanged.

Oral contraceptives also affect the incidence of migraine attacks. Some migraine sufferers find their attacks are worsened while they are on birth control pills. Others find that they are not affected, and a small percent report improvement. Yet, some women even without any predisposition to migraine develop it while on the Pill, and nearly three-quarters find their headaches disappearing after they stop taking the Pill.

Diagnosis

When a headache does not respond to relaxation, rest, sleeping, simple self-medication such as aspirin and non-steroidal anti-inflammatory drugs available over-the-counter, cold compresses on the head or relaxation in a dark room, medical assistance should be sought. During a complete physical and neurological examination, the physician will ask about the history of the headaches, the period of time they have been occurring, when they occur, the circumstances at the time and how long they last.

Diagnostic techniques may include use of computerized tomography scanning (CT scanning) or magnetic resonance imaging (MRI).

Diagnosis is necessary before an individual takes any medication for headaches. Medications that help tension headaches will not help severe migraine headaches, and drugs targeted to relieve migraine headaches may not help any other type. Also, it is important that one does not overmedicate for headaches and bring on other side effects from medications.

Therapies for Headaches

Treatments for headaches include non-pharmacological treatments, such as biofeedback, meditation and relaxation techniques, as well as prescription medications. In the mid-1990s, a medication became available in tablet form (sumatriptan succinate) that is a highly selective serotonin receptor agonist for the treatment of migraine with or without aura. It is not used for cluster headache.

For migraine or vascular headaches, medication is targeted toward altering the responses of the vascular system to stress, hormonal changes, noise and other stimuli. Such medications affect the dilation reaction of the blood vessels. Ergot, a naturally occurring substance that constricts blood vessels and reduces the dilation of arteries, has historically been a popular medication. Ergot may be given by inhalation, injection, orally or rectally. Some people find that if they take the ergot medication early enough, in the pre-pain stages, of an attack they can abort their headaches or at least reduce their intensity.

Some vascular headaches are helped with prophylactic (preventive) measures. The drug of choice for prevention of migraine in carefully selected patients is propranolol. Propranolol is a vasoconstrictor that can be taken daily for as long as six months. This drug may slow down the vascular changes that occur during the migraine attack; it is frequently prescribed for some individuals who have headaches more than once each week. Propranolol has an advantage over ergot medications in that rebound headaches are not brought on by the discontinuation of propranolol.

Medication for muscle contraction headaches are directed toward relieving muscular activity and spasm. Analgesics (pain relievers) commonly used are aspirin, dextropropoxyphene and ethoheptazine. Injection with anesthetics and corticosteroids may be helpful.

For treating cluster headaches, the choice of medications depends on the frequency and severity of headaches, as well as the response to previous treatments. Some drugs used include ergotamine, methysergide, cyproheptadine, lithium and steroids, as well as oxygen inhalation and histamine desensitization. These treatments should only be used under the careful guidance of a physician who is familiar with their use.

In depressed individuals, some antidepressant drugs may provide relief from headaches including migraine; examples are the monoamine oxidase inhibitors (MAOIs), such as phenelzine sulfate.

Complementary Therapies

A wide variety of complementary therapies may be helpful for headache sufferers. Some individuals experience relief with their use and without medication, while other use them in conjunction with medication. When individuals consider alternative therapies, they should be discussed with the attending physician. Although some people can relieve their headache pain with alternative therapies, for others these therapies act as an adjunct or complement to pharmacological therapy, making the sufferer more receptive to medical treatment.

Biofeedback involves teaching a person to control certain body functions through thought and willpower with feedback from an electronic device.

Meditation (also known as transcendental meditation) is a technique of inward contemplation that helps some people relieve anxieties and in turn relieve some headaches using relaxation. During meditation, the mind as well as other organs in the body slow down, heart rate decreases, breathing becomes slower and muscle tensions diminish.

Acupuncture has been successfully used to treat some headache sufferers. Acupuncture probably works because the needle insertions somehow stimulate the body to secrete endorphins, naturally occurring hormonelike substances that kill pain. Acupressure involves pressing acupuncture points with hands, and can be done by a professional as well as a trained lay person.

For information:

American Association for the Study of the
  Headache
19 Mantua Road
Mt. Royal, NJ 08061
Phone: (609) 423-0043
Web site: www.aash.org

National Headache Foundation
5252 N. Western Avenue
Chicago, IL 60625
Phone: (773) 878-7715
Web site: www.headaches.org

See also ACUPRESSURE; ACUPUNCTURE; ANXIETY; BIOFEEDBACK; BOREDOM; CAFFEINE; COMPLEMENTARY THERAPIES; COPING; DEPRESSION; DIVORCE; GUIDED IMAGERY; HANGOVER; HALLUCINATIONS; HYPNOSIS; MEDITATION; MENOPAUSE; PERFECTION; PHARMACOLO-

GICAL APPROACH; PUBERTY AND PUBERTY RITES; RELAX-
ATION; TEMPOROMANDIBULAR JOINT SYNDROME.

Diamond, Seymour. *The Hormone Headache: New Ways to
  Prevent, Manage, and Treat Migraines and Other
  Headaches.* New York: Macmillan, 1995.
Kahn, Ada P. *Stress A to Z: The Sourcebook for Facing Every-
  day Challenges.* New York: Facts On File, 2000.
Inlander, Charles B., and Porter Shimer. *Headaches: 47
  Ways to Stop the Pain.* New York: Walker and Com-
  pany, 1995.
Maas, Paula, and Deborah Mitchell. *The Natural Health
  Guide to Headache Relief: The Definitive Handbook of Nat-
  ural Remedies for Treating Every Kind of Headache Pain.*
  New York: Pocket Books, 1997.

healing touch   See THERAPEUTIC TOUCH.

health maintenance organization (HMO)   See
MANAGED CARE.

heart attack   See ANGINA PECTORIS.

helplessness   A feeling that one cannot do anything by oneself or for oneself; a common symptom
of depression. Helplessness often goes along with
hopelessness. It is a feeling of being "stuck" and
that there is "no way out." Individuals who feel
this symptom severely should seek mental health
counseling.

  See also DEPRESSION; LEARNED HELPLESSNESS;
LEARNED OPTIMISM.

help lines   See HOT LINES; SELF-HELP GROUPS; SUP-
PORT GROUPS.

herbal medicine   Use of a plant or a plant part
valued for its medicinal, savory or aromatic qualities. Herbalism gained popularity in the United
States toward the end of the 20th century. Estimates are that Americans spend more than 1 billion dollars on herbal remedies in a year; many
people seek these alternative remedies to relieve
anxieties and other mental health concerns.

  Herbal medications are deeply rooted in most
folk medicine traditions and have played an important role in the evolution of modern medicine and
pharmacology. For example, when the Pilgrims

landed in Plymouth in 1630, they set up herb gardens that contained the medicinal varieties brought
from England. The settlers soon discovered that the
Native Americans had their own healing plants,
including cascara sagrada and goldenseal. According to the World Health Organization, 80 percent of
the earth's population uses some form of herbal
therapy.

  Many contemporary medications are based on
specific herbs but are manufactured from synthetic
substances believed to be more effective than the
natural herbs. Still, herbal therapies remain a
major component of Ayurvedic, homeopathic and
other alternative approaches.

  Herbal products are marketed in the United
States as foods, and are permitted by the Food and
Drug Administration provided that the products do
not make any therapeutic claims. Herbal products
are sold "over-the-counter" and are not subject to
the same safety and efficacy standards that apply to
prescription medications. Herbal packaging labels
rarely contain guidelines regarding indications for
proper use. As with any medication, herbal remedies are best used under the guidance of a knowledgeable individual, called an herbalist.

CONSIDERING HERBAL REMEDIES FOR MENTAL HEALTH CONCERNS

- See a physician first for serious conditions. Do not attempt
  to self-medicate
- Consider the sources of your products; select reputable
  brands
- Choose reliable forms such as tinctures or freeze-dried, as
  powdered forms may lose potency upon exposure to air
- Overdosing can have harmful effects. Take recommended
  dosages at suggested intervals.
- Watch for reactions; if unwanted reactions occur, stop the
  medication.

For information:

The Herb Research Foundation
1007 Pearl Street, Suite 200
Boulder, CO 80302
Phone: (303) 449-2265

  See also AYURVEDA; COMPLEMENTARY THERAPIES;
FOLK MEDICINE; HOMEOPATHY.

Barrett, Bruce, David Kiefer, and David Rabago. "Assessing the Risks and Benefits of Herbal Medicine: An

Overview of Scientific Evidence." *Alternative Therapies* 5 no. 4 (July 1999) 1:40–49.

Chevallier, Andrew. *The Encyclopedia of Medicinal Plants.* New York: Houghton Mifflin, 1996.

Evans, Michael F., and Katie Morgenstern. "St. John's Wort: An Herbal Remedy for Depression?" *Canadian Family Physician* 43 (Oct. 1997): 1735–1736.

National Women's Health Report. "Alternative Therapies and Women's Health." Washington, D.C.: National Women's Health Resource Center, May/June, 1995.

Schar, Douglas. *The Backyard Medicine Chest: An Herbal Primer.* Washington, D.C.: Elliott & Clark Publishers, 1995.

heredity Transmission of traits as well as disorders through genetic mechanisms. Some mental disorders are hereditary; researchers have found that depression, particularly bipolar disorder, obsessive-compulsive disorder, alcoholism and panic disorder occur more frequently in some families than others, as well as in identical as opposed to fraternal twins, suggesting a hereditary vulnerability for the illness.

See also PANIC DISORDER.

heroin A controlled narcotic that has no legitimate medical use in the United States. Because tolerance to heroin develops rapidly, it is one of the most addictive drugs known. Heroin addiction is a strong physiological and psychological dependence characterized by tolerance and, when discontinued, withdrawal syndrome. Heroin abuse is a major health problem in many countries. It is a major sociological and economic problem as well as a personal danger for the user. A major danger to heroin users is an overdose from an unexpectedly pure sample, which, if untreated, can cause depressed breathing, possible convulsions, coma or death.

Sharing of contaminated needles for injection also poses a risk of transmitting diseases such as AIDS and hepatitis. Children of pregnant addicts are born addicted and suffer acute withdrawal upon birth, including irritability, tremors and anxieties.

Heroin is synthesized from morphine, which originates from opium poppies cultivated in Southeast Asia, Southwest Asia and Latin America. Most illicit heroin is in the form of a powder, which may vary in color from white to dark brown. Another form called "black tar" or "tootsie roll" is of substantially higher purity and is thus more potent.

Heroin is usually sold on the street in small bags, cellophane envelopes or foil packages. These are called "nickel" or "dime" bags. Pure heroin is rarely sold on the street. Usually it is "cut" with diluents such as sugar, starch and powdered milk, making it between 4 and 6 percent pure. Street heroin has been known to be cut with toxic substances.

Heroin can be combined with water, "cooked" down and injected. It can also be sniffed or smoked, both of which are becoming increasingly more common methods of administration.

Adapted from *Media Resource Guide on Common Drugs of Abuse.* Public Relations Society of America, National Capital Chapter, Fairfax, Va., September 1990.

high blood pressure The term "blood pressure," as used in medicine, refers to the force of blood against the walls of one's arteries; the force is created by the heart as it pumps blood through the body. As the heart pumps or beats, the pressure increases; as the heart relaxes between beats, the pressure decreases. High blood pressure (hypertension) is the condition in which blood pressure rises to and remains at an unhealthy high level.

High blood pressure is an important individual and public health issue because it affects as many as 25 percent of the adult population in the United States. High blood pressure has been associated with the stresses resulting from certain negative emotions or aggressive and hostile behaviors. Although the degree of stress is difficult to assess objectively, acute and probably chronically stressful situations can result in an elevation of the blood pressure. Certain individuals are overreactive to stress, and they may suffer more than others when confronting certain situations. Individuals with high blood pressure have higher irritability levels, more guilt feelings and increased psychic distress.

There are many studies of the effects of psychological factors such as stress, psychological or personality characteristics and life events on blood pressure. A problem with these studies has been the difficulties of assessing and determining whether the psychosocial factors are causes or consequences of high blood pressure. It is possible that the process of labeling or treating a person with blood pressure elevation can induce a stressful psychological change, thereby increasing hypertension.

Diagnosing High Blood Pressure

According to the National Heart, Lung and Blood Institute, high blood pressure is more likely to develop in people with a family history of high blood pressure, those who are overweight, eat a high-salt diet, drink excessively and/or are physically inactive.

In its early stages, high blood pressure does not usually produce any symptoms; for this reason it is sometimes called "the silent killer." Many people who have high blood pressure feel just fine.

High blood pressure is usually diagnosed during an office visit to a physician. The physician uses a stethoscope and a sphygmomanometer, an inflatable cuff attached to a device that measures blood pressure. With each heartbeat, blood is pumped through the arteries and veins. The force with which blood pushes against the artery walls creates blood pressure, which is represented by two numbers. The top number, systolic pressure, indicates the maximum pressure with which blood pushes against the arteries during a heartbeat. The lower number, diastolic pressure, indicates pressure against the arteries when the heart is at rest. Normal or healthy blood pressure is in the 80 to 120 range. If the reading regularly hits 140/90, one is said to have high blood pressure.

High blood pressure usually starts when arteries become too narrowed or constricted, which impedes the flow of blood. High pressure in these damaged arteries makes them susceptible to the build up of fatty, cholesterol-containing deposits, a condition known as atherosclerosis. If the blood vessels feeding the heart become blocked and/or hardened, a person may suffer chest pain (known as angina) or may have a heart attack. When the blood supply to the brain is disrupted, a stroke may occur. Other effects may be kidney failure and eye damage.

"White Coat Hypertension"

Some individuals actually show elevations in their blood pressure when visiting a physician's office. Their blood pressure is generally normal but increases in the presence of physicians and other health care professionals. This is because these individuals feel stressed and fearful of doctors or the surroundings, such as laboratories where they might encounter needles or blood testing devices. They may be inadvertently diagnosed with high blood pressure.

Physicians who understand this phenomenon usually take the patient's blood pressure at the end of the visit as well as at the beginning, and they also take a careful history to determine the effects of the patient's phobias on the blood pressure.

Treating High Blood Pressure

Non-drug measures can help many people control their high blood pressure. In many cases, however, other measures may be recommended along with medication because they are beneficial for overall good health. Helpful techniques include biofeedback; breathing; guided imagery; hypnosis; relaxation; and t'ai chi.

SELF-HELP TIPS FOR REDUCING HIGH BLOOD PRESSURE

- *Stress control:* Training in relaxation techniques and use of biofeedback helps some patients handle stressful life situations in more constructive ways.
- *Weight reduction:* Some overweight people can reduce their blood pressure by losing excess weight.
- *Salt restriction:* In combination with medication, salt restriction is often helpful.
- *Restriction of dietary cholesterol:* High blood level of cholesterol, coupled with high blood pressure, can damage arteries.
- *Restriction of alcohol consumption:* Drinking should not exceed two ounces of 100-proof liquor, eight ounces of wine or 24 ounces of beer a day.
- *No smoking:* Nicotine directly affects the heart and blood vessels, producing acute increases in blood pressure. Independent of high blood pressure, smoking can damage arteries.

Many activities that reduce stress, including aerobic exercise, running, biking, walking, and swimming, also reduce both systolic and diastolic blood pressure. The American College of Sports Medicine (ACSM) recommends aerobic activities three to five days a week for 20 to 60 minutes per workout at intensities 40 percent to 80 percent of maximum effort.

However, the ACSM advises people with high blood pressure to avoid high-intensity strength training (weight training), because it temporarily elevates blood pressure whether one has high blood pressure or not.

Role of Nutrition

Maintaining a proper diet can be beneficial in treating high blood pressure, according to a review in the *Archives of Family Medicine* (August 14, 1995). Claude K. Lardinois, M.D., University of Nevada School of Medicine, conducted a study to determine the efficacy of nutritional factors in preventing high blood pressure, as well as their role in the treatment of individuals with established high blood pressure.

The study found that weight reduction, sodium chloride restriction and avoidance of excessive alcohol consumption appear to be the best nutritional approaches to the treatment of high blood pressure. "The role of dietary alterations of fiber, calcium, magnesium, potassium, dietary fats, carbohydrates and protein is less convincing. Unfortunately, much of the available data are insufficient to make a final recommendation regarding a potential role for these alterations in the prevention and treatment of high blood pressure," said Dr. Lardinois.

Weight control is important because the prevalence of high blood pressure is 50 percent higher among overweight adults than among adults of normal weight; 33 percent of people who have high blood pressure are overweight. Overweight individuals have a twofold to sixfold increased risk for developing high blood pressure. Modest weight loss can favorably affect high blood pressure.

Drug Treatment for High Blood Pressure

Taking medication for high blood pressure is stressful for some individuals because many medications cause side effects or other problems that complicate treatment. These effects may include fatigue, sexual impotence and dizziness. A study in the *Journal of the American Medical Association* (June 14, 1985) reported that of the 3,844 patients being treated for high blood pressure, 9.3 percent stopped their drug treatment because of "definite" or "prob-able" side effects, and an additional 23.4 percent stopped drug treatment because of "possible" side effects.

In some cases, one drug will maintain blood pressure control over time. More often, one drug controls is for a time; then a second or third may be needed. High blood pressure can be controlled, as long as some of the following appropriate medicines are taken:

Diuretics act on the kidneys, causing them to flush out salt and water. As fluid in the blood vessels goes down, pressure goes down.

Beta blockers act on the heart, reducing the rate at which it beats and the amount of blood it pumps; with less output, pressure drops.

Vasodilators relax the small arteries, reducing their resistance to blood flow, causing blood pressure to go down.

Sympathetic inhibitors act on the sympathetic nervous system and also relax the arteries, keeping pressure down.

Calcium channel blockers lower the levels of calcium in the blood vessel muscle cells. This relaxes the vessels, and pressure drops.

ACE inhibitors work in a unique way in the body. They have been shown to be effective in controlling high blood pressure, usually without causing some of the troublesome side effects caused by older drugs. ACE inhibitors interrupt a chemical chain reaction in the body that causes blood pressure to rise. The kidney triggers the process by releasing an enzyme called "renin" into the blood stream. As part of the chain reaction, the lungs produce an enzyme called ACE (angiotension-converting enzyme). The presence of ACE leads to the production of another chemical that raises pressure. ACE inhibitors bind up ACE, interrupting the chemical chain and maintaining more normal pressure.

Alpha blockers and central alpha agonists keep blood vessels open by blocking the action of certain nerves.

For information:

American Heart Association
7320 Greenville Avenue
Dallas, TX 75231
Phone: (214) 373-6300

National Heart Lung and Blood Institute
9000 Rockville Pike
Bethesda, MD 20892
Phone: (301) 496-4236

See also BIOFEEDBACK: BREATHING; COMPLEMEN-
TARY THERAPIES; DIZZINESS; EXERCISE; GUIDED IMAGE-
RY; GUILT; HYPNOSIS; IMPOTENCE; PERSONALITY; PETS;
RELAXATION; STROKE; T'AI CHI; TYPE A PERSONALITY.

Kerman, D. Ariel. *H.A.R.T. Program: Lower Your Blood
Pressure Without Drugs.* New York: HarperCollins,
1992.
Lardinois, Claude K. "Role of Nutrition in Treating
Hypertension." *Archives of Family Medicine* (Aug. 14,
1995.)
Pickering, Thomas G. et al., "How Common Is White
Coat Hypertension?" *Journal of the American Medical
Association* (Jan. 8, 1988): 225–228.

hippocampus   See ADRENAL CORTEX.

HIV   See ACQUIRED IMMUNODEFICIENCY SYNDROME;
HUMAN IMMUNODEFICIENCY VIRUS.

**HIV/AIDS Treatment Information Service
(ATIS)**   A free telephone reference service for
health care providers, as well as people living with
HIV disease. Many people find relief from some of
the psychological stresses of living with HIV disease
when they get answers to their questions and
sources for further information. During 1995, its
first year, the staff responded to more than 10,000
calls.

The HIV/AIDS Treatment Information Service is
sponsored by the Agency for Health Care Policy and
Research, Centers for Disease Control and Preven-
tion, Health Resources and Services Administration,
National Institutes of Health and the Substance
Abuse and Mental Health Services Administration.
The service is offered through the Centers for Dis-
ease Control National AIDS Clearinghouse.

Reference specialists answer questions about the
latest treatment options, provide customized data-
base searches and link callers to other HIV/AIDS
information resources. Through the service, callers
can acquire copies of the latest federally approved
treatment guidelines, including recommendations
for HIV counseling and voluntary testing for pregnant women, guidelines for prevention of opportunistic infections in persons infected with HIV and
study results concerning anti-HIV therapy, which
lowers the risk of AIDS and death in patients with
intermediate-stage HIV disease.

In late 1995, the treatment service developed
the *Glossary of HIV/AIDS-Related Terms* to help people understand the technical terms related to HIV,
its associated treatments and the medical management of related conditions. To obtain a copy of the
Glossary, or to obtain information on new treatment
guidelines, phone: (800) HIV-0440.

See also HUMAN IMMUNODEFICIENCY VIRUS.

HMO   See MANAGED CARE.

hobbies   Activities people engage in because they
want to, not because they have to for economic
reasons. They are sources of satisfaction, relaxation, relief from the stresses of everyday life and
avenues toward improvement of mental health for
many people. People who look forward to retirement do so because they will have more time for
hobbies. Choosing hobbies is up to each individual,
although in many cases they bring people with
common interests together. For many people, col-
lecting things like antiques is a hobby.

According to Allen Elkin, Ph.D., director, Stress
Management and Counseling Center, New York
City, "people who derive most of their identity
from their profession are going to need other
sources of self-esteem when they leave that profession behind." People who have hobbies usually
have a consuming interest in their chosen activity.
Many former workaholics find satisfaction in a
hobby that forces them to concentrate and be
patient, such as building a model train, bird watching or producing clay sculptures.

Winston Churchill is said to have commented
on hobbies: "The cultivation of a hobby and new
forms of interest is a policy of first importance . . .
to be happy and really safe, one ought to have at

least two or three hobbies." Churchill painted and also wrote a book, *Painting as a Pastime*.

See also RELAXATION; RETIREMENT; SELF-ESTEEM; VOLUNTEERISM.

Godbey, Geoffrey, and John Robinson. *Time For Life: The Surprising Ways Americans Use Their Time*. University Park: Pennsylvania State University Press, 1997.
Kanfer, Stefan. "The Art of Having Fun." *Modern Maturity* (Oct. 1995).

holiday depression A low mood swing experienced during a period of the year in which holidays occur or on the holidays themselves. Some single and widowed individuals experience holiday depression because they feel alone and lonely on holidays and see the rest of their society in the celebratory mood with families around them. This type of depression often occurs when an individual has been uprooted from his or her family and moved elsewhere for employment or other reasons. Some individuals in family settings experience mood shifts out of nostalgia for lost loved ones or for circumstances that existed earlier in their lives. Some people who know that they will be alone on holidays avoid their holiday depressive episodes by planning ahead to take a trip to an interesting place, engage in some enjoyable activity with a group, or invite other people without families to share holiday activities together. Some individuals who know they will be alone on holidays volunteer their services to hospitals or shelters for the homeless so that others may be with their families. Feeling that one is helpful to others is a way of combating the low mood.

The depressed mood is usually brought about by holidays under such circumstances and disappears after the holiday season. However, when the depressive mood does not improve as the calendar rolls on, the individual should seek counseling from a mental health professional.

See also DEPRESSION; SEASONAL AFFECTIVE DISORDER.

holistic medicine A shift in belief systems from the dualistic mind/body split toward a view of mind, body and spirit as being closely connected. It has come to mean a specific way of thinking and practicing the art and science of medicine, for dealing with illness and relieving stress. Practitioners of holistic medicine view the individual as a totality, rather than as a headache to be relieved or a backache to be cured.

See also AYURVEDA; COMPLEMENTARY THERAPIES; HERBAL MEDICINE; HOMEOPATHY; MIND/BODY CONNECTIONS; PSYCHONEUROIMMUNOLOGY.

Williams, Allison. "Therapeutic Landscapes in Holistic Medicine." *Social Science and Medicine* 46 no. 9 (May 1998): 1193–1203.

Holmes, Thomas H., III (1918–) A neuropsychiatrist who researched the effects of stressful life change events on health status. He is known for devising a social adjustment rating scale along with Richard H. Rahe, M.D., another researcher in the area of life changes, as a predictor of illness.

See also LIFE CHANGE SELF-RATING SCALE.

homelessness Mental health concerns of homeless people range from solving practical everyday problems such as finding enough food to serious disorders such as substance abuse, depression and schizophrenia. Physical as well as mental health problems are intensified by homelessness; conversely, homelessness precipitates health problems. Because of the nature of the population, it is difficult to assess the numbers of homeless people and their characteristic mental health problems and for society to provide care for them.

Problems in providing mental health care for the homeless are related in part to reluctance of the people to present themselves for care as well as the poor funding of community mental health centers. Since the psychiatrically impaired homeless often avoid contact with the health care system, mobile outreach services in some communities are an important way to help these individuals obtain food, clothing and medical and psychiatric care.

Many emergency department physicians are the primary care physicians for the poor and homeless population. These physicians often provide care for poor children and adolescents, the elderly, victims of rape and domestic violence and drug abusers.

A survey of homeless adults living in beach areas near Los Angeles revealed a high rate of prior psychiatric hospitalization. The survey covered 529 people who had spent the previous night outdoors, in a shelter, in a hotel or in the home of a relative with whom they did not expect to stay very long. Sixty-four percent of the people interviewed were white; 73 percent were men. They had been homeless for an average of two years. Altogether, 44 percent had been in hospitals for psychiatric reasons, including alcoholism and drug dependence. Twenty-one percent had made an outpatient visit for a mental or emotional problem within the past year. Forty-one percent had never used mental health services.

The worst symptoms were noted in the hospitalized group. They were more suicide attempts, daily drinking and delirium tremens. Seventy-six percent of the hospitalized group and 48 percent of the others had been arrested. People who had been hospitalized were more likely to be living in shelters. The 41 percent who had never used mental health services had been homeless about half as long as the rest and were least likely to be sleeping outdoors. Surprisingly, they scored at the same level as the general population on a questionnaire estimating well-being.

Mental health professionals agree that to address the complex needs of those categorized as homeless persons requires a multi-disciplinary approach. Social services are needed for the short-term and long-term provision food, housing and entitlement services. Networks must be developed to enable access for those people to specialty medical services, emergency food pantries, transportation, overnight shelter and respite care for children while the parent negotiates the systems. Churches often provide for emergency needs and long-term support. Legal services are needed to advocate for the rights and entitlements. Children who are homeless require interaction with school systems, health care providers, day-care centers and often child protective services to promote health and prevent further illness or trauma.

Gelberg, Lillian; Lawrence S. Linn; and Barbara D. Leake. "Mental Health, Alcohol and Drug Use and Criminal History among Homeless Adults." *American Journal of Psychiatry* 145 (Feb. 1988).

McFarland, Gertrude K., and Mary Durand Thomas. *Psychiatric Mental Health Nursing.* Philadelphia: J. B. Lippincott, 1991.
Council on Long Range Planning and Development. "The Future of Psychiatry." *Journal of the American Medical Association* 264, no. 19 (Nov. 21, 1990).

homeopathy   A system to promote healing based on a philosophy of not bombarding the body with medications, but stimulating and assisting the body to heal itself, using the smallest amount of medication possible. Many people use homeopathic remedies to prevent, reduce and alleviate stress. Homeopathy is considered by many to be a complementary therapy.

Homeopathy uses medicines made from plants, minerals, animals, animal substances and chemicals. Whereas some conventional medications suppress symptoms and the body's immune response, occasionally causing unfortunate reactions to drugs or drug interactions, homeopathic practitioners prescribe only one medication at a time and claim that there are rarely, if ever, unwanted side effects. Homeopathic medicines are produced in accordance with processes described in the *Homeopathic Pharmacopoeia of the United States.*

A person-oriented instead of disease-oriented system, homeopathy allows practitioners to treat patients based on their symptoms, rather than relying solely on diagnostic techniques. Homeopathic practitioners seek to find *causes,* as well as to treat symptoms; this is often done in a holistic way by talking extensively with the patient to obtain a complete health and psychosocial history. In this regard, homeopathy has a characteristic in common with the Chinese belief that the best doctors do not use medicine; homeopathic practitioners heal by giving guidance for healthful living.

Homeopathy is used for a wide variety of chronic and acute problems. These include (but are not limited to) anxieties, allergies, digestive problems, gynecological conditions and skin diseases. Many homeopathic remedies can be self-prescribed and purchased over-the-counter. However, as with any medication, it is prudent to consult a practitioner who is knowledgeable about the subject. Such individuals can be located through reputable local homeopathic pharmacies or the National

Center of Homeopathy, Alexandria, Virginia, or the International Foundation for Homeopathy, Seattle, Washington.

The practice of homeopathy came to the United States in the early 1800s. By the mid-1800s, several medical colleges, including the New England Female Medical College, taught homeopathy. Around 1900, there were 22 homeopathic medical colleges, and one out of five doctors used homeopathy. However, by 1920, only 15 colleges remained. The decline in use of homeopathy in the United States came along with medical science's increasing view of the body as a mechanistic device, the advent of medical specialization, development of other prescription drugs and medicinal technology and opposition from the American Medical Association. The American Foundation for Homeopathy began teaching homeopathy as a post-graduate course for doctors in 1922. Today, courses are offered by the National Center for Homeopathy.

In recent years, interest in homeopathy has increased along with widening interest in holistic medicine and complementary therapies. Homeopathy may appeal to many people because only natural substances are used as medications. Remedies include substances that can be dissolved in a liquid medium; they do not consist of metals and salts because these are not dissolvable. Remedies are ground together ten times for ten minutes, a process that releases subatomic energy. For an inexplicable reason, once diluted beyond the twelfth dilution, nothing is found under a microscope. Also, because medications are so diluted, possibilities of side effects are reduced. Some homeopathic practitioners in the United States also use other adjunctive therapies such as spinal manipulation and nutritional counseling in addition to this type of medication.

The largest use of homeopathic medications is in India, but it is also popular in France and England and becoming popular in Australia and Germany. In Switzerland and Germany, homeopathic practitioners work under the direction of doctors of medicine. Family physicians in France prescribe homeopathic medicines. A survey in the *British Medical Journal* (June 7, 1986) indicated that 42 percent of British physicians refer patients to homeopathic physicians. According to *Everybody's Guide to Homeopathic Medicines* (1991), members of the English royal family are homeopathic medicine users and the queen of England is the patron of the Royal London Homeopathic Hospital and the British Homeopathic Association.

Another Homeopathic Technique: Bach Flower Remedies

Bach flower remedies are so-called after Edward Bach (1886–1936), a British bacteriologist and homeopath. Flower remedies are a branch of homeopathic medicine, said to be useful in acute situations. He developed a system of 38 flower remedies for 38 different emotional states, based only on a person's psychological symptoms. It is distinct from homeopathy because more than one Bach remedy is prescribed at a time.

For information:

International Foundation for Homeopathy
2366 Eastlake Avenue E, #301
Edmonds, WA 98020
Phone: (206) 776–4147

National Center for Homeopathy
801 North Fairfax Street, Suite 306
Alexandria, VA 22314
Phone: (703) 548-7790

See also ANXIETY; COMPLEMENTARY THERAPIES; HOLISTIC MEDICINE.

Merz, Beverly, ed. "Complementary Therapies: Homeopathy" *Harvard Women's Health Watch* 4, no. 5 (Jan. 1997).

Cummings, Stephen, and Dana Ullman. *Everybody's Guide to Homeopathic Medicines.* New York: Jeremy Tarcher/Perigree Books, 1991.

Thomas, Patricia, ed. "Homeopathy: Is Less Really More?" *Harvard Health Letter* 20, no. 7 (May 1995).

homeostasis The body's tendency to maintain a steady state, despite stressful external changes. The physical properties and chemical composition of body fluids and tissues tend to remain remarkably constant; however, when our self-regulating powers fail, often because of repeated stress, the individual's health is threatened.

In the late 19th century, Claude Bernard, a French physiologist at the College de France in

Paris, taught that one of the most characteristic features of all living beings is their ability to maintain the constancy of their internal composition, despite changes in their surroundings. Walter B. Cannon, a Harvard physiologist, named this power to maintain constancy "homeostasis," which can be translated as physiological "staying power or self-preservation."

Coping with stress and disease involves a fight to maintain the homeostatic balance of our tissues, despite damage. Hans Selye, the Austrian-born Canadian pioneer in stress research, discussed the concept of homeostasis in his landmark works, *The Stress of Life* (originally published in 1956) and *Stress Without Distress* (1978). He said that the nervous system and the endocrine system play particularly important parts in maintaining resistance during stress. They help to keep the structure and function of the body steady, despite exposure to stress-producing (stressor) agents, such as nervous tension, wounds, infections or poisons. He explained this steady state as a function of homeostasis.

See also COPING; GENERAL ADAPTATION SYNDROME; MIND/BODY CONNECTIONS; SELYE, HANS; STRESS.

Selye, Hans. *Stress Without Distress.* New York: J. B. Lippincott, 1974.
———. *The Stress of Life,* rev. ed. New York: McGraw-Hill, 1978.

homesickness See MIGRATION; NOSTALGIA.

homosexuality Sexual activity between members of the same sex, ranging from sexual fantasies and feelings through kissing and mutual masturbation, to genital, oral or anal contact. A male individual who practices homosexuality is termed a homosexual; a female homosexual is referred to as a lesbian. Both male and female homosexuals are sometimes referred to as gay.

It seems that the term "homosexuality" was coined in 1969 in a pamphlet by Karoly Maria Bankert. During the 19th century, other terms were proposed, including "homoerotic" (aroused by the same sex) and "homophile" (lover of the same sex). Cunnilingus between two women was called sapphism after the ancient Greek poet Sappho; lesbianism came from the Greek island of Lesbos where she lived.

Fear of or prejudice against homosexuals is known as homophobia.

homosexual panic Homosexual panic (Kempf's disease) is a panic attack that develops from a fear or delusion that one will be sexually assaulted by an individual of the same sex. The term, coined by Edward Kempf, an American psychiatrist (1885–1971), in 1920, also applies to the fear that one is thought to be homosexual. This feeling occurs more often in males than females. There may be depression, conscious guilt over homosexual activity, agitation, hallucinations and ideas of suicide. This type of panic attack may develop after many varied life circumstances, such as a loss of or separation from an individual of the same sex to whom one is emotionally attached, or after failures in sexual performance, illness or extreme fatigue.

See also BISEXUALITY; GAY LIBERATION; LESBIANISM; SEXUAL FEARS; SEXUALITY.

Campbell, Robert J. *Psychiatric Dictionary.* New York: Oxford University Press, 1981.
Kite, Mary E., and Kay Deaux. "Gender Belief Systems: Homosexuality and the Implicit Inversion Theory." *Psychology of Women Quarterly* 11 (1987).
Mahoney, E. R. *Human Sexuality.* New York: McGraw-Hill, 1983.
Owen, William F., Jr. "Medical Problems of the Homosexual Adolescent." *Journal of Adolescent Health Care* 6 (1985).
Wyers, Norman L. "Homosexuality in the Family: Lesbian and Gay Spouses." *Social Work* (Mar.–Apr. 1987).

hope A feeling about the uncertainty of the future in a positive, optimistic and, in some cases, unrealistic way. Imagination, seeing alternatives and the ability to create wishes are important in maintaining a hopeful attitude. Scientists have long recognized the power of hopeful feelings in physical health. In controlled experiments, patients who received placebos frequently reported feeling better and, at times, have unaccountably improved. A hopeful attitude is helpful in maintaining good mental health, because the opposite of hope is hopelessness, a characteristic of depression that correlates to the development of heart disease as well as earlier death in cardiac patients.

In a Gallup poll published in 1990, Americans were hopeful and optimistic about their own futures but pessimistic about the future of society. Participants in the survey looked forward to improvement in their finances, career and general quality of life to the extent that the hopeful outnumbered the pessimistic eight to one. Adults over age 50 were less hopeful about their personal futures. The greatest optimism was among the young, the educated and those who were financially secure. In seeming contradiction, the survey showed attitudes of pessimism in regard to society as a whole. Many said that inflation and unemployment would increase and that there will be little progress with regard to such problems as homelessness and drug addiction.

There are elements of fear and prayer in a hopeful attitude. For example, one World War II veteran said: "I flew 30 missions in a bomber. As the going got rougher, I would just hope all the harder that we would get out of harm's way. Fear motivated the hoping and where hoping ends and prayer begins, I don't know." From his concentration camp experiences of the 1930s and 1940s, Victor Frankl developed the philosophy that where there is life there is hope and that hope is essential to continue living.

In Christianity and other religious thought, hope is considered to be a virtue. Religious groups encourage hopeful feelings through concepts such as the coming of the Messiah or the second coming of Christ, life after death and the forgiveness of sins.

See also DEPRESSION; HOPELESSNESS.

hopelessness   A state of mind in which one feels that it is impossible to deal with life, that situations have no solutions. The person may see only limited or no available desirable personal alternatives. There may be feelings of emptiness, pessimism and being overwhelmed. Nothing matters to the person who feels hopeless, and the individual "gives up."

Hopelessness is a characteristic of depression. A hopeless person is passive and lacks initiative. Such an individual may not be able to reach a desired goal, accept the futility of planning to meet goals,

have negative expectations of the future, perceive a personal loss of control and see "no way out." Successful treatment of depression with medication and certain types of psychotherapy can reverse this profound state of hopelessness.

Feelings of hopelessness may lead to addiction or suicide. Hopelessness sometimes results from false or unrealistic expectations. For example, the hopeless person may feel that he or she should be able to accomplish anything and everything and descends into despair upon failure. Some individuals with depression feel that nothing they do will work out and that they are powerless.

Hopeless feelings sometimes result from magnifying events to the extent that everything and everyone seem to be insurmountable obstacles in relation to the self. Still, another type of magnification results in despair when people and events are idealized. For example, a new friend may be thought to be perfect, or an upcoming vacation is planned to run a smooth course. When the friend proves to have perceived personality flaws or when bad weather spoils the vacation, the individual who is the most unrealistically idealistic may begin to lose hope about any friends or any vacation.

Hopelessness may also result from a sense of being trapped in a negative set of circumstances from which there is no escape. When presented with a task that must be performed but seems to be impossible, a sense of frustration and futility leads to hopelessness. Prisoners and members of social and ethnic groups that suffer discrimination frequently feel so limited that their lives become hopeless. In societies that practice hexing and voodoo, victims sometimes become ill and die because they see themselves as literally having no future. In some of these situations—when victims are convinced that the hexing was a mistake and that the curse is lifted—health is recovered.

Confusion also leads to a sense of hopelessness, as it contributes to an individual's feeling of loss of control. What is important to understand is that hopelessness is a subjective state, related to the way an individual perceives his or her prospects. It is potentially reversible even though the hopeless person always has "reasons" to justify the hopelessness.

See also DEPRESSION; LEARNED OPTIMISM.

hormone replacement therapy   See MENOPAUSE.

hormones   Chemical messengers produced by various organs and tissues that regulate or modulate effects elsewhere throughout the body. Hormones produced by the brain are known as neurohormones; they are produced by neurons known as neuroendocrine transducers, which release a hormone in response to activation at the synapses of neurotransmitters.

Examples of hormones are cortisol, estrogen, insulin and epinephrine. Hormones control many body functions, including growth, sexual development and the body's response to illness.

See also CORTISOL; ENDOCRINE SYSTEM; EPINEPHRINE.

hospice   An organization that provides care and assistance through several mental and physical health disciplines for the terminally ill and their families. The hospice movement started in the middle of the 19th century in Ireland but did not attract attention in the United States until the 1960s. Hospices may be part of a hospital complex or separate institutions. They may supply both inpatient and home care. Hospice care usually involves the joint efforts of physicians, mental health professionals, nurses, social workers, chaplains and volunteers. Many hospice patients suffer from cancer and AIDS. Hospice treatment only begins when the patient's chances of survival are nonexistent and life expectancy is short. Long-term degenerative neurological illnesses are not usually treated in a hospice setting. Hospice treatment concentrates on relieving the symptoms of the patient and providing psychological comfort and support rather than further attempts at curing the disease, which, particularly in cancer cases, may actually increase the patient's discomfort. Hospice programs also assist families with practical and psychological concerns during the terminal illness and may provide continuing service for a time following the patient's death.

See also ACQUIRED IMMUNODEFICIENCY SYNDROME; DEATH; TERMINAL ILLNESS.

Kitch, D. L. "Hospice." In *Encyclopedia of Psychology,* vol. 2, edited by Raymond Corsini, New York: Wiley, 1984.

Zimmerman, Jack. *Hospice.* Baltimore: Urban and Schwarzenberg, 1986.

hospitalization   The stress of illness is often intensified by the threat of being in a hospital, a prospect that most people find anxiety-producing from beginning to end.

Stress starts with the need for a second medical opinion which, unless there is an emergency, is often a requirement of medical insurers before commitment to a hospital can be made. Stress then follows patients to the hospital registration desk, where the approach of many admissions personnel to the gathering patient information does little to make people feel comfortable.

Loss of privacy, another key stressor, begins at the very moment patients exchange their clothes for hospital gowns and settle down in rooms shared with at least one or more strangers, more or less sick than they. It is further compounded by the number of visitors they or their roommates may have—people who talk loudly as they spill into all corners and all sides of what can be too-small hospital rooms. In teaching hospitals, the stress continues when doctors and interns gather around patients' beds to discuss clinical aspects of the illness, sometimes as if the patients didn't exist or weren't right there in the bed.

Stress escalates when the loss of privacy combines with the loss of control patients experience as they are thrown into the uneven rhythm of the hospital routine—being aroused at early hours for medication before a change in shifts occurs, moving on stretchers or in wheelchairs from one end of the hospital to another, waiting in drafty corridors for countless tests and X rays, buzzing for nursing assistance, having unappealing meals served at hours when they may not be hungry and facing constantly changing caretakers and variations in the delivery of care. The most serious sources of hospitalization stress is being in pain and having to rely on others for help in controlling that pain. A device that allows patients to control the intake of pain medication has alleviated this problem for some.

Today, patients waiting to receive various transplants—heart, lungs, kidney and liver—experience an additional aspect of stress regarding the arrival of the vital organ. The lists of those needing transplants far exceeds their availability, and for some there is little likelihood of a match. Questions also arise concerning the criteria for the lists and for those who are given priority. An example of that arose in 1995, when baseball star Mickey Mantle received a transplant a short time after a diagnosis was made.

Stress follows all patients out of the recovery room—with regulations concerning how long their hospital stays can be. In 1995, length of hospitals stays became a major issue in connection with the birth of babies. It was felt by some that first-time mothers were being sent home too soon and were often both mentally and physically ill-prepared to take care of a baby. For other mothers, the added stress of taking care of older children along with the responsibilities of a newborn before they have fully recovered their strength awaited them.

The shortened hospital stays of the later 1990s increased the anxiety of most patients. Much of the time needed for rehabilitation and recovery now is spent outside of the hospital, which puts a good deal of the burden of care on patients' families. For those without families, other means of home care must be found and questions of how the costs of this care can be met must be answered.

Lastly, there is the stress on the family and friends related to hospitalization of the dying—ethical questions relating to withdrawal of nourishment and treatment particularly when there are no directions from the patient.

See also ANXIETY; AUTONOMY; CONTROL; DEATH; END OF LIFE ISSUES; PAIN; PERSONAL SPACE.

hostages Hostages are usually victims who are subjected to isolation, confinement and sometimes mental and physical torture. They may be blindfolded, kept in darkness and have their ears covered. The sensory deprivation experience may produce hallucinations. Their captors frequently keep them in a state of uncertainty about their fate. Some hostages have become paranoid and depressed and have developed feelings that their country and families have forgotten them. An odd familiarity occasionally develops between terrorist and hostage, especially given that both are in dangerous situations. Some hostages have even developed hostile feelings toward the government and agencies who are attempting to rescue them. Patty Hearst, the heiress who was kidnapped in February 1974 by the Symbionese Liberation Army, became interested in their cause and joined the group in bank robberies and other illegal activities until the leaders were killed and she was captured and imprisoned.

Readjustment to normal life after their release, though welcome, is sometimes difficult for hostages. Many experience nightmares, insomnia, bouts with abnormal fears, depression and feelings of rage and helplessness for some time. There have been cases of suicide. Mental health professionals are gaining understanding of the state of mind of former hostages through experience. Current thinking is that a regulated "decompression period" helps former hostages adjust to normal life and to being back with their families.

Following the Persian Gulf War during 1991, several hostages were released after long years of captivity. Interviewed in *Psychiatric News*, Richard Rahe, M.D., director of the Nevada Stress Center at the University of Nevada School of Medicine and a former Navy psychiatrist with extensive experience working with hostages and disaster victims, said, "People who do well have done well in the past with stress. They have had adequate-to-good childhoods. They did well in captivity. They passed through depression, past themselves, to helping others. They turned the experience into a positive one, by reviewing their lives, making positive changes."

Dr. Rahe also said that survivor guilt is common, as are recriminations about the way they might have behaved in captivity, and many are angry toward their families or the government for not doing enough to help them. At greatest risk of developing full-blown post-traumatic stress disorder (PTSD) are those people already having symptoms and those without a good support system.

In advising therapists regarding hostages, Dr. Rahe suggested dealing with the PTSD only if it becomes chronic. Rather, he suggested they deal with the day-to-day issues.

Elmore Rigamer, M.D., chief psychiatrist at the U.S. State Department, was quoted in *Psychiatric News* (Jan. 4, 1991) regarding the "keys to staving off deterioration" in a hostage situation. "Mastery" and "connectedness" are the keys to overcoming psychological hurdles associated with having been a hostage. Mastery (a sense of control) and connectedness (feeling accurately informed) are both important for hostages and their families. As Dr. Rigamer said, "The ones who were able to take control of themselves will do wonderfully. The more feeling of loss of control, the worse. In therapy we go over and over what happened, and imagine what they would like to have done that gives them a post-facto mastery and catharsis."

Dr. Rigamer emphasized the psychological value of relaying information to hostages and families during and after the crisis. He said that during the crisis he spent as much time as he could on the telephone with State Department hostages in Baghdad and Kuwait and their families back home, clearing up rumors and giving out information. Being in communication increases one's sense of mastery, which helps prevent PTSD in both the hostages and their families.

In *Psychiatric News* (Jan. 4, 1991), Thomas M. Haizlip, M.D., director of the Child Psychiatry Division at the University of North Carolina at Chapel Hill, outlined seven stages of mastery that he believes are applicable to both the hostages and their families:

1. Discriminating between good and bad forces
2. Coping by knowing what to do if it ever happens again
3. Putting your life back in order
4. Dealing with survivor guilt (having left some people and worldly goods behind)
5. Realizing that healthy people are willing to "seal it over" and taking advantage of a two- to three-week "window" after the experience, when willingness to talk is greatest
6. Hooking up any symptoms with the event, rather than further repressing
7. Recognizing that many people do not want help because they feel they themselves are important dispensers of help

Many of these stages are also applicable after other life traumas, such as witnessing or being a victim of a crime or family violence.

See also ANXIETY; BRAINWASHING; CONTROL; DEPRESSION; POST-TRAUMATIC STRESS DISORDER; TERRORISM.

Kahn, Ada P., and Jan Fawcett. *The Encyclopedia of Mental Health.* New York: Facts On File, 1993.
Haizlip, Thomas M. "Hostages." *Psychiatric News* (January 4, 1991): 18.

hostility   A persistent attitude of deep resentment and intense anger. It may be the result of stressful situations, and it can also cause stress for the individual. The hostile person may have an urge to retaliate against a person or situation. During some situations of intense frustration, deprivation or discrimination, feelings of hostility may be a normal reaction. However, hostile attitudes also may occur during anxiety attacks, in obsessive-compulsive disorder or depression. Some people who have anti-social personalities frequently have hostile attitudes.

At best, hostile people are simply grouchy. At worst, they are consumed by hatred. A hostile person may have a tense-looking face and body. They are easily excitable. They seem to have a chip on their shoulders and a bitterness toward the world. They may be sarcastic, moody and aggressive when they feel challenged.

For many individuals, the stresses of hostilities can be worked out with through exercise, better communication skills, behavior therapy, use of meditation and relaxation and psychotherapy.

See also AGGRESSION; ANGER; ANXIETY; BEHAVIOR THERAPY; COMPLEMENTARY THERAPIES; DEPRESSION; EXERCISE; FRUSTRATION; MEDITATION; OBSESSIVE-COMPULSIVE DISORDER; PERSONALITY; PSYCHOTHERAPIES; RELAXATION; TYPE A PERSONALITY.

Friedman, Howard S. *The Self-Healing Personality.* New York: Henry Holt, 1991.

hot flashes   A common symptom of menopause experienced by many women before menstrual periods stop and after cessation of menses. Hot flashes are disturbing to a woman's sense of well-being because they are unpredictable. A hot flash is a sudden feeling of warmth occurring on the face, chest or entire body. The woman's body may become flushed, and patches of redness may appear on her chest, back, shoulders and upper arms. As her body temperature readjusts, she may perspire profusely and have a cold, clammy sensation. Episodes may last from seconds to minutes. As sweat evaporates, the body temperature decreases, which sometimes causes chills or the cold, clammy sensation. Many women say that the worst aspect of hot flashes is that it makes them feel out of control of their bodies and interferes with their sense of mental well-being. Previous generations of women were sometimes told that hot flashes were "all in their head" and that menopause was expected to be a time filled with bizarre behavior and delusions.

Modern women know that hot flashes are not a threat to health; however, they may make a woman uncomfortable and even anxious about having one in social or professional situations. Because hot flashes may occur during the night and disrupt sleep, women experiencing hot flashes may become irritable, tired and depressed. In a 1986 survey (Kahn and Holt), typical complaints about hot flashes included waking up at night drenched in sweat, ruining clothes from perspiration, feeling embarrassed at flushing and shivering with no control and being intolerant of heat or cold. Many women find their bodies unable to deal comfortably with even slight variations in temperature.

Some women have hot flashes several times a day, once a week or less frequently. For most women, hot flashes are self-limiting symptoms and disappear without any treatment. However, there is some disagreement concerning when hot flashes stop. According to a report in the *Journal of the American Geriatric Society* (Sept. 1982), they usually stop within one to five years, yet some women report that they had hot flashes over a 10-year period.

Causes

Understanding why hot flashes happen helps women cope with the anxieties produced by the anticipation of flashes. A hormone known as luteinizing hormone (LH) rises after menopause. Before menopause, it is the substance that helps trigger ovulation. LH "surges" seem to set off hot flashes by dilating surface blood vessels. Hormonal changes associated with the hot flash may also be due to nerve activity in the hypothalamic area that controls temperature and anterior pituitary function.

Medical and Mental Health Help

When hot flashes occur so often that a woman frequently cannot get a good night's sleep, if they interfere with sexual activity or work or if they make her chronically exhausted and depressed, medical assistance should be sought. Hot flashes are often treated with hormone replacement therapy and alternatives including sedatives and anticholinergic agents (substances that block or interfere with transmission of certain impulses in the parasympathetic nervous system).

Self-helps

Many women overcome their fears of being out of control of their bodies and their hot flashes by developing a series of self-help techniques. The following are some recommendations regarding hot flashes based on a survey of 967 women in 1987:

- Air stuffy rooms, keep a window open if one is too warm. Layer clothing. A suit with a lightweight blouse gives the wearer more flexibility than a wool dress.
- Wear a cotton (or other absorbent material) blouse under a sweater. Avoid wearing a sweater next to the skin.
- For desk workers, use a small desktop fan.
- During a hot flash, do not overreact. By keeping calm, others will not pay attention.
- Learn relaxation techniques to feel in control of the situation.
- Regular exercise will tone the vascular system and may help a woman feel better.
- Keep weight down. Slender women seem to have less erratic estrogen production and hence less erratic experiences with hot flashes.

See also AGING; CLIMACTERIC; MENOPAUSE.

Kahn, Ada P., and Linda Hughey Holt. *The A to Z of Women's Sexuality.* Alameda, Calif.: Hunter House, 1992.

———. *Midlife Health: A Woman's Practical Guide to Feeling Good.* New York: Avon Books, 1989.

hot lines   Throughout the United States, hot lines cover many mental health and related concerns. The numbers available for information and help are often toll-free and usually operate on a 24-hour basis. Most city telephone directories include a list of some of the available hot lines.

A listing of national self-help groups can be obtained by writing to:

St. Clares—Riverside Medical Center
Dept. P
1 Indian Road
Denville, NJ 07834
Phone: (201) 625-6000

See also SUPPORT GROUPS.

human immunodeficiency virus (HIV)   The virus responsible for causing the infection that leads to acquired immunodeficiency syndrome (AIDS). When the virus was first isolated in the early 1980s, it was known as HLTV-III. The virus is transmitted by direct exchange of body fluids, such as blood or semen, or by using contaminated needles for illicit drug use. Many individuals have anxieties about contracting the virus by eating in restaurants in which infected individuals work or by sending their children to a school that an infected child is known to attend. In most cases, these anxieties are unfounded, as, according to research reports, the virus does not survive outside the body. As of the early 2000s, casual contact through sharing utensils or towels or even kissing has not been shown to transmit the virus.

The virus is found in semen; the most common form of semen transmission in the United States is anal intercourse, during which tears of and bleeding from the delicate rectal lining can occur. The vaginal wall is tougher and less prone to tear and bleed, but sperm does travel through the uterus into the abdomen as a result of sexual intercourse. It has been reported that women have a seven to 10 times greater likelihood of infection from vaginal intercourse than men.

Individuals who suspect their partners of having outside, high-risk sexual contacts, such as homo-sexual men or prostitutes, should seek medical advice about screening for and preventing transmission of the HIV virus. Use of condoms during sexual intercourse is promoted as a way to prevent the transmission, yet it is known that they are not 100 percent safe. Distribution of condoms in schools to young people in areas of high prevalence of the infection in the 1990s caused controversy among parents and educators but was viewed as one step toward slowing down the rapid rise of the infection among young people.

See also ACQUIRED IMMUNODEFICIENCY SYNDROME (AIDS); HOMOSEXUALITY.

Kahn, Ada P., and Linda Hughey Holt. *Midlife Health: A Woman's Practical Guide to Feeling Good.* New York: Avon Books, 1989.

humanistic psychology   An approach to understanding human nature, behavior and mental health that focuses on an individual's personal experience. The American Association for Humanistic Psychology was founded in 1962 by Carl Rogers, Abraham Maslow, Kurt Goldstein, Rollo May and others. Humanistic psychology emphasizes individual choice, creativity, valuation, self-realization and the development of each person's potential.

Humanistic psychologists believe that people have a hierarchy of many needs, beginning with physiological needs, as well as those for safety, love, "belongingness," self-esteem, to know and understand and, finally, self-actualization.

Humanistic psychology differs from the Freudian approach, which suggested that sexual drive is the motivating force, and behavioral psychology, which explains behavior as a result of various environmental relationships.

See also SELF-ESTEEM.

humor   A balanced sense of humor is an aspect of good mental health. Ancient scholars understood the role of humor in good health. The Book of Proverbs says: "A merry heart doeth good like a medicine." Conversely, many individuals who suffer from depression lose their sense of humor, and few things make them smile or laugh. Studies in the late 20th century suggested that an ability to enjoy humor and to laugh has effects on mental as well as physical health.

For most people, humor and laughter usually provide a helpful release of tension and anxieties. Laughter may actually ease pain and may help the respiratory system by exercising the lungs. Laughter and other positive emotions may influence the immune system, possibly by stimulating production of certain hormones.

Shared humor relieves anxiety in stressful group situations, such as delayed airplanes or trains, and also relieves stress that results from boredom. At times when it seems that nothing is left to talk about, familiar topics can be renewed by employing humor.

Some therapists employ humor to momentarily relieve depression during therapy sessions. One technique is known as paradoxical therapy, in which the therapist gives the individual new perspectives on his or her problems by exaggerating them to the point of making them seem funny. The therapist assigns the individual to be depressed or anxious at a certain time of day. Sometimes the silliness of such situations helps alleviate the individual's depressed or anxious feelings.

Humor is a universal language and has universal appeal. The basis for much humor is that we are prepared for one thing and something else happens. Although we are startled, we know there is no danger and we release our surprise in laughter. Thus a story with an unexpected ending or a game of peek-a-boo for an infant can bring about a laughter response.

See also LAUGHTER.

Fry, William F., and Waleed A. Salameh, eds. *Handbook of Humor and Psychotherapy.* Sarasota, Fla.: Professional Resources Exchange, 1987.
Morreall, John. *Taking Laughter Seriously.* Albany: State University of New York, 1983.
Ziv, Avner. *Personality and Sense of Humor.* New York: Springer Publishing Co., 1984.

Hunter's syndrome   A form of mental retardation caused by the X-linked recessive gene. There may be moderate to severe developmental delay.

See also MENTAL RETARDATION.

Huntington's disease (Huntington's chorea)   A hereditary progressive brain disease that causes involuntary movements and dementia. Due to a single autosomal dominant gene, the disease was first described by George Huntington (1815–1916), an American neurologist, in 1972.

The average age of onset is 35. In early stages, the individual may have symptoms that appear to be anxiety and depression. There is moodiness, irritability and a poor ability to concentrate or remember.

According to the Alzheimer's Disease and Related Diseases Association, a family history of the disease, recognition of typical movement disorders and CAT brain scanning provide evidence for a diagnosis of Huntington's disease (HD). A genetic marker liked to the Huntington gene has been identified and further research is under way.

Sedative drugs help some individuals. The movement disorders and psychiatric symptoms seen in HD can be controlled by drugs, but there is no treatment available to stop the progression of the disease. Developments in understanding of human genetics in the early 2000s continue to give researchers more information on this somewhat rare disease.

See also ALZHEIMER'S DISEASE.

Hurler syndrome   A form of mental retardation that causes severe and progressive developmental delay, caused by a genetic deficiency.

See also MENTAL RETARDATION.

hyperactivity   Mental and physical restlessness. Hyperactive children have unlimited energy and short attention spans, are prone to temper tantrums and seem to require little sleep. The condition is more common in male children. Until their disorder is understood, many are considered unmanageable or troublemakers by teachers and parents. There is a difference of opinion regarding causes of hyperactivity. Some physicians say hyperactive behavior may be due to minimal brain damage that cannot be detected by any diagnostic tests or due to birth trauma. Others attribute hyperactivity to food allergies. Diagnosis requires careful evaluation and is usually made before the child is seven years old; children so diagnosed exhibit at least six months of disruptive behavior.

Some physicians prescribe a stimulant medication called Ritalin (methylphenidate hydrochloride) or Dexedrine (dextroamphetamine sulfate) for hyperactivity, which makes hyperactive children more manageable and able to concentrate better. The drugs may work by diminishing the brain's excess of natural stimulants and replacing them with milder, synthetic ones. Stimulant medications should be used cautiously because they can be addictive in young adults.

Therapy may include psychotherapeutic counseling, meeting with parents and teachers and participating in support groups for parents and children. Coping with a hyperactive child requires a great degree of understanding and patience.

Hyperactivity in children is also known as attention-deficit hyperactivity disorder (ADHD).

See also ATTENTION-DEFICIT HYPERACTIVITY DISORDER.

hypersomnia Excessive daytime sleepiness and an inability to wake up quickly. This can be seen in one form of depression, which also may manifest in increased eating and weight gain, as opposed to another form associated with insomnia, weight loss and agitation-anxiety. Patients with sleep apnea syndrome or narcolepsy may also show excessive daytime sleepiness.

See also DEPRESSION; NARCOLEPSY; SLEEP.

hypertension See HIGH BLOOD PRESSURE.

hyperthyroidism Overactivity of the thyroid gland, which causes an increase of all chemical reactions within the body, affecting mental as well as physical processes. It is more common in women than men.

Because some of the symptoms of hyperthyroidism seem similar to those of anxiety and depression, an evaluation by a physician is essential to make a careful diagnosis.

Normally, thyroid gland activity is controlled by a hormone produced in the pituitary gland. Even when normal levels of hormone are produced, the thyroid gland itself continuously produces quantities of its own hormone, thyroxin.

Symptoms of hyperthyroidism include anxiety, tiredness with an inability to sleep, shakiness, trembling and insensitivity to cold and perspiration when others are comfortable. There may be irregular and fast heartbeat, palpitations, a fluttering feeling in the chest and breathlessness after mild exertion.

Individuals who have hyperthyroidism may eat more and lose weight, muscles may waste away, and women may have absent or scant menstrual periods. The thyroid gland in the neck may enlarge (goiter). In severe cases, eyes may look wide open and protrude, leading to blurred or double vision.

Hyperthyroidism is treated with medications containing antithyroid drugs, with surgery to remove a lump in the thyroid gland or, in some cases, most of the gland. More commonly, sufferers take a drinkable form of radioactive iodine, which acts on the glandular tissue in the thyroid gland to control the overactivity of the cells.

Underactivity of the thyroid gland is known as myxedema. Individuals with underactive thyroid glands feel tired much of the time. This condition, too, can mimic or mask depression and needs careful diagnosis.

Recent research has shown the presence of subtle abnormalities of thyroid function in clinical depression.

See also HYPOTHYROIDISM.

hyperventilation Deep and fast breathing, sometimes referred to as overbreathing. Some individuals who have panic attacks and phobias react with hyperventilation, which in turn makes them fear that they are dying or having a heart attack. While individuals who overbreath feel short of breath and breathe deeply and faster to get more air into their lungs, they are really taking in too much air. This breathing pattern makes them feel worse, as it removes too much carbon dioxide from the blood; some is needed in the body to perform efficiently.

Overbreathing leads to rapid heartbeat, lightheadedness, dizziness, sweating and numbness or tingling in the hands and feet. Fainting sometimes occurs; hyperventilation may be mistaken for a heart attack. At the least, it exacerbates the individual's anxiety level.

When an individual has a dizzy spell or feels the effects of hyperventilation, breathing into a paper bag for a few minutes can help restore the balance of oxygen and carbon dioxide in the blood. When some of the exhaled carbon dioxide from the bag returns to the lungs, the individual will begin to breathe more normally again.

Relaxation therapy, including breathing instruction, helps some individuals who suffer from panic attacks and other anxiety disorders.

According to sex researchers William Howell Masters and Virginia Johnson, hyperventilation is a reaction of women and men during the late plateau phase of sexual intercourse. The physiological intensity and duration of the reaction indicate the degree of developing sexual tension.

See also BREATHING; RELAXATION TRAINING.

hypnosis (hypnotherapy) A type of attentive, receptive and focused concentration accompanied by a diminished awareness of environmental stimuli. In a therapy situation utilizing hypnosis, the patient cooperates with the therapist to utilize this form of intense concentration to facilitate and accelerate reaching particular therapeutic goals. Individuals cannot be hypnotized against their will, but some individuals are more or less capable of achieving a hypnotic trance. Hypnosis has been described in detail in the writings of Sigmund Freud.

Hypnosis is sometimes used to relieve specific symptoms such as insomnia, anxiety, conversion reactions, phobias and pain and well as to control habits, such as smoking, nail biting and overeating. While hypnosis has limitations as a therapy, many clinicians believe that hypnosis can be helpful when used selectively.

Therapy with hypnosis involves teaching the individual self-hypnosis techniques so they can induce a trancelike state in themselves and use suggestions that help them restructure their thinking regarding the condition for which they are seeking help. For example, in management of pain, hypnosis helps to block the perception of pain by drawing the individual's attention away from it.

Self-hypnosis is sometimes used with anxiety reactions to promote relaxation on cue in fearful situations. In general, autohypnosis by itself will not significantly relieve anxiety responses. It can, however, be used as a supplement to behavioral therapy to make images more vivid and to heighten one's ability to concentrate.

hypnotic drugs Short-acting drugs that induce sleep by depressing the central nervous system. An example of a hypnotic drug is sodium secobarbital (Seconal). In the past, hypnotics were sometimes prescribed for individuals who were anxious and could not sleep soundly. Because of possibilities for abuse of drugs in the category of hypnotics, they are no longer widely prescribed. Tranquilizers or benzodiazepine drugs are now more commonly prescribed as sleep-inducing medications in individuals with anxieties.

See also ANXIETY; ANTIANXIETY MEDICATIONS; TRANQUILIZER DRUGS.

hypochondriasis An overconcern or preoccupation with one's health problems that may be real or imaginary. Some individuals (hypochondriacs) become extraordinarily concerned with their heartbeat, digestion or minor physical abnormalities, such as a skin blemish. People who are hypochondriacs often have symptoms of anxiety, depression and obsessive-compulsive personality traits.

hypoglycemia A reduced amount of glucose in the blood, which can produce nervousness, trembling and some symptoms mimicking anxiety disorders.

hypomanic episode An episode in which symptoms are similar to those in a manic episode but less severe. In a manic episode, the individual has a period in which the predominant mood is elevated, expansive or irritable to such an extent that functioning and social activities are impaired. The individual with a manic episode may need hospitalization to avoid harm to self and others, while those with hypomanic episodes may exhibit poor judgment but usually do not require hospitalization, unless it is necessary for the depression that almost inevitably follows the manic or hypomanic episode.

See also BIPOLAR DISORDER; MANIC-DEPRESSIVE ILLNESS.

hypothalamus   The coordinating center of the brain. It is a small area located above the pituitary gland, with nerve connections to most other areas of the nervous system. It controls the sympathetic nervous system (which in turn controls the inner body organs). During excitement or fear, the brain sends signals to the hypothalamus, which initiates a chain of activity, including faster heartbeat, faster breathing rate and increased blood flow to the muscles (the fight or flight response). The hypothalamus also controls reactions that cause sweating or shivering, stimulates appetite and thirst, regulates sleep, motivates sexual behavior and determines emotions and moods; it also indirectly controls many of the endocrine organs, which secrete hormones.

See also BRAIN; BRAIN CHEMISTRY.

hypothyroidism   Underactivity of the thyroid gland and below-normal production of thyroid hormones, which stimulate energy production from sugar. Symptoms of lack of the hormone may include muscle weakness, a slow heart rate, dry, flaky skin, hair loss and a deep and husky voice. The disorder is diagnosed by tests to measure the level of thyroid hormone in the blood. Treatment consists of replacement therapy with the thyroid hormone thyroxin. Depression may be associated with thyroid hypofunction.

See also HYPERTHYROIDISM.

hysterectomy   Surgical removal of the uterus. It is an operation that causes many women emotional upheaval and, for some, physiological concerns. The word "hysterectomy" comes from the Greek work *hystera,* meaning "woman."

The first successful hysterectomy in the United States was performed in 1853. More than 650,000 American women undergo hysterectomies each year, nearly one-quarter of whom are over age 50.

There is a great deal of confusion among the public over the precise meaning of hysterectomy. A better understanding contributes to better psychological acceptance of the event. A "total" hysterectomy refers to removal of the uterus and cervix. "Partial" refers to removal only of the body of the uterus. If the fallopian tubes and ovaries are removed, the procedure is called a "total hysterectomy bilateral salpingoophorectomy." A hysterectomy can be done vaginally or via an abdominal incision.

Some women experience sexual dysfunction following hysterectomy. Women who had preexisting sexuality problems are more likely to develop postoperative problems than are women who enjoyed a healthy sex life prior to surgery. Sexual problems can result from underlying poor self-concept; a woman who equates sexuality with fertility may feel like "less of a woman" without a uterus; a woman who has been raised to think sex is evil unless aimed at procreation may feel guilty about sexual activities following hysterectomy. Some women experience painful intercourse after a hysterectomy; this can be due to vaginal dryness if the ovaries were removed or due to loss of some of the lubricating glands.

Part of female orgasm consists of rhythmic uterine contractions; while women still experience orgasm, some women are aware of a difference in internal sensations with orgasm.

However, many women experience an improvement in sexual relations if the hysterectomy successfully treated a painful condition such as endometriosis or if a bleeding problem made sexual activity messy or distasteful.

See also DEPRESSION.

Kahn, Ada P., and Linda Hughey Holt. *The A to Z of Women's Sexuality.* Alameda, Calif.: Hunter House, 1992.
Rosenfeld, Nancy, and Dianna Bolen. *Just as Much a Woman.* Rocklin, Calif.: Prima, 1999.

hysteria   A medical diagnostic term for illnesses characterized by emotional outbursts and transformation of unconscious conflicts into physical symptoms, such as pain, paralysis or blindness. The term encompasses a wide range of symptoms that are usually attributed to mental stress. Derived from the ancient Greek word *hysteron,* meaning "uterus," the term was first used to refer only to diseases of women that ancients explained arose from problems in the uterus. Until the late 1800s, when Sigmund Freud presented a case of male hysteria, the illness was considered solely a female problem.

Psychiatrists say that the term is no longer helpful in diagnosis, and symptoms formerly grouped under this term are now included in more specific diagnostic categories such as conversion disorder, dissociative disorders, somatization disorder and factitious disorder.

Mass hysteria refers to the psychological spread of symptoms (for example, itching, nausea or fainting) from person to person. This situation occurs in schools or institutions in response to group tensions or worries, such as worries about the threat of toxins in the water supply.

See also FREUD, SIGMUND.

iatrogenic psychiatric disorder Symptoms that mimic psychiatric disorders induced by prescribed medications. This seems to happen more in elderly individuals than in younger people. For example, patients treated with diuretics for hypertension may have a potassium deficiency that produces fatigue, appearing to be depression; propranolol may have a similar effect. Digitalis toxicity and phenytoin (Dilantin) toxicity can induce fatigue and mental confusion that may mimic depression, psychosis or dementia. Anxiolytic drugs and hypnotic drugs can also produce symptoms that appear to be a psychiatric disorder, such as confusion, lethargy or withdrawal. Sometimes the diagnosis of a psychiatric condition due to prescribed drugs can be made from the individual's history. In other cases, laboratory tests are needed.

See also PHARMACOLOGIC THERAPY in BIBLIOGRAPHY.

Andreason, Nancy C., and Donald W. Black. *Introductory Textbook of Psychiatry.* Washington, D.C.: American Psychiatric Association, 1991.

id According to Sigmund Freud, the id consists of human instincts and the energy associated with them. He believed that there were no conflicts within the id and that all functions existed side by side to fulfill the id's aims. When the newborn has to obtain substances from the environment to survive, aims are met by initiating activity such as breathing, crying or sucking. When conflicts occur between the internal and external realities, one portion of the id was modified to become the ego, which would deal with the conflicts between the internal and external worlds and mediate between what the individual needed and what was possible.

See also EGO; FREUD, SIGMUND.

ideas of influence Ideas that a source, such as a radio or television broadcast, speaker, animal or voice is telling one what to do or is influencing behavior. The individual takes these messages seriously and does not question the fact that no one else hears them. This symptom is often a characteristic of schizophrenia.

See also DELUSION; IDEAS OF REFERENCE; PARANOID; SCHIZOPHRENIA.

idealization A mental mechanism in which the person attributes exaggeratedly positive qualities to the self or others.

ideas of reference Insignificant remarks, statements or events interpreted by the individual to have some special meaning to him or her. For example, one who walks into a room and sees people laughing may think they are laughing at her or him. For another individual, items read in the newspaper or heard over the news on television are thought to have some special meaning for that person. The individual may be suspicious but recognizes that the ideas may be erroneous. When the individual truly believes that the statements or events refer to him or her, this is considered a delusion of reference. Ideas of reference are a characteristic of paranoid schizophrenia.

See also PARANOID; SCHIZOPHRENIA.

identification A defense mechanism, an unconscious process, by which one patterns oneself after some other person. Identification plays a major role in the development of personality, specifically the superego. This is different from role modeling, which is a conscious process.

See also DEFENSE MECHANISMS; SUPEREGO.

idiot savant   An individual who shows general low mental ability but exhibits high ability in the areas of music, art, mathematics, geography, the calendar, motor coordination or extrasensory perception. Idiot savants are also called "autistic savants" by some authorities. Others feel that their behavior stems from retardation rather than autism.

Holmes, D. L. "Idiot Savant," In *Encyclopedia of Psychology,* vol. 2, edited by Raymond J. Corsini. New York: Wiley, 1984.

illiteracy   Illiteracy is a social problem in the United States and a personal problem for many individuals. Those who cannot read have a poor self-image and have difficulty obtaining employment with which to support themselves and their families. Illiterates or those who read very poorly feel inferior and frequently develop techniques to hide or compensate for their lack of reading ability. Embarrassment may also keep them from seeking help for their problem.

It is estimated that 75 percent of unemployed Americans are illiterate. Recently the New York Telephone Company had to test 60,000 people on an entry level exam to hire 3,000 employees. One major corporation had to use graphics on its assembly line to compensate for workers' inability to read simple phrases. As jobs become more technical and the economy shifts from an industrial to service base, more jobs will require skills beyond the ninth grade level, compared with the fourth grade level skills typical after World War II. In 1986, a National Advisory Council on Adult Education survey showed that 40 percent of all armed service enlistees read below a ninth grade level. Illiteracy is strongly related to poverty, crime and drug use. About 75 percent of adult prison inmates are functionally illiterate.

A large segment of the illiterate population is afflicted with learning disabilities. According to a study undertaken in 1987 by the Federal Interagency Task Force, 12 million to 24 million Americans have learning disabilities that make it difficult for them to learn to read. Complicating this problem is the issue of whether illiteracy in itself constitutes a learning disability.

illusion   A distorted sensation, perception or memory, based on misinterpretation of a reality. For example, one may interpret seeing a pen or pencil as a dangerous knife. Optical illusions occur in daily life. An example is a narrow road that appears to come together ahead; or, when one is anxious and waiting, one may think that an hour has passed when only a few minutes have gone by. Illusions are usually brief and can be understood upon explanation. They may occur with anxiety or tiredness, as a reaction to drugs, as a result of certain forms of brain damage or in delirium tremens.

See also DELIRIUM TREMENS.

imagery   See GUIDED IMAGERY.

imaging techniques   See BRAIN IMAGING.

imipramine hydrochloride   The original tricyclic antidepressant drug (trade name: Tofranil), which is effective in treating depressive episodes of major depression and bipolar, dysthymic, panic and phobic disorders. Like other drugs in its class, imipramine may take up to three to four weeks to become effective. It is quite toxic in an overdose and may produce seizures or serious cardiac arrhythmias.

See also ANTIDEPRESSANT MEDICATIONS; TRICYCLIC ANTIDEPRESSANTS; PHARMACOLOGICAL APPROACH.

immune system   Cells and proteins that work to protect the body from possibly harmful microorganisms such as viruses, bacteria and fungi. The immune system is involved in problems of allergies and hypersensitivity, rejection of tissues after grafts and transplants and probably cancer.

Defects in the immune system cause the body's own proteins to be misidentified as antigens, and the body then attacks them, resulting in autoimmune disorders.

Suppression of the immune system can occur as an inherited disorder or after infection with certain viruses, including HIV (the virus that causes AIDS), resulting in lowered resistance to infections that are usually resisted and to the development of malignancies. There is evidence that severe stress and depression may inhibit normal immune function, but it has not yet been proven that the reduced function measured is of clinical significance. This research continues and may show that pathological stress responses and moods affect physical health.

Many people believe that a positive mental attitude can influence the immune system in a positive way.

See also HUMAN IMMUNODEFICIENCY VIRUS; IMAGERY.

implosive therapy (implosion)   A technique used in behavioral therapy in which the individual imagines an intense anxiety-producing situation for long periods of time without escaping. Developed by Thomas G. Stampfl, an American psychologist at the University of Wisconsin, this procedure is designed to eradicate the avoidance response that feeds the anxiety.

See also BEHAVIORAL THERAPY; CATHARSIS; PSYCHOTHERAPIES.

impotence   The inability of a male to complete sexual intercourse due to partial or complete inability to achieve or maintain an erection. Short episodes of erectile impotence are common and should not be a cause for undue concern by the man or his partner. In certain situations, such as times of stress or after drinking too much alcohol, many men experience temporary erectile impotence. Chronically impotent men, however, are continually unable to have an erection.

It is estimated that 10 million American men have erectile impotence and consequent mental health problems of frustration, embarrassment and irritability.

Scientific and medical views vary regarding the numbers of those afflicted with psychological and physiological impotence. Recent research, according to Surgitek/Medical Engineering Corporation, indicates that nearly 50 percent of impotent men suffer from physiological problems, with a large number afflicted with irreversible organic impotence.

The penis contains two cylindrical chambers filled with tiny, spongelike compartments. When a man becomes sexually aroused, his nervous and circulatory systems cause microscopic valves in the penis to open, filling the spongy erectile tissues with eight times the normal amount of blood, resulting in erection.

Impotence may take the form of low interest in sexual activity, premature ejaculation, coitus without ejaculation or erectile capacity only with prostitutes. Impotence differs from sterility, which means that a person is not capable of producing a child.

Although some men believe that liquor and drugs make them more potent, two of the most common causes of impotence are heavy cigarette smoking and excessive consumption of alcohol. Nicotine constricts blood vessels and can impair sexual function.

Sex researchers Masters and Johnson have given the label primary impotence to the condition of never having had an erection, and secondary impotence to the condition of having had an ability in the past to have an erection but no longer being able to do so. There are multiple causes of impotence. Some of the most common causes include illnesses such as diabetes, which effects the nervous and vascular supply to the penis; circulatory problems, such as arteriosclerosis; neurological disorders resulting from diabetes; Parkinson's disease; multiple sclerosis; prostate surgery; injury to the nerves, spinal cord or brain; hormonal abnormalities, such as thyroid disease or decreased testosterone; and medications, such as antihypertension drugs, which affect nerve function. Emotional factors, such as marital stress or depression, also affect impotence. It was once thought that psychological factors caused most impotence, but with increasing medical knowledge, the proportion that can be explained on physiological grounds is increasing.

It is important for a man suffering from impotence to have a thorough checkup for physical as well as emotional causes of impotence by a knowledgeable physician and/or sex therapist. Treatment may be as simple as treatment of the disease or elimination of the drug causing it, or as complicated as surgical implantation of a prosthesis.

Sex therapy is helpful to many men. It can often be as simple as helping him relax during sexual activity.

Diagnosing the causes of impotence involves a battery of sophisticated physical and psychological tests conducted with the impotent man and, in some cases, his partner. The physical examination includes blood, hormone and circulation tests, neurological studies and tests on penile blood pressure and temperature, among others.

An important test to distinguish organic from psychological impotence is the Nocturnal Penile Tumescence (NPT) Test, in which erections that occur during sleep are measured. A normal man has between two and five erections while asleep, each lasting from five minutes to half an hour. In the test, which can be conducted in sleep laboratories or the home, an electronic device is used to record changes in penile size. An insufficient number of nocturnal erections may indicate a physical problem.

See also MASTERS, WILLIAM H.; SEX THERAPY.

impulse control disorders   Several mental health disorders in which individuals are unable to resist an impulse or temptation that is harmful to themselves or to others. These disorders include kleptomania (shoplifting, stealing), pathological gambling and pyromania (setting fires). Some people are arrested for stealing and setting fires before a mental diagnosis is made. Individuals with these disorders should seek psychotherapy before their compulsions interfere with the rest of their lives in a personal or legal sense.

Other impulse disorders may involve violent suicidal or self-mutilatory behavior. Evidence is developing that impulse disorders may be related to decreased serotonin levels in the brain.

See also GAMBLING; SEROTONIN.

incest   Sexual intercourse between closely related individuals, within degrees wherein marriage is prohibited by law or custom. Almost all societies have some incest taboos. In some societies sexual intercourse between cousins or between uncles and nieces, aunts and nephews, is prohibited. In the United States, father-daughter, mother-son and brother-sister seem to be the most heinous infraction of mores. When sexual relations occur against a person's will, even with a

family member, the situation is considered sexual abuse. Many family members do not report such abuse to authorities out of fear of reprisal from the family member, fear of being abandoned or other reasons.

Vidmar, Lou Ann Lalani. "A Multidimensional Psychotherapy for Women Incest Victims." Thesis, Rosemead School of Psychology, 1985.

indecision   See DECISION MAKING.

indigestion   A variety of symptoms brought on by eating, including flatulence, heartburn, abdominal pain and nausea. It causes a burning discomfort in the stomach because the individual has eaten too much or too fast, or because the food consumed was too rich, spicy or fatty. Nervous indigestion is a common cause of stress. This stress generally results from anything that causes anger, anxiety, pain and fear. Stage fright, going for a job interview or going on a first date are sometimes stressful situations that can cause indigestion.

To keep stress levels in line, eat a balanced diet. Allow plenty of time for eating. Limit foods that cause indigestion; eat small meals four times a day. Get adequate sleep and practice deep breathing, visualization and other stress-reducing techniques.

Belching

Belching, or common burping, comes from the swallowing of air or from gas in the stomach caused by the chemical reactions of food and digestive juices. Many individuals feel stressed by the embarrassment that results from belching in a social situation or public place. To overcome the embarrassment, as well as the source of the problem, careful attention to diet may make a difference. Also, taking more time to select foods carefully and eat slowly may reduce the incidence of this annoying reaction.

Belching may occur more frequently when an individual feels stressed because he or she either eats too fast or selects foods that contribute to heartburn, bloating and belching. In addition to diet, relaxation techniques may be useful.

Bloating

The term bloating applies to the full, distended feeling in the abdomen which occurs after overeating. Many people react to stressful situations by overeating, eating too fast or eating spicy or greasy foods, all of which contribute to bloating. The discomfort causes further stress, as bloating leads to belching or burping, which can be socially embarrassing.

TIPS TO RELIEVE ANXIETY DUE TO BLOATING

- Relax before eating; eat and drink slowly.
- Limit foods/beverages that contain air, such as carbonated drinks, baked goods, whipped cream and soufflés. Don't smoke, chew gum, suck on hard candy or drink through straws or narrow-mouthed bottles.
- Correct loose dentures.
- Eat fewer rich foods, such as fatty meals, fried food, cream sauces, gravies and pastries.
- Don't lie down immediately after eating.
- Don't try to force yourself to belch.

See also ANGER; ANXIETY; FEAR; IRRITABLE BOWEL SYNDROME; NAUSEA; NUTRITION; PAIN; RELAXATION; STAGE FRIGHT.

Kahn, Ada P. *Stress A to Z: The Sourcebook for Facing Everyday Challenges.* New York: Facts On File, 2000.

inferiority complex First described by Carl Jung, an inferiority complex is a feeling of very low self-esteem and that other people are better looking, better achievers or more successful than oneself. Some children develop an inferiority complex because they are the victims of bullies as they are growing up. Other children do so because their parents have not encouraged them or belittle or overcriticize all their efforts. In some families one child may be compared unfavorably with another; this can lead to an inferiority complex. Some people have inferiority complexes because of their body image. Many people learn to raise their self-image during psychotherapy.

See also COMPLEX; SELF-ESTEEM.

infertility An inability to become pregnant and give birth to a child. Usually the diagnosis of infertility is made when a couple fails to conceive after at least one year of sexual intercourse without contraception; some reproductive endocrinologists make this diagnosis after six months. Infertility is often a cause of anxiety and stress for many couples, particularly those who have delayed marriage and childbearing until their late thirties. This frustrating and often anguishing problem affects about 15 percent of all couples of childbearing age.

According to William W. Hurd, assistant professor of obstetrics and gynecology, University of Michigan Medical Center, Ann Arbor, about one in 10 couples are considered "subfertile," which means that their chances of having a baby without professional intervention are slim. The infertility rate increases dramatically with age; couples between ages 30 and 35 have a 33 percent chance of being subfertile, and the odds jump to 50 percent by the time they reach 40. The probability of becoming pregnant the "old-fashioned" way is less than 10 percent among couples age 40 and older.

Reasons why subfertility increases with time are largely based on changes that take place in a woman's body as she ages. For example, older ovaries produce less fertility-enhancing hormones. Additionally, middle-aged ova are not as receptive to sperm penetration, and they tend to be spontaneously aborted once fertilized. During the 1980s, the number of American married couples unable to conceive diagnosed with an infertility problem rose from 15 percent to 20 percent. Infertility is touching an increasing number of young people whose reproductive systems have been damaged by chronic infections and sexually transmitted diseases such as gonorrhea and chlamydia.

According to Dana A. Ohl, M.D., assistant professor of surgery, Section of Urology, University of Michigan Medical Center, Ann Arbor, anabolic steroids, which can lower sperm count drastically and sometimes irreversibly, will also leave an indelible mark on infertility statistics in the years to come; young men in high school who use steroids will find difficulty in impregnating their wives five to 10 years from now.

Infertility does not always mean that conception is impossible. Many people with reproductive problems eventually have babies. According to the Center for Assisted Reproduction (CFAR), Northwestern University, Chicago, medicine has made great strides in the area of infertility in the last generation. Forty years ago, physicians had neither the knowledge base nor the technology to offer infertile couples a lengthy list of options. Adoption was the principal and many times painful alternative. Doctors knew little then about the value of fertility drugs to stimulate ovulation or laparoscopy to view the pelvis and correct problems of the reproductive organs. They had not yet imagined the diagnostic and therapeutic value of in vitro fertilization (IVF), which moves the actual fertilization of the egg from the fallopian tubes inside the woman to a glass petri dish inside the laboratory.

Today there are advances in at least seven areas that might affect fertility: ovulation, cervical, uterine and endometrial, tubal, pelvic and sperm. In diagnosing infertility, CFAR physicians look at the seven medical factors that, alone or in tandem, could prevent pregnancy. They want to know, for example, if the ovaries release an egg each month and, along with it, the necessary amount of hormones to allow for implantation. They also want to know if the male partner's sperm is of sufficient volume, motility and quality to fertilize an egg.

In approximately 40 percent of infertility cases, the problem is solely female; in another 40 percent it is solely male; in 17.5 percent of the cases, it involved both partners. In the remaining 3.5 percent of cases, infertility is never explained.

While infertility problems were once considered the woman's domain, today sperm production and motility, hormonal imbalances, anatomical factors, infections and inflammatory diseases are known to affect a man's ability to father a child. Some men perceive their condition as a threat to their masculine identity, which they may associate with their sexual prowess. One of the best ways to get men to accept infertility is to encourage them to talk about their condition, both with their partners and with supports groups. For women, the inability to have a child can attack the depths of femininity.

According to Ann Colston Wentz, M.D., CFAR, research has never established that stress causes infertility but rather that the reverse is true. When a couple is infertile, however, the partners become frustrated, anxious, hostile and angry. They question their own sexuality, and their infertility becomes one of the greatest stressors of their lives.

However, according to Dr. Hurd, some researchers have reported a correlation between stress reduction and increased fertility. When couples consciously stop trying for a while and replace their anxiety with relaxation, pregnancy rates have actually been shown to increase. A study compared the effects of relaxation therapy on infertility. Researchers took 100 people with unexplained infertility and did relaxation therapy on half of them. That half had a higher pregnancy rate than the half that did not have such therapy.

The stress of infertility can also result in sexual problems, such as low or nonexistent sexual desire. Fortunately, for most couples, this is usually a situational problem; when the infertility is resolved, the desire problem goes away.

According to Sally A. Kope, M.S.W., a senior clinical social worker in the Department of Obstetrics and Gynecology, University of Michigan Medical Center, in couples facing ongoing infertility, symptoms of overt depression can occur, including frequent crying, poor concentration and difficulty completing tasks. Such symptoms often resolve, however, as soon as the couple starts taking control of their future, even if it is the decision to stop trying so hard to have a baby.

Couples interested in exploring how medical technology can help them conceive should contact a local medical center for names of physicians who specialize in infertility or reproductive endocrinology.

See also PREGNANCY.

Corson, Stephen L. *Conquering Infertility: A Guide for Couples.* New York: Prentice-Hall Press, 1990.

Finn, Kristen Lidke. "Beating the Biological Clock: The Fertile Territory of Assisted Reproductive Technology." *Health Feature Service,* University of Michigan Medical Center Health News Service, Ann Arbor (Aug. 1991).

Hintz, Christine A. ". . . And Baby Makes Three." *Northwestern Perspective,* Chicago (fall 1991).

informed consent Agreement to a treatment plan for physical or emotional disorders. For example, one must give informed consent before undergoing electroshock treatment. If one is incompetent to sign a form indicating consent, another individual may do so. Elements of informed consent include:

- Adequate and accurate knowledge and information must be given to the patient.
- The patient has the legal capacity to consent.
- Consent is voluntarily given without coercion.

The term also refers to the right of the health care professional to release information learned during visits only with the consent of the patient.

See also GUARDIANSHIP; LEGAL ISSUES.

inhalants   Substances that can be inhaled through the nose or "huffed" by mouth. Like anesthetics, inhalants slow down the mind and body. Common inhalants include paint thinner, gasoline, spray paint, glue, kerosene and other solvents, amyl and butyl nitrate, aerosol sprays and nail polish remover.

Amyl nitrate and butyl nitrate, respectively nicknamed "snappers" or "poppers" and "locker room" or "rush," are liquids that produce highs that last up to several minutes after they are inhaled. Other than amyl nitrate, which has a legitimate use for heart patients, inhalants do not have an approved medical use.

Among the effects of inhalants are "sudden sniffing death" (a form of acute cardiac arrest) and breathing difficulties, headaches, vomiting, diarrhea and impaired reflexes. Some inhaled materials coat the lung tissue and may cause severe or even fatal pneumonia. Solvent use has been linked to kidney failure and other problems. Users can become dependent on inhalants and suffer painful symptoms of withdrawal if they stop using them. Inhalant users may appear to be alcohol intoxicated and may black out, have panic attacks or become disoriented or aggressive.

See also SUBSTANCE ABUSE.

Adapted from *Media Resource Guide on Common Drugs of Abuse*. Public Relations Society of America, National Capital Chapter, Fairfax, Va., September 1990.

inhibition   The inner restraint that prevents individuals from carrying out any mental or physical activity. As a psychoanalytic term, inhibition means unconsciously restraining instinctual impulses. People who have many inhibitions are often shy and withdrawn, whereas extroverted

personalities are usually less inhibited. Some individuals who are extremely inhibited about certain areas of their life and activities may develop social phobias. These can be overcome with a variety of therapies, including behavioral therapy. Some people have inhibitions related to sexual activity; sex therapy helps some people in this area of life.

See also PHOBIA; SEX THERAPY.

inkblot test   See RORSHACH TEST.

insanity   The legal term for a severe mental illness that renders the person incapable of managing his or her own affairs in a competent manner. The definition of insanity and its legal aspects vary among states in the United States. Aspects of the definition may include guardianship, lack of responsibility for contracts or crimes and inability to distinguish between right and wrong.

A person can be mentally ill or have an addiction problem but not be found legally insane as a defense for a felony. Most states require that it be proved that as a result of a mental disease (for example, schizophrenia, organic psychosis) or defect (mental retardation) an individual did not recognize the wrongfulness of the act or was unable to conform his or her behavior to the requirements of the law.

See also GUARDIANSHIP; LEGAL ISSUES.

insanity defense   See LEGAL ISSUES.

insomnia   Insomnia, the inability to sleep or stay asleep, is usually a symptom of other disorders. Among the most prevalent of the causes is a history of stress, recent grief or mental disorders such as anxiety or depression. According to a study reported in *Canadian Family Physician* (Feb. 1992), insomnia occurs in up to 35 percent of those patients who have depression, anxiety and mania. Certain prescription drugs (antihypertensives, antiasthmatics) along with caffeine, nicotine and alcohol are believed to account for another 12 percent of cases of insomnia. While alcohol helps some people fall asleep more easily, they awaken in about four hours with rebound insomnia. Other causes of insomnia include tolerance to, or withdrawal from, sedative-hypnotics, restless leg syndrome and sleep apnea.

See also ANTIDEPRESSANT MEDICATIONS; ANXIETIES; DEPRESSION; SLEEP.

Harrison, Pam. "Insomnia Not a Diagnosis but a Complaint." *Canadian Family Physician* 38 (Feb. 1992).

instinct　An innate urge. Humans have needs for food, warmth, love and sex, but the instinct for survival is probably the strongest. An instinct is different from a reflex, which is an involuntary response to a stimulus, such as slowing down at the sound of a railroad train whistle. Sigmund Freud saw life as a contest between the two most important instincts, Eros—the life instinct, a positive creative force—and Thanatos—the death instinct, which is negative and destructive.

See also FREUD, SIGMUND.

insulin-shock therapy (insulin-coma therapy)　A treatment for severe mental disorder, such as schizophrenia, consisting of intramuscular administration of insulin, which results in a short-term hypoglycemia coma. The treatment is rarely used now because it has been replaced by electroconvulsive (electroshock) therapy and psychoactive drugs, which are less dangerous and more effective.

See also ELECTROCONVULSIVE THERAPY.

integration　A psychiatric term referring to the developmental process in which separate personality characteristics, experiences, abilities and values are brought together. A "well-integrated person" is one who functions well in various relationships and at various levels. In the layperson's language, such a person is "all together."

intelligence　An ability to understand concepts and reason them out. Intelligence involves many factors, including speed of thought, learning and problem solving. It also includes the meaning of words, fluency with words, working with numbers, visualizing things in space, memory and speed of perception.

Intelligence can be rated on a continuum, from highly gifted (IQ over 140) people on one end to mentally retarded people on the other.

See also INTELLIGENCE TESTS.

intelligence tests　Tests planned to provide an estimation of a person's mental capabilities. The result of standard tests is known as intelligence quotient (IQ). In recent years, there has been criticism of the use of intelligence tests as the basis for predicting whether a person can cope with certain jobs or pass certain examinations. Some say standardized tests are biased regarding gender and race. In any event, intelligence tests are useful in assessing effects of brain disease and in assessing the nature of a child's problem so that effective remedial instruction can be initiated.

There are many different tests; the most widely used is the Wechsler Adult Intelligence Scale (WAIS) and the Wechsler Intelligence Scale for Children (WISC). These are divided into sections relating to words and actions. Another test is the Stanford-Binet Test, the original of which was devised in 1905 by Alfred Binet (1857–1911), a French psychologist. Other tests focus on testing one particular aspect of intelligence. For example, the Goodenough-Harris test assesses performance by asking a child to draw a picture of a man. In scoring, details such as proportion of the body and details of clothing are counted.

Scoring of intelligence tests is usually based on mental age (MA) in relationship to actual chronological age (CA), as intelligence usually increases with maturity.

See also MENTAL RETARDATION.

intergenerational conflicts　Intergenerational conflicts result in particular threats to good mental health within the family. Because people live longer, it is not unusual to have family members representing as many as three or four generations interacting. Having more than two of those generations living under one roof is less likely to occur today than in earlier times, but it is generally agreed that generational conflicts are often due to living together in one residence. However, no matter how close or far apart the generations live, as long as they continue to meet and share holiday and other family celebrations, some areas of intergenerational conflict, often labeled as a generation gap, will persist.

"Generation gap" refers to the inability to communicate, viewing the same phenomenon with opposite conclusions, insensitivity to the feelings of others and criticism of one's feelings and beliefs. In multi-generational families, the issue that most often involves all generations in areas of disagreement is behavior.

Some young people often carry a stereotype of older adults as "living in the past," overly conservative and unable to understand either being young or how much things have changed. While many young people admire and love older people and in specific instances (parents, relatives, friends, teachers) even use them as role models, the stress-filled intergenerational conflicts persist.

A good deal of stress emanating from middle-aged and older adults toward the young is, in fact, due to the overpowering youth culture of the 1990s and early 2000s. In addition, older people's view of the younger generation may be colored by their own feelings of self-achievement and life satisfaction. When they feel good about themselves, they are more likely to have higher expectations of the younger generation.

See also BABY BOOMERS; COMMUNICATION; ELDERLY PARENTS; LISTENING; PUBERTY AND PUBERTY RITES.

intimacy   A very close association and friendship between individuals. Emotional intimacy can exist between lovers, friends, siblings or children and parents. There is evidence that intimacy can be linked to good health, but when a relationship turns sour and the intimacy disappears, it can be a threat to good mental health for many people.

Good Health and Close Relationships

Evidence suggests that when individuals have happy relationships, the likelihood of disease and complications from disease is far less, according to Len Sperry, M.D., Duke University Durham, North Carolina. A five-year study found that unmarried heart patients who did not have a confidant were three times more likely to die from cardiac disease

than those who were married or had a close friend. Similar findings were presented in a Canadian study of 224 women with breast cancer. Seven years after they had been diagnosed, 76 percent of the women with at least one intimate relationship survived. The explanation for this, Sperry says, is that feeling cared about and important helps maintain a person's optimism in times of stress. These emotional boosts translate into a strong immunity that helps fight disease.

The Stress and Fear of Intimacy

Author of the book, *Too Close for Comfort: Exploring the Risks of Intimacy,* Geraldine Piorkowski, Ph.D., explored the theory that the fears and stresses of intimacy can be healthy when they are realistic and protective of the self. Piorkowski suggests that individuals reflect and learn from past experiences, schedule enough time to develop these relationships, be willing to share feelings with others, work at relationships but allow for failures and be on intimate terms with more than one person.

PRESERVE GOOD MENTAL HEALTH WITH INTIMATE RELATIONSHIPS

- Don't plunge in. Relationships should develop slowly.
- Autonomy is important; don't lose control of your own needs.
- Don't expect perfection in yourself or the other person.
- Set boundaries and recharge; use periods of distance to strengthen your sense of self.
- Accept criticism, rejection and disappointment as a fact of life.
- Maintain a life away from the relationship.

Dr. Piorkowski comments, "There is a level of imperfect intimacy that is good enough to live and grow on. In good-enough intimacy, painful encounters occasionally occur, but they are balanced by the strengths and pleasures of the relationship. There are enough positives to balance the negatives. People who do well in intimate relationships don't have the perfect relationship, but it is good enough."

Cyberspace Relationships

More and more people are developing relationships on-line. They meet in chat rooms, and, for more intimacy, carry on communication through e-mail and exchange photos via the Internet. There's also an addictive quality to conversing on-line, which makes it easy to get too close too quickly. Some people lie about themselves, thereby wasting the other person's time and destroying their intimacy. There is also a real danger involved in cyberspace relationships: Pedophiles use chat rooms to find their next victims, marriages have ended and murders have been committed—all in the name of intimacy.

Piorkowski, Geraldine K. *Too Close For Comfort: Exploring the Risks of Intimacy.* New York: Plenum Press, 1994.

introversion A personality characteristic marked by self-reliance and a preference for working or doing recreational activities alone. This is in contrast to extroversion, a characteristic of a more outgoing character. Introverts may be preoccupied with their own inner thoughts and feelings rather than with other people. Introverts tend to be rather contemplative and sensitive people and may seem aloof to others.

involutional melancholia An obsolete term referring to a depressive disorder that was commonly believed to affect people, particularly women, at mid-life and after. Today it is diagnosed as major depression.

See also CLIMACTERIC; MENOPAUSE.

iproniazid Known by the trade name Marsalid, this drug was one of the first in the monoamine oxidase (MAO) inhibitor class. It is no longer used in the United States.

See also ANTIDEPRESSANT MEDICATIONS; DEPRESSION; MONOAMINE OXIDASE INHIBITORS.

irrational beliefs Ideas that are unreasonable and unrealistic; such ideas are characteristic of some mental illnesses. For example, mentally ill persons frequently have unrealistic concepts such as a feeling that everyone is or should be paying attention to them or that they are being persecuted (paranoia). They may feel that they are being poisoned or that the government or other powerful organizations are eavesdropping or tapping their telephone. Some people who are not mentally well

may develop fixations and feel that they have personal relationships with movie stars, political figures or other celebrities. These fixed beliefs are considered delusions.

Experiences and ideas that cannot be proved rationally are also present in the population that does not have mental disorders. According to a recent Gallup poll, one out of four Americans believes in ghosts, and 55 percent of Americans believe in the devil. One in four Americans feels that he or she has had a telepathic experience, and 17 percent believe that they have been in touch with someone who has died. While only 18 percent of the population admits to being very or somewhat superstitious, another 16 percent admits to a slight level of superstition. Black cats crossing the path leads the list of experiences to be avoided, followed by walking under a ladder.

See also DELUSION; SUPERSTITION.

Gallup, George, Jr., and Frank Newport. "Belief in Psychic and Paranormal Phenomena Widespread among Americans." *Gallup Poll Monthly* (Aug. 1990).

irritable bowel syndrome (IBS) A chronic disorder of the colon. Most IBS symptoms are related to an abnormal movement pattern of the colon. In people who have IBS, the muscle of the lower portion of the colon contracts abnormally. An abnormal contraction, or spasm, may be related to episodes of crampy pain. Sometimes the spasm delays the passage of stool, leading to constipation. At other times, the spasm leads to more rapid passage of feces, or diarrhea.

Though IBS can cause a great deal of discomfort, it is not serious and does not lead to any serious disease. However, for some people it can be disabling. Some people may be afraid to go to dinner parties, seek employment or travel on public transportation. However, with attention to proper diet, stress management and sometimes medication prescribed by a physician, most people with IBS can keep their symptoms under control.

Because doctors have been unable to pinpoint its organic cause, IBS has often been considered to be caused by emotional conflict or stress. Many individuals who suffer from anxiety disorders, panic attacks or panic disorder also suffer from IBS.

In addition to stress, there are other contributing factors. For example, eating causes contractions of the colon. Normally, this response may cause an urge to have a bowel movement within 30 to 60 minutes after a meal. In people with IBS, the exaggerated reflex can lead to cramps and sometimes diarrhea.

Stress also stimulates colonic spasm in people with IBS. This process is not clearly understood, but scientists point out that the colon is partially controlled by the nervous system. Mental health counseling is sometimes helpful for alleviating the symptoms due to IBS. However, according to the American College of Gastroenterology, this does not mean that IBS results from a personality disorder.

Self-help Relief from IBS

For many people, eating the proper diet helps lessen IBS symptoms. Before considering a change in diet, one should note whether any particular foods seem to cause distress; these facts should be discussed with a physician. If dairy products cause symptoms to flare up, one can try decreasing the amount consumed at any one time. Yogurt can be a satisfactory substitute.

Dietary fiber, present in whole grain breads and cereals and in fruits and vegetables, also has been shown to be helpful in lessening IBS symptoms. High-fiber diets keep the colon mildly distended, which helps to prevent spasms from developing. Some forms of fiber also keep water in the stools, thereby preventing hard, difficult-to-pass stools from forming. High-fiber diets may cause gas and bloating; however, over time, these symptoms may dissipate as the digestive tract becomes used to the increased fiber intake.

Large meals may also cause cramping and diarrhea in some people. Eating smaller meals more frequently, or eating smaller portions of foods at mealtimes (especially foods that are low in fat and rich in carbohydrates and protein), may also help alleviate symptoms.

Pharmacologic Therapy

Some doctors prescribe a combination of antispasmodic drugs and tranquilizers to help relieve symptoms. The major concerns in drug therapy of IBS are dependency on the medication and the effects the disorder can have on lifestyle. In an effort to regulate colonic activity or minimize stress, some patients become dependent on laxatives or tranquilizers. If this becomes the case, the physician should try to withdraw the drugs slowly.

See also ANXIETY; GUIDED IMAGERY; MEDITATION; RELAXATION.

Cunningham, Chet. *The Irritable Bowel Syndrome (I.B.S.) and Gastrointestinal Solutions Handbook.* Leucadia, Calif.: United Research Publishers, 1995.

Kahn, Ada P. *Stress A to Z: The Sourcebook for Facing Everyday Challenges.* New York: Facts On File, 2000.

Tannenhaus, Norra. *Learning to Live with Chronic IBS.* New York: Dell, 1990.

isocarboxazid An antidepressant drug in the monoamine oxidase inhibitor (MAOI) class (trade name: Marplan). It is effective in the treatment of major depression, dysthymic disorder and atypical depression. It is also useful in the treatment of panic disorder and the phobic disorders. All MAOIs can produce serious adverse reactions; patients should be supervised closely and must follow a special diet and avoid certain foods and medications that can cause a reaction.

See also ANTIDEPRESSANT MEDICATIONS; DEPRESSION; MONOAMINE OXIDASE INHIBITORS; TYRAMINE.

isolation See LONELINESS.

Janimine Trade name for imipramine hydrochloride, a tricyclic antidepressant drug. Imipramine is the prototype of the tricyclic antidepressants and is effective in the treatment of depressive episodes of major depression and bipolar, dysthymic, panic and phobic disorders.

See also ANTIDEPRESSANT MEDICATIONS; IMIPRAMINE HYDROCHLORIDE.

Japan, stress in See KAROSHI.

jealousy An emotion that encompasses a continuum of envy, reduction in self-esteem and hostility toward another. Jealousy is a feeling that some infants experience when a new sibling arrives. In adults, jealousy occurs when one's mate has a relationship with another individual, or in a divorce situation when one partner feels abandoned because his or her partner has been attracted to another individual. Sexual jealousy, real or imagined, can trigger abuse of a spouse. Sexual jealousy is also referred to as the "Othello syndrome," which may be a type of delusional disorder, and has been reported to respond to medication therapy.

Homosexual jealousy may be more common among males than among female homosexuals, possibly because they are in a fairly closed community with some degree of social prejudice against it.

See also EMOTIONS.

Buunk, Bram, and Ralph B. Hupka. "Cross Cultural Differences in the Elicitation of Sexual Jealousy." *Journal of Sex Research* 23, no. 1 (Feb. 1987).

jet lag A disruption of one's body rhythms (circadian rhythms) resulting from traveling through several time zones within a short span of time. It takes many individuals several days to readjust their sleep schedule, appetite and ability to concentrate well while recovering from jet lag.

See also CIRCADIAN RHYTHMS.

Wingler, Sharon. *Travel Alone & Love It: A Flight Attendant's Guide to Solo Travel.* Willowbrook, Ill.: Chicago Spectrum Press, 1996.

job change Making the transition into a new position, whether continuing to work for the same company or for a new one. Both situations can be a challenge to good mental health, and both have pros and cons. Coming from the outside means the individual does not have to worry about managing coworkers or friends. However, when the individual does not have a mentor or friend in a new company, he or she has no one to rely on or explain corporate policies and politics. Starting out fresh also means not knowing what employees are good at, who the hard workers are and who sloughs off.

Promotion, whether from within or without, can also significantly raise stress levels because it raises fear of incompetence and fear of failure. Usually these fears and stresses will go away once the new position is mastered and evidence of success becomes visible.

Job Change and Savings

Changing jobs, traditionally confined to the youngest workers in the labor force, is growing more common among experienced managers and the result may be a serious depletion of retirement savings and anxieties about money, according to Challenger, Gray & Christmas Inc., an international outplacement firm that tracks workplace trends, in *What's Next?: Challenger Workplace Outlook, 2001.*

Challenger statistics show that jobless managers and executives, average age 45, have had four or more jobs during their careers. With a new job every four or five years, there is not much time to build a nest egg, especially since many corporate retirement programs are based on a vesting schedule. For example, an employee with two years on the job may only receive 20 percent of the contributions into his or her retirement fund.

The problem is exacerbated by the fact that many job switchers do not properly transfer employer-retirement savings when switching jobs. One recent poll found that more than two-thirds of job changers take cash payouts on their 401k plans, which, when withdrawn before the age of 59 1/2, result in as much as a 40 percent loss in one's nest egg due to penalty fees and taxes.

See also JOB SECURITY; WORKPLACE.

Snyder, Don J. *The Cliff Walk: A Memoir of a Job Lost and a Life Found.* Boston: Little, Brown, 1997.

job security   Lack of job security is a major cause of instability and stress for workers throughout the world. This was not an issue or concern 30 to 40 years ago. Then, many employers had implicit or explicit long-term employment contracts with their workers, contracts that emphasized management's commitment and pledge to minimize the need for layoffs. Wages and job benefits increased over the years, and it was not unusual for the company to pay the total cost of employees' health care and charge minimally for family coverage. This job security led workers to expect to remain in their jobs for many years; it was not unusual for workers to devote their entire working lives to one company, retiring with the traditional gold watch and company pension.

During the later 1990s and early 2000s, downsizing, layoffs, mergers and other organizational changes have greatly altered the job security picture. Employers are no longer sharing their wealth; raises and employee benefits have been scaled back. Full-time jobs are harder to find.

Job cuts in 2001

For an unprecedented third consecutive month, job cut announcements exceeded 100,000 as U.S. employers in February 2001, announced 101,731 planned job cuts, nearly triple the figure from the previous year.

In a report issued on March 5, 2001, Challenger, Gray & Christmas, Inc., an international outplacement firm that tracks workplace trends, said that the February 2001 job cuts increased 187 percent from February 2000 (35,415).

In 1998, when 677,795 job cuts, a decade high, were announced, the monthly average was 56,483.

In addition to the option of operating their own business, suggestions in *Money* include considering oneself a free agent or skilled artisan; set new professional goals; look for new jobs while still employed; build portable skills; set up a board of directors (network) made up of five to 10 trusted colleagues, clients, former bosses and other professionals who know your track record, as well as opportunities available in the industry, to use as references and mentors; create an escape hatch (options, lateral moves, further education) and be ready to accept change.

See also JOB CHANGE; LAYOFFS; WORKPLACE.

Alderman, Lesley. "Here's How You Can Work on Job Security." *Money* (Sept. 1995).

journal keeping (journaling)   Writing things is practical advice for dealing with confusion and problems. Writing can put the individual close to or further from his concerns. Writing and reading what has been written sometimes exposes one's subconscious, suppressed feelings that can be dealt with more constructively when they are recognized. In this sense a diarist may get closer to himself and better understand self-motivations.

Some mental health professionals say that symptoms such as anxiety, depression and apathy are actually masks for envy, jealousy and rage turned inward at the self. Writing may help to get to the core of such feelings by bringing some of the repressed thoughts and attitudes into the open and eliminating some of the restrictions that sap energy and limit productivity. Some diarists have found it useful to write a portrait of a person whom they envy or who has angered them. The portrait sometimes reveals qualities of their own (which they see in the other person) that they wish to either develop or change.

The cathartic effect of writing involves a distancing from negative feelings and experiences. Once the feelings or experiences are described on paper, the writer frequently has a sense of being rid of them, of being ready to go on to something else. Simply the act of writing may also give a sense of control, a way of giving some order and manageability to problems. List making in a diary has also been found to be a good way of setting goals and giving order to what may seem to be an enormous or chaotic task. Keeping a journal has also been useful for the person who is attempting to control addictive or obsessive behavior. The diary not only improves self-understanding and serves as a way to record progress, but it also gives the individual something she can refer to when she wants a drink or a cigarette or is about to give in to a desire to overeat.

Journal keeping is used by many support groups for overeaters, as well as those who wish to stop smoking or drinking. Writing in a journal or diary also serves the obvious purposes of recording the events and impressions of the day and of improving writing style.

See also CONTROL; EATING DISORDERS; SUPPORT GROUPS.

Adams, Kathleen. *Journal to the Self.* New York: Warner Books, 1990.
Baldwin, Christina. *One to One: Self-understanding Through Journal Writing.* New York: M. Evans, 1977.
Rainer, Tristine. *The New Diary.* Los Angeles: J. P. Tarcher, 1978.

juvenile delinquency   See CONDUCT DISORDER.

Kabat-Zinn, Jon, Ph.D. Founder and director of the Stress Reduction Clinic, University of Massachusetts Medical Center, Worcester, where he is also an associate professor of medicine.

He is the author of popular books about mental health, including *Mindfulness Meditation in Everyday Life* (1993) and *Full Catastrophe Living: Using the Wisdom of Your Body and Mind to Face Stress, Pain and Illness* (1991).

Dr. Kabat-Zinn is a proponent of mindfulness meditation, a more than 2,000-year-old Buddhist method of living fully in the present. This approach offers a unique way to cope with stress and illness because mindfulness meditation can help induce deep states of relaxation and, at times, directly improve physical symptoms.

Other forms of meditation involve focusing on a sound or the sensation of breath leaving and entering the body; anything else that comes up in the mind during meditation is seen as a distraction to be disregarded. Mindfulness, on the other hand, is "insight" meditation. It encourages one to note any thoughts and observe them nonjudgmentally, moment by moment, as they occur in one's awareness. This practice of observing thoughts, feelings and sensations can help one become calmer and have a broader perspective on one's life. It involves a significant commitment to oneself; it is a way of life.

In his writings, Dr. Kabat-Zinn explains how to live in the moment by taking up such techniques as "non-doing," trust and concentration. He shows readers meditation postures and describes ways to meditate, including visualizing mountains and lakes and concentrating on walking or standing.

Like many mind/body techniques, mindfulness has just begun to be explored scientifically. Typically, the training program for mindfulness medita-tion lasts eight weeks. Controlled studies are investigating whether mindfulness meditation can influence the healing process and help in treating many diseases.

For further information:

Stress Reduction Clinic
University of Massachusetts Medical Center
55 Lake Avenue North
Worcester, MA 01655
(508) 856-1616

See also COMPLEMENTARY THERAPIES; MEDITATION; RELAXATION.

Kabat-Zinn, Jon. *Full Catastrophe Living: Using the Wisdom of Your Body and Mind to Face Stress, Pain and Illness.* New York: Delacorte, 1991.
———. *Wherever You Go, There You Are: Mindfulness Meditation in Everyday Life.* New York: Hyperion, 1994.

karoshi Karoshi, or "death from overwork," has become synonymous with stress in Japan. In an article in *Alternative Therapies* magazine (July 1995) C. Frank Lawlis, Ph.D., wrote "People [in Japan] are literally dying at their workstations. It appears that their entire physiological system collapses or shuts down."

Lawlis drew from a 1989 study by Chiyoda Fire and Marine Insurance, Ltd., one of the top insurance carriers in Japan. Chiyoda, which covers more than 100,000 Japanese corporations, conducted a major study on the health problems Japanese people are likely to encounter. One important conclusion of the study was that stress played a major role in 40 percent of the health problems.

In 1997, Dr. Katsuo Nishiyama of Japan, published a paper in the *International Journal of Health Services* (February 4, 1997) in which he reviewed the history of karoshi and progress to stop the increase in the disease. The process of work intensification, he said, has resulted in night shift work, increased scheduled and unscheduled overtime and holiday work and formal and informal functions during off-work time. A low base pay forces people to work hard to get extra benefits. Low allowances for overtime, night shifts and other additional hours drive workers to work longer hours and more nights and holidays.

According to Nishiyama, three psychosocial components lead to excessive job strain: psychological job demands, work control and work related social support. Workers in high demand, low control and low social support jobs are at increased risk for developing and dying of cardiovascular disease. However, he suggests that karoshi should not be thought of as a solely Japanese phenomena. Workers in other countries who are exposed to a similar system of work organization and management philosophy also report stress related symptoms. Types of disorders thought to be stress related in the West include elevated blood pressure, digestive system disorders, work related musculoskeletal disorders, depression, anxiety and certain behaviors such as drug and alcohol use.

See also ACCULTURATION; CROSS-CULTURAL INFLUENCES; WORKPLACE.

kinesics The study of communication as expressed through facial expression and other body movements. Theories and techniques of studying this type of nonverbal communication were developed by Ray L. Birdwhistell (1918–   ), who found that certain gestures and expressions were specifically male or female and also related to regional and national groups. Body language also changes with mood, health, age and degree of tension or relaxation. Birdwhistell developed his theories with the use of photography and with a notation system of symbols called kinegraphs to describe gestures and expressions.

See also BODY LANGUAGE.

Birdwhistell, Ray L. *Kinesics and Context*. Philadelphia: University of Pennsylvania Press, 1970.

kleptomania An overwhelming desire to steal or to pick up things that do not belong to oneself. An example is shoplifting, which accounts for countless lost millions of dollars' worth of merchandise from retail businesses around the world. Kleptomania may be a form of compulsion, similar to compulsive gambling in some cases. Some kleptomaniacs are highly professional people and, when apprehended, have no explanation for their behavior. Some kleptomaniacs perform their compulsion frequently; others are very selective and only do it when they believe that they will not be caught. Many famous and highly respected people are arrested in the United States every year for petty thievery, some of which may be compulsive.

See also OBSESSIVE-COMPULSIVE DISORDER.

Klonopin Trade name for the benzodiazepine medication clonazepam.

See also BENZODIAZEPINE MEDICATIONS; PHARMACEUTICAL APPROACH.

Kohut,   Heinz (1913–1981) Austrian-born American psychoanalyst. His work combined an interest in neurology, neuropathology and literature that led him to psychoanalysis. He developed a "self psychology" theory that challenged many of the theories of Sigmund Freud. Although Freudian in his training, Kohut differed with Freud's concept of sex and aggression as the basis of human emotion and personality structure. Instead he explored his interest in the narcissistic personality, which he felt was caused by social and family pressures rather than Oedipus conflict. Those who have followed his teachings and applied his theories in working with patients are known as Kohutians. His major works include *The Analysis of the Self* (1971), *The Restoration of the Self* (1977) and *The Search for the Self* (1978).

Kohut also differed from contemporary mental health practitioners and aroused criticism by being supportive to his patients rather than using the usual confrontational, challenging methods common in the field. Kohut was born in Vienna; in the United States he worked at the University of Chicago hospitals and the Institute for Psychoanalysis of Chicago.

The Heinz Kohut Archives were established in 1991 at the Institute for Psychoanalysis. For details on the archives, contact:

Kohut Archives
Institute for Psychoanalysis
180 North Michigan Avenue
Chicago, IL 60601
Phone: (313) 726-6300

See also FREUD, SIGMUND; NARCISSISM; PSYCHO-
ANALYSIS; PSYCHOTHERAPIES.

"Heinz Kohut, Whose 'Self' Theory Challenged Freud's,
   Is Dead at 68." *New York Times Biographical Service,*
   Oct. 1981.

Korsakoff's syndrome (psychosis)   An organic
syndrome that occurs in some chronic alcoholics,
in some individuals who have severe head trauma
and in several other conditions, such as prolonged
infections, metallic poisoning or brain tumor. It
was described in 1898 by Sergei Korsakoff
(1854–1900), a Russian neurologist. Major symptoms include amnesia, confusion, confabulation
(made-up stories) and disorientation.

kundalini   See YOGA.

labile A term used in medical reports and records meaning likely to undergo change, or unstable. In mental health, the term is sometimes used to refer to emotional instability. Blood pressure that has a tendency to fluctuate is sometimes described as labile.

laboratory tests A variety of different tests are available to determine medical conditions (such as thyroid deficiency) that may contribute to depression, anxiety and other conditions that may detract from good mental health. Tests involve analyzing chemicals in the blood and/or urine or measuring brain waves.

The metabolism of the brain is separate from body metabolism to a great extent because of the existence of a physiological blood brain barrier that selectively allows chemicals to pass from the blood to the brain and back. There are presently no reliable tests for clinical use. Many tests used for research in mental illness have been advocated as useful, but none has been established as clinically useful to diagnose mental illness.

Tests of certain chemicals in cerebrospinal fluid, blood or urine, in response to the administration of challenges by single doses of hormones or chemicals that react in the brain, are producing new knowledge about some of the biochemical factors in some mental illnesses.

Neurological tests such as electroencephalograms, CAT (computerized axial tomography) scans and MRI (magnetic resonance imaging) are used to rule out neurological causes. "High-tech" research instruments, such as PET (positron emission tomography) scanning, allow for measurement of chemical changes in the human brain, while magnetic resonance spectroscopy (MRS) is able to measure chemical changes in certain brain regions.

Illness such as manic-depression, major depression, panic disorder and obsessive-compulsive disorder have shown changes from normal function in PET scans.

See also BLOOD TESTS; COMPUTERIZED AXIAL TOMOGRAPHY (CAT); ELECTROENCEPHALOGRAM.

lactate-induced anxiety See SODIUM LACTATE INFUSIONS.

latency (latency stage) A term relating to the stage of psychosexual development when sexual interest is repressed and sublimated. During this period, the child controls his or her energies and drives in socially acceptable ways, such as school work and group activities. For example, the child focuses attention on peer activities with members of his or her own sex. During this period, the child learns basic patterns of relating to people and the environment that will carry over when adult relationships are established. This stage lasts approximately from the fourth or fifth year until the onset of puberty.

latent content See DREAM ANALYSIS; DREAMING.

laughter A reaction of amusement and joy. Laughter is an involuntary sign indicating instant pleasure. As we laugh at a comic situation or funny story, we retreat temporarily from the reality of the seriousness of the adult world. A good laugh can help individuals relieve worries and stress. An ability to laugh easily is related to one's sense of humor. Often, a good sense of humor can help individuals deal with difficult situations in a sensible, more relaxed manner. Being able to maintain one's sense of humor can help one cope better with a chronic disease, for example. Some individuals suffering from depression lose their ability to laugh and see any humor in their lives or around them.

At times, laughter may also be a sign of defense against feelings of self-consciousness or embarrassment. An ability to laugh at oneself can be helpful, if not overdone. Some individuals find it difficult to laugh at themselves because they cannot acknowledge that they have either made a mistake or have done something "stupid."

There may be some physiological benefits from laughter. A good hearty laugh increases heartbeat, respiratory activity and oxygen exchange and may enhance the body's ability to fight inflammation. Laughter, like exercise, may also stimulate the brain to produce endorphins, which may increase one's sense of physical and mental well-being.

The late Norman Cousins (1912–1990), former editor of the *Saturday Review* and later a member of the faculty of the medical school at the University of California at Los Angeles, used laughter's curative power to help himself recover from a degenerative disease of the body's connective tissue.

The following are a few excerpts from Cousins's *Anatomy of an Illness,* in which he described the benefits of laughter:

> I made the joyous discovery that ten minutes of genuine belly laughter had an anesthetic effect and would give me at least two hours of pain-free sleep . . . Exactly what happens inside the human mind and body as the result of humor is difficult to say. But the evidence that it works has stimulated the speculations not just of physicians but of philosophers and scholars over the centuries.

While fighting ankylosing spondylitis, Cousins checked out of the hospital and spent weeks watching Marx Brothers movies and other comedies. He attributed his recovery to the positive feelings that laughter aroused in him.

Excessive giggling or totally inappropriate laughter or smiling may be symptoms of a form of schizophrenia (hebephrenic).

For information:

International Laughter Society
16000 Glen Una Drive
Los Gatos, CA 95030
Phone: (408) 354-3456

See also HUMOR; SCHIZOPHRENIA.

Peter, Laurence J. *The Laughter Prescription: The Tools of Humor and How to Use Them.* New York: Ballantine Books, 1982.
Provine, Robert R. "Laughter." *American Scientist* 84, no. 1 (Jan.–Feb. 1996).
Roach, Mary. "Can You Laugh Your Stress Away?" *Health* (Sept. 1996).

lay analyst   Any nonmedical individual who performs psychoanalysis; such a person is trained in the theory and practice of psychoanalysis but does not have a medical degree.

See also PSYCHOANALYSIS.

layoffs   Layoffs, or reductions in force (RIFs), have become common occurrences for many employers. The potential for this occurring affects everyone and is a threat to good mental health. In the early 2000s, there seems to be no job security, and the large organization that took care of its workers is a thing of the past.

An example of a major national corporation implementing massive layoffs is AT&T: Early in January 1996, AT&T announced that it would eliminate 40,000 jobs by 1998. In November 1996, AT&T offered buyouts to more than 70,000 workers, but only 6,500 accepted. Of the 40,000 jobs to be eliminated, about 75 percent had to be cut by layoffs.

The AT&T cutback was the third-largest in corporate America in three years. In 1993, IBM did away with 63,000 jobs, and Sears, Roebuck and Co. announced the demise of 50,000 jobs, including jobs connected to its catalog, known as the Big Book.

During the recession years of the 1980s, job reduction was blamed on national and international business conditions. In the early 2000s, more and more companies are reducing their workforces in order to save money (after merger or acquisition) or to realize productivity gains.

Layoffs also are due to plant closings, work slowdowns and corporate downsizings. Being laid off is different from being fired, though the individual will probably feel the same stress. When workers are fired, it is because their performance is lacking; when layoffs occur, performance is rarely cited.

Typically, there are five emotional stages that follow a termination, and they are not unlike those felt at the time of any major loss:

Stage One—Denial: *It must be some mistake, this can't be happening to me.*

Stage Two—Self-Blame: *I must have done something wrong. How did I screw up?*

Stage Three—Anger: *Why did management do this to me?*

Stage Four—Depression: *It's not worth getting out of bed in the morning.*

Stage Five—Acceptance: *What happened may be for the best.*

On virtually every indicator of mental and physical health, job loss due to layoffs has a negative impact. People who lose their jobs are often anxious, depressed, unhappy and, in general, dissatisfied with their lives. They have lowered self-esteem, are short-tempered and are fatalistic and pessimistic about the future. Thus, job loss is clearly hard on one's health, and it is important to get control over one's life and one's stress after a job loss.

See also JOB SECURITY; SELF-ESTEEM; WORKPLACE.

Kahn, Ada P. *Stress A to Z: The Sourcebook for Facing Everyday Challenges.* New York: Facts On File, 2000.

L-dopa See LEVODOPA.

lead poisoning Lead poisoning is very harmful to young children. If they accidentally eat paint chips containing lead, they may develop severe learning disabilities. However, if detected early enough, lead poisoning can be treated, Lead encephalopathy is a brain disorder seen in children who eat lead-containing paint. Symptoms include convulsions, mania, delirium and coma. (Lead encephalopathy can also occur in adults who inhale tetraethyl lead in gasoline fumes.)

learned helplessness A term developed during the 1970s by Martin Seligman (1942–) to refer to a feeling of helplessness and stifling of motivation caused by exposure to aversive events over which the individual has no control, sometimes leading to depression.

When individuals believe they have no control over their situation, they feel powerless and helpless. Having no ability to gain praise or positive reinforcements, they become passive and nonassertive. Under these circumstances, tendencies toward depression increase. The situation develops sooner or later in individuals who experience their efforts having no positive effect on a negative or painful situation.

This researcher said that self-initiated behavior is learned and that hindrance to initiation contributes to the helpless feeling the individual develops over time. However, there is emerging evidence that the development of learned helplessness or resistance to this development in experimental animals may be controlled by a genetic trait and modified by drugs used to treat depression.

See also LEARNED OPTIMISM.

learned optimism An attempt to identify habits of thinking that lead to negative feelings and giving up (learned helplessness), coined by Martin Seligman (1942–) and reverse them so that when under stress or facing a failure, an individual may persist or fight back and not "give up." Examples of such negative beliefs are: (1) If I fail, it is always my fault. (2) If I fail in one area, I will fail in others. (3) If I fail now, I will continue to fail. Seligman attempts to show how reversal of these responses can produce learned optimism. Seligman expounded on this theory in his book *Helplessness: On Depression, Development, and Death* (San Francisco: W. H. Freeman, 1975).

See also LEARNED HELPLESSNESS.

learning disabilities A group of psychological and neurological disorders that interfere with learning or make learning impossible. Children with learning disabilities are often taunted by their peers, which further reduces their sense of self-esteem and motivation. Learning disorders are generally difficult to diagnose; after diagnosis, children should be observed and taught by specialists in their education. Such disabilities include problems in learning caused by defects in speech, hearing and memory but do not include disabilities due to emotional or environmental deprivation or to poor teaching.

There are some specific learning disabilities. For example, dyslexia is difficulty reading; dyscalculia is an inability to perform mathematical problems; and dysgraphia refers to writing disorders. Specific learning difficulties in children of normal intelligence may be caused by forms of minimal brain dysfunction, which may be inherited.

Children with minimal or borderline mental retardation generally have difficulty learning.

See also ATTENTION-DEFICIT HYPERACTIVITY DISORDER (ADHD); HYPERACTIVITY; MENTAL RETARDATION.

Grey House Publishing. *The Complete Learning Disabilities Directory.* Lakeville, Conn.: Grey House Publishing, 1994.
Hall, David. *Living With Learning Disabilities: A Guide for Students.* Minneapolis: Lerner Publications, 1993.

legal issues   Many legal issues are involved in mental health care. As consumers become more aware of the standard of care required for mental health disorders, increasing attention is focused on issues including clients' rights, confidentiality between therapists and patient, competency of the mentally ill, the insanity defense, competency to stand trial, malpractice by health care practitioners and sexual misconduct by a therapist. Dying with dignity is also considered a legal issue, as a living will and a durable power of attorney are legal documents that can be enforced by courts of law.

Clients' Rights and Civil Rights

In 1986 the Protection and Advocacy Bill for Mentally Ill Individuals was enacted in the United States, which covers areas such as access to records and protection from abuse and neglect. Many states have laws stating rights of patients while hospitalized for psychiatric illnesses. The only right one loses under such circumstances is the right to liberty.

Confidentiality

Confidentiality is the duty of a mental health practitioner to keep certain information from disclosure. This duty is usually governed by state laws but is also covered under many codes of ethics followed by health care workers. Confidentiality assures that client information is not used for personal gain or curiosity and that it is shared only among other individuals involved in the care of that client.

The concept of privileged communication involves statements between certain individuals, such as husband-wife, priest-penitent or psychiatrist-client, whom the law protects from disclosure. Some states have strict confidentiality laws relating to psychiatric hospitalizations; some states recognize nurse-client privilege.

Exceptions to confidentiality and professional privilege include allegations of child abuse, threats voiced to a therapist by a client toward himself or against a third person and a client's waiver of confidentiality and privileges by filing of a lawsuit or for medical insurance reimbursement. In most states, information regarding child abuse must be disclosed to proper authorities. In some cases, nonreporting of such information may be a criminal offense.

TESTS FOR INSANITY (M'NAGHTEN RULE)

The individual suffered from a mental condition that affected his reason, and he was unaware of the nature and quality of his act or that his act was wrong.

Irresistible impulse rule
The individual either met the M'Naghten test or in response to an irresistible impulse also lacked criminal responsibility even though he or she knew the wrongfulness of the act.

Durham rule
The acts were the product of a mental disease or defect.

American Law Institute
The individual was suffering from a mental illness at the time of the act and was unable to appreciate the wrongfulness of the act or was unable to conform behavior to requirements of law.

Mental health practitioners have a duty to use reasonable care to protect possible victims if they believe that their patients have intentions to kill or otherwise harm themselves or others. This protection may take the form of notifying police or other authorities.

Clinical information must be disclosed if an individual is in a court of law for a hearing on involuntary commitment or a guardianship proceeding.

In addition, when a client brings a lawsuit in which his or her own mental status is an issue, medical information from a health care practitioner may be brought before the court. In such an event, the individual waives the right to confidentiality.

Insanity Defense

In some cases, a pretrial order may require that the defendant's mental condition at the time the crime was committed be assessed. Several tests are used to determine "sanity."

Competency to Stand Trial

Competency to stand trial refers to the mental condition of a defendant at the time of a criminal trial. If an individual is judged not competent to stand trial, he or she will be given immediate mental health treatment, with the main goal to restore competency. Such treatment may include medication, individual and group therapy and education about courtroom proceedings.

The rules for competency vary from state to state; however, a widely used assessment includes whether the client has an ability to assist the attorney with the defense, an ability to understand the nature and consequences of the charge and an ability to understand courtroom procedures.

Sexual Misconduct of Mental Health Practitioners

Sexual relationships in a therapist-client relationship are unethical behavior and a criminal offense on the part of the therapist, who is presumed to be "taking advantage" of the patient. In some cases, sexual relations have been considered rape. In the early 1990s, cases came to light in which the therapist included "sexual therapy" as part of psychotherapy and the client brought charges against the therapist.

Least Restrictive Alternative

Least restrictive alternative is a concept emphasized during the 1960s which says that less treatment rather than more is the most desirable objective, with the minimum level of restrictions on the patient's freedom.

This concept led to housing mentally retarded individuals within communities rather than segregating them in institutions.

McFarland, Gertrude K., and Mary Durand Thomas. *Psychiatric Mental Health Nursing.* Philadelphia: J. B. Lippincott, 1991.

lesbianism   Female homosexuality. The term is derived from the name of the Greek island of Lesbos, home of the poetess Sappho. Women who practice lesbianism (lesbians) prefer women as sexual partners, although some lesbians also have or have had heterosexual partners. Lesbians as well as homosexual men are referred to as part of the "gay community."

Lesbian sexual expression includes caressing, kissing, mutual masturbation and oral-genital contacts. Tribadism is the term for a practice in which one woman lies above the other, simulating coitus while the genitals are mutually stimulated. Masters and Johnson were among the first to write about sexual dysfunctions in homosexuals and included some lesbians in their study of anorgasmia.

Many lesbians have taken an active role in the "gay liberation" movement during the 1970s and 1980s, encouraging homosexuals to meet and discuss important issues and provide a political organization to work toward legal change and fight job discrimination. The National Gay Task Force is the clearinghouse for these groups and provides information on local organizations. The most well-known lesbian organization is the Daughters of Bilitis (founded in 1956).

Lesbian couples have become parents (comothers) through artificial insemination and adoption. Lesbian relationships have been depicted in art, for example, in Rubens's *Jupiter and Callisto,* and in films, such as Bergman's *Persona* (1967).

For information, contact:

The National Gay Task Force
80 Fifth Avenue
New York, NY 10011
Phone: (212) 741-1010

See also HOMOSEXUALITY.

Harris, Mary B., and Pauline H. Turner. "Gay and Lesbian Parents." *Journal of Homosexuality* 12, no. 2 (winter 1985/6): 101–113.

Jay, Karla, ed. *Dyke Life: From Growing Up to Growing Old, a Celebration of the Lesbian Experience.* New York: Basic Books, 1995.

McDaniel, Judith. *The Lesbian Couples Guide: Finding the Right Woman and Creating a Life Together.* New York: HarperPerennial, 1995.

Polikoff, Nancy. "Lesbian Mothers, Lesbian Families: Legal Obstacles, Legal Challenges." *Review of Law and Social Change* Vol. 14 (1986): 907–914.

Slater, Suzanne. *The Lesbian Family Life Cycle.* New York: Free Press, 1995.

leukotomy, leucotomy (prefrontal lobotomy)
A surgical procedure on the brain in which certain nerve pathways in the prefrontal lobes are severed from the rest of the brain as therapy to reduce violent behavior and treat severe resistant forms of depression, psychosis and obsessive-compulsive disorder. However, since the advent of better methods of psychotherapy and improved pharmacologic means, this treatment is rarely used.

More specific procedures involving less brain tissue destruction and side effects have been developed in a neurosurgical procedure called cingulotomy.

levodopa (trade names: Dopar, Larodopa) Levodopa is beneficial in both Parkinson's disease and postencephalitic parkinsonism. All major Parkinson's symptoms may be ameliorated, particularly bradykinesia, rigidity and, to a lesser extent, tremor. Balance, posture, gait and handwriting improve promptly; mood may be elevated. Although all intellectual functions may improve initially, this effect is often transient. Mental deterioration and dementia may develop during long-term therapy. It has not been established whether mental changes reflect progression of degenerative disease or are a direct effect of levodopa.

See also PARKINSON'S DISEASE.

American Medical Association. *Drug Evaluations Annual, 1991.* Chicago: AMA, 1991.

libido A term derived from the Latin words for "desire, lust" commonly used for sexual desire or "love energy." An active libido is generally considered a sign of good mental health, particularly in younger, healthy individuals. In some individuals, libido wanes with age but not necessarily so in every case.

Sigmund Freud used the term to relate to human drives including the sexual instinct, love-object seeking and pleasure. To Freud, libido was one of two vital human instincts, the drive toward self-preservation and the drive toward sexual gratification. According to Freud, when an individual represses libido because of social pressures, ongoing repression leads to personality changes and to anxieties.

Freud's original concept was expanded by Carl Jung to relate to term to the general life force that provides energy for all types of activities, including sexual, social, cultural and creative.

Loss of libido is one of the most frequent problems sex therapists encounter. It is one of the more difficult problems to treat, as the cause is often an underlying physical, emotional or psychological problem and not correctable by simple behavioral approaches.

Loss of libido occurs in men and women during many illnesses, including depression, alcoholism and drug addiction. Stress and overwork can cause loss of libido, as can certain medications or loss of an appropriate partner.

See also DEPRESSION; FREUD, SIGMUND; SEX THERAPY.

Librium Trade name for chlordiazepoxide hydrochloride, a widely prescribed sedative-tranquilizer containing a benzodiazepine derivative. It is used to reduce anxieties and tension and to treat or prevent withdrawal symptoms during alcoholic withdrawal and detoxification treatment. It should not be taken with alcohol or other central nervous system depressants. Physical and psychological additive effects and dependency can develop. Overdoses can result in drowsiness, confusion, reduced reflexes and possibly coma.

See also ANTIANXIETY MEDICATIONS; BENZODIAZEPINE MEDICATIONS.

life change events See GENERALIZED ADAPTATION SYNDROME; LIFE CHANGE SELF-RATING SCALE; SELYE, HANS.

life change self-rating scale The original life change rating scale was developed as a predictor of illness based on stressful life events by authors Thomas H. Holmes and Richard H. Rahe and presented at the Royal Society of Medicine in 1968. Many variations of this type of rating scale have been used to help individuals determine their composite stress level over the course of the past year.

To take this test, mark any of the changes listed below that have occurred in your life in the past 12 months. Your total score indicates the amount of stress you have been subjected to in the one-year period. Your score may be useful in predicting your chances of suffering illness in the next two years due to physiological effects of serious mental health challenges.

LIFE CHANGE SELF-RATING SCALE	
Event	Value
Death of spouse	100
Divorce	73
Marital Separation	65
Death of close family member	63
Personal injury or illness	53
Marriage	50
Fired from work	47
Marital reconciliation	45
Retirement	45
Change in family member's health	44
Pregnancy	40
Sex difficulties	39
Addition to family	39
Business readjustment	39
Change in financial status	38
Death of close friend	37
Change to different line of work	36
Foreclosure of mortgage or loan	30
Change in work responsibilities	29
Son or daughter leaving home	29
Trouble with in-laws	29
Outstanding personal achievement	28
Spouse begins or stops work	26
Starting or finishing school	26
Change in living conditions	25
Trouble with boss	23
Change in residence or school	20
Change in recreational habits	19
Change in church or social activities	19
Change in sleeping habits	16
Change in eating habits	15
Vacation	13
Christmas season	12
Minor violation of the law	11
Your total score:	======

What Your Score Means

A total score less than 150 may means you have a 27 percent chance of becoming ill in the next year. If your score is between 150 and 300, you have a 51 percent chance of encountering poor health. If your score is more than 300, you are facing odds of 80 percent that you will become ill, and as the score increases, so does the chance that the problem will be serious. To avoid these consequences, pay attention to the amount of relaxation and stress relief you get.

See also RELAXATION; STRESS.

*Adapted from Holmes and Rahe, Life Change Measurements as a Predictor of Illness, proceedings, Royal Society of Medicine, 1968.

Kahn, Ada P. *Stress A to Z: A Sourcebook for Facing Everyday Challenges*. New York: Facts On File, 2000.

light therapy See SEASONAL AFFECTIVE DISORDER.

limbic system The part of the parasympathetic nervous system that controls expression of emotional behavior, including sweating, trembling, breathing, alterations in facial expression, drives such as attack (fight or flight), defense, thirst, hunger and sexual motivation.

See also BRAIN.

listening Hearing with thoughtful attention is a skill necessary for good communication between individuals. It is an active process in which one gives complete attention to both what the other is saying and how they are saying it. According to Deborah Tannen, author of *Talking from 9 to 5: How Women's and Men's Conversational Styles Affect Who Gets Heard, Who Gets Credit and What Gets Done at Work*, "Listening taps two important areas, gathering information and developing relationships." Active listening can reduce the stress of communication not only in business but in one's personal life as well.

By using nonverbal gestures such as a nod of the head or a smile, active listeners can convey concern and reinforce or encourage the other's verbalizations. Listeners contribute by asking good questions, providing feedback on what they hear and seeking consensus or pointing out differences of opinion within a group. A person feels listened to when more than just their ideas get heard; as a consequence, they feel valued and will contribute a lot more to the conversation.

LISTENING SKILLS FOR BETTER MENTAL HEALTH

- Focus on the speaker; use eye contact. Keep interruptions, such as phone calls and other conversations, down to a minimum.
- It helps to question the speaker. You can gently guide a conversation, show that you are interested in what he or she is saying and indicate what you might want to learn.
- Don't judge the person speaking; concentrate on the information he or she is presenting.

See also BODY LANGUAGE; COMMUNICATION.

Nichols, Michael P. *The Lost Art of Listening.* New York: Doubleday, 1995.

Tannen, Deborah. *Talking from 9 to 5: How Women's and Men's Conversational Styles Affect Who Gets Heard, Who Gets Credit and What Gets Done at Work.* New York: William Morrow, 1994.

literacy See ILLITERACY.

lithium carbonate (trade names: Eskalith, Lithane, Lithonate, Lithotabs) A therapeutic agent that counteracts mood changes and is considered to be the only specific antimanic drug for the prophylaxis (prevention) and treatment of bipolar disorder. Acute hypomanic and manic episodes respond to lithium, but combined therapy with an antipsychotic agent may be preferred to control behavior initially. Lithium may be effective in maintenance therapy for major depression, although antidepressants are preferred. Lithium carbonate is also used in preventing cluster headache in some people.

The antimanic action of lithium is not fully understood, but it seems to act by altering the metabolism of norepinephrine in the brain, thus altering the chemical balance within certain nerve cells. Synthesis and release of acetylcholine are depressed. Because lithium interferes with calcium, the release of many neurotransmitters, including monoamines, is diminished.

Lithium has little effect on otherwise healthy patients except for mild sedation, and it has an antiadrenergic or anticholinergic action. In normal individuals, lithium produces mild subjective feelings of lethargy, inability to concentrate and possibly a decrease in memory function; slow waves in the electrocardiogram increase.

Lithium salts were used during the 1940s as a sodium chloride substitute for cardiac patients on salt-free diets, but its use was stopped when severe side effects and deaths were reported. Then, in the late 1940s, Australian researchers noted that lithium had certain tranquilizing properties; lithium safely quieted manic patients to whom it was administered. However, because of known toxic effects of lithium, interest in it dropped for almost a decade. In the 1950s and 1960s, some European studies led to increased acceptance of lithium in European psychiatric practices as safe and effective therapy for manic-depressive illness. In the 1970s, lithium began to be used in American practice after the need for careful monitoring a blood levels to overcome side effects was understood. Recent studies from Europe have raised the possibility that lithium therapy may reduce the risk of suicide in patients with bipolar disorder or recurrent major depression.

See also ANTIDEPRESSANT MEDICATIONS; BIPOLAR DISORDER; HEADACHES; MANIC-DEPRESSIVE ILLNESS; NOREPINEPHRINE; TRICYCLIC ANTIDEPRESSANT.

CHECKLIST FOR PATIENTS TAKING LITHIUM

- Take medication regularly as prescribed.
- Obtain regular blood tests for lithium levels.
- Have the physician take blood tests for lithium levels 12 hours after the last dose.
- Inform the physician if other medications are being taken, as they can change lithium levels.
- Notify the physician whenever there is a change in diet, since it may cause the lithium level in the body to change.
- Advise the physician about any changes in frequency of urination, diarrhea, vomiting, excessive sweating or illness; further adjustments in dosage may be necessary.
- If planning to become pregnant, advise the physician.
- It takes time for mood swings to be completely controlled by lithium; be patient and continue taking the medication until advised otherwise by the physician.

SOURCE: Roesch, Roberta. *Encyclopedia of Depression.* New York: Facts On File, 1990.

American Medical Association. *AMA Drug Evaluations Annual, 1991.* Chicago: AMA, 1991.

living will   See END OF LIFE ISSUES; LEGAL ISSUES.

lobotomy   A surgical procedure on the brain in which certain nerve pathways from the frontal lobes are cut in an attempt to change behavior.
See also LEUKOTOMY.

locus coeruleus   A small area in the brain stem containing norepinephrine neurons that is considered to be a key brain center for anxiety and fear.
See also ANXIETY; BRAIN.

logotherapy   An approach to the spiritual and existential aspects of mental disorders, developed by Victor Frankl, a German-born American psychiatrist (1905–1997).
See PSYCHOTHERAPIES.

loneliness   A state of mind and a unique set of circumstances, not to be confused with being alone. An element in loneliness is the lack of control or choice in being alone. For example, a happily married woman who moves to a new city because of her husband's career may feel lonely. She will be cut off from her previous network of acquaintances and very much on her own while he is welcomed by his new colleagues and absorbed in his new position. On the other hand, those who have chosen lifestyles and careers that require isolation and independence sometimes profit from, rather than resent, solitude. Lifelong conditioning may also make solitude attractive and even essential to some people. For example, only children, who have had to rely on their inner resources since childhood, are disproportionately present among astronauts and writers.

The potential for loneliness is strong in adolescence, when teenagers long to be part of their peer group and are deeply wounded by slights and rejections. Conditions such as mental or physical handicaps and language or ethnic barriers sometimes produce isolation that results in loneliness.

Loneliness sometimes results from a sense of loss, a feeling that the past was better than the present. A 1990 Gallup poll showed that loneliness is most common among the widowed, separated and divorced. Over half of this group felt lonely "frequently" or "sometimes," compared with 29 percent of the married participants. Adults who had never married fell in between. According to the survey, women are more likely to be lonely than men, possibly not because they genuinely have less companionship but because they place more importance on friendship and are more willing to confess to being lonely.

Money played a role in the Gallup survey as a preventive for loneliness. The survey showed 27 percent of adults with incomes over $50,000 are "frequently" or "sometimes" lonely, compared with 46 percent of those whose incomes were under $20,000.

Lonely people behave in different ways. Some fit the shy, retiring stereotype often assigned to the lonely. Others compensate for their feelings by trying to become the life of the party, throwing themselves into frenetic activity or by accumulating possessions.

Loneliness is often a factor in depression, drug addiction and alcoholism.
See also DEPRESSION.

Beck, Alan, and Aaron Katcher. *Between Pets and People: The Importance of Animal Companionship.* New York: Putnam, 1983.
Padus, Emrika. *The Complete Guide to Your Emotions and Your Health: Hundreds of Proven Techniques to Harmonize Mind and Body for Happy, Healthy Living.* Emmaus, Pa.: Rodale Press, 1992.
Wilson, Marlene. *You Can Make a Difference!* Boulder, Colo.: Volunteer Management Associates, 1990.

longitudinal study   A study in which the same group of individuals are observed and characteristics are noted at two or more different points in time. For example, in a longitudinal study of a group of depressed patients taking the same drug, their responses to the drug therapy will be measured at two or usually more points in time. Much research on pharmacologic treatment of mental health disorders is based on longitudinal studies. They are often submitted as evidence of drug efficacy when applications for approval of drug products are submitted to the U.S. Food and Drug Administration.

lorazepam Generic name for the benzodiazepine medication Ativan.

See also BENZODIAZEPINE MEDICATIONS; PHARMACEUTICAL APPROACH.

love object The person in whom one invests affection, devotion and usually sexual interest.

LSD See LYSERGIC ACID DIETHYLAMIDE.

L-tryptophan An essential amino acid found in eggs, turkey, milk, beans and wheat that human bodies use to manufacture proteins. The human brain uses L-tryptophan to manufacture serotonin, an amine transmitter. When the diet does not include an adequate amount of L-tryptophan, brain serotonin levels fall; some have speculated that this may contribute to depression and some anxieties. During the 1970s and 1980s, many individuals obtained L-tryptophan as an over-the-counter medication in tablet, capsule and powder form as a sleep aid and relaxant. The product was withdrawn from the market in 1989 when the Food and Drug Administration found that there may be a link between consumption of L-tryptophan supplements and an outbreak of a rare blood disorder (eosinophilamyalgia syndrome).

See also ANTIDEPRESSANT MEDICATIONS.

Kahn, Rene S., and Herman G. M. Westenberg. "L-5-Hydroxytryptophan in the Treatment of Anxiety Disorders," *Journal of Affective Disorders* 8 (1985).

Ludiomil Trade name for the tricyclic antidepressant medication maprotiline.

See also ANTIDEPRESSANT MEDICATIONS; PHARMACOLOGICAL APPROACH; TRICYCLIC ANTIDEPRESSANTS.

lumbar puncture See BRAIN.

lump in the throat Many individuals have experienced this unpleasant sensation at some time as part of an anxiety reaction. It feels like there is something to swallow, but the sensation does not go away upon swallowing. It may often feel difficult to swallow. Some individuals have this feeling before a stressful event, such as a public appearance, and are concerned that they not be able to speak appropriately. Relaxation and breathing techniques can help overcome this feeling. The medical term for lump in the throat is globus hystericus.

See also ANXIETY; STRESS.

lunacy An obsolete term meaning insanity. The term "lunacy" derives from the word *luna*, meaning "moon" in Latin. Ancients believed that phases of the moon could bring on mental illness and that as the moon waxed and waned, mental illnesses came and went. Until the 20th century, individuals with mental problems were referred to as lunatics, and mental hospitals were referred to as lunatic asylums.

See also INSANITY.

lysergic acid diethylamide (LSD) LSD is a very potent, odorless and colorless chemical hallucinogen that was first synthesized in the late 1930s. Effects of LSD can last from two to 12 hours and may include impaired judgment of time, distorted visual perceptions and hallucinations. LSD causes dilated pupils, elevated body temperatures and high blood pressure. Psychological reactions include suspicious behavior, fear, confusion, anxiety, loss of control and flashbacks. Flashbacks are common over a period of several years after the drug was consumed.

LSD is also known as acid and microdot and is usually found in liquid form, which is placed on a sugar cube or on blotter paper and then digested.

See also FLASHBACKS; HALLUCINATION; HALLUCINOGENS.

Media Resource Guide on Common Drugs of Abuse. Public Relations Society of America, National Capital Chapter, Fairfax, Va., September 1990.

magic An ability to exert control over human affairs and the forces of nature. Practitioners of magic may be known as witch doctors, wizards, diviners, wise women, witches, sorcerers or magicians. Magic may also fall within the bounds of religious practice and may include contact with supernatural forces. Historically, the mental health of those who practice magic, as well as those who believe in it, has been challenged or questioned by less believing individuals.

The ability to practice magic has often been thought to be inborn or hereditary. Magical arts are often acquired secretly in an individual manner with the aspiring magician progressing ever higher in his art in his own way rather than being taught in the usual manner. The ability to practice magic is thought by some to be amoral. Magical spells may be used to create or destroy; they may also have a preventive, protective nature. An evil spell may be cast without the victim's knowledge to keep her from hiring a more powerful sorcerer. For victims of magic who are aware of the spell, it may become a self-fulfilling prophecy, since in civilizations in which magical beliefs are strong, simply the knowledge of being bewitched is enough to make the victim weaken and, sometimes, die. In such cases it is the power of suggestion that is the strong force at work.

Early humans and the classical civilizations believed in and practiced magic. Christianity has both used and rejected magical beliefs and practices. Early Christians gained power by claims that their mystical ceremonies and rituals were superior to those of pagans. Later Christianity rejected magic as a vestige of paganism and an attempt to interfere with God's will. During the Middle Ages various temples and secret societies preserved magical beliefs and practices. The scientific, rational philosophies of the 17th and 18th centuries caused magic to fall into disrepute. In the 19th century, Aleister Crowley and a fraternal group, the Hermetic Order of the Golden Dawn, revived interest in magic. An interest in magic resurged again with the religion of neo-pagan witchcraft, which forbids the use of magic for other than beneficial purposes.

Throughout history, magic has been used as an explanation for things that cannot be seen or answered logically. Individuals seeking answers become believers.

"Magic," In *Harper's Encyclopedia of Mystical and Paranormal Experience*. edited by Rosemary Ellen Guiley. San Francisco: Harper, 1991.

magical thinking The conviction that thinking equates doing. It is characterized by a lack of realistic relationship between cause and effect. This occurs most often in children's dreams in some cultures and in some seriously ill patients.

magnetic resonance imaging (MRI) See BRAIN IMAGING.

mainstreaming An educational technique that involves placing students who are handicapped or exceptional in other ways as much as possible with normal students in an environment that offers as few restrictions as possible. Mainstreaming programs allow for a flexible assessment of each child's needs with the consultation of a variety of support personnel, such as school psychologists, to give each child an individual program that will suit his needs and specific disabilities and talents. This concept also calls for frequent assessment of a child's progress in consultation with his parents.

See also MENTAL RETARDATION.

"Least Restrictive Environment," "Mainstreaming," In *American Educator's Encyclopedia*. edited by Edward L. Dejnozka. Westport, Conn.: Greenwood Press, 1982.

major affective disorders   A term referring to disorders characterized by noticeable and persistent mood disturbances, such as depression, mania or bipolar disorder. These disorders may be episodic or chronic.

See also AFFECTIVE DISORDERS; BIPOLAR DISORDER; BRAIN CHEMISTRY; DEPRESSION; MANIC-DEPRESSIVE ILLNESS.

major depression   The term used to indicate a clinical depression that meets specific diagnostic criteria regarding duration, functional impairment and involvement of several physical and mental symptoms.

See also ANTIDEPRESSANT MEDICATION; BRAIN CHEMISTRY; DEPRESSION.

malingering   Purposeful pretense of physical or psychological symptoms for a particular reason, such as to obtain time off from work or to avoid a family affair. This differs from factitious disorders, in which one pretends illness for no reason other than to gain attention. This also differs from hypochondriasis, in which the person is obsessed with her own physical condition and believes that she has symptoms.

See also MUNCHAUSEN'S SYNDROME.

managed care   A term covering many varieties of health insurance, including health maintenance organizations (HMOs) and preferred provider organizations (PPOs). The premise on which HMOs is based is that insurance companies provide specified services for a prepaid fee for an enrolled population. In many cases, employers and employees share the costs for coverage of employees and their families. HMOs and other forms of managed care are also available to retirees as a supplement to Medicare. Enrollment in managed care plans rose significantly after a 1973 federal law paved the way for insurance companies to finance and deliver health care. In 1996, about 60 percent of Americans were enrolled in some sort of managed care

health plans, up from 36 percent in 1992. The increase is due in large part to employers shifting their workers away from the traditional, and considerably more expensive, "fee for service" health insurance plans.

Critics of HMOs claim limitation of choices regarding doctors, while proponents claim higher quality and closer monitoring of care. Some managed care plans have physicians as their employees, while other plans compensate physicians on a "capitation," or the number of patients which they serve, basis.

As health care costs spiraled upward, health plans became the subject of criticism for enacting limits on what managed care would cover. In most cases, managed care plans limit the number of mental health visits for which a patient may be covered.

In the early 2000s, HMOs have been touted for bringing affordable health coverage to a wide range of consumers, as well as criticized for cutting costs by limiting treatment options and patient choice. Doctors and patients increasingly are seeking new ways to regulate the managed care industry by giving patients new rights, including the ability to sue their health plans. Controversy continues over how to protect patients without further driving up already expensive health care costs.

mania   A mental disorder characterized by periods of elation, overactivity or irritability. Mania usually occurs in conjunction with moods of depression, and when the two occur at intervals in the same individual, the disorder is known as manic-depressive illness.

A manic individual will show an abnormal increase in activity and believe that he is capable of achieving any goal. There may be a grandiose sense of knowing more than others around, extravagant spending of money, little need for sleep, increased appetite for food, alcohol and sex or inappropriate bursts of laughter or anger. Severe mania may result in violence, and hospital admission is often required. Relatively mild symptoms are known as hypomania.

The first appearance of manic attacks is usually before age 30 and may last for a few days or several months. When attacks begin after age 40, they may be more prolonged. Mania often runs in families and may be genetically transmitted.

Treatment of mania includes the use of antipsychotic drugs; relapses are prevented with the use of lithium.

See also ANTIDEPRESSANT MEDICATIONS; ANTIPSYCHOTIC MEDICATIONS; LITHIUM CARBONATE.

manic-depressive disorder A mental disorder characterized by disturbances of moods, including depression, mania (unipolar) or a swing between the two states (bipolar disorder). In the manic state, the individual is excessively elated, agitated and hyperactive and has accelerated thinking and speaking.

In the manic phase, overactivity may be due largely to extra amounts of the neurochemical dopamine in parts of the brain.

Depression is more common than mania, affecting about one in 10 men and one in five women at some time in their lives. Mania (unipolar or bipolar) affects only about eight per 1,000 people, men and women equally. More than 80 percent of patients recover from this disorder.

Severe manic-depressive illness often requires hospitalization. Antidepressant drugs or electroconvulsive therapy are sometimes used in treating depression. Antipsychotic drugs are used to control the symptoms of mania. To prevent relapse, lithium is often used. When taking lithium as advised by their physician, many people who have manic-depressive illness can lead healthy, well-balanced lives.

See also AFFECTIVE DISORDERS; ANTIDEPRESSANT MEDICATIONS; BIPOLAR DISORDER; LITHIUM CARBONATE; MANIA.

manic episode See MANIA; MANIC-DEPRESSIVE DISORDER.

MAOIs See MONOAMINE OXIDASE INHIBITORS.

MAO Inhibitors See MONOAMINE OXIDASE INHIBITORS.

maprotiline An antidepressant drug (trade name: Ludiomil). The pharmacologic and clinical profiles, as well as efficacy, resemble those of imipramine. This drug principally blocks the neuronal uptake of norepinephrine; it has relatively weak serotonergic activity.

See also ANTIDEPRESSANT MEDICATIONS; TRICYCLIC ANTIDEPRESSANT MEDICATIONS.

marijuana Marijuana is a drug derived from the plant *Cannabis sativa*. Marijuana's effects vary considerably, depending on the personality and health of the user, frequency and circumstance of use, potency and other factors. The larger the dose, the greater the hypnotic effects and the loss of psychomotor functions. Marijuana use intensifies sensory experiences, including seeing, hearing, tasting and touching. The user may feel relaxed or, less commonly, anxious, fearful and distrustful. Sustained mental effort may be difficult for marijuana users; they are easily distracted and often cannot complete a thought.

Problems associated with chronic marijuana use include decreased blood supply to the heart; damage to the lungs and pulmonary system; impaired sexual development and fertility; damage to the immune system; and "amotivational" syndrome, which includes low motivation, loss of attention, impaired communication skill, lethargy and impaired learning ability. Marijuana impairs motor ability and judgment, increasing the likelihood of accidents. Marijuana adversely affects the user's ability to drive because of impaired perception and reaction time. Marijuana smoke contains more cancer-causing agents than tobacco smoke.

Marijuana use during pregnancy is associated with low birth weight and body length, prematurity and a range of other problems. Marijuana is also transmitted in breast milk.

Marijuana is an ongoing problem for law enforcement officials as well as mental health workers who treat drug abusers. Most of the marijuana consumed in the United States comes from Colombia, Mexico, Jamaica and Thailand. It is also cultivated domestically.

Medical Use of Marijuana

Many results of studies have been published indicating the positive effects that marijuana can have for people facing debilitating conditions such as cancer and glaucoma. Marijuana has proven to be useful in helping control pain and also to help with side effects of treatments such as chemotherapy. Some AIDS patients who have "wasting syndrome" find that marijuana use increases their appetites with effective health benefits.

A March 1999 Gallup poll found that 73 percent of respondents in the U.S. would vote for making marijuana legally available for doctors to prescribe in order to reduce pain and suffering.

In the last 20 years, 36 states have passed some form of legislation recognizing the medical value of marijuana. In 1996, voters in Arizona and California passed laws allowing the medical use of marijuana. In 1998 Alaska, Washington State, and Oregon passed medical use of marijuana laws, in 1999 Maine passed a similar law and in 2000 Hawaii passed such a law through the legislature.

See also SUBSTANCE ABUSE.

Grinspoon, Lester. *Marijuana: The Forbidden Medicine.* New Haven: Yale University Press, 1997.
Media Resource Guide on Common Drugs of Abuse. Public Relations Society of America, National Capital Chapter, Fairfax, Va., September 1990.
Potter, Beverly A. and Dan Joy. *The Healing Magic of Cannabis.* Berkeley, Calif.: Ronin Publishing, 1998.
Randall, Robert C. *Marijuana Rx: The Patient's Fight for Medicinal Pot.* New York: Thunder's Mouth Press, 1998.
Zimmerman, Bill. *Is Marijuana the Right Medicine for You?: A Factual Guide to Medical Uses of Marijuana.* New Canaan, Conn.: Keats, 1998.

marital rape   See RAPE, RAPE PREVENTION AND RAPE TRAUMA SYNDROME.

marital therapy   Therapy for individuals in a troubled marriage. This may involve couples therapy or therapy for the individuals alone. The therapy may be aimed at overcoming specific problems, such as coping with the other's depression, or at saving a marriage that might end in divorce. Marital therapy may involve only psychological counseling or sexual therapy or a combination of both.

See also BEHAVIORAL THERAPY; DIVORCE; FAMILY THERAPY; MARRIAGE; SEX THERAPY.

Marplan   Trade name for the monoamine oxidase antidepressant medication known as isocarboxazid.

See also ANTIDEPRESSANT MEDICATIONS; MONOAMINE OXIDASE INHIBITORS (MAOIS).

marriage   Lifelong emotional and legal commitment to another individual. Some form of marriage has been present in all cultures, and most societies have considered marriage necessary for a satisfying adult life. Romance, mutual selection and compatibility are generally considered less important in other cultures than in the modern Western world. In some societies, couples are promised to each other as children or even before birth. Family or tribal relationships and economic considerations quite often take precedence over individual wishes. Some arranged marriages result in lifelong loving relationships, while others lapse into marriages of convenience and for procreation, with one or more of the spouses acquiring other romantic and sexual partners.

Marriage ceremonies may be lengthy and complex or very simple. Most marriage ceremonies involve, or are followed by, a meal or the ceremonial consumption of food. Ceremonies are frequently a blend of religious observance and superstition or folk culture.

Monogamy, the marriage of one man with one woman, is the common form of marriage in the Western world. Polygyny, the union of one man and several wives, is practiced in some African tribes and Islamic cultures. In Tibet, one woman may have several husbands who are brothers. The Catholic church and other religious groups consider members of religious orders married to their divine being. Many religious groups have prohibitions against marrying outside the group. Most cultures prohibit incest to some degree.

In her early 1980 work, *Outrageous Acts and Everyday Rebellions,* feminist Gloria Steinem issued a veiled warning that the reason that women are not attracted to gambling is that the uncertainties and precariousness of marriage satisfy most women's gambling instincts. However, in the face of recent reports showing the statistical difficulty of acquiring a husband and of career possibilities opened up by the women's movement, women still seem to favor marriage as a way of life. A Gallup poll in 1987 showed that only 8 percent of the women surveyed thought that being a single career woman was an ideal way of life, approximately the same percentage as when the question was asked in 1975. Another Gallup poll indicated what may be a return to a more conservative approach to marriage and sexual relationships. Whether a product of a heightened national interest in religion, an overall conservative trend or fears about sexually transmitted disease, the segment of the population who believe that premarital sex is wrong rose from 39 percent in 1985 to 46 percent in 1987.

Opposites may attract, but they probably will not marry or stay married, according to researchers. People do tend to marry within their own social and educational groups, although tendencies to marry within religious groups are crumbling. This may be due in part to the fact that modern American life brings people of differing religions together but somewhat segregates by social and educational status. People who "marry down" in social, financial or educational terms quite often acquire a more physically attractive or personable spouse than if they married at their level.

Dissolution of Marriage Rising

A 1980s statistical projection predicted that four out of 10 marriages of the 1970s would end in divorce. Marriage has undergone great stress and strain in the last 30 years. From a romantic commitment that was entered into for life and was almost a social requirement in the 1950s, traditional marriage became a subject that aroused feelings of rebellion and disdain in the late 1960s and 1970s as divorce became more common and socially acceptable and premarital sex became more common. Young people experimented with communal arrangements or simply lived together without benefit of marriage vows.

Because so many traditional monogamous marriages have resulted in divorce, many individuals have experimented with alternative marital-sexual relationships. Recently the possibility of marriages between homosexual couples has become an issue.

Open Marriage. This emphasizes equality and flexibility in female roles in the marriage and includes an agreement not to be emotionally, socially or sexually exclusive. The concept was espoused by Nena and George O'Neil in their book *Open Marriage* (1972). Disadvantages of this system include possibilities for jealousy and fear of losing one's spouse. Although this system attracted attention, it was largely discarded as generally unworkable for most couples.

Group Marriage. A term for "multilateral" marriage. This involves a group of individuals with some type of marriage ties to one another. For example, each person may be married to at least two others in the group. Sexual activities with each of one's spouses occur on a rotation schedule. Group sex is uncommon.

Swinging. A married couple's sharing sexual activities with another couple or couples. A pair may switch partners with another married couple, or a married couple may engage in sexual activities with a single female, single male or an unmarried couple. Recreational swingers are primarily interested in sexual activities without close friendships or involvement with their sexual partners. "Utopian" swingers seek sex activity as well as close interpersonal relationships.

Swinging first gained public attention during the 1950s (then known as "wife swapping"). There have been magazines and clubs devoted to swinging. Major reasons for dropping out of swinging are jealousy, the threat to marriage and the threat of sexually transmitted diseases and even acquiring the HIV virus or AIDS.

Child Marriage. A marriage between an adult (usually male) and a minor female is known as child marriage. Historically, some parents permitted daughters to marry older men in order to provide support.

Fear of marriage is known as gamophobia or gametophobia. In the late 1980s and early 1990s, many young people developed a fear of commitment and have thus avoided marriage until their late thirties. Marriage later in life brings with it the stress of the "biological clock" for women and increased anxieties about becoming mothers before they are too old.

For information:

American Association of Marriage and
  Family Therapy
1717 K Street NW, Suite 407
Washington, D.C. 20006
Phone: (202) 429-1825

See also DIVORCE; LIVE-IN; REMARRIAGE; STEPFAM-
ILIES; LOVE.

Gottman, John Mordechai. *Why Marriages Succeed or Fail:
  What You Can Learn From the Breakthrough Research to
  Make Your Marriage Last.* New York: Simon & Schus-
  ter, 1994.
Roloff, Tamara L., and Mary E. Williams, eds. *Marriage
  and Divorce.* San Diego: Greenhaven Press, 1997.
Simpson, Eileen B. *Late Love: A Celebration of Marriage
  After Fifty.* Boston: Houghton Mifflin, 1994.
Stack, Steven. "Marriage, Family and Loneliness: A
  Cross-National Study." *Sociological Perspectives* 41, no.
  2 (1998): 415–432.
Steinem, Gloria. "Night Thoughts of a Media Watcher."
  Outrageous Acts and Everyday Rebellions (New York:
  New American Library, 1983): 370–381.

Marsalid   See IPRONIAZID.

masked depression   A depression that a person
hides behind a facade of appearing to be well. These
individuals outwardly do what they think is
expected of them while inwardly feeling hopeless
and even suicidal. They may have little facial ani-
mation and appear to have a fixed expression,
showing little emotion. The terms "depressive equivalents," "affective equivalents," "hidden depression" and "missed depression" are also used for this
situation. Many health care professionals feel that
"borderline depression" may be categorized as
masked depression.

See also DEPRESSION; MANIC-DEPRESSIVE DISORDER.

masochism   A desire to be abused either physically or emotionally. It is often used to refer to
achievement of sexual excitement by means of
one's own suffering. The condition can be life
threatening if individuals increase the degree of
their masochistic acts. The term was derived from
the name of the 19th-century Austrian novelist
Leopold von Sacher-Masoch.

See also SADISM; SADOMASOCHISM.

massage therapy   Massage therapy is a form of
body therapy in which the practitioner applies
manual techniques—the kneading, stroking and
manipulation of the soft tissues of the body, skin,
muscles, tendons and ligaments—with the intention of positively affecting the mental health and
physical well-being of the client. Massage therapy
helps many people relieve stress and body aches
caused by tension and anxieties.

A professional massage increases blood flow and
relaxes muscles. Massage therapy can provide anything from soothing relaxation to deeper therapy
for specific physical problems. It can aid in recovery
from pulled muscles or sprained ligaments. Massage therapy can also ease many of the uncomfortable stresses of childbearing, the discomforts of
back pain and exhaustion, as well as the pains of
certain repetitive stress injuries related to on-the-
job activities.

According to the American Massage Therapy
Association (AMTA), once the massage is underway, many beneficial reactions are set in motion.
Massage therapy can hasten the elimination of
waste and toxic debris stored in muscles, increase
the interchange of substances between the blood
and tissue cells and stimulate the relaxation
response within the nervous system. In addition,
responses to massage therapy can help to
strengthen the immune system, improve posture,
increase joint flexibility and range of motion and
reduce blood pressure.

Types of Massage

The most universally understood Western form of
massage is Swedish, also called Esalen. It consists of
many types of strokes: gliding the hand across the
skin, kneading, lifting, squeezing and grasping the
muscles, gentle pushing, friction, vibration,
jostling, rocking and percussion (hacking, chopping
and rapid pounding).

Eastern massage, sometimes referred to as shiatsu or acupressure, involves pressing at certain
points along invisible energy meridians that run
through the body; the practitioner looks for tight
spots, knots or anything that interferes with the
flow of energy.

Deep tissue massage uses slow strokes and deep
finger pressure to combat aching muscles. Sports

massage is a combination of stretching and Swedish or deep-tissue massage performed before or after strenuous exercise.

Reflexology, or the massaging of the hands, feet and ears, is based on the belief that specific areas govern all parts of the body. For example, the tips of the toes correspond to the head, while the inside arch of the foot reflects the spine. The theory is that by stimulating the nerve endings of the different organs in the body, changes can be affected.

Choosing a Massage Therapist

According to the American Massage Therapy Association (AMTA), a qualified massage therapist should have a solid foundation in physiology and be knowledgeable about the inner workings of the body. Therapists from an accredited school have usually completed 500 hours of training, including classes in anatomy, first aid and cardiopulmonary resuscitation.

The American Massage Therapy Association, founded in 1943, is the largest and oldest national organization representing the profession. Membership in the AMTA is limited to those who have demonstrated a level of skill and expertise through testing and/or education. All AMTA therapists must agree to abide by the AMTA Code of Ethics.

According to the AMTA, their membership increased from under 5,000 in 1986 to more than 20,000 in 1994.

Experiencing a Massage

Most massage therapists work in small, semi-dark rooms, with soft music of the client's choice playing. Some therapists offer a choice of scented candles. The massage therapist leaves the client alone to undress and lie down on a padded massage table. During the massage, the entire body is draped in a sheet; only the portion currently being worked on is exposed. Quiet is an essential feature of the massage experience. While conversation with the therapist may be limited, a person should speak up if experiencing discomfort, feeling hot or cold, desiring more or less pressure or wanting more attention paid to a certain area of the body.

Massage is "productive down time." During the massage, the body becomes very heavy and sinks into the table. As the therapist's hands locate areas of tension, the individual consciously tries to let go and relax these areas. He or she lets go of a desire to control movement and allows the therapist to move limbs into whatever position is required.

Patricia Deer, a certified massage therapist and owner of Energy Breaks, Chicago, says that a good neck and shoulder massage may contribute toward better mental performance, as well as relief of stress. One study reported that people who received 15-minute seated massages during their workday showed brain-wave patterns consistent with greater alertness. Those people were also able to complete arithmetic problems twice as fast and with half the errors as they did before the massage. "Employers are increasingly recognizing the benefits of 'mini-tune-ups' for people who sit at desks or computers for much of the day," says Deer.

Massage Therapy and Hospitalized Patients

Some acute care and long-term facilities are instituting therapy programs to support their patients' health, healing and quality of life. Researchers at the University of Colorado conducted a project to uncover and elucidate a range of patient outcomes of a therapeutic massage program within an acute care setting. Narrative data were coded into eight categories (pain, sleep, tension/anxiety, body awareness, physical functioning, psychological support, enhancing healing and value). Selected patient responses were included to elaborate the meanings of these categories. The most frequently identified outcomes were increased relaxation (98 percent), a sense of well-being (93 percent) and positive mood change (88 percent). More than two-thirds of the patients attributed enhanced mobility, greater energy, increased participation in treatment and faster recovery to massage therapy. The study supported the value of the hospital-based massage therapy program and uncovered a range of benefits of massage therapy. Recommendations for further study were indicated.

For information:

American Massage Therapy Association
800 Davis Street, Suite 100
Evanston, IL 60201
Phone: (847) 864-0123

See also ACUPRESSURE; BODY THERAPIES; COMPLE-
MENTARY THERAPIES; MIND-BODY CONNECTIONS;
REFLEXOLOGY; RELAXATION; ROLFING; SHIATSU; STRESS.

Shulman, Karen R. and Gwen E. Jones. "The Effectiveness of Massage Therapy Intervention on Reducing
Anxiety in the Workplace." *Journal of Applied Behavioral Science* 32, no. 2 (June 1996): 160–173.
Smith, Marlaine C. et al. "Benefits of Massage Therapy
for Hospitalized Patients: A Descriptive and Qualitative Evaluation." *Alternative Therapies* 5, no. 4 (July
1999): 64–71.

mass hysteria Mass hysteria, also known as epidemic anxiety, is a condition in which many people
are simultaneously affected by extreme, often
unfounded anxiety. Mass hysteria was recognized
during the latter part of the Middle Ages, when
whole groups of people were affected by similar
anxieties—for example, dance manias involving
raving, jumping and convulsions. Some thought
they had been bitten by a tarantula (a spider) and
would jump up and run out to dance in the street.
This activity became known as tarantism in Italy
and St. Vitus's Dance in the rest of Europe.

Another example of mass hysteria occurred during the 16th century when individuals imagined
themselves as a wolf and then acted like one. In the
1950s, there was also a mass hysteria incident in
the state of Washington involving the pitting of
auto windshields. Groups of people feared that the
pitting (a normal phenomenon) had developed
from radioactive material in the air.

See also ANXIETY; EPIDEMIC ANXIETY.

masturbation Sexual self-stimulation for gratification and pleasure and usually to orgasm. The
usual method is massaging the penis or clitoris with
the hand. In previous generations, parents warned
young people against masturbation, suggesting that
doing so would lead to acne, impotence, insanity or
worse consequences. Thus, many people who
believed that they were going against cultural
mores developed anxieties and guilt about the
practice. Now it is considered normal behavior,
particularly among teenagers and those without
sexual partners. Masturbation can be done on oneself and can also be performed on another person.

In the 1960s, Alfred Kinsey said that more than
90 percent of men reported masturbatory experiences in their adolescence. In the early 1980s,
Shere Hite, an American researcher on female sexuality, reported that about 82 percent of American
women masturbate.

Sex therapists during the latter part of the 20th
century use masturbation as a technique to instruct
clients in learning to know what pleases them so
that they can later instruct a partner.

Compulsive masturbation is an obsessive urge to
masturbate without sexual feeling or satisfaction.
Such an individual may substitute masturbation for
lack of social satisfaction, to compensate for shyness or an inability to establish relationships with
the opposite sex or to relieve anxieties.

See also SAFE SEX; SEX THERAPY; SEXUAL DYSFUNC-
TION.

Kahn, Ada P., and Linda Hughey Holt. *The A to Z of
Women's Sexuality.* Alameda, Calif.: Hunter House,
1992.

mathematics anxiety Stress related to the practical applications of mathematics in everyday life,
such as counting small change or reading timeta-
bles. Additionally, math anxiety occurs because
mathematics is an abstract science and many people have difficulties understanding abstractions.

Simply balancing a checkbook causes many
individuals to perspire and experience a more rapid
heartbeat. Many students who are good in all other
subjects experience feelings of discomfort in math
classes. There is no clearcut explanation for this.
The individual may be unsure of his or her abilities
regarding adding and subtracting, or there may be
a fear of making a mistake. In a school setting,
making a mistake when called upon can be embarrassing.

Medicaid A federal-state medical assistance program authorized in 1965 to pay for health care services used by people defined as medically needy or
categorically needy. The latter type of persons are
low-income aged, blind, disabled, first-time pregnant women or families with dependent children.
Medically needy persons are any of the above
whose incomes are above eligibility limits for the

categorically needy but who have high medical expenses that reduce their resources below established limits.

See also MEDICARE.

Medicare A nationwide, federally administered health insurance program authorized in 1965 to cover the cost of hospitalization, medical and mental health care and other related services. Eligible persons must be over age 65, receive Social Security, or suffer from end-stage renal disease. Medicare consists of two separate but coordinated programs: hospital insurance (Part A) and supplementary medical insurance (Part B). Health insurance protection is available to insured persons without regard to income.

Medicare intermediaries or carriers are fiscal agents (typically Blue Cross plans or commercial insurance firms) under contract to the Health Care Financing Administration for administration of specific Medicare tasks. These tasks include determining reasonable costs for covered items and services, making payments and guarding against unnecessary use of covered services for Medicare Part A payments. Intermediaries also make payments for home health and outpatient hospital services covered under Part B.

See also MEDICAID.

Health Care Financing Administration. *Medicare & You 2000.* Washington, D.C., 2000.

meditation A learned technique to relieve stress and improve mental health involving deep relaxation brought on by focusing attention on a particular sound or image and breathing deeply. One directs thoughts away from work, family, relationships and the environment. During meditation, the heart rate, blood pressure and oxygen-consumption rate decreases, temperature of the extremities rises and muscles relax.

Meditation also has been shown to reduce a number of medical symptoms and improve health-related attitudes and behaviors. People with heart disease, hypertension, cancer, diabetes and chronic pain have reported feeling more self-confident, more in control in their lives and better able to mange stress after mastering the meditation tech-

nique. Meditation has been used successfully by individuals who have panic attacks and panic disorder.

Meditation may bring out increased efficiency in the body by eliminating unnecessary expenditures of energy. Individuals who practice meditation sometimes report a beneficial surge of energy marked by increased physical stamina, increased productivity on the job, the end of writer's or artist's "block" and the release of previously unsuspected creative potential.

Learning to Meditate for Better Mental Health

Meditation is a very self-disciplined routine that provides a way to learn more about one's thoughts and feelings. Simple procedures can be learned easily. The basics include sitting in a quiet room with eyes closed, breathing deeply and rhythmically with attention focused on the breath. Also, there may be a focus on either a special word, or "mantra," such as "peace" or "om," which one repeats over and over again; others find steadily watching an object, such as a candle flame for a 20-minute period once or more daily, equally effective.

Meditation relies on the close links between mind and body. When one meditates, the alpha brainwaves indicate that the body is relaxed and free from physical tension and mental strain. Biofeedback monitoring has indicated that meditation encourages the brain to produce an evenly balanced pattern of alpha and theta brain wave rhythms. This means that the body is relaxed and the mind is calm yet alert. The "relaxation response" sets in—the physical opposite of the tension that results from stress.

Individuals who meditate frequently report that they are more aware of their own opinions after beginning meditation. They are not as easily influenced by others as they were previously and can arrive at decisions more quickly and easily. They may be more self-assertive and more able to stand up for their own rights effectively. Additionally, researchers have shown that the meditating person may become less irritable in his or her interpersonal relationships within a relatively short period of time after beginning meditation.

Types of Meditation

Modern meditation techniques are derived from spiritual practices in Eastern cultures dating back more than 2,000 years. Traditionally, the benefits of the techniques have been defined as spiritual in nature, and meditation has constituted a part of many religious practices. In the latter part of the 20th century, however, simple forms of meditation have been used for stress management with excellent results. Contributing to the rising interest is the fact that these meditation techniques are related to biofeedback (which also emphasizes a delicately attuned awareness of inner processes) and to the muscle relaxation and visualization techniques used in behavior therapy.

There are two basic types of meditation: *concentration* and *insight*. Concentration types, such as transcendental meditation, often use a special sound or silently repeated phrase to focus attention and to screen out extraneous thoughts or stimuli. Insight-oriented meditations, such as mindfulness meditation, accept the thoughts and feelings that arise from moment to moment as objects of attention and acceptance. The goal of mindfulness is an increased awareness of what is happening in one's mind and body at that particular moment. Recognition and acceptance of present reality provides the basis for changes of attitudes and conditions.

SITUATIONS IN WHICH MEDITATION MAY IMPROVE MENTAL HEALTH

- Tension or anxiety
- Chronic fatigue
- Insomnia and hypersomnia
- Abuse of alcohol or tobacco
- Excessive self-blame
- Chronic sub-acute depression
- Irritability, low tolerance for frustration
- Strong tendencies to submissiveness
- Difficulties with self-assertion
- Prolonged bereavement reactions

See also BEHAVIOR THERAPY; BENSON, HERBERT; BIOFEEDBACK; COMPLEMENTARY THERAPIES; GUIDED IMAGERY; KABAT-ZINN, JON; PANIC ATTACKS AND PANIC DISORDER; RELAXATION; STRESS; TRANSCENDENTAL MEDITATION.

Benson, Herbert. *The Relaxation Response.* New York: William Morrow, 1975.

Chopra, Deepak. *Creating Health: How to Wake Up the Body's Intelligence.* Boston: Houghton Mifflin, 1991.
———. *Creating Affluence: Wealth Consciousness in the Field of all Possibilities.* San Rafael, Calif.: New World Library, 1993.
Kabat-Zinn, Jon. *Full Catastrophe Living: Using the Wisdom of Your Body and Mind to Face Stress, Pain and Illness.* New York: Delacorte, 1991.
———. *Wherever You Go, There You Are: Mindfulness Meditation in Everyday Life.* New York: Hyperion, 1993.
Kerman, D. Ariel. *The H.A.R.T. Program: Lower Your Blood Pressure Without Drugs.* New York: HarperCollins, 1992.
Mahesh Yogi, Maharishi. *Science of Being and Art of Living: Transcendental Meditation.* New York: Meridian, 1995.

medulla oblongata   See BRAIN.

megalomania   Exaggeration of one's own abilities or importance. Megalomania may become a delusion that one is someone famous. It may also take the form of becoming involved in some grandiose activity, such as renting an amusement park for a party. Although megalomania is not considered a mental disorder by itself, it may be an aspect of mania or manic behavior in manic-depressive illness.

See DELUSION; MANIA; MANIC-DEPRESSIVE ILLNESS.

melancholia   An old term meaning depression. It is derived from the Greek word meaning "black bile." Ancients believed that an excess of black bile caused low moods. The term "melancholia" is used currently to refer to certain symptoms that occur during severe depression, such as loss of pleasure in most activities and lack of reaction to pleasurable stimuli.

See also AFFECTIVE DISORDERS; DEPRESSION.

memory   An ability to retain, remember and call up information presented through the senses. For example, memories of smell, touch and taste are placed in several places in the brain, awaiting a similar stimulus, such as the smell of a familiar food, to reactivate the memory.

Verbalizing the memory involves finding the right words, which then calls into play the entire left side of the brain, where words are stored. All parts of the brain are required for comprehension and storage of memory.

Minor memory difficulties may be caused by depression, grief, fatigue, stress, illness, medication, alcohol or just simply trying to remember too much at once. Minor memory difficulties do not mean that the person is not mentally well.

Individuals have recall in various steps. Immediate recall involves remembering from a few seconds to a few minutes; an example is remembering a phone number long enough to write it down. Short-term recall involves memory from a few minutes to a few days. Long-term memory refers to memory from a few days to a few years.

According to Sid Gilman, M.D., professor and chairman of the Department of Neurology at the University of Michigan Medical Center, Ann Arbor, memory is a cell-to-cell transmission of information across a synapse that has both electrical and chemical properties. This interaction and transmitting across cell walls takes place in a split second.

Many individuals are less able to remember certain types of information as they get older. The term "age-associated memory impairment" (AAMI) is used to describe minor memory difficulties that come with age. When the person is relaxed, he or she will be able to remember the forgotten material with no difficulty. There is no treatment for AAMI, but written reminders, lists, using association to remember names and allowing more time to remember may be helpful.

According to Stanley Berent, Ph.D., neuropsychologist at the University of Michigan, Ann Arbor, individuals should seek professional help for memory difficulties if they feel uncomfortable, anxious or fearful because of the loss, if they feel out of touch with reality because they cannot remember what day of the week it is or where they are or if they feel that forgetting things is upsetting their role as a parent or grandparent.

See also ALZHEIMER'S DISEASE; DEMENTIA.

Kra, Siegfried J. *Aging Myths: Reversible Causes of Mind and Memory Loss.* New York: McGraw-Hill, 1985.
Mark, Vernon H. *Reversing Memory Loss; Proven Methods for Regaining, Strengthening, and Preserving Your Memory.* Boston: Houghton Mifflin, 1992.

menarche   The first menstruation, usually occurring when a girl is between 11 and 17, which marks the onset of female puberty. It is a time characterized by changes in body shape and increased interest in young men and sexual matters. Many young women do become sexually active during these years, and many pregnancies result in unwed mothers.

See also MENSTRUATION.

meninges   See BRAIN.

menopause   Cessation of menses (menstrual periods). Because menopause occurs at mid-life, when women have many psychosocial concerns as well as those of their bodies, it is often a time filled with stress, conflict and challenges. In past generations, the "change of life" was considered to be a time when women would be naturally irritable and even irrational. Many of women's complaints around the time of menopause were written off by doctors as being "all in their head." Now, however, it is recognized that other issues in a woman's life at this time contribute to her mental health in addition to changes in hormonal levels.

Menopause occurs in the United States between age 50 and 51; in the United Kingdom, about a year earlier. Menopause is brought on when a woman's ovaries stop producing eggs (ovulating) and monthly bleeding from the uterus ceases. During the climacteric, a time period when gradual hormonal changes occur before and after menopause itself, the ovaries gradually produce less estrogen and progesterone. Women face many health care controversies around the time of menopause. A major one is the issue of hormone replacement therapy, which, at the beginning of the 1990s, is still controversial. While some authorities say that hormone replacement therapy can be a preventive for osteoporosis and heart disease, others caution that there may be cancer-related risks. However, advances in hormone replacement therapy have made them safer to use with fewer side effects. Hormone replacement therapy helps many women who have hot flashes and vaginal dryness. However, differences of opinion regarding hormone replacement therapy by experts leave many women feeling confused and in search of additional opinions. The number of educational programs featuring speakers on the topic of menopause and hormone replacement therapy is testimonial to the interests and confusion pertaining to the subject.

Women develop many mental health concerns around the time of menopause. One is a feeling that they are no longer attractive to men; another is a feeling of loss because they are no longer able to bear children. They may be divorced, widowed, facing a husband's (or their own) retirement, dealing with grown children who have returned home or anticipating financial difficulties due to an inflationary economy. All of these factors contribute to a woman's mental outlook; when irritability and depression occur, they should not be confused with effects of hormonal changes.

Physiological problems interfere with women's feeling of mental well-being, too. Hot flashes plague many women, and they feel embarrassment when they occur. Vaginal dryness that occurs along with diminishing estrogen levels contributes to painful sexual intercourse and hence reduced interest in sexual activity. What a husband or lover may interpret as lack of interest may actually be physical discomfort and fear of painful intercourse.

See also CLIMACTERIC.

Kahn, Ada P., and Linda Hughey Holt. *Midlife Health: A Woman's Practical Guide to Feeling Good.* New York: Avon Books, 1989.

Kahn, Ada P., and Linda Hughey Holt. *Menopause: The Best Years of Your Life.* London: Bloomsbury Publishing, 1987.

menstruation (menstrual period) Uterine bleeding that commonly occurs approximately once a month between puberty and menopause. Historically, for many women the onset of menstruation (menarche) has been filled with anticipation, wonder, awe and sometimes fear. Menstruation marks the beginning of physical adulthood for women, as bearing children becomes possible after menarche. Many young women become pregnant shortly after the onset of menstruation, with, in many cases, unwanted children.

Menstruation consists of periods of bleeding (menstrual periods) that occur in most (but not all) women every 28 days. Although the blood flow usually lasts about four to five days, it can last fewer or more and still be considered within the range of normal.

Menstruation is the removal of products from the uterus that are prepared each month as a uterine lining to provide for a potential pregnancy. At the same time, the ovary ripens an egg (ovum) each month and releases it (ovulation) so that it can be fertilized and implanted in the uterus. If fertilization does not occur, the uterus empties and these cyclical preparations begin again. Blood loss during each period averages about 25 cc (about one ounce) but can vary from a third of an ounce to almost two ounces.

Menstruation usually begins two weeks after ovulation if the egg is not fertilized. Duration between two menstrual periods can vary from three to five weeks. When a woman experiences irregular ovulation, irregular menstruation may be the only symptom she notices.

Menstruation is caused by cyclic fluctuation of the hormones estrogen and progesterone. During a "typical" menstrual cycle, ovarian estrogen is produced in response to stimulation from the pituitary hormones FSH (follicle stimulating hormone) and LH (luteinizing hormone). Estrogen builds up the uterine lining. At midcycle, ovulation occurs in response to an "LH surge," and the ovary forms a small cyst called a corpus luteum in the area of cells (called a follicle) that had surrounded the egg or ovum. These cells produce progesterone, which causes structural changes in the uterine lining.

If the ovum is fertilized and implants in the uterine lining, menstruation does not occur; hence, a missed menstrual period is a common signal of pregnancy. If the ovum is not fertilized, the uterine lining is sloughed off approximately two weeks after ovulation, resulting in a few days of vaginal bleeding. An artificial menstrual flow can be induced by giving a woman estrogen and progesterone; this is commonly done in the form of birth control pills or hormone replacement therapy.

Premenstrual Syndrome (PMS). Many women are more irritable or depressed just before and during a menstrual period. Some notice annoying bloating, fluid retention, breast tenderness and headaches. Most women cope successfully with these symptoms by getting a little extra rest, limiting or decreasing salt intake and recognizing the temporary nature of these annoyances. Women who have excessive premenstrual symptoms should bring them to the attention of a physician. Therapy used may involve vitamin supplements, progesterone injections, the drug bromocriptine, antidepressants or tranquilizers and oral contraceptives.

Some women who have migraine headaches find that their onset is associated with their menstrual periods. Newer prophylactic (preventive) therapies for migraine headaches can help many women with this problem.

Mental Health Concerns
About Menstruation

Fear of menstruation is known as menophobia. Some uninformed young women may become anxious about menstruation because they have not learned about their bodies. Because blood flow is usually a signal of physical injury, and a common fear among young children, adolescent girls may become alarmed at the first sight of monthly bleeding with the onset of menstruation. Some women who fear menstruation reflect anxiety felt by their mothers and generations of women before them; they feel shame if men around them are aware that they are menstruating.

In some cultures, menstruating women are excluded from society during their periods. Over centuries, concerns regarding menstruation have included the notions that sexual intercourse during menstruation is harmful to both men and women's health and that deformed children may result from intercourse during this time. Anxieties surrounding menstruation can be overcome with education, information and reassurance that monthly periods are a normal part of the female life cycle.

Protecting one's clothing and hiding the fact that a woman is having her menstrual period have been concerns among women for generations. At one time "sanitary supplies" were sold only in drug stores and wrapped in plain wrapping paper. Women were embarrassed to ask their husbands, fathers or brothers to buy these supplies for them. The most common ways of disposing of menstrual

fluid is the use of externally worn sanitary napkins (in Britain, known as sanitary towels) or internally worn tampons. Commercially prepared sanitary napkins developed during the early 20th century after generations used cloth bandages, towels, and absorbent rags, washed and reused. Today sanitary napkins are available in many sizes and styles, to accommodate all body sizes and types of menstrual flow.

Internally worn tampons can be used by young women from the start of menstruation. Many mothers of young daughters are concerned that use of a tampon interferes with "virginity." Physicians say that virginity is intact until one's first act of sexual intercourse. The hymeneal ring, a tissue between the internal and external genital organs, is usually large enough to admit a tampon, which has been slightly lubricated for easier insertion. Many young women find tampons a neater way to deal with menstruation and a way to avoid external irritation of the genital area with a napkin or pad. Many women of all ages use tampons or napkins for different rates of menstrual flow at different times. In fact, some women, during periods of heavy flow, use a tampon and a napkin at the same time.

During the 1980s, concern about a condition called toxic shock syndrome—a serious infectious disease—caused many women to stop using tampons. However, with proper attention to hygiene and frequent replacement of tampons, women need not fear toxic shock syndrome. In addition, some of the materials used in tampons have been changed by the manufacturers, making them safer for use.

Sexual Intercourse During Menstruation

For aesthetic reasons, many couples abstain from sexual intercourse during a woman's menstrual period. Some men and women find sexual activity distasteful during this time, while some women enjoy the closeness and support of their mate. There is no medical reason to avoid intercourse; the woman will not be injured by the thrusting of the penis, and the man will not "catch" anything from the woman. If a couple desires to have sexual intercourse during menstrual bleeding, preparations, such as putting a heavy towel under her buttocks, will prevent soiling the bedclothes with blood. Some women report that sexual activity during menstruation—particularly leading to orgasm—actually relieves cramps and menstrual discomforts.

Menstruation and Psychotropic Drugs

In many women the menstrual cycle influences the pharmacokinetics of psychotropic medications. According to Margaret F. Jensvold, director of the Institute for Research on Women's Health, Washington, D.C., physicians should select medication doses with regard for the menstrual cycle. In an article in *Psychiatric News* (Oct. 4, 1991), Jensvold advised that premenstrual or menstrual symptoms should not be confused with drug effects, and she suggested that the issue of constant or periodic dosage is understudied. Jensvold referred to some case reports of women with bipolar disorder whose symptoms recurred relative to their menstrual cycles. One woman on a constant lithium dosage had premenstrual recurrence of bipolar symptoms and a premenstrual serum level drop premenstrually. With an increased dose for a week premenstrually, her serum levels remained constant and prevented the premenstrual recurrence of bipolar symptoms, giving her good control of the symptoms.

Another case was reported of a woman with bipolar disorder who became hypomanic early in each menstrual cycle and depressed in the latter part of the cycle, with relief at onset of menses. Her serum lithium levels were lowest while she was hypomanic, highest when she was depressed and intermediate when she was feeling well and calm (euthymic).

There may be a subgroup of women who have bipolar disorder whose mood and lithium levels vary with the menstrual cycle. However, it raises the question of whether lithium levels varied with the menstrual cycle or with the pathological state. To address that question, a study in 1990 looked at six women taking birth control pills and six women not taking birth control pills; all were asymptomatic. Lithium levels after a single dose were the same through all phases of the menstrual cycle on or off birth control pills.

Bipolar disorder is equally common in women and men, but rapid cycling bipolar disorder (more than three mood switches per year) is much more common in women. In a study of 52 people with rapid cycling bipolar disorder, 92 percent were women. There was not one woman whose rapid cycling was related to her menstrual cycle. In another case, in 1983, moods of women with bipolar illness cycled with their menstrual cycles but sometimes became out of synchronization with their cycles.

These reports suggest that for a subgroup of women with bipolar disorder, their illness may cycle relative to the menstrual cycle and they may show changes in lithium levels relative to their menstrual cycle. Once such a pattern is identified, a clinician can adjust treatment across the menstrual cycle to give a woman better control. However, this does not apply to all women with bipolar disorder. Changes in bipolar disorder do not always occur in relation to the normal menstrual cycle. It is still unclear why the mood cycle goes out of synchronization with the menstrual cycle at times. Clinicians should consider each woman an individual case and determine how individual differences in the menstrual cycle affect medications.

See also HEADACHES.

Beauvoir, Simone de. *The Second Sex.* New York: Modern Library, 1968.

Delaney, Janice et al. *The Curse, a Cultural History of Menstruation.* New York: E. P. Dutton, 1976.

Douglas, Mary. "Menstruation," In *Man, Myth and Magic,* vol. 7, edited by Yvonne C. Deutch. New York: Marshall Cavendish, 1983.

Holt, Linda Hughey, and Melva Weber. *Guide to Woman Care.* New York: The American Medical Association and Random House, 1984.

Kahn, Ada P., and Linda Hughey Holt. *Midlife Health: A Woman's Practical Guide to Feeling Good.* New York: Avon Books, 1989.

Sarafino, Edward P. *The Fears of Childhood.* New York: Human Sciences Press, 1986.

Weideger, Paula, ed. *Menstruation and Menopause: The Physiology and Psychology, the Myth and the Reality.* New York: Knopf, 1976.

mental health   Mental health refers to an individual's ability to negotiate the daily challenges and social interactions of life without experiencing undue emotional or behavioral incapacity; mental health is more than just the absence of mental disorders. It can be affected by many factors, ranging from exogenous stresses that are difficult to manage to biologic defects or organic diseases that impair brain function.

Many approaches have been proposed to reduce the impact of mental health problems. Stress, whether stemming from life events, chronic strain or environmental pressures, is associated with biologic changes linked to cognitive, emotional and behavioral dysfunctions. Healthful habits, such as good nutrition and adequate amounts of exercise and relaxation techniques, may be useful in helping to relieve stress. Because people with low levels of control over their environment (actual or perceived) appear to be at greater risk, interventions have also been directed at increasing individuals' resources and coping skills through education and social support. For those needing more aggressive attention, medical interventions are available that include use of psychotherapies, antidepressant drugs and a variety of other techniques such as biofeedback and meditation.

Developmental delays in childhood and specific skill disorders have also been linked to learning and adjustment problems in adolescence and early adulthood. Early interventions with parents and children that address prenatal care, parental skills and remedial help in early school programs may help prevent developmental problems and their progression to mental health problems.

mental illness   An illness that affects or is manifested in a person's brain. It may affect how the person thinks, behaves and interacts with other people. The term encompasses many psychiatric disorders that vary in severity.

Since the 1980s, research has led to advancements in diagnosis and treatment of many mental illnesses. Where once mentally ill people were hospitalized because they were disruptive or feared to be harmful to themselves or others, today most people who suffer from a mental illness, including those disorders that can be extremely debilitating, such as schizophrenia, can be treated effectively and lead full lives.

Mental illnesses are described and categorized in the book *Diagnostic and Statistical Manual of Mental Disorders, Fourth Edition,* published by the American Psychiatric Association. Among the most commonly known psychiatric disorders are depression, manic depression, bipolar disorder, anxiety disorders, generalized anxiety disorder, specific phobias, social phobia, panic disorder, agoraphobia, obsessive-compulsive disorder, schizophrenia and other psychotic disorders (such as delusional disorder), substance abuse and disorders related to substance abuse, delirium, dementia (including Alzheimer's disease), eating disorders, sleep disorders, attention-deficit/hyperactivity disorder, learning disorders, sexual disorders, dissociative disorders and personality disorders (such as borderline personality disorder and antisocial personality disorder).

Mental illness is not a weakness or defect in character. Mental illnesses are real illnesses that require and respond well to treatment.

See also AGORAPHOBIA; ALZHEIMER'S DISEASE; ANXIETY DISORDERS; BIPOLAR DISORDER; DEPRESSION; DIAGNOSTIC AND STATISTICAL MANUAL OF MENTAL DISORDERS; PHARMACOLOGICAL APPROACH; SCHIZOPHRENIA.

mental retardation   A particular state of functioning, characterized by limitation in both intelligence and adaptive skills, that begins in childhood. As defined by the American Association on Mental Retardation, mental retardation is characterized by significantly subaverage intellectual functioning, which exists concurrently with related limitations in two or more of the following applicable adaptive skill areas: communication, home living, community use, health and safety, leisure, self-care, social skills, self-direction, functional academics and work. Mental retardation manifests before age 18.

The American Association on Mental Retardation is an international multidisciplinary association of professionals. The Association has had responsibility for defining mental retardation since 1921. The AAMR promotes progressive policies, sound research, effective practices, and universal human rights for people who have intellectual disabilities.

The Arc of the United States represents more than seven million children and adults with mental retardation and related developmental disabilities and their families. With chapters across the United States, the Arc is active in legislative lobbying as well as providing resources for the public.

For information:

American Association on Mental Retardation
444 North Capitol Street NW, Suite 846
Washington, D.C. 20001-1512
Phone: (202) 387-1968
Fax: (202) 387-2193
Web site: http://www.aamr.org

The Arc of the United States
1010 Wayne Avenue, Suite 650
Silver Spring, MD 20910
Phone: (301) 565-3842
Fax: (301) 565-5342
E-mail: Info@thearc.org

Association for Retarded Citizens (ARC)
P.O. Box 6109
Arlington, TX 76005
Phone: (817) 640-0204

National Down Syndrome Congress
1800 Dempster
Park Ridge, IL 60068-1146
Phone: (708) 823-7550

mentor An older, more experienced and higher-ranking individual in an organization or field who promotes the career of a younger, lower-ranking person with assistance and advice. Mentors serve as teachers and role models and have been shown to be a key element in the rise to success. Although they are not necessarily close friends of their proteges, friendships may develop. They serve to make the protege comfortable in the field or corporate structure. A mentor may also use his or her influence directly to promote the protege's career. For this reason, mentors are rarely in a direct line of authority over the protege because of the problems of jealousy and resentment from colleagues. The mentor offers support to the protege in terms of professional decisions or crisis.

Most mentor relationships grow somewhat spontaneously out of work situations and usually start with requests for advice or help. Frequently neither side is precisely aware when the relationship started. A mentor is usually drawn to a younger employee because of his or her talent, ambition and interest in the field or organization. Although the benefits to the protege are obvious, there are also definite benefits to the mentor, most obviously a sense of generosity and satisfaction. A mentor may also be at a point in her career when she has reached the pinnacle but feels the need for further accomplishment. In acquiring a protege, a mentor also gains support for her ideas or programs within the organization. She may also accumulate information from the lower-ranking person about problems or other matters within the organization that could not be acquired through more formal methods.

Mentor relationships may also benefit the organization. For example, proteges are integrated into the organization in a way that enhances formal training and are groomed for higher positions. Relationships with mentors provide for longevity and lower employee turnover and promote communication and understanding among the different levels in an organization.

With all of their benefits, there are also problems inherent in the mentor-protege relationship. For example, a male-female relationship may turn into a romance or at least give the appearance of doing so. Even without this element, the relationship may promote envy or charges of favoritism. A mentor-protege relationship is inherently temporary, since the object for the protege is advancement in the organization; but one of the two may hang on and become dependent on the relationship in a destructive way. The protege may also experience difficulties if the relationship is interrupted because the mentor is transferred or becomes ill or unable to function for some other reason. Either side may also fall in the corporate opinion if one makes a blunder or performs poorly.

Collins, Nancy W. *Professional Women and Their Mentors.* Englewood Cliffs, N.J.: Prentice-Hall, 1983.

meperidine The generic name for an analgesic (pain-relieving) drug (trade name: Demerol). It has effects similar to those of morphine and is widely used in anesthetic premedication, in balanced anesthesia and with caution in obstetric analgesia. The dosage of meperidine should be reduced when antipsychotic agents, sedative-hypnotics or other drugs that depress the central nervous system are given concurrently. There can be adverse reactions in individuals who use meperidine at the same time as monoamine oxidase inhibitors.

meprobamate The generic name for an antianxiety drug (trade names: Equanil, Meprospan and Miltown). While useful in treatment of anxiety, it is less effective than the benzodiazepine drugs.

See also BENZODIAZEPINE MEDICATIONS.

Meprospan Trade name under which the antianxiety drug meprobamate is marketed.

See also ANXIETY; MEPROBAMATE.

mercury poisoning Inhalation of mercury vapor is a common cause of mercury poisoning that may result in shortness of breath and alter brain and kidney damage. Mercury poisoning in the brain may cause uncoordination, tremors, excitability and, in severe cases, impairment of vision and a type of irreversible dementia. Mercury encephalopathy is a type of brain damage that can occur.

The expression "mad as a hatter" arose because many hatmakers often suffered from mental confusion, slurred speech and tremors as a result of inhaling poisonous mercury-laden vapors while making felt hats.

Treatment of mercury poisoning includes use of agents to help the body excrete the mercury rapidly; in some cases dialysis (to purify the blood) is performed.

See also DEMENTIA.

mescaline A hallucinogenic drug obtained from the Mexican peyote (peyotl) cactus. Effects of the drug generally last for four to eight hours and include changes in thought and mood, a sense of being in touch with the unknown and an altered sense of time. Frightening experiences or thoughts may lead an individual to panic and injury. Use of mescaline can be addictive.

See HALLUCINOGENS; PEYOTE; SUBSTANCE ABUSE.

methadone A synthetic pain-killing narcotic that resembles morphine. It is used to relieve withdrawal symptoms in individuals undergoing a supervised morphine or heroin detoxification program, as it causes only mild symptoms when withdrawn.

methamphetamines Stimulants available by prescription for limited medical purposes such as narcolepsy and certain cases of obesity. In some case these drugs are diverted from the legitimate market. The most common forms are white powders, pills or "rock." This class of stimulants is swallowed, injected into veins or inhaled through a tube into the nose. Ice is a rock form of methamphetamines that is ingested via smoking, which magnifies the drug's effects.

These stimulants affect the central nervous system to produce feelings of increased alertness and an enhanced sense of well-being. Best known for their appetite suppressant abilities, stimulants also increase blood pressure and respiratory rates. Some individuals use these drugs to stay awake for long periods of time. Significant adverse effects include dizziness, headaches, blurred vision, loss of coordination, nervousness, irritability and tremors. Acute anxiety and paranoia are not uncommon. The "crash" following amphetamine use can lead to suicidal behavior. Street names include speed, uppers, pep pills, bennies, dexies, meth, crystal, black beauties and crank.

See also SUBSTANCE ABUSE.

Media Resource Guide on Common Drugs of Abuse. Public Relations Society of America, National Capital Chapter, Fairfax, Va., September 1990.

MHPG test See 3-METHOXY-4-HYDROXYPHENYL-GLYCOL.

mid-life crisis A term given to life stresses that occur at or around middle age. Men and women both may experience mid-life crises. In a sociological sense, these occur as individuals realize that they have reached the prime of their lives and begin to question whether or not they have achieved their goals, reset goals and, in some cases, turn their lives in new directions. In physiological terms, mid-life crises occur as people realize that they no longer have the physical strength and stamina that they had when they were younger. For women, menopause marks the end of their child-bearing years. Many men and women begin to fear that they are losing their attractiveness and sex appeal. Many turn to cosmetic surgery to relieve aging lines, give more character to their chins or remove excess body fat. Some people focus more on their body shape and embark on strenuous courses of exercise at health clubs and gyms in an effort to retard effects of aging.

The term "mid-life crisis" is really a misnomer for many psychological stresses that occur in the 45–60 age range. Such stressors include children growing up and leaving home, married children returning home with their own children, facing job loss, facing forced retirement, divorce, widowhood, loss of a sex life because of lack of a partner, seeking a new partner and adjusting to a second marriage and a set of secondhand problems with another's children or parents and caring for aging parents. While some blame psychological distress in women on decreasing hormonal levels, these psychosocial factors should not be discounted.

See also CLIMACTERIC; EMPTY NEST SYNDROME; MENOPAUSE; STRESS.

Kahn, Ada P., and Linda Hughey Holt. *Midlife Health: A Woman's Practical Guide to Feeling Good.* New York: Avon Books, 1989.

migraine headaches   See HEADACHES.

migration   Migration has a profound impact on an individual's mental health. Leaving one's country sets in motion a mourning process similar to that which occurs after losing a person.

Sigmund Freud stated: "Mourning is regularly the reaction to the loss of a loved person, or to the loss of some abstraction which has taken the place of one, such as one's country, liberty, an ideal, and so on." The loss of one's country resembles the death of a person, and depending on the age at the time of loss, it may even more closely parallel a developmental loss, particularly the emotional detachment from parents in late adolescence.

The mourning process may include three stages. The first is dominated by separation anxiety, grief and efforts to recover the object. Retrieval has been given up in the second stage, when the focus is no longer on the lost object. It is accompanied by pain, despair and even depression. The third phase heralds reorganization, which may include maintaining values and pursuing goals that have developed in association with the lost object.

As early as 421 B.C., Euripides, in *Medea,* wrote: "There is no sorrow above the loss of a native land." At first sight, loss of country might appear clearer and less complicated in the event of involuntary emigration; however, it is no less true of the voluntary emigrant. The latter may, through a reversal mechanism, feel abandoned. The feeling of abandonment may be reinforced at times by relatives and friends who feel abandoned themselves and resent the person leaving. Although the newcomer may appear to adjust to a new life in the new country more and more, at the same time he or she may be longing for the old country and idealize it as a result.

He may have fantasies of "bringing it back," in this case taking himself back to it. The disillusionment may be intense when the immigrant decides to return to live in his homeland and finds that the country he left is no longer there. His relationship with the country is fixated at the time of his emigration. Subtle external signs of this fixation may include dated use of the language. Return to the homeland may be the moment of truth when disavowal of the loss no longer works, and depression may follow.

Culture Shock

Another aspect of migration is culture shock, which can be described as the result of a sudden change of an average, expectable environment to a strange and unpredictable one. The impact of the violent encounter with the new environment, combined with the mourning process set in motion by the loss, causes a threat to the newcomer's identity. The sense of the continuity of the self, as well as the sense of self-sameness, is threatened. Concomitantly, the consistency of one's own interpersonal interactions is disrupted. No longer is there the same confirmation of one's identity in interaction with the environment. One's national identity is hardly thought of as an issue while in one's own country, but an American in a hostile country would be likely to be acutely aware of his nationality. National symbols such as the flag and national anthem would take on added significance. But even in a more friendly foreign country, one's sense of national identity is heightened and may be threatened. Many environmental clues that normally confirm one's identity are absent and have been replaced by unfamiliar phenomena, including language, architecture, manner of dress, food, music and smell.

One means of coping is to try to translate the unfamiliar into the familiar. For example, an individual from a forested country may look at tall buildings in a city and say that tall buildings look like the forest. A similar mechanism may have been at work when early settlers chose an area that was physically like the one they left, thus reducing the psychologically "unsettling" effect of beginning a new life in a strange environment.

The country and its physical environment—the nonhuman aspect—constitute a separate object the person relates to, and a separate object that needs to be mourned when it is left behind. Common usage confirms its object status; one speaks of one's fatherland or motherland. In 63 B.C., Cicero already recognized this when he said, "Our country is the common parent of all." The process of mourning one's country may be the focal point in the migration process and may be parallel to—or at times interchangeable with, depending on the developmental level—the late-adolescent developmental process of decreasing dependency and preoccupation with idealization of the parents of childhood. Idealization of the lost object, be it a dead parent or a lost country, is common.

Certain cultural or basic aspects of the native country, such as food, may be glorified. Social gatherings with compatriots, at which traditional foods are eaten, have a quality of the funeral meal after the death of a mother or father, at which siblings gather and reminisce about that parent. In this case, they reminisce about the beloved country. These gatherings thus become part of a lifelong mourning process.

Returning to visit the lost country turns one into a visitor, in many ways similar to visiting the parental home when one is no longer a child. Moreover, just as an adolescent may begin to see

his own family more clearly when he gets to know other families, the immigrants may see his native country in a different light once he becomes familiar with the new country.

It is tempting to use the image of adoption, particularly when birth mother and country of birth so closely parallel each other. Yet in some ways, what happens is more like entering a stepfamily. Unlike an adoptive family that may be eagerly awaiting the arrival of the adopted child, a stepfamily is more likely to have strong ambivalent feelings about the new arrival. The latter is also true of the receiving country, which may be quite ambivalent about new arrivals.

See also NOSTALGIA.

De Vryer, Miepje A. "Leaving, Longing, and Loving: A Developmental Perspective of Migration." *Journal of American College Health* 38 (Sept. 1989).

Silove Errick, Ingrid Sinnerbrink, and Annette Field. "Anxiety, Depression and PTSD in Asylum Seekers: Associations with Pre-Migration Trauma and Post-Migration Stressors. *British Journal of Psychiatry* 170, no. 4 (April 1997): 351–357.

milieu therapy A complex approach to the care of individuals using environment or aspects of the environment in ways to promote mental health and change behaviors of clients involved. It includes a structuring of the physical and social environment of a mental health treatment program so that every interaction and activity is as therapeutic as possible for the patient. Milieu therapy is used in a variety of community and institutional settings.

Milieu therapy revolves around the idea that an individual's mental health difficulties in relating to others often contribute to the development of problems in responding and adapting to the environment. An increasing awareness of basic psychosocial principles can aid the individual in making more positive adaptations.

Milieu therapy stresses the patients' responsibilities not only in their own care but also in the care of their peers. Whether milieu therapy is used in a facility depends on the resources of the facility, type of client population and their length of stay. Milieu programs are generally characterized by commitment, democracy, engagement, communalism and humanitarianism.

See also BEHAVIORAL THERAPY.

Miltown   A trade name under which the antianxiety drug meprobamate is marketed.

See also ANXIETY; MEPROBAMATE.

mind/body connections   Links between the mind, brain and other organ systems. Research studies have demonstrated that both psychological and physical stress have effects on health. Increasingly, physicians are recognizing that behavior therapy and complementary therapies, such as guided imagery, relaxation, biofeedback and hypnosis, are useful adjuncts in the comprehensive care of many patients, many of whom have mental health concerns.

The term "mind/body medicine" relates to many treatments and approaches ranging from meditation and relaxation training to social support groups planned to engage the mind in improving physical as well as emotional well-being.

According to Herbert Benson, M.D., author of *The Relaxation Response*, "too often in the practice of modern medicine, the mind and body are considered to be separate and distinct, which is not in our best interests. Because of specialization, patients are no longer treated as whole persons. Instead, we are separated into groups of organs and specific symptoms are not considered in context."

In *The Mind/Body Effect*, Dr. Benson emphasizes the need for practicing behavioral medicine, which incorporates the principles of medicine, physiology, psychiatry and psychology. Patients should be viewed in their entirety with the realization that what happens in their mind has direct bearing on the state of their physical health. Dr. Benson also makes it clear that psychological factors often induce physical ailments. He indicates that in extreme cases, fear and a sense of hopelessness can even induce death.

Many conditions have been found to respond to such techniques of behavior and complementary therapies when they are used alone or in combination with standard medical and surgical treatments;

these conditions include high blood pressure, coronary artery disease, cancer, chronic pain, temporomandibular joint (TMJ) syndrome, headaches and irritable bowel syndrome.

ADVANTAGES OF MIND/BODY THERAPIES FOR BETTER MENTAL HEALTH

- Can be used along with standard medical practices
- Financial cost of procedures is low
- Physical and emotional risk is minimal; potential benefit is great
- Many can be taught by paraprofessionals
- No high-tech interventions
- May improve quality of life by reducing pain and symptoms for people with chronic diseases
- May help control or reverse certain underlying disease processes
- May help prevent disease from developing

See also BEHAVIOR THERAPY; BIOFEEDBACK; COMPLEMENTARY THERAPIES; GUIDED IMAGERY; HEADACHES; HIGH BLOOD PRESSURE; HYPNOSIS; IRRITABLE BOWEL SYNDROME; KABAT-ZINN, JON; MEDITATION; PAIN; PSYCHONEUROIMMUNUNOLOGY; RELAXATION; SIEGEL, BERNIE; SOCIAL SUPPORT SYSTEM; SUPPORT GROUPS; TEMPOROMANDIBULAR JOINT SYNDROME; WEIL, ANDREW.

Benson, Herbert. *The Relaxation Response*. New York: Avon Books, 1975.
———. *Beyond the Relaxation Response*. New York: Berkeley Press, 1985.
———. *The Mind/Body Effect: How Behavioral Medicine Can Show You the Way to Better Health*. New York: Simon & Schuster, 1979.
Borysenko, Joan. *Minding the Body, Mending the Mind*. New York: Bantam, 1988.
Kerns, Lawrence L. "A Clinician's Guide to Mind-Body Treatments." *Chicago Medicine* 97, no. 22 (Nov. 21, 1994).
Locke, Steven, and Douglas Colligan. *The Healer Within*. New York: New American Library, 1984.
Palley, Regina. "Emotional Processing: The Mind/Body Connection." *International Journal of Psychoanalysis*. 79, no. 2 (April 1998): 349–362.

mindfulness meditation   See also COMPLEMENTARY THERAPIES; KABAT-ZINN, JON; MEDITATION; MIND/BODY CONNECTIONS.

minor tranquilizers   Drugs used to reduce low levels of anxiety. An example is the benzodiazepine class of drugs. See also SUBSTANCE ABUSE.

miscarriage   Spontaneous loss of a pregnancy before the fetus is capable of surviving outside the uterus; it is also known as spontaneous abortion. Many women who experience miscarriage experience symptoms of grief and depression for a period of time after the event. A woman will feel the loss, even though the child was never born and she never saw the child. Family and friends seem less sympathetic toward women who have suffered miscarriages than those whose babies are stillborn or die in early infancy. Many are encouraged to try to achieve another pregnancy very soon. Those who do often overcome their depressed feelings; but with those for whom another pregnancy is difficult to achieve, regrets about the lost pregnancy may linger. Women who experience miscarriage can mentally accept the situation better when they understand the physiology involved in the process. Early miscarriages are usually the result of defects in the fetus. Later miscarriages, which occur in the middle trimester, are more likely to be caused by an incompetent cervix, uterine abnormalities, toxemias or preexisting chronic material disease.

Normal exercise does not usually induce miscarriage. Most women who have been tennis players, hikers or swimmers are advised by their obstetricians to continue exercising throughout their pregnancy (or until the last two months). Women who miscarry after some strenuous activity may feel guilty and believe that they induced the miscarriage. Usually this is not the case.

Habitual abortion is a term used when a woman has miscarried three or more consecutive times. The first sign of the possibility of miscarriage is vaginal bleeding, with or without cramping. Not all vaginal bleeding indicates miscarriage. Some bleeding may be associated with implantation, or it may come from the vagina, vulva or cervix. If bleeding occurs from the uterus without any dilation of the cervix, and usually without pain, the situation is termed threatened abortion. Treatment includes rest and waiting to see what happens. With appropriate medical care, cases of threatened abortion can be salvaged, and many women have healthy babies who were in the "threatened" stage during pregnancy.

In a later miscarriage, when the placenta and embryo are totally evacuated, the term used is complete abortion. When placental tissue remains in the uterus, the term is incomplete abortion, and the tissue must be removed by curettage. Late miscarriage may be the most difficult for a woman (and the infant's father) to accept. If she has had good medical care and has taken good care of herself, she should not feel that anything she did or did not do induced the miscarriage.

See also POSTPARTUM DEPRESSION; PREGNANCY.

mitral valve prolapse (MVF)   A heart defect that has sometimes been linked with anxiety. In this condition, the mitral valve does not close sufficiently and blood is forced back into the atrium as well as through the aortic valve. About 40 percent of normal adults have MVP.* The condition can lead to a feeling of palpitations, anxiety and difficult breathing. Research to study the relationship between anxiety disorders and mitral valve prolapse has unequivocally demonstrated that MVP is not a precursor to, cause of or even related to panic and agoraphobia. While there is some symptom overlap, the overwhelming majority of MVP reactors do not develop panic or anxiety. However, individuals who have an anatomic vulnerability of their mitral valves may develop prolapse as a result of increased demands placed on their cardiovascular systems by anxiety.

See also PANIC ATTACK.

*Marks, Isaac M. *Fears, Phobias and Rituals.* New York: Oxford University Press, 1987.
Mazza, Dominic et al. "Prevalence of Anxiety Disorders in Patients with Mitral Valve Prolapse." *American Journal of Psychiatry* 143, no. 3 (Mar. 1986).

modeling   A behavioral therapy technique in which the individual learns by observation without reinforcement from a therapist. The troubled individual watches someone else perform a particular action, such as riding up and down in an elevator (in the case of an elevator phobic person), and then gradually becomes able to perform the action without fear. In a traditional learning sense, modeling is a form of social learning; children learn appropriate culturally acceptable behaviors in this way from their parents.

See also BEHAVIORAL THERAPY; ANXIETIES AND ANXIETY DISORDERS in BIBLIOGRAPHY.

money Money is such a practical matter and so consistently present in daily life that many people never identify their real feelings about it and what it symbolizes. For some, money arouses feelings of envy, possibly one reason that those who have it may be reluctant to discuss it and those who lack it may pretend that they are well off. Parents may be reluctant to reveal financial matters to their children, which may lead them to fantasize that they are quite well off or in serious financial straits or simply lead to the impression that money is a taboo subject.

Western tradition offers two conflicting messages: self-denial, generosity, spirituality and antimaterialism; and the opposite spectrum, the capitalistic, materialistic, hardworking influence of the Protestant work ethic. The practical solution seems to be that it is good to have money but not to flaunt it or overly discuss it.

In 1913 Sigmund Freud wrote, "Money questions will be treated by cultured people in the same manner as sexual matters, with the same inconsistency, prudishness and hypocrisy." As the end of the 20th century approaches, society has lost a good deal of reluctance to discuss sex openly and honestly, but issues involving money are still handled carefully. For example, a question about the price of a friend's coat or furniture might be asked indirectly or with elaborate apologies or not asked at all, even though owning clothes and furniture is really not as personal and private a matter as sexual activity.

Money may not bring happiness, but it is strongly associated with powerful forces of love, freedom and power. To some extent, fear of success may be a fear of giving up love. Some people associate being on their own financially with giving up a childlike, dependent role in which someone cares for them and loves them to such an extent that they may sabotage or ignore their own abilities in favor of letting someone else be the boss or handle their finances. Shopaholics, people who are addicted to purchasing and spending, often try to overcome depression and buy love for themselves to compensate for not being loved or for actual abuse early in their lives.

Money buys freedom from daily cares and from the fear of economic disaster. However, it may make some people feel constricted and unworthy to the extent that they may embark on spending sprees because they feel undeserving of inherited wealth or even money that they themselves have earned.

Immortality, the ultimate power, is frequently associated with money. In addition to the power that money bestows in normal day-to-day life, a man or woman who is wealthy enough to endow social institutions, build a lavish home and pass money along to heirs really does seem to live beyond physical death.

The very rich are a minority and may experience the same feelings of isolation and alienation that other minorities experience. Middle- and upper-middle-class children sense that both rich and poor children are different and may reject them for that reason. Marriage among the wealthy is often riddled with divorce and extramarital affairs, possibly because the marriages are frequently entered into for financial rather than emotional reasons. If both spouses are affluent, each may go his or her own way and never have to form the cooperative team of middle-class life. By "marrying down" a wealthy person may acquire a more attractive spouse than he might reasonably expect if only relying on his own personal qualities; but day-to-day living may make some of the challenges this type of relationship difficult.

Children of the wealthy may experience a conflicted type of upbringing in which one or both parents may be absent or preoccupied a good deal of the time. The child may be looked down upon if she seems less than likely to live up to the larger-than-life achievements and reputation of her family. Further complicating the life if the "poor little rich girl"—or boy—is that when help with psychological problems is sought, it may be less effective because of a variety of difficulties than for a person of average background. Mental professionals may be somewhat envious or intimidated when dealing with a wealthy family. A "fast track" life is not conducive to consistent treatment. Additionally, the patient or his family has the resources to shop around for a therapist who tells them what they want to hear, since the truth is often as difficult for other family members as for the patient to accept.

See also SHOPAHOLISM.

Damon, Janet. *Shopaholics.* Los Angeles: Price Stern Sloan, 1988.
Krueger, David, ed. *The Last Taboo.* New York: Brunner/Mazel, 1986.

monoamine oxidase inhibitors (MAOIs)   A class of antidepressant drug that reduce excessive emotional fluctuations and may stabilize brain chemistry by inhibiting action of monoamine oxidase, which in turn inactivates norepinephrine. The more mood is elevated, the more norepinephrine becomes available in the sympathetic nervous system. Examples of MAOIs include isocarboxazid, phenelzine sulfate and tranylcypromine sulfate. Persons taking MAOIs should avoid foods containing tyramine.

Tricyclic antidepressants are a newer form of antidepressant medication, but MAOIs are in widespread use, too.

See also ANTIDEPRESSANT MEDICATIONS; NOREPINEPHRINE; SYMPATHETIC NERVOUS SYSTEM.

moods   Emotions that determine how a person feels. Examples of moods include sad, glad, angry, or happy. Moods can be characterized as follows:

Dysphoric: An unhappy or sad mood, such as depressed, anxious or irritable.
Elevated: A more cheerful than usual mood.
Euphoric: A feeling of extreme well-being; this occurs in manic-depressive disorder. This type of mood is beyond what most people rate as simply "feeling good."
Euthymic: Feeling good; absence of depressed or elated mood, and feeling able to cope with life.
Irritable: A feeling of internal tension and being easily annoyed and provoked to anger.

See also AFFECTIVE DISORDERS; DEPRESSION; MANIC-DEPRESSIVE DISORDER.

American Psychiatric Association. *Diagnostic and Statistical Manual of Mental Disorders,* 4th ed. Washington, D.C. 1994.
Justice, Blair. *Who Gets Sick: How Beliefs, Moods and Thoughts Affect Your Health.* Los Angeles: J. P. Tarcher, 1988.
Kals, W. S. *Your Health, Your Moods and the Weather.* Garden City, N.Y.: Doubleday, 1982.

mood disorders   According to the American Psychiatric Association's *Diagnostic and Statistical Manual of Mental Disorders,* mood disorders include disorders that have a disturbance in mood as the predominant feature. Mood episodes include major depressive episode, manic episode, mixed episode and hypomanic episode. Also categorized as mood disorders are major depressive disorder, dysthymic disorder and bipolar disorder.

See also AFFECTIVE DISORDERS; BIPOLAR DISORDER; DEPRESSION; DYSTHYMIC DISORDER; MANIA.

American Psychiatric Association. *Diagnostic and Statistical Manual of Mental Disorders,* 4th ed. Washington, D.C. 1994.
Fawcett, Jan, Bernard Golden, and Nancy Rosenfeld. *New Hope for People with Bipolar Disorder.* Roseville, Calif.: Prima Publishing, 2000.

morals   Accepted and excepted norms of behavior and social values within a culture. Mental health professionals believe that a child's moral sense is at first simply a response to authority and to his feelings that what he is told about right and wrong is quite fixed and almost sacred. At early stages a child is unable to comprehend that others have the feelings that he has and is unable to discipline himself or anticipate the outcome of his actions. Moral development continues through childhood as the child gradually comes to recognize that others feel pain and deprivation as he does until he actually develops an ability to put himself in the situation of others and to supply his own set of rules to govern his behavior. The development of the capacity to feel guilty for wrongdoing parallels this tendency to internalize feelings of morality.

According to a 1989 Gallup poll, the American public is becoming more concerned with morals. As part of a survey of social values, participants were asked to rate the importance of following a strict moral code. The number of participants who felt that it was very important to follow a strict moral code climbed from 47 percent in 1981 to 60 percent in 1989. Of the women surveyed, 66 percent thought that a strict moral code was important, as compared with 54 percent of the men.

The survey did not attempt to define specific areas of morality, which are outgrowths of cultural values and may actually be in conflict in the same culture. Even as basic an issue as preservation of life is open to moral conflict. For example, controversy has arisen over the right of terminally ill patients to die and to request painless methods of euthanasia from physicians. Advocates and opponents of birth control and abortion continue to argue the sanctity of life against the mental and physical welfare of the mother and the environment and social problems presented by added unwanted children to the population.

Kohlberg, Lawrence. "Moral Development." In *International Encyclopedia of the Social Sciences,* vol. 10, edited by David S. Sills, New York: Macmillan, 1968.
Leach, Penelope. "Discipline and Self-Discipline," in *The Child Care Encyclopedia.* New York: Knopf, 1984.
"Social Values, Public Values and Intangible Assets More Than Material Possessions." *Gallup Report* (Mar./Apr. 1989).

mothers Qualities of mothers traditionally include protecting and caring for offspring. Mothers give the infant and child emotional warmth as well as sensory stimulation, both of which are necessary for the child to develop a sense of self-worth and an ability to deal effectively with the environment. Mother love is the natural protective and possessive affection a mother displays toward her child. This feeling may be instinctive, but it is also reinforced by pressures of the social group, which expects mothers to nurture their offspring with tenderness.

If television situation comedies reflect reality, mothers have changed, or possibly the audience has grown more realistic and tolerant—even admiring—of different types of mothers. For example, in the 1950s and early 1960s, television mothers were always present in the home, dispensing maternal wisdom and feminine charm while well dressed and adorned with neat pearl necklaces. Title roles in the mid-1990s are occupied by wisecracking, tougher, thoroughly flawed but likable characters. Some fit unwed motherhood into their lifestyles with help from friends and colleagues. Typically, television mothers in the 2000s are working mothers.

Many women undertake the double role of having a career as well as family out of economic necessity. However, a Gallup poll measured a growing tendency to perceive this as desirable despite the conflicts. Between 1975 and 1987 the percentage of women polled who felt that having marriage, children and a full-time job was not only possible but also a preferable way of life rose from 32 percent to 43 percent. However, women still tend to be saddled with family and social responsibilities. Even men who are willing to stay home with a sick child or leave work punctually because of a family obligation may not be met with an understanding or positive attitude from an employer or colleagues. Working mothers must not only get themselves to work; they quite often have to adapt their schedules to getting their child to a care facility or home. Some mothers of school-age children may have to deal with the uncertainties of having "latch key" children. Careers may have to be adapted to eliminate travel and situations that keep the mother inaccessible by telephone. Hobbies, interests or just having time for oneself are almost nonexistent on such a schedule. Faced with these pressures, more women are expressing an interest in limiting their family to one child. Beginning in the late 1970s many women tried to "have it all"—meaning marriage, family and career—but later felt constantly pressured by all factors. During the 1990s, some working women opted for less aggressive career tracks so that they could spend more time with their families and have better mental health.

Motherhood may serve many purposes other than the simple desire for a child. A child may seem to be the solution for a troubled marriage, or even a less than certain suitor. Women may expect their child to succeed where they have failed and may live vicariously through their offspring. Faced with her older children maturing and the threat of no longer being needed, some women will have another child rather than explore the next phase of life. Women may also work out conflicts and problems in the relationships with their own parents through their children.

Regardless of how good the relationship between mother and child, a mother must at times scold, correct and attempt to control the child's behavior. Many mental health professionals feel that the legendary "wicked stepmother" is actually a veiled symbol for the angry disciplinarian that all mothers must at some time seem to be to their children.

In her landmark work *The Second Sex,* Simone de Beauvoir succinctly summarized the experience of motherhood as "a strange mixture of narcissism, altruism, idle day-dreaming, sincerity, bad faith, devotion and cynicism," adding her observation of the still stranger paradox that while women have generally been considered less talented, emotionally stable and more frivolous and petty than men, the education and training of the next generation has been left almost entirely in their hands.

See also MARRIAGE; OEDIPUS COMPLEX; REMARRIAGE; STEPFAMILIES; SURROGACY.

Beauvoir, Simone de. *The Second Sex.* New York: Modern Library, 1968.

Jetter, Alexis, Annelise Orleck, and Diana Taylor, eds. *The Politics of Motherhood: Activist Voices From Left to Right.* Hanover, N.Y.: University Press of New England, 1997.

Leach, Penelope. *The Child Care Encyclopedia.* New York: Knopf, Alfred A. 1984.

"U.S. Women Endorse Jobs, Marriage and Children." *Gallup Report* (Dec. 1987).

mothers-in-law In some families, mothers-in-law present in-law problems, with conflict often arising between daughter-in-law and husband's mother. In other young couples, the conflict is between husband and wife's mother because of the young bride's continuing dependence on her mother. In some cases, sources of these conflicts may be children's repressed resentments of their own parents being projected toward in-laws; ethnic, social and religious differences; or the mother-in-law's own difficulty in adjusting to the departure of her children and the aging process.

Mother-in-law jokes abound. While some jokes probably reflect some underlying social truths, many people actually have excellent relationships with their in-laws, particularly as the in-laws become grandparents and share in the joy of child-rearing.

See also MOTHERS; PARENTING.

Kahn, Ada P., and Linda Hughey Holt. *The A to Z of Women's Sexuality.* Alameda, Calif.: Hunter House, 1992.

motion sickness A feeling of queasiness, nausea and dizziness that occurs when one is on a moving vehicle, such as a car, boat or airplane. About a third of the population develops motion sickness during a car trip on a bumpy road. Another third requires more unstable conditions, such as a ride aboard a pitching boat, to become upset. The other third sometimes thinks that motion sickness is all in the sufferer's mind; these individuals are not very sympathetic to sufferers.

Motion sickness is a very real event for sufferers and seems to happen when the central nervous system cannot reconcile conflicting signals coming from the inner ear, the eyes and the rest of the body. There may be heat rushes and cold sweats, headaches, drowsiness and vomiting, followed by lethargy and dehydration. Symptoms usually disappear shortly after one leaves the moving vehicle. Many individuals have experienced motion sickness while on a boat, but shortly after they get on land, they are able to enjoy eating a normal meal.

For those who suffer from motion sickness, here are some helpful hints:

Keep your eyes on the horizon.

Take deep breaths of fresh air.

Avoid drinking alcohol before a trip.

Do not overeat before a trip.

If you are in a car, stop occasionally, get out and stretch.

A number of over-the-counter medications are available to help prevent motion sickness. They work by depressing signals from the inner ear and by quieting the gastrointestinal tract and decreasing nausea. Most of these preparations should be taken an hour or so before departure.

For some, the power of suggestion is helpful. Keeping busy is also helpful. Often the same individual who feels ill as the passenger does not develop motion sickness if he is the driver. If a person has suffered from motion sickness before, she will become apprehensive about going on the same vehicle again. Just the fear of developing motion sickness and the concentration on waiting for symptoms to occur may be enough to trigger an attack.

See also CENTRAL NERVOUS SYSTEM.

mourning   See GRIEF.

MRI   See BRAIN IMAGING; MAGNETIC RESONANCE IMAGING.

multi-infarct dementia   The second most common cause of dementia, after Alzheimer's disease. It differs from Alzheimer's disease in its history and concomitant symptoms. Symptoms of vascular disease, both within and outside the brain, are characteristic of multi-infarct dementia. Characteristics are variable among individuals and may include aphasia, amnesia, agnosia, apraxia or slowness, depression, emotional liability, forgetfulness and reduced cognitive function. There may be a past or recent history of transient ischemic episodes (small strokes), high blood pressure and cerebrovascular disease.

In some cases, infarctions may be visible on computerized tomograms of the head, but they may be too small to be radiologically visualized. In cases of vascular dementia, electroencephalography may be useful in revealing multifocal slowing.

No therapy has proved efficacious for this disorder. However, treatment is usually directed at improving the underlying condition; speech and language therapy may help improve dysarthria and aphasia.

Because of the vascular nature of this disorder, there are several theoretical implications. If predisposing conditions can be diminished, the progression of dementia may be slowed, if not stopped. In the future, studies may give some clues about possibilities of pharmacologic agents to enhance cerebrovascular circulation or decrease the propensity for thrombotic or embolic episodes that may alter the course of this type of dementia.

See also ALZHEIMER'S DISEASE; DEMENTIA.

Cummings, Jeffrey L. *Clinical Neuropsychiatry.* Orlando: Grune & Stratton, 1985.

David, Kenneth; Howard Klar; and Joseph T. Coyle. *Foundations of Psychiatry.* Philadelphia: W. B. Saunders, 1991.

multiple personality disorder (MPD)   A severe chronic dissociative disorder characterized by a disruption of memory and identity. Dissociation is the process during which a set of ideas and feelings loses most of its relationship with the rest of the personality, functioning somewhat independently.

See also DISSOCIATIVE DISORDERS.

multiple sclerosis (MS)   A progressive disease of the central nervous system in which scattered patches of the protective covering of nerve fibers in the brain and spinal cord are destroyed, causing symptoms ranging from numbness and tingling to paralysis and incontinence. Severity of the disease varies among individuals. Although causes are unknown, it is thought to be an autoimmune disease, in which the body's defense system treats some of its own parts as foreign matter and destroys them. Another theory is that it is a virus picked up by a susceptible person during early childhood and develops later on.

There may be a genetic factor in the disease, a relatives of affected people are eight times more likely than others to contract the disease. It is five times more common in temperate zones than in the tropics. The ratio of women to men with the disease is three to two.

Researchers are still seeking a cure for MS, and sufferers are encouraged to lead as active a life as their disabilities allow and to keep a positive mental attitude. Physical therapy helps many maintain their mobility. For some individuals, corticosteroid drugs are prescribed to relieve symptoms of an acute attack.

MS is a disease that affects families and family relationships, as other individuals may be called on to become a caregiver at any time. A good communication system within the family network is essential as the disease progresses, so that understanding and empathy can be expressed openly.

See also CAREGIVERS; CENTRAL NERVOUS SYSTEM; CHRONIC ILLNESS; PAIN.

Munchausen's syndrome A form of chronic disorder in which the individual complains of physical symptoms that are pretended or self-induced; the disorder is also known as factitious disorder. Such individuals want attention and want to be taken care of. Many are repeatedly hospitalized for investigation of a variety of ailments.

The name for the syndrome comes from the 19th-century Baron von Munchausen, who was known for tall tales and fanciful exaggeration.

Individuals with this syndrome may complain of dizziness, pain in the abdomen, skin rashes and fever. They usually invent a dramatic history to gain attention and entry into a hospital; many have detailed medical knowledge on which to base their stories. Physicians must be aware of this syndrome to help such individuals avoid having surgery and other unnecessary procedures performed that ultimately might be harmful.

The incidence of this syndrome is unknown, probably because many cases go undetected. In one study involving fever of unknown origin, up to 10 percent of the fevers were diagnosed as factitious. Factitious symptoms can occur in almost any organ system, and the various symptoms produced are limited only by the imagination of the patient.

muscle relaxants Pharmacological agents that act on the central nervous system or its associated structures to reduce muscle tone and spontaneous activity. Many people experience tense, tight or strained muscles as a result of stress or injury, and some resort to these prescription medications instead of or in addition to using mind/body techniques for relaxation. Many skeletal muscle relaxants also function as minor tranquilizers.

See also MIND/BODY CONNECTIONS; RELAXATION.

music therapy Music therapists admit they do not know precisely why music produces such powerful effects, but they contend the benefits are unmistakable. According to Donna Devall, a social worker in Washington, D.C., "music is a way to connect" and of "getting through" to people who are otherwise unreachable. Songs embody life experiences and bring back memories of courtship, a wedding or even wartime. In many nursing homes, individuals who have been very untalkative and unresponsive may start to tap their foot, hum or sing to music, particularly live music that they are watching being performed.

According to Oliver Sacks, an American neurologist, author of *The Man Who Mistook His Wife for a Hat* and pioneer in developing therapies, music organizes motor functions, thus smoothing out, for example, the uncontrolled movements that afflict patients with Parkinson's disease or enabling people with speech losses to sing the words to familiar melodies.

Using music as a healer is not new. According to Greek mythology, Apollo was god of both music and medicine. His son, Aesculapius, who became god of medicine, cured mental diseases with song and music. Plato, the Greek philosopher, believed that music influenced a person's emotions and character. According to the Bible, David's harp playing relieved King Saul's melancholy (depression). During the Middle Ages, music was used to exhaust crowds of people suffering from mass hysteria; the music probably encouraged them to continue dancing until they were exhausted. In his plays, Shakespeare referred to the healing powers of music. The first English-language book on music as therapy, *Medicina Musica,* was written in the early 1700s by Richard Browne, an apothecary. Browne said music could "soothe turbulent affections" and calm "maniacal patients who did not respond to other remedies."

Music therapy was used in the early part of the 19th century in the form of brass bands for patients with the then-identified mental disorders, including anxiety. In the 20th century, particularly during World War II, many American psychiatric hospitals began active music therapy programs. In 1950 the National Association for Music Therapy (NAMT) was organized; in 1954, the NAMT recommended a curriculum for preparation of music therapists. Subsequent organizations of music therapists were formed in Europe, South America and Australia.

Music is no substitute for conventional treatment. Its benefits may end almost as soon as the music ends. However, when used in conjunction with other therapies, it may be useful and get results other therapies cannot.

Music Therapy and Alzheimer's Disease

Researchers at the University of Miami School of Medicine and Michigan State University reported on a study to assess the effects of a music therapy intervention on concentrations of melatonin, norepinephrine, epinephrine, serotonin and prolactin in the blood of a group of patients with Alzheimer's disease. Blood samples were obtained before initiating therapy, immediately at the end of four weeks of music therapy sessions and at a follow-up six weeks after cessation of the sessions. Changes in melatonin, norepinephrine, epinephrine, serotonin and prolactin following music therapy were notable. Melatonin concentration in serum increased significantly after music therapy and was found to increase further at the six week follow-up. A significant increase was found between baseline values and date recorded after the music therapy sessions, as well as at the six week follow-up. Norepinephrine and epinephrine levels increased significantly after four weeks of music therapy, but they returned to pre-therapy levels at the six week follow-up. Serum concentration of prolactin and platelet serotonin levels remained unchanged after four weeks of music therapy and at the six week follow-up. The researchers' conclusion was that the increased levels of melatonin following music therapy may have contributed to the patients' relaxed and calm mood.

HOW MUSIC CAN IMPROVE MENTAL HEALTH

- Heart rate acceleration is correlated with loudness, tempo and musical complexity; heart rate deceleration is correlated with resolution of musical conflict, decreasing loudness and slowing tempo.
- Stimulative music increases heart rate; sedative music decreases heart rate.
- Rock music leads to heart deceleration.
- Tachycardia (fast heartbeat) is associated with driving rhythms and increasing dynamics; bradycardia (slow heartbeat) is associated with changes in rhythm, texture and dynamics.

- Sedative music significantly increases finger temperature.
- Blood pressure is affected by music listening, but the type of music that affects these changes is unknown. Music is effective in reducing blood pressure in essential hypertensives.
- Music that is enjoyed increases respiration.
- Music decreases stomach acid production.
- Popular music produces more electroencephalograph (EEG) changes than classical music, particularly in middle-aged subjects. Popular music causes a decrease in blood flow to the brain in young adults; classical music promotes brain blood flow enhancement in middle-aged subjects.

See also COMPLEMENTARY THERAPIES; EMOTIONS; PAIN; STRESS.

Aldridge, David. "The Music of the Body: Music Therapy in Medical Settings." *ADVANCES, The Journal of Mind-Body Health.* 9, no. 1 (Winter 1993).

Blascovich, Allen K., and J. Blascovich. "Effects of Music on Cardiovascular Reactivity among Surgeons." *Journal of the American Medical Association* (1994): 882–4.

Crowley, Susan L. "The Amazing Power of Music." *Bulletin,* American Association of Retired Persons, (Feb. 1992).

Kuman, Adarsh M., Frederick Tims, Dean G. Cruess et al. "Music Therapy Increases Serum Melatonin Levels in Patients with Alzheimer's Disease." *Alternative Therapies* 5, no. 6 (Nov. 1999): 49–57.

mutism Inability or refusal to speak, which may occur as a symptom of severe manic-depressive illness, catatonic schizophrenia and a rare form of conversion disorder.

As a childhood disorder, elective mutism may start before the child is five years old. Although the child understands language and is able to speak properly, he only nods his head and gestures. Mild retardation or the anxiety of leaving home for school may contribute to the condition.

Treatment for mutism varies, depending on the underlying cause.

See also DEPRESSION; SCHOOL PHOBIA; SEPARATION ANXIETY.

nail biting One of a group of habits including thumb sucking and hair pulling that may continue because of their routine, unconscious nature without a real continuing underlying cause. Nail biting is a difficult habit to break. Many nail biters are embarrassed by their habit.

Mental health professionals say that nail biting is a soothing or stimulating habit that helps children deal with anxiety or boredom but exact causes are not known. Nail biting does not really correlate with specific personality qualities despite the stereotype of the nervous nail biter. There seems to be a slight hereditary tendency to nail biting, but this is difficult to establish because family members are prone to mimic one another's habits. A nail-biting parent is likely to have trouble correcting a nail-biting child. Nail biting is a somewhat universal habit that seems to have no relationship to sex, race or intelligence, although more women than men seek help to break the habit. It is estimated that over 50 percent of the population has had the nail-biting habit at some point in life. About 20 to 25 percent of adults are nail-biters. Nail biting usually starts in childhood after the age of three and frequently ends in adolescence when peer pressure and personal grooming become important.

See also ANXIETY; PEER GROUP; PEER PRESSURE.

narcissism An exaggerated feeling of self-love. A narcissistic person may overestimate her capacities, so that she feels omnipotent and demands extreme amounts of attention and admiration from others. While initially they may seem charming, people who have excessive narcissistic traits lack empathy for others. Any criticism may lead to rageful feelings in such individuals. While appearing to have exaggerated positive self-esteem and confidence, the highly narcissistic individual in fact suffers from low self-esteem and emptiness, which lead them to have difficulty being alone and to require constant applause and adulation by others. The term comes from Narcissus, a character in Greek mythology who fell in love with his own image reflected in the water. Excessive narcissism is termed narcissistic personality disorder.

See also EGO; PERSONALITY.

narcolepsy Dropping off to sleep at inappropriate times, such as while walking, driving a car, eating or carrying on a conversation. Narcolepsy occurs three or four times more often among men than women. The causes are unknown, but it is suspected that narcolepsy is related to some malfunction of the sleep-controlling centers of the hypothalamus, a part of the brain. Narcolepsy may follow sudden emotional experiences, such as laughter or crying. The narcoleptic person may have a few or dozens of sleep episodes every day, becoming unconscious for two or three minutes or for hours. There are no ill effects unless the sleep attacks cause an accident.

Methylphenidate (Ritalin) is considered one standard medication for this condition. It increases alertness and reduces sleep attacks.

See also SLEEP.

narcotic drugs Drugs prescribed by physicians to produce sleep and relieve pain. Alcohol, cocaine and opium, plus its derivatives, heroin, morphine and codeine (the opiates), are all narcotics. When used to excess, they produce euphoria, addiction and both physical and psychological dependence. Unconsciousness caused by narcotics is known as narcosis.

See also SUBSTANCE ABUSE.

Nardil   Trade name for the monoamine oxidase inhibitor antidepressant medication phenelzine.

See also ANTIDEPRESSANT MEDICATIONS; MONOAMINE OXIDASE INHIBITORS; PHARMACOLOGICAL APPROACH.

National Alliance for Research on Schizophrenia and Depression (NARSAD)

A privately funded organization that raises and distributes funds for scientific research regarding prevention, causes, treatments and cures of severe mental illnesses, primarily schizophrenias and depressions.

Formed in 1986, the NARSAD complements federal funding efforts of the National Institute of Mental Health (NIMH). For example, NARSAD has established an award process to identify promising research and enable investigators to obtain necessary funding to initiate research rather quickly. The group's Scientific Council, composed of distinguished psychiatric researchers, solicits and evaluates research proposals and responds to grant requests.

For information, contact:

National Alliance for Research on
   Schizophrenia and Depression
60 Cutter Mill Road, Suite 404
Great Neck, NY 11021
Phone: (516) 829-0091
Fax: (516) 487-6930
Web site: www.narsad.org

National Alliance for the Mentally Ill

A national organization composed of family members of patients with serious mental illnesses. Chapters of AMI provide local forums for sharing information with members who give one another encouragement and support and raise hopes through diminishing feelings of isolation.

For information, contact:

National Alliance for the Mentally Ill
2101 Wilson Boulevard, Suite 302
Arlington, VA 22201
Phone: (703) 524-7600 or (800) 950-6264
Fax: (703) 524-9094
Web site: www.nami.org

National Depressive and Manic-Depressive Association (NDMDA)

A national association that recognizes the biochemical nature of bipolar and unipolar affective disorders and the disruptive psychological impact of the illnesses on patients and families. Its purpose is to provide personal support and direct service to persons with major depression or manic-depression and their families; to educate the public concerning the nature and management of these disorders; and to help patients suffering with depression and manic-depression gain access to effective care.

Membership in the group provides not only information and support but also a source of realized self-esteem and dignity for those suffering from depressive disorders and their families.

In addition to the service aspect of local chapters, the national organization fights the stigma associated with mental illness, promotes funding for research to improve diagnosis and treatment and lobbies for adequate insurance coverage for the treatment of these disorders. The association also gives an annual research award to a research investigator contributing to improved treatments, as well as the Dr. Jan Fawcett Humanitarian Award to individuals who have contributed to the goals of the organization.

There are chapters throughout the United States and Canada.

For information contact:

NDMDA
730 North Franklin Street, Suite 501
Chicago, IL 60610
Phone: (800) 826-3632 or (312) 642-0049
website: www.ndmda.org

See also AFFECTIVE DISORDERS; BIPOLAR DISORDER; DEPRESSION; MANIC-DEPRESSIVE DISORDER.

National Foundation for Depressive Illness

A group of lay and professional people organized to advance private and public education about depression and its treatment. There is an 800 number that gives a recorded message concerning symptoms of depression and offering to send a list of local referrals and literature.

For information, contact:

National Foundation for Depressive Illness, Inc.
P.O. Box 2257
New York, NY 10116
Phone: (800) 248-4344
Web site: www.depression.org

See also DEPRESSION; MANIC-DEPRESSIVE DISORDER.

National Institute of Mental Health (NIMH)   A U.S. government agency that supports and conducts research concerning prevention, diagnosis and treatment of mental illnesses. Studies bring hope to individuals with mental health problems, to those at risk of developing problems and to concerned families and friends. NIMH is part of the Alcohol, Drug Abuse and Mental Health Administration, a component of the U.S. Department of Health and Human Services.

For information, contact:

National Institute of Mental Health
6001 Executive Boulevard
Bethesda, MD 20892
Phone: (800) 421-4211
Web site: www.nimh.nih.org

National Institute on Drug Abuse   A part of the U.S. Alcohol, Drug Abuse and Mental Health Administration (ADAMHA). Its function is to provide leadership, policies and goals for governmental work in preventing, controlling and treating narcotic addiction and drug abuse and in rehabilitating affected individuals.

For further information, contact:

National Institute on Drug Abuse
6001 Executive Boulevard
Bethesda, MD 20892
Phone: (800) 644-6432
Web site: www.nida.nih.gov

National Mental Health Association   A voluntary nongovernmental organization for the prevention of mental illness and promotion of mental health, with more than 650 chapters nationwide. Goals of the organization include protecting the rights of people with mental health problems, educating the public about mental health and promoting research concerning all aspects of mental health.

For information, contact:

National Mental Health Association
1021 Prince Street
Alexandria, VA 22314-2971
Phone: (800) 969-6642
Fax: (703) 684-5968
Web site: www.nmha.org

See also DEPRESSION; MANIC-DEPRESSIVE DISORDER.

naturopathy   This form of alternative medicine is based on two principles: The accumulation of waste products and toxins in the body cause disease, and symptoms of disease are the body's way of trying to get rid of these substances. Proponents believe that nature heals itself by strengthening the healing powers within and that individuals can do the same by dealing with the factors that potentially hinder wellness. In addition to the accumulation of waste products and toxins, these hindrances include bodily structural imbalances, emotional stressors and detrimental lifestyles.

The goal of naturopathy therapy is to free the body to heal itself by enhancing its self-healing power. Practitioners agree that the ultimate goal of any type of wellness is for the practitioner to encourage the body's own life force to operate more efficiently within the individual. He or she may encourage the individual to use many techniques for controlling stress and promoting wellness, including nutritional and herbal supplements, breathing and exercise programs and meditation.

For information:

American Association of Naturopathic
   Physicians
P.O. Box 20386
Seattle, WA 98102
Phone: (206) 323-7610

See also COMPLEMENTARY THERAPIES; BREATHING; EXERCISE; HERBAL MEDICINE; MEDITATION; NUTRITION; STRESS.

nausea   A feeling of sickness in the stomach as if one may have to vomit. There may be dizziness, lightheadedness or sweating along with nausea. Some individuals experience nausea when coming into contact with a food associated with an anxiety-producing experience recalled from the past. Other individuals experience nausea before certain events, such as before a public appearance for speaking or performing. Some develop nausea before playing in a sports event or before taking tests. Such nausea can be overcome with behavioral therapy techniques. However, in all cases of repeated nausea, physical causes should first be ruled out. Some medications may produce nausea as a side effect in susceptible individuals.

See also BEHAVIORAL THERAPY.

Marks, Isaac M. *Fears, Phobias, and Rituals.* New York: Oxford University Press, 1987.

near-death experiences Certain sensations and out-of-body experiences are common to many people who have come close to dying but have been revived. After observing similar phenomena in several patients and hearing reports of other near-death situations, Raymond Moody, a physician, coined the phrase "near-death experience" and described his findings in his work *Life after Life,* published in 1975. His work encouraged people to talk more freely about such experiences.

In 1982, a Gallup poll showed that 8 million adult Americans had survived what they considered to be a near-death experience. There are common elements in many of these near-death experiences. Many subjects describe a sensation of floating above their own body watching attempts to resuscitate. Some have convincingly described visiting their families in other parts of the hospital and have recounted details of their clothing and conversations that they could not have known without a genuine out-of-body experience.

A common element is a sense of peace, joy, freedom from pain and reluctance to return to life to the extent that some become angry at their physician for reviving them. Many describe an experience of entering a lighted tunnel and of contact with beings who are surrounded by light, some of whom are family and loved ones who have died. Some recount a nonjudgmental review of their life and an encounter with a supreme being who is a projection of their religious beliefs. Despite a sense of reluctance to return to life, many later see the experience as a glimpse into another world that they accept with gratitude. The experience seems to be as common to the nonreligious as to the religious but frequently results in an increased interest in spiritual, metaphysical matters. Many report a stronger belief in the afterlife and an increase in psychic abilities.

Skeptics of the near-death experience point to the fact that these sensations take place when the body is in the grip of its own chemical response to stress and also frequently influenced by drugs such as painkillers, tranquilizers and anesthetics. To refute near-death experience claims, some researchers have reproduced similar sensations in laboratory situations using drugs. One researcher concerned with psychological similarities among subjects of near-death experiences found a high incidence of childhood abuse and neglect.

Moody, Raymond. *The Light Beyond.* Toronto: Bantam Books, 1988.
"Near Death Experience," In *Harper's Encyclopedia of Mystical and Paranormal Experience* edited by Rosemary Ellen Guiley. San Francisco: Harper, 1991.

nervous A nonmedical term and form of anxiety referring to feelings of restlessness, apprehension, irritability, fearfulness and tension. The word "nervous" derives from Sigmund Freud's theory that neurological weaknesses (neurasthenias) develop as a result of unconscious conflicts. When people say they have "nervous symptoms," they usually mean that they have anxieties. Nervousness is a normal symptom under many circumstances, such as the first day of school, the first day of a new job, approaching the platform to deliver a speech, trying to catch a train at the last minute, having an important meeting with a boss or walking into a room full of strangers. Nervousness is related to social phobia in that social phobics display nervousness about certain situations; the phobic, however, carries the nervousness and anxieties to such an extreme that he begins to avoid the circumstances that make him fearful and nervous.

Individuals who occasionally have bouts of nervousness need not fear that they are having a nervous breakdown. As long as they feel that they are coping well with their situation and keep their emotions under control, their equilibrium will probably return soon.

A "nervous stomach" refers to feelings of abdominal discomfort, nausea and diarrhea that happen to many people when they feel nervous or anxious. Nervous stomach is also a common symptom of irritable bowel syndrome and panic attack.

A "nervous habit" refers to involuntary twitches and facial tics and voluntary habits such as nose picking, thumb sucking and nail biting. These habits are thought to be a means of relieving stress and anxieties. Nervous habits increase during periods of stress.

See also ANXIETY; ANXIETY DISORDERS; IRRITABLE BOWEL SYNDROME; STRESS.

nervous breakdown   A nonmedical term applied to any one of several mental health disorders in an acute phase. The term applies when one loses control of his emotions so that he is no longer able to control his behavior. Popularly, the term is applied to severe anxieties as well as more severe psychoses. The individual suffering the breakdown feels that his emotions are out of control, and perhaps a better term would be "emotional breakdown." The individual may be unable to sleep, will have little interest in eating, may cry frequently and may become fearful or severely depressed. Physical symptoms may be fast heartbeat, dizziness, headaches, fainting and sweating palms. These symptoms will interfere with activities of daily living as well as work.

Many individuals experience some of these symptoms for brief periods of time. It is when they last for a long time that they produce a breakdown.

Avoiding an emotional breakdown can be best accomplished by developing an ability to share one's feelings and emotions with another person. Just talking to another person helps many people get their life situation in a better focus before their emotional system goes on overload and breaks down.

Many breakdowns occur at times of transition and change, such as adolescence, middle age, entering or graduating from school, marriage, divorce and parenthood. At times of transition a person is more insecure and hence more vulnerable to emotional swings.

See also ANXIETY DISORDERS; DEPRESSION; STRESS.

nervous habits   Habits include both involuntary (twitches and facial tics) and voluntary behaviors (nose picking, thumb sucking and nail biting). These habits may be a reaction to stress or a means of relieving anxieties for some people. If the individual has a strong desire to overcome these nervous habits, behavioral therapy techniques will help in some cases.

See also ANXIETIES; HABITS; HAIR PULLING; NAIL BITING; OBSESSIVE-COMPULSIVE DISORDER; STRESS.

Woods, Douglas W., and Raymond G. Miltenberger. "Are Persons with Nervous Habits Nervous? A Preliminary Examination of Habit Function in a Nonreferred Population." *Journal of Applied Behavior Analysis* 29 no. 2 (summer 1996): 259–261.

nervous system   See BRAIN; CENTRAL NERVOUS SYSTEM.

neuroimaging   See BRAIN IMAGING; POSITRON EMISSION TOMOGRAPHY.

neuroleptic   A medication that helps to relieve psychotic symptoms (antipsychotic drugs) such as delusions or hallucinations, schizophrenia and mania.

See also ANTIPSYCHOTIC MEDICATIONS; HALLUCINATION; SCHIZOPHRENIA.

neurological examination   To help physicians diagnose conditions affecting the nervous system, brain and spinal cord, several types of imaging techniques may be used after a complete general physical examination. These techniques include magnetic resonance imaging and computerized axial tomography (CAT). Angiography (X-ray imaging to show blood vessels) may also be used.

See also ALZHEIMER'S DISEASE.

neurology   The branch of science that studies the human nervous system, including the brain and the spinal cord. The medical specialist within this field is a neurologist. In the last few decades, advances have been made in neurology, and now, with improved understanding of the biochemical and structural bases of neurological disorders, new treatments have been developed, including drug treatment for some forms of dementia, surgical removal of tumors and repair of damaged nerves.

See also PARKINSON'S DISEASE.

neuromyasthenia   Disease of the nerves and muscles. The term is sometimes used synonymously with chronic fatigue syndrome.

See also CHRONIC FATIGUE IMMUNE DYSFUNCTION SYNDROME; CHRONIC FATIGUE SYNDROME.

neuron   A nerve cell. The central nervous system has billions of neurons that act in various combinations to initiate all human actions and thoughts. Neurons trigger the release of neurotransmitters, which may then cause an endocrine gland to release a hormone, or a muscle cell to contract. Different stimuli activate types of neurons. For example, sensory neurons may be aroused by a physical stimulus, such as a bright light or intense cold.

Babies are born with their total number of neurons, and the number decreases thereafter. Neurons can be damaged or obliterated by disease, injury or persistent alcohol abuse. Consequently, loss of neurons interferes with mental as well as physical capacities.

See also NEUROTRANSMITTERS.

neuropsychiatry   The branch of medicine dealing with the relationship between symptoms of mental illness and distinct neurological disorders. Such disorders are usually forms of brain disease, such as temporal lobe epilepsy, tumors or infections. Neuropsychiatry emphasizes the interplay of neurological, psychodynamic, genetic and environmental factors. New neurodiagnostic technology has allowed psychiatric diagnoses and treatment to become more specific, while providing a means for testing neurobiologic hypotheses. Neuropsychiatry uses diagnostic techniques drawn from neurology, behavioral neurology and neuropsychology in combination with traditional methods of interviewing and mental status evaluation to study mental health conditions associated with brain abnormalities. Basic sciences related to neuropsychiatry include neuroanatomy, neurochemistry, neurophysiology, neuropathology, neuroimmunol-

ogy and behavioral genetics. Clinical sciences related to neuropsychiatry include general psychiatry, psychopharmacology, behavioral neurology, neuropsychology, neuroendocrinology and neuroimaging.

See also NEUROPSYCHOLOGICAL TESTING.

neuropsychological testing   A method of further evaluating a patient's cognitive functioning. A neuropsychologist (specialist trained in neuropsychology) administers a group of cognitive tests to the patient. Reasons for neuropsychological testing may include gathering additional data in support of a possible diagnosis, localizing cognitive deficits picked on another examination, determining a cognitive baseline against which future testing can be compared to document improvement or deterioration, or to determine the severity of an injury or deficit. Testing is also used to facilitate rehabilitation plans, to assess treatment effect and to determine whether preexisting deficits could be contributing to a current clinical problem.

Common neuropsychological tests used in evaluating adults include intelligence tests, achievements test, attention surveys and tests relating to abstraction, memory, language ability, calculation ability, visual-spatial thought and motor skills.

See also NEUROPSYCHIATRY.

neurosis   An old term for a variety of mental health disorders including agoraphobia, anxiety, panic attacks, panic disorder, phobias, depression, dysthymia, hypochondria and obsessive-compulsive disorder. Historically, some of these conditions have been referred to as neurotic disorders (now an obsolete term).

See AGORAPHOBIA; ANXIETY DISORDERS; DEPRESSION; DYSTHYMIA; HYPOCHONDRIASIS; OBSESSIVE-COMPULSIVE DISORDER; PANIC ATTACKS AND PANIC DISORDER; PHOBIA.

neurosurgery   The medical specialty concerned with the surgical treatment of disorder of the central nervous system, including otherwise untreatable pain. Conditions more commonly treated by neurosurgery include tumors of the brain, spinal cord or meninges (membranes that surround the brain and spinal cord); certain abnormalities of the blood vessels that supply the brain, such as an aneurysm (bulge in a weak point of an artery); and bleeding inside the skull. Neurosurgery is also sometimes used in certain types of epilepsy and nerve damage caused by accidents or illness.

See also BRAIN.

neurosyphilis When syphilis is untreated, it can result in an infection of the brain or spinal cord. Symptoms may include poor coordination of leg movements when walking, urinary incontinence and pains in the limbs and abdomen. Brain damage may result in dementia, muscle weakness and extensive neurological damage, which is sometimes referred to as general paralysis of the insane.

Syphilis is considered a sexually transmitted disease (formerly known as venereal disease) and contracted through sexual intercourse and can also exist at birth (congenital syphilis). The drug of choice for treatment of syphilis is penicillin, although other medications are also used. However, organ damage already caused by the disease cannot be reversed.

See also SEXUALLY TRANSMITTED DISEASES.

neurotransmitters Chemical messengers released by neurons. The neurotransmitters norepinephrine and seratonin have been closely linked with depression. Neurotransmitters help transfer nerve impulses from one cell to another.

See also BRAIN CHEMISTRY.

nicotine dependence Nicotine is the main substance responsible for dependence on tobacco. Nicotine in tobacco smoke passes into the bloodstream after inhaling; in chewing tobacco the nicotine is absorbed through the lining of the mouth. In habitual smokers, nicotine increases the heart rate, narrows blood vessels, raises blood pressure, stimulates the central nervous system, reduces fatigue, increases alertness and improves concentration. Regular smoking results in tolerance, and a higher intake is required to bring about the desired effects.

See also SMOKING; SUBSTANCE ABUSE.

nightmare A dream during the night characterized by frightening elements. Usually people awaken immediately after a nightmare with a clear recollection of the dream and a feeling of intense uneasiness. Many normal children have nightmares after witnessing a frightening movie or after a day filled with great excitement, such as a first day of school or an important community event. Usually children outgrow nightmares and, when they do occur, can distinguish a dream from reality and are less frightened.

Individuals who have witnessed a crime, been a victim of a crime or served in a battle (among many causes) may experience post-traumatic stress disorder and also experience nightmares as part of that disorder. They may relive their experience in the nightmare and wake up just as frightened as they felt when the event or period of time was happening.

Nightmares usually occur during REM (rapid eye movement) sleep and during the later part of the sleep during the night.

Children are more likely to experience nightmares when they have a cold or other infection, if their breathing is impaired or when they are separated from their parents. Adults taking certain medications, such as beta blockers and benzodiazepine drugs, have been known to have nightmares as a side effect.

Nightmares can usually be remembered upon awakening the next morning, whereas night terrors tend to be forgotten.

See also BEHAVIORAL THERAPY; DREAMING; NIGHT TERROR; POST-TRAUMATIC STRESS DISORDER.

Marks, Isaac. *Fears, Phobias and Rituals.* New York: Oxford University Press, 1987, p. 393.

night terror (sleep terror) An intense nightmare from which the sleeper, usually a child, awakens screaming in terror, disoriented, agitated and difficult to comfort. Episodes usually occur about half an hour to three and a half hours after falling asleep. These may occur between age four and seven and usually diminish in early adolescence. Such episodes are frightening to parents and should be discussed with the pediatrician. Usually the dreamer does not recall the event upon awakening the next morning.

When adults experience night terrors, the episodes may be part of an anxiety disorder. In addition, nightmares of people who have post-traumatic stress disorder may at times be classified as terrors because they are so vivid and frightening.

See also DREAMING; NIGHTMARE; SLEEP.

noncompliance The simple behavioral act of either not doing what is one element of a regimen, or doing that which is proscribed.

Compliance is extremely important in mental health care because of the complications that may result from the presence of a chronic mental illness that is not treated in an optimal manner. For example, some people deviate from their prescription regimen or do not take their medication at all. Mental health care practitioners face a challenge to increase patients' informed decision making as well as compliance. They constantly strive to determine methods for measuring compliance as well as develop more acceptable treatments.

According to Raymond A. Ulmer, Ph.D., director of the Noncompliance Institute of Los Angeles (established in 1976), the 10 problem areas of compliance (noncompliance) are:

1. Meeting medical appointments with physician
2. Reporting for diagnosis and treatment
3. Proper taking of medications
4. Avoiding drug abuse
5. Avoiding alcohol use
6. Following smoking recommendations
7. Following dietary suggestions
8. Following work recommendations
9. Conforming to exercise suggestions
10. Proper rest

The Noncompliance Institute of Los Angeles is an organization that works with patients and health care professionals to achieve greater compliance. According to a study conducted by the institute, noncompliant patients have twice as many complications as a compliant patient and cost four times as much to treat.

For further information, contact:

Noncompliance Institute of Los Angeles
6411 W. Fifth Street
Los Angeles, CA 90048
Phone: (213) 553-7387

See also COMPLIANCE.

non-REM sleep See SLEEP.

norepinephrine One of several neurotransmitters (also known as noradrenaline). Norepinephrine is a biogenic amine that transmits electrochemical signals from one brain cell to another. It is responsible for signaling many major functions, including wakefulness, learning, memory and eating. Norepinephrine can signal excitation or inhibition; it causes increased pulse and blood pressure. The level of norepinephrine in the brain may be associated with depression and manic states. One theory is that depression may result from too little norepinephrine and mania results from too much. Serotonin, another neurotransmitter, may also bring about depression when in short supply.

See also BIPOLAR DISORDER; DEPRESSION; NEUROTRANSMITTERS; SEROTONIN.

Norpramin Generic name for the tricyclic antidepressant medication desipramine.

See also ANTIDEPRESSANT MEDICATIONS; PHARMACEUTICAL APPROACH; TRICYCLIC ANTIDEPRESSANTS.

nortriptyline A tricyclic antidepressant drug, marketed under the trade names Aventyl and Pamelor. Nortriptyline is as effective as imipramine in the treatment of depressive episodes of major depression and bipolar disorder; it also may be useful in the depressive periods of dysthymic disorder and in atypical depression.

See also ANTIDEPRESSANT MEDICATIONS; DEPRESSION; PHARMACOLOGICAL APPROACH.

Griest, J. H., and J. W. Jefferson. *Depression and its Treatment: Help for the Nation's #1 Mental Problem.* Washington, D.C.: American Psychiatric Association, 1984.

nostalgia A longing to return to a place where one may have emotional ties, for example, to a home or to a native country. Nostalgia is related to feelings of isolation in the adopted location. According to Miepje DeVryer, writing in the *Journal of American College Health* (Vol. 39, Sept. 1989), nostalgia should be distinguished from homesickness, which tends to be resolved by returning "home." By contrast, in nostalgia, the longing or yearning is for a lost past without a desire to actually return. It is characterized by a bittersweet feeling, painful on the one hand, pleasurable and soothing on the other; these feelings combine with memories of the past. In nostalgia, the memories are consistently of places and nonhuman experiences, not of people.

See also MIGRATION.

nutrition Good mental and physical health depends on good nutrition. The body and mind need many nutrients to function optimally. Factors that affect one's nutrition involve emotional, biologic, cognitive and sociocultural aspects. However, at times of certain mental or physical illnesses, nutrition may be less than optimal. For example, a severely depressed individual may have little interest in eating and lose weight, or an individual with a chronic illness such as cancer may have little appetite because of chemotherapy.

Alcoholism and substance abuse can suppress the appetite, leading to a decrease in food intake. Additionally, excessive alcohol intake impairs liver and pancreatic functioning and often results in gastric inflammation. There may be nutrients taken in by the alcohol abuser that are malabsorbed; vitamin B complex, magnesium, zinc, folic acid and vitamin K are just a few examples.

Severe anxiety and stress can interfere with an individual's ability to meet optimal nutritional needs. For example, severe anxiety increases the release of epinephrine and norepinephrine. These hormones shunt blood from the digestive organs to the muscles, heart and brain. In addition, during stress, the body prepares itself for fight or flight. The body's response to stress is to fuel itself for this response, and the body increases its release of glucocorticoids as well as growth hormone. Glucocorticoids increase glucose production, while growth hormone decreases the effectiveness of insulin in glucose metabolism. Decreased blood flow, along with the increased glucose production, creates a state of anorexia in which the individual has a decreased intake of essential nutrients.

Psychotropic medications can contribute to inadequate nutrition for some individuals. For example, dry mouth, a side effect of some medications, may make eating less pleasurable than usual. Other side effects that interfere with one's ability to maintain good nutrition include glossitis (inflammation of the tongue), nausea, abdominal pain, vomiting and diarrhea.

Mental impairment, caused by organic mental disorders, alcohol and other drug use or mental retardation, can result in an inability to make decisions about eating. The lack of judgment may be reflected in inappropriate selection or preparation of meals. Memory impairment associated with some of these disorders may cause one to forget to eat—even after frequent reminders—or forget that one has already eaten, and eat a second meal.

In today's society, many homeless and destitute individuals do not have adequate nutrition. Social isolation, inadequate financial resources and lack of food storage and preparation facilities offer the potential for inadequate nutrition.

Emphasis on thinness in our society has led many to poor nutritional habits in an effort to lose weight. Hence one's perception of body image may also interfere with proper nutritional intake.

See also EATING DISORDERS.

nutritional disorders Some psychiatric symptoms can be brought on by nutritional disorders. For example, thiamine deficiency may lead to Wernicke-Korsakoff syndrome and Korsakoff's syndrome, an amnestic disorder. Pernicious anemia can also produce dementia. Pellagra (niacin deficiency), a major problem in underdeveloped countries, shows a dramatic response to niacin, even when mental changes have been present for a long time.

See also NUTRITION; WERNICKE-KORSAKOFF SYNDROME; KORSAKOFF'S SYNDROME.

nymphomania A female compulsion including an excessive or insatiable desire for sexual stimulation and gratification. This desire may be expressed not only in seeking frequent sexual intercourse but also in frequent masturbation. Psychoanalytic explanations for this disorder include denial of homosexual tendencies, attempts to disprove frigidity, a reaction to seduction in childhood or an outlet for emotional tension.

Feminists say that nymphomania is a sexist term for women who have an excessive desire for sexual activity.

See also SEXUAL DYSFUNCTION.

Kahn, Ada P., and Linda Hughey Holt. *The A to Z of Women's Sexuality.* Alameda, Calif.: Hunter House, 1992.

obesity   Obesity, a state of being overweight, affects an individual's self-esteem, feeling of attractiveness and one's mental well-being. Obesity can lead to social withdrawal or to constant binge-dieting. Many psychological factors are often associated with an individual's obesity. For example, one might overeat because of persistent emotional tension, use food as a substitute for satisfaction in a sexual relationship or because of sexual frustration.

Obesity can result from certain endocrine diseases (for example, hypothyroidism or hyperadrenal function, also known as Cushing's disease). There is an ongoing controversy about whether subtle biochemical or metabolic differences not yet specified may lead to obesity in some individuals.

Obesity can affect a woman's or man's enjoyment of sexual activities, as some grossly overweight individuals have difficulty in finding a comfortable position during a sexual relationship.

Obesity is also a risk factor for many diseases, including diabetes, heart and kidney disease and some forms of cancer.

For information:

American Society of Bariatric Physicians
5600 S. Quebec, Suite 1600
Englewood, CO 80111
Phone: (303) 779-4833

National Association to Aid Fat Americans
P.O. Box 188620
Sacramento, CA 95818
Phone: (916) 443-0303

See also BODY IMAGE; EATING DISORDERS; SELF-ESTEEM.

Merz, Beverly, ed. "Obesity Drugs Redux." *Harvard Women's Health Watch* IV, no. 6 (Feb. 1997).

object relations   A psychiatric term referring to the emotional bonds between one person and another, as contrasted with interest in and love for the self. The term is usually used with regard to the capacity to love and react appropriately to others' love.

obscenity   Words, gestures, drawings, stories, films or sexual behavior (such as exhibitionism and voyeurism) that are considered repulsive and revolting because they grossly violate the norms of "good taste" in a particular society or group of individuals. Historically, many jokes regarding sexuality have been considered obscene. However, general ideas of obscenity change with cultures, the times and the setting. In the 1950s, television broadcasts could not portray a couple in a double bed; anything closer than a married couple in twin beds was considered "obscene." Some people consider nudity obscene; others do not. Bare breasts might seem obscene in a "girly" show but not on a sculpture in an art museum. Hence, obscenity is defined by cultural standards.

obsessive-compulsive disorder (OCD)   An anxiety disorder characterized by a person's obsessions, which are repeated intrusive, unwanted thoughts, that may lead to carrying out ritualized, compulsive acts. This disorder affects 2.4 million Americans and is a cause for stress for the sufferer, as well as family members, coworkers, and friends.

OCD may come on suddenly, often beginning in early childhood, around ages eight to 10. The disorder is twice as prevalent in the general population as panic disorder or schizophrenia. OCD is partly inherited and partly the result of environmental factors. Personality traits of orderliness and cleanliness are said to be related to OCD, and certain brain disorders can result in compulsive behavior.

Obsessions

Obsessions come into the mind involuntarily and recur. Sufferers are not able to ignore them; they consider these thoughts, such as fear of being infected by germs or dirt, or constant doubt about turning the coffee pot off or locking the front door, senseless and somewhat unpleasant but nevertheless unrelenting and unstoppable.

Compulsions

A normal lifestyle routine is impossible for many OCD sufferers because they constantly repeat rituals that take up considerable time. People who have OCD are aware that their compulsions and rituals are irrational, but they cannot help themselves. Some are ashamed of their actions and hide them from family and friends, often delaying treatment for years.

Hand washing, checking and counting are the most common compulsions among people with this disorder. Other types of rituals relate to fastidiousness and perfection, such as cleaning the house, showering, repeating names or phrases, hoarding, avoiding objects and performing tasks extremely slowly and repeatedly.

OCD and Depression

Researchers speculate that OCD may be closely associated with depression. Some individuals experience only OCD, while others suffer from both OCD and depression. Many OCD sufferers have symptoms associated with depression, such as guilt, indecisiveness, low self-esteem, anxiety and exhaustion. The link between OCD and depression is borne out by laboratory tests on patients who have the two illnesses. For example, obsessive-compulsives, like some people who have depression, do not stop producing dexamethasone, a steroid naturally produced in the body, during a dexamethasone suppression test. When the steroid is injected into the body, the body should stop producing dexamethasone on its own. OCD patients continue to make the steroid. Also, obsessive-compulsive, like depressed people, show an abnormal lapse in the time it takes between first falling asleep and the first dream (normally from one to two hours). When researchers looked at the immediate family members of people suffering from OCD, they found a high percentage had depression or manic-depressive disorder; this connection indicates a possible genetic link. Also, some scientists theorize that OCD may be learned from a depressed or compulsive family member.

Pharmacological and Behavior Therapies

Pharmacological approaches include the use of prescription medications for some individuals. Researchers have learned that medications that affect the serotonergic system (such as clomipramine and fluoxetine) can be useful in relieving symptoms in some patients.

Behavior therapy is one of the most effective treatments for OCD. During therapy sessions, the person is exposed to situations that cause extreme

BEHAVIOR THERAPY FOR OCD		
Technique	Action Experienced	Anticipated Effect
Prevention of response	Individual gradually delays performing ritual for longer intervals	Helps reduce compulsion
Thought stopping	Individual tries to voluntarily interrupt obsessive thoughts	Helps decrease obsessions
Imagery	Individual is encouraged to imagine being exposed to feared situation and prevent an unwanted response	Help decrease obsessions and anxiety
Modeling	Therapist actively models response	Alters patient's unwanted behaviors to more acceptable ones
Exposure	Individual is gradually exposed to the feared thought or object	Reduces anxiety; decreases obsessions and compulsions

stress and anxiety and provoke compulsive behaviors. The individual is not allowed to go through the usually performed rituals, such as excessive hand washing after handling money. This technique works well for people whose compulsions focus on situations that can be easily recreated. For those who follow compulsive rituals because they fear catastrophic events that cannot be recreated, individuals must rely more on imagination, guided imagery and other visualization techniques.

For information, contact:

Anxiety Disorders Association of America
11900 Parklawn Drive, Suite 100
Rockville, MD 20852
Phone: (301) 231-9350
Fax: (301) 231-7392
Web site: www.adaa.org

Obsessive-Compulsive Disorder Foundation
P.O. Box 60
Vernon, CT 06066
Phone: (800) 639-7462

See also ANXIETY DISORDERS; BEHAVIOR THERAPY.

American Psychiatric Association. *Obsessive Compulsive Disorder.* Washington, D.C.: American Psychiatric Association, 1988.
Kahn, Ada P. Stress *A to Z: The Sourcebook for Facing Everyday Challenges.* New York: Facts On File, 2000.
Pigott, Terasa A., and Sheila Seay. "Pharmacotherapy of Obsessive-Compulsive Disorder." *International Review of Psychiatry* 9, no. 1 (March 1997): 133–147.

Oedipus complex   The Oedipus complex, originally described by Sigmund Freud, is a crucial component of Freudian thinking. The concept comes from the Greek myth about Oedipus, who unwittingly killed his father and married his mother. Freud saw this myth as representing every small boy's unconscious sexual attachment and desire for his mother and jealousy and rivalry with his father.

Freud believed that a boy who does not successfully rechannel such urges may be tormented, leading to anxieties and other mental health problems. He also hypothesized that as children develop, they come to identify with the parent of the same sex and are later able to make sexual attachments with members of the opposite sex outside the family. A young child represses these feelings and keeps them in the unconscious out of fear of displeasure or punishment by the parent of the same sex.

In its original use, the term applied only to a boy or man and his relationship with his mother. The term "Electra complex" applied to girls and women and their relationships with their fathers.

The Oedipus complex may influence young men in their choice of wives. Some choose women just like their mothers, and some choose the exact opposite. Other men look for older women in whom they see a mother figure. Overall, the Oedipus complex is one of the most well-known terms left in the legacy of Freudian thinking.

See also ELECTRA COMPLEX; FREUD, SIGMUND.

Stone, Evelyn M., ed. *American Psychiatric Glossary,* 6th ed. Washington, D.C.: American Psychiatric Press, 1988.

ohashiatsu   A form of therapy based on the same system of Eastern medicine as acupuncture; useful for relief of stress for some people. Ohashiatsu addresses the body's energy meridians and the points along those meridians called *tsubos.* Instead of using needles, however, the practitioner of ohashiatsu uses hands, elbows and sometimes even knees as tools. The goal is to achieve a feeling of deep relaxation, harmony and peace.

Ohashiatsu adds psychological and spiritual dimensions to traditional shiatsu, by incorporating Zen philosophy, movement and meditation to balance the energy of body, mind and spirit.

See also ACUPUNCTURE; BODY THERAPIES; COMPLEMENTARY THERAPIES; MEDITATION; MIND/BODY CONNECTIONS; RELAXATION; SHIATSU.

only children   The concentrated attention and love that an only child usually receives from parents has both advantages and disadvantages. Only children have a strong sense of security and all family resources devoted to developing their talents, but they may be handicapped when the need to become independent and strike out for themselves arises. The only child may have less privacy, the burden of trying to fulfill high expectations and an unrealistic sense of what the world is like because of undivided parental attention. Only children rarely get away with behavioral transgressions because there is no one else to blame for mundane events such as mud on the carpet, but they are never blamed for what someone else did. Adult life—in which it is very possible to be blamed for things done by others but also to get away with undesirable behavior—may come as a shock to only children.

On the other hand, some only children experience a type of deprivation because the home remains adult-centered. Parents may continue a romantic, exclusive relationship because one child requires less change than two or more. For example, adult standards of cleanliness, quiet and neatness that would be difficult to preserve with two or more children may stay intact. Parents of one child may be less likely to plan vacations and other recreation around the child because they are in the majority.

Only children frequently not only live in an adult-centered home but in many cases have relatively older parents. The fact that the child has to learn early to be a "little adult" helps to prepare for adult life but may make the child quieter and more sophisticated, and therefore such a child may seem somewhat unusual to other children.

While their parents age, only children are in a unique position. They have to deal with their aging problems with no help from siblings. The problems may burden such children while their own families and occupational responsibilities are at their peak.

Only children share some attributes with older children. They have parents who have no experience in parenting. As more children arrive, parents may become more realistic and mellow regarding childlike behavior, but the only child does not get the benefit of this attitude. Firstborns and only children tend to be achievers and score higher on intelligence tests, particularly in the area of verbal ability. Other children in the family constellation may share the only child experience. Mental health professionals believe that any child with an age difference of seven years or more from the closest sibling or even a single girl in a family of boys or vice versa may have the experience and outlook of an only child.

Despite possible disadvantages of being an only born, the only child usually learns to tolerate and even enjoy solitude and to develop inner resources. Only children frequently enter fields that require them to work in an independent, solitary manner. In many cases, only-born women seem to adapt to widowhood better than women who had many siblings. As an only child, the young women learned to fill their time without others around.

Numbers of only children are increasing and will probably continue to do so in the Western world. A number of factors have contributed to the increasing number of couples who produce only one child. Improved birth control techniques and legal abortions have given couples control of family size. More frequently than in the past, divorce brings the growth of a family to a halt. It has become less common for a financially established man to marry a younger woman with many child-bearing years ahead of her. In general, couples are marrying later; the emphasis on women's education and careers means that a woman may postpone childbearing until one child is the only biologic possibility. Additionally, women often feel that juggling career and motherhood is easier with only one child. The simple cost of raising and educating more than one child may be prohibitive, particularly in urban areas where comfortably housing a family of more than three can be quite costly.

Limiting families to one child is not an entirely new phenomenon. During the Depression, one out of four children were only children. During the Baby Boom, the ratio dropped to one in 10. In the 1980s, the Census Bureau found that the number of married women expecting to have only one child was 11 percent of the population, compared with 7 percent in 1960.

See also BIRTH ORDER.

open marriage   An arrangement in which both partners agree to accept the freedom of their spouse to have extramarital sexual activity. Success of an open marriage depends on an equal desire by both partners to maintain the arrangement. Each partner in an open marriage may have sexual and emotional needs that cannot be satisfied within a monogamous relationship.

The concept of open marriage increased in popularity during the 1960s but decreased during the

1980s along with the spread of sexually transmitted diseases (STDs) and acquired immunodeficiency syndrome (AIDS).

See also MARRIAGE.

opioid substance abuse   In the 1980s, there were nearly 500,000 opioid addicts in the United States. Opioid substances include many opium-related compounds. In addition to the natural alkaloids of opium, morphine and codeine, there are important synthetic derivatives such as heroin, hydromorphone hydrochloride (trade name: Dilaudid), oxycodone (trade name: Percocet) and oxymorphone hydrochloride (trade name Numorphan), as well as purely synthetic opioids such as meperidine (trade name: Demerol), methadone (trade name: Dolopine), pentazocine (trade name: Talwin) and dextropropoxyphene hydrochloride (trade name: Darvon). Men outnumber women by three to one among narcotic addicts, and addiction is more prevalent among people between the ages of 18 and 25. Few addicts manage to break the habit, and recidivism is estimated to be as high as 90 percent. Some health care professionals who have ready access to narcotics become addicted to them.

Serious complications of opioid addiction include infection, suicide and homicide. In the 1990s, the spread of the AIDS virus through shared needles made heroin addiction a major risk factor for contracting the virus.

Mental health professionals treat many addicts for their addictions in hospital emergency rooms when they are experiencing overdose or withdrawal symptoms as well as in outpatient settings.

See also SUBSTANCE ABUSE.

oral character   A psychoanalytic term for personality patterns that derive from experiences during the oral phase of psychosexual development. This theory suggests that a child who experiences adequate sucking satisfaction and attention from the mother during this period will develop a friendly, optimistic, cooperative and generous outlook on life. However, if the child is not satisfied during the oral sucking and biting stage, the individual may become hostile, overly competitive, aggressive and critical.

See also PSYCHOSEXUAL DEVELOPMENT.

Orestes complex   A psychiatric term referring to a son's repressed impulse to kill his mother, or the actual act of killing his mother (matricide). The term is derived from the myth of Orestes, who killed his mother, Clytemnestra, and her lover.

See also COMPLEX.

organic approach   A concept that mental and physical disorders have a biochemical or biologic basis. For example, those who hold this view point to evidence that manic-depressive disorder, schizophrenia and anxiety disorders occur because of biochemical disturbances in the nervous or glandular system. While there may be growing evidence of organic or biologic factors in certain forms of mental illness, it is understood by most psychiatrists that most organic disorders represent an interaction of psychological factors or stresses with a biologic vulnerability, which is also true of many medical disorders such as myocardial infarction (heart attack).

See also BIOLOGICAL MARKERS; DEPRESSION.

organic brain syndrome   See BRAIN SYNDROME, ORGANIC.

orgasm   The climax or peak of intense pleasure during sexual activity. It is the third stage of the sexual response cycle, after excitement and the plateau stage. Orgasm is the culmination of sexual tension in muscle contractions, which force out accumulated blood from erect and engorged genital tissues. This is usually accompanied by a feeling of intense pleasure. There may be a momentary feeling of clouding of consciousness.

In women, an orgasm usually involves a series of rhythmic muscular contractions, each lasting about a second, of the lower vagina and surrounding tissues and may involve uterine contractions. In males, ejaculation from the penis occurs. The focus of the male orgasm is the penis, prostate gland and seminal vesicles. During orgasm, blood pressure and heart rate usually increase.

Orgasm is a very individual experience. Feelings based on mutual warmth and understanding between the two individuals are important factors for women in achieving sexual gratification. Variations in orgasm are reported by different women, and the experience differs in one woman at different times. With sexual stimulation, some women experience more than one orgasm; such multiple orgasms may occur as close together as only a few minutes. Although there is wide variation among individuals, according to sex researchers Masters and Johnson, women take longer on average to reach orgasm than men, 15 minutes as opposed to three minutes.

For some women, penile thrusting is not enough to bring them to the point of orgasm; many achieve orgasm most easily by stimulation of the clitoris either by hand (hers or her partner's) or during oral or vaginal intercourse. A woman's partner often cannot tell if a woman's orgasm is occurring. With communication between partners, they can achieve mutual intensification of the experience.

According to Freud's dual-orgasm theory, there are two types of female orgasm, the "mature" vaginal orgasm and the "immature" clitoral orgasm. In their 1966 work, Masters and Johnson reported that there is only one type of female orgasm, with the clitoris as the center of sensation. Since that time, some sex researchers agreed that the most likely stimulation to create arousal to orgasm is direct stimulation of the clitoris. Other researchers say women achieve orgasm without direct stimulation of the clitoris, and not all women respond to only clitoral stimulation.

According to E. R. Mahoney, in *Human Sexuality* (1983), orgasm by clitoral stimulation is typically described as very intense, sharp and ecstatic, while orgasm by means of deep vaginal penetration is described as more internal, soothing, subtle and full.

Some women report that regular sexual stimulation that stops short of orgasm results in pelvic discomfort. However, many women enjoy sexual activity without orgasm. Some women who have lost sensation in the lower part of their body enjoy sexual stimulation of various erogenous areas of their body. Other women report that orgasm can relieve the pelvic congestion associated with menstrual cramps.

The term "frigidity" is used to refer to the condition of never achieving an orgasm during sexual activity. The term "female orgasmic dysfunction" is currently used to refer to difficulty in achieving orgasm.

Orgasmic Dysfunction

Inability to reach orgasm through physical stimulation. Masters and Johnson, in their major 1966 work *Human Sexual Response,* described two types. Primary orgasmic dysfunction meant that the woman never had an orgasm through any physical contact, including masturbation. Situational orgasmic dysfunction meant that the woman had at least one instance of orgasm through physical contact. Orgasmic dysfunction is not limited to females.

Orgasmic Reconditioning (Orgasmic Reorientation)

A technique used in sex therapy in which fantasies or illustrative representations are used to arouse the patient, who then engages in masturbation until sexual climax is reached. Later, these stimuli are replaced by more conventional heterosexual representations just before orgasm and at progressively earlier points, in order to develop normal arousal patterns.

See also CLITORIS; FRIGIDITY; MALE SEXUAL DYSFUNCTION; MASTURBATION; SEX THERAPY.

Kahn, Ada P., and Linda Hughey Holt. *The A to Z of Women's Sexuality.* Alameda, Calif.: Hunter House, 1992.

orthopsychiatry   An interdisciplinary approach to mental health emphasizing child development and family life. Social workers, pediatricians, psychiatrists, psychologists, sociologists and nurses collaborate in studying and treating emotional and behavioral problems before they become severe and disabling.

orthostatic   A term relating to standing erect. For example, orthostatic hypotension refers to a drop in blood pressure when one rises from a lying or sitting position. The individual may experience dizziness or lightheadess; falls are sometimes attributed to orthostatic hypotension.

See also HIGH BLOOD PRESSURE.

over-the-counter medications (OTC) Medications that may be purchased without a prescription from a physician. Many remedies for colds, headaches and minor pains are available without a prescription. Medications that require prescriptions are known as ethical drugs.

pain A sensation that can range from mild discomfort to an unbearable and excruciating experience. How one perceives pain is a very individual matter. The term "pain threshold" applies to the level at which individuals become very uncomfortable from a similar level of unpleasant stimulation. Fear and anxiety are often associated with pain, because a pain may signal a problem of unknown origin and unknown outcome. Unexplained pain seems more stressful than a pain for which a diagnosis can be made.

How individuals relate to pain and express pain may be affected by their upbringing and culture. For example, in Western society, many men were raised to endure mild pain, such as athletic injuries, while women were asked to rest upon the slightest suggestion of pain. Men were told that uncomplaining endurance of pain was "manly."

Drugs that relieve pain are known as analgesic drugs. They usually help in relieving mild pain such as headache, toothache or dysmenorrhea (menstrual pain). The most widely used drugs in this group are acetaminophen and aspirin. Mild to moderate pain, such as that caused by sports injuries or arthritis, is often treated with a nonsteroidal anti-inflammatory drug (NSAID). Severe pain caused by kidney stones, a serious injury, a surgical procedure or cancer may be treated with a narcotic analgesic. Non-drug treatments include massage, ice packs or hot packs. Recurrent or chronic pain is sometimes relieved by acupuncture, acupressure or hypnosis; biofeedback also helps some individuals. Laughter has been known to ease pain. People who are depressed are more likely to interpret pain as more serious than those who feel good about themselves and their life situations.

In *Mental Medicine Update* (1995), Robert Ornstein, Ph.D., and David S. Sobel, M.D., stated that 10 to 30 percent of Americans suffer from chronic or recurrent pain, which extracts a heavy toll on health, ability to work, and sense of well-being. While feelings of anxiety, frustration and loss of control and confidence can amplify the experience of pain, it does not mean that the pain is not "real"; it just means that these emotions make it worse. In addition to physical treatment of pain, the authors suggested behavioral self-management that includes mind-body strategies such as relaxation techniques, support group therapy and biofeedback training; the practice of complimentary therapies allows those suffering chronic pain to become partners in the pain treatment.

SELF-HELPS FOR PAIN CONTROL

- Identify small steps toward independence from pain, such as accepting the pain and not blaming others for your problems.
- Track pain levels and activities with awareness of the difference between physical pain sensations and emotional pain distress.
- Check the "costs/benefits" in relation to participation in family activities, work, play and relationships with people.
- Express feelings and anxieties; learn ways to decrease anger responses.
- Block negative thoughts; use relaxation techniques to fight the chronic stress of sleep disturbance, fatigue, poor concentration, increased muscle tension, anxiety, depression and loss of self-control—all of which amplify pain.
- Distract yourself by focusing on the environment, singing or using imagery to concentrate on pleasant, dramatic and healing thoughts.
- Indulge in healthy pleasures and fun.
- Focus on the pain, as well as the thoughts and feelings that accompany the pain.
- Reclaim an active life by setting short- and long-term goals.
- Exercise on a regular basis, gradually increasing the amount. Modify how you use your body during lifting, bending, sitting and other physical activities and what you

SELF-HELPS FOR PAIN CONTROL (continued)

are using for physical support—chairs, height of desks and counters, wrist bands and other methods.

• Prepare for flareups by knowing the specific pain relievers that work best for you.

For information:

American Academy of Pain Medicine
5700 Old Orchard Road
Skokie, IL 60077
Phone: (847) 966-9510

American Pain Society
P.O. Box 186
Skokie, IL 60076
Phone: (847) 475-7300

Pain Management Guidelines
Agency for Healthcare Policy Research
P.O. Box 8547
Silver Spring, MD 20907
Phone: (800) 358-9295

See also ANXIETY; BIOFEEDBACK; COMPLEMENTARY THERAPIES; DEPRESSION; GUIDED IMAGERY; HEADACHES; HYPNOSIS.

Ford, Norman D. *Painstoppers: The Magic of All-Natural Pain Relief.* West Nyack, N.Y.: Parker Publishing, 1994.
Ornstein, Robert, and David Sobel. "Rx: Managing Chronic Pain." *Mental Medicine Update* IV, no. 1 (1995).

palpitations   An awareness that the heart is beating faster than normal or skipping beats. This occurs during and after exercise or in stressful or feared situations. If the feeling lasts for several hours or recurs over several days, or if it causes chest pain, breathlessness or dizziness, a physician should be consulted as soon as possible. Palpitations may be caused by a cardiac arrhythmia, usually premature ventricular beats or contractions (PVB) or mitral valve prolapse, which usually do not require treatment; if severe, these may require further diagnosis or treatment. If palpitation episodes are brief, they are probably within the range of normal. Rarely, some medications can produce palpitations from PVBs. Some cases of mitral valve prolapse require treatment. Persistent palpitations or tachycardia can be evaluated by a family physician, general internist or specialist in cardiology.

Palpitations often occur during panic attacks or as a phobic reaction to a feared stimulus. For example, a person who is phobic about dogs may experience palpitations just at the sight of a dog walking on the street. Although the dog is on a leash and does not seem aggressive, the phobic individual may experience palpitations along with sweaty palms, weak knees and dizziness.

Those who experience palpitations may fear that they are having a heart attack or that they are going to die. Just thinking these thoughts and becoming afraid of imagined consequences can cause the palpitations to increase.

Symptoms of anxiety, such as palpitations, are treated with behavioral therapy, cognitive therapy and, in some cases, drug therapy.

See also ANXIETY DISORDERS; ANXIOLYTIC DRUGS.

Pamelor   Trade name for the tricyclic antidepressant drug nortriptyline.

See also ANTIDEPRESSANT MEDICATIONS; PHARMACOLOGICAL APPROACH; TRICYCLIC ANTIDEPRESSANTS.

panic attacks and panic disorder   A panic attack is a short period (five to 10 minutes) of suddenly occurring intense fear or discomfort, usually for no apparent reason. The feeling may be caused by stress, but it also causes extreme stress in the affected individual because it is usually accompanied by a fear of dying, a sense of imminent danger or impending doom and an urge to escape.

Panic attacks are considered one of several anxiety disorders. They can occur in a variety of anxiety disorders, such as panic disorder, agoraphobia, social phobias and post-traumatic stress disorder.

The word panic is derived from the name "Pan," whom Greeks worshiped as their god of flocks, herds, pastures and fields. Pan loved to scare people and make eerie noises to frighten those who passed by; the fright he aroused was known as "panic."

Diagnosing Panic Attacks

To be diagnosed as a panic attack, possible organic causes must first be ruled out. The panic incident must include at least four or more of the characteristic symptoms: a sense of breathing difficulty, palpitations or rapid heartbeat; sweating; trembling or shaking; feelings of smothering or choking; chest pains, nausea or abdominal distress; dizziness or lightheadedness; paresthesia and chills or hot flashes.

Hyperventilation (fast, shallow breathing) worsens the symptoms and leads to a pins and needles sensation and a feeling of derealization or depersonalization. These symptoms are usually the result of underlying emotional conflicts, such as fear of being trapped or loss of emotional support.

According to the *Diagnostic and Statistical Manual of Mental Disorders* (4th ed., 1994) (DSM-IV), the first attack typically occurs in individuals in their late teens. Initially, attacks are unexpected and do not occur immediately before or upon exposure to a stressful situation, such as a simple phobia or social phobias. Later, in the course of the disorder, certain situations may be identified with causing a panic attack, such as crossing a bridge or being on an escalator. Once a panic attack has occurred in a particular setting, the individual may become fearful that it will happen again and tend to avoid that situation.

Panic Attacks in Context

When a health professional assesses the significance of the problem, it is important to determine the context in which it occurs. According to *DSM-IV*, three characteristic types of panic attacks relate in different ways to the onset of the attack and the presence or absence of situational triggers:

Unexpected panic attack: The onset of the attack is not associated with any situational trigger.
Situationally bound attack: The attack almost invariably occurs immediately upon exposure to, or in anticipation of, the stressful situational trigger.
Situationally predisposed panic attack: More likely to occur upon exposure to the situational cue or trigger, but it is not invariably associated with the cue and does not necessarily occur immediately after exposure to the stressful factor.

Panic Disorder

When panic attacks recur frequently and disrupt an individual's life, the condition is known as panic disorder. Sufferers (1 to 2 percent of the population) may have attacks ranging from two or three a day to two to four times a week. This type of disorder tends to run a fluctuating course and worsens when the individual comes under stress. Panic disorder usually begins during periods of choices, transitions, separation and added responsibilities. There is often a family history of panic disorder. For example, first-degree relatives of patients with panic disorder are at a markedly higher risk of developing the disorder (15 to 20 percent compared to 1 percent in the general population).

In diagnosing panic disorder, the essential feature is the presence of recurrent, unexpected panic attacks followed by at least one month of persistent concern about having another panic attack, worry about the possible implications or consequence of the attacks or a significant behavioral changed related to the attacks.

Personality Characteristics

Personality characteristics of those who have panic disorder vary considerably. However, H. Michael Zal, a clinical professor of psychiatry at the Philadelphia College of Osteopathic Medicine, has observed some common factors. Additionally, cross-sectional studies of persons with panic disorder or agoraphobia have demonstrated personality traits of dependency, avoidance, low self-esteem and interpersonal sensitivity. One common attribute shared by panic-prone people includes placing a great value on control. Any loss or threatened loss of control, particularly in changes in their lifestyles, causes them to feel anxious and stressed. According to Dr. Zal, panic-prone people overvalue their independence and feel great discomfort in acknowledging their dependencies. They are often reluctant to accept help and prefer to help others. Known to repress feelings, they feel anxious when their emotions surface. As perfectionists and compulsive individuals, they have high expectations of themselves and others.

It is difficult to estimate how many men suffer from panic disorder because men may attempt to mask their symptoms by drinking alcohol. This type of self-medication can develop into a secondary problem. Many men go to family physicians, see multiple specialists or end up in emergency rooms, all the while thinking they have physical disorders. They complain of lower gastrointestinal problems, which are sometimes a symptom of panic disorder. When the panic disorder is treated, these gastrointestinal symptoms disappear.

Treating Panic Disorder

Treatment for the stresses that come with panic disorder may involve cognitive therapy, behavior therapy or medical therapy. Often a combination of treatments is specifically chosen for each patient. Treatment begins with education about the illness and encouragement to reenter those situations that the person has come to avoid. Cognitive therapy (changing how they think and dealing with their feeling of anxiety) helps for some individuals. For others, behavior therapy (changing how they act in response to certain situations and using desensitization techniques to gradually expose sufferers to the situations they have avoided) is useful.

During the late 1990s, alprazolam (trade name: Xanax) was the first medication approved in the United States for panic disorder. Previously, various studies indicated that tricyclic antidepressant drugs (such as imipramine) provided an effective, safe treatment for panic disorder. However, those medications typically take three to six weeks for noticeable improvement, and side effects, including anxiety symptoms, occur in up to one-third of the patients. Other drugs used are the SSRIs, (selective serotonin reuptake inhibitors) such as Zoloft and Prozac.

Three-quarters of patients who have to take drugs will need long-term drug therapy, while another 25 percent will not be helped regardless of how long they take drugs. Overall, a quarter of the patients who do take drugs are helped permanently and will not have to continue with medication.

How Family Members Can Help Panic Disorder Sufferers

Treatment for panic disorder is not limited to medical or psychotherapeutic intervention. Family members can help in recognizing panic disorders by being alert to the individual's level of anxiety. Because symptoms can be hidden, repeated avoidance of situations is often the best clue. Family members can give the sufferer support, be good listeners and talk openly and constructively among each other. Instead of enabling the person to avoid a situation, family members can help him or her make a small step forward by finding something positive in that effort. Most importantly, family members should be patient and accepting and not sacrifice their own lives nor build resentment toward the sufferer.

For information:

Anxiety Disorders Association of America
11900 Parklawn Drive, Suite 100
Rockville, MD 20852
Phone: (301) 231-9350

National Mental Health Association
1021 Prince Street
Alexandria, VA 22314
Phone: (800) 969-NMHA or (800) 969-6642

See also AGORAPHOBIA; ANXIETY DISORDERS; BEHAVIOR THERAPY; CONTROL; HYPERVENTILATION; PALPITATIONS; PHOBIA; POST-TRAUMATIC STRESS DISORDER; SELF-ESTEEM; TACHYCARDIA.

American Psychiatric Association. *Diagnostic and Statistical Manual,* 4th ed., rev. Washington, D.C.; 1994.
Kahn, Ada P. "Panic Attacks" and "Family Members Can Help Sufferers Cope with Attacks." *Chicago Tribune* (June 23, 1991).
Norton, G.R. et al. "Panic Disorder or Social Phobia: Which Is Worse?" *Behavior Research Therapy* 34, no. 3 (1996): 273–276.
Zal, H. Michael. *Panic Disorder: The Great Pretender.* New York: Insight Books, Plenum Press, 1990.

paranoia   A pervasive and unwarranted tendency to interpret the actions of others as deliberately demeaning or threatening. For example, a paranoid person may question loyalty of employees or friends. In new situations, a paranoid individual may read hidden meanings into remarks or events. These individuals are quick to anger and are reluctant to confide in others because they fear that information may be used against them.

Many normally healthy individuals have paranoid tendencies at certain times and under certain circumstances, some of which may be warranted. However, when carried to extreme, paranoid tendencies are considered paranoid personality disorder. This term is applied to persistent, nonbizarre delusions that are not due to any other mental disorder, such as schizophrenia or a mood disorder. Common types of delusions are erotomanic, grandiose, jealous and persecutory. Erotomanic delusions are that one is loved by another, usually a famous or important person. Grandiose delusions commonly take the form of the person's being convinced that he or she possesses some great talent or has made some important discovery for which he or she will be recognized. Jealous delusions involve feelings that one's spouse or lover is unfaithful (Othello syndrome).

Persecutory delusions are the most common type and usually involve a single theme or series of themes, such as being spied on, cheated, followed, poisoned or drugged. Small slights may be exaggerated and become the focus of a delusional system. Elderly patients with dementia, as they see themselves losing control of their life and decisions, may accuse loyal and helpful children of stealing their funds or savings.

Additionally, there are somatic delusions (or paranoias) in which individuals have a delusion about their body or parts of their body, for example, that they have a foul odor emanating from their breath, that certain parts of the body are not functioning or that they have an internal parasite.

Paranoid disorders are slightly more common in females than males. They usually begin in middle or late adult life but can begin at a younger age. In most studies, average age of onset has been found to be between 40 and 55.

Paranoid schizophrenia is a type of schizophrenia in which extreme delusions are related to a single theme; unlike undifferentiated schizophrenia, paranoid schizophrenia may develop in the late twenties or thirties.

See also AGORAPHOBIA; BODY IMAGE; DELUSION; IDEAS OF REFERENCE; SCHIZOPHRENIA.

paraphilias Psychosexual disorders in which an individual requires unusual or bizarre acts or images for sexual excitement. They include specific types, such as coprophilia (feces), exhibitionism, fetishism, frotteurism (rubbing), klismaphilia (enema), mysophilia (filth), necrophilia (corpses), pedophilia (children), sexual masochism, sexual sadism, telephone scatalogia (lewdness), transvestitism, voyeurism, urophilia (urine) and zoophilia (animals).

Imagery may take one of many forms, including preference for inhuman objects, such as animals or clothes of the other sex; sexual activity involving real or simulated humiliation or suffering, such as bondage or whipping; or repetitive sexual activity with nonconsenting partners.

Some cultures view any form of paraphilia as abnormal; other cultures are accepting of forms that do not involve victimization of others or interfere with satisfying sexual relationships. For example, many men who are transvestites (cross-dressers into women's clothes) may enjoy perfectly satisfying sex lives. In a sexually permissive society this may not be problematic behavior, whereas in a restrictive culture this could be considered abnormal behavior. However, behavior patterns such as pedophilia can lead to molestation of young children; such victimization that can result in long-term damage to the child is not a harmless sexual variant.

Kim, Peggy Y., and J. Michael Bailey. "Sidestreets on the Information Superhighway: Paraphilias and Sexual Variations on the Internet." *Journal of Sex Education and Therapy* 22 no. 1 (June 1997): 35–43.

parapsychology A branch of psychology concerned with events and experiences that cannot be explained by scientific method; also known as extrasensory perception (ESP). Examples of such phenomena are paranormal experiences, such as telepathy—in which one communicates thoughts to another—or clairvoyance, an ability to mentally see events from afar.

parasomnia A type of sleep disorder including conditions such as nightmares, sleep terrors and sleepwalking. These conditions are particularly common in children.

See also NIGHTMARE; NIGHT TERROR; SLEEP; SLEEPWALKING.

parenting Caring for and nurturing children. The term "parenting" is also applied to the situation when middle-aged adults care for their own aging parents. Of all the roles in life, parenting is one of the most important, yet one for which there is the least preparation. Individuals become parents at the time of the birth of their infant (or at the time of adoption), usually with little instruction or experience. Parenting roles and relationships never stop, no matter how old the children are.

Parenting skills throughout life include the basics of feeding and bathing as well as the psychological nurturing necessary to encourage the child to grow into a communicative, socially adjusted individual. As the child ages, parents become role models. They provide basic teaching about moral and ethical values held by the family and the culture within which the family lives. They must also be disciplinarians, which involves daily training by actions, words and examples to influence their children's behavior. Rewarding acceptable behavior helps reinforce good conduct on the children's part; withholding rewards helps reduce unwanted behaviors if conduct is unacceptable. Teaching compliance with rules begins as soon as an infant gets out of his or her crib. When the baby begins to crawl, safety rules must be enforced. At the toddler stage, information regarding social skills has to be communicated.

Parenting involves dealing with family disputes, including sibling rivalry. While parents try to avoid playing favorites by treating all their children alike, sometimes they do not treat the children the same without conscious effort. Birth order may affect the way children are treated, as well as family circumstances when the child arrives.

Parenting involves responding to problems and concerns of children, both physical and mental. One example of coping with children's concerns is dealing with troubling nightmares. Usually nightmares of small children can be related to some exciting event, such as going to a frightening movie or having started a new school or in a new classroom. If a parent does not respond with comfort to the cries of a child with a nightmare, just the sound of his or her own voice will add to the terror the child feels upon awakening. Permitting a child to keep a small light on may allay many fears of young childhood.

As children grow, parents teach them about sexuality. Parents should be open to questions and give children the amount of information they can assimilate at the time. Children are naturally curious and may ask questions about sexuality as soon as they can talk. As they grow older, they can understand more information. With young people becoming sexually active at an early age plus the spread of AIDS and sexually transmitted diseases, it is imperative that children receive as much information about their bodies and sexuality as soon as they are interested and able to understand. Although still controversial, the topic of sex education is still taught in many schools, starting from kindergarten on up.

As children become adults, the parenting role often becomes one of friend and companion. Many adult children and their parents enjoy sports activities, traveling and hobbies, whether they live nearby or in distant cities. Characteristics of their relationship while the children were young, such as open and honest communication, carry over into late life. These qualities make for good relationships between adult children and their parents.

When young people leave home, some parents are faced with the "empty nest" and no longer feel needed. While this may be a time of loneliness for some parents, it is also a time in which the parents can explore their own interests, further their educations and enjoy the intimacy they shared as newlyweds.

Since the mid-1980s, in the United States, there has been a trend concerning grown children who leave home and then return, some divorced and with children; for many, this is occurring out of economic necessity. Some families cope well with this multigenerational situation, but others find that it produces constant stresses and strains. Generally, if communication between the child and parents was good before he or she left home, problems occurring in the new situation can be dealt with happily. Parents in this situation need to remember that the children are adults and should not be treated like children.

See also BIRTH ORDER; EMPTY NEST SYNDROME; SIBLING RIVALRY; STRESS.

paresthesia Numbness or tingling. This symptom may occur during a panic attack or phobic reaction, along with dizziness and weakness in the knees. It can also occur as the result of vitamin deficiencies.

See also ANXIETY DISORDERS; PANIC ATTACK; PANIC DISORDER.

pargyline Generic term for the monoamine oxidase inhibitor Eutonyl.

See also ANTIDEPRESSANT MEDICATIONS; MONOAMINE OXIDASE INHIBITORS; PHARMACOLOGICAL APPROACH.

Parkinson's disease (PD) A disease in which individuals lack the substance dopamine, which is involved in the control of muscle activity by the nervous system. Tremor, stiffness and slowness are characteristic features of Parkinson's disease. Speech may be slow, and movement may be difficult to initiate. Late in the course of the disease some individuals develop dementia. According to the Alzheimer's Disease and Related Disorders Association, some Parkinson patients develop Alzheimer's disease and some Alzheimer patients develop Parkinson symptoms. Drugs for PD may improve the motor symptoms but may not improve the mental changes that occur. Research on drugs for PD has also encouraged research on Alzheimer's disease.

See also ALZHEIMER'S DISEASE.

Parnate Trade name for the monoamine oxidase inhibitor tranylcypromine.

See also ANTIDEPRESSANT MEDICATIONS; MONOAMINE OXIDASE INHIBITORS; PHARMACOLOGICAL APPROACH.

partial hospitalization Treatment at a mental hospital or another treatment facility for a number of hours each day but without an overnight stay. Many mental health services are offered through partial hospitalization, also referred to as day treatment or partial care.

passive-aggressive personality disorder A disorder characterized by being aggressive in a quietly passive way. For example, while outward aggression shows itself in a loud voice and possibly with physical force, passive aggression is more calculated and done quietly. A passive-aggressive act may be one in which a person gives another directions to find a place but purposely leaves out an important detail. Another such act might be deliberately being late, causing others to wait and miss a train or other important opportunity. Characteristics of this personality disorder include putting off or forgetting to do a chore or being purposefully inefficient. This procrastination or inefficiency gets in the way of job promotion and social acceptability.

Passive-aggressive characteristics may be caused by hidden aggression.

See also AGGRESSION; DEPRESSION; PERSONALITY.

pathological gambling An inability to resist the impulse to gamble, despite the outlook for serious adverse consequences.

See GAMBLING.

Pavlov, Ivan Petrovich (1849–1936) Russian physiologist known for learning theories based on conditioning techniques.

In experiments with dogs, Pavlov gave them food (unconditioned stimulus) and simultaneously range a bell. The dogs, in an unconditioned response, salivated at the scent of food. After many trials, the dogs salivated at the sound of the bell. They had learned a conditioned response to a conditioned stimulus. This became known as Pavlovian conditioning and became the basis for teaching and reinforcing behavior. According to Pavlovian theory, learning is the response to an external events, or stimulus, to which a person or animal becomes accustomed or conditioned.

pavor nocturnus See NIGHT TERRORS; NIGHTMARES.

Paxil Trade name for the antidpressant medication paroxetine.

Paxipam Trade name for the benzodiazepine drug halazepam.

See also BENZODIAZEPINE DRUGS; PHARMACOLOGICAL APPROACH.

PCP Phencyclidine, a hallucinogen. It was first developed as a human anesthetic, but human use was discontinued because of severe side effects.

Later it became commercially available for veterinary use; however, this was discontinued in the late 1970s. Thus, virtually all PCP available in the United States is produced clandestinely.

PCP's effects vary based on the amount ingested. Sensory changes are often accompanied by slurred or blocked speech and a loss of coordination that may be accompanied by a sense of strength and invincibility. PCP can produce psychoses indistinguishable from schizophrenia. Because PCP causes disorientation, some users suffer accidents—even fatally—and others become violent.

Available in tablets and capsules, PCP is most widely used in powder and liquid forms, applied to leafy materials such as parsley, mint, oregano and marijuana and then smoked. PCP is known by many street names. The most common are angel dust, supergrass, killer weed, K.J. crystal, embalming fluid, rocket fuel and sherms.

See also SUBSTANCE ABUSE.

Media Resource Guide on Common Drugs of Abuse. Public
    Relations Society of America, National Capital Chapter, Fairfax, Va., September 1990.

Peck, M(organ) Scott (1936–) American psychiatrist, lecturer and author of several best-selling books including *The Road Less Traveled: A New Psychology of Love, Traditional Values and Spiritual Growth* (1978) and *The Road Less Traveled and Beyond* (1997). He received his M.D. degree from Case Western Reserve University and his A.B. from Harvard University. Peck postulates that when an individual accepts the inherent stresses in life, he or she can transfer weakness into strength through self-discipline and love. This "real love" is "an act of the will to extend oneself for the purpose of nurturing one's own or another's spiritual growth." For many years, Peck has had an interest in the growing interface between religion and science.

See also FAITH; GENERAL ADAPTATION SYNDROME; HARDINESS; PRAYER; RELIGION.

Peck, M. Scott. *The Road Less Traveled and Beyond.* New
    York: Simon & Schuster, 1997.
————. *The Road Less Traveled: A New Psychology of Love,
    Traditional Values and Spiritual Growth.* New York,
    Simon & Schuster, 1978.

peer group A like-age group that influences one's self-concept, self-esteem, attitudes and behavior. Peer group relationships are important to children as well as adults. While teenagers look to one another for acceptance and approval, so do adults seeking to make new friends, and same-level employees in a workplace.

Although peer relationships are most obviously important to adolescents, peers are actually crucial to psychological development throughout life. Children were once thought to be most highly influenced by adults; however, modern thinking recognizes the importance of the peer group to childhood. Through peer relationships, children learn to cooperate, work together, handle aggressive impulses in nondestructive ways and explore differences between themselves and their friends. Children who do not learn to combat loneliness by fitting into a peer group may develop emotional problems later in life. For adults, the increasing mobility that often cuts them off from family and longtime friends has made the development of peer relationships through work or other activities extremely important.

See also PEER PRESSURE.

peer pressure Peer pressure begins to dominate life in adolescence. Teenagers want to "fit in" and feel that they belong to the group they choose. They react to the confusing physical changes and approaching adult responsibilities by extremely close bonding with members of their own age group. Fads in music, language and clothing become extremely important and are accepted and discarded quickly as teenagers try to meet conventions established by their peer group. The rallying cry of teenagers is often "everybody's doing it" (or "everyone has it"). Parents frequently become distressed by this peer influence. They may feel left out of activities and decisions from which their child now excludes them in favor of peers. They may also fear that the influence of friends may lead to genuinely damaging activities such as experimenting with drugs, smoking, drinking, criminal behavior, irresponsible sexual activity or dropping out of school.

Some children who feel "different" from their peers have some difficulties "fitting in." Such children may be those who are in recently divorced families, in recently "merged" families with two sets of parents, or adopted children of single parents.

See also ADOPTION; PARENTING; PEER GROUP; REMARRIAGE; SELF-ESTEEM; STEP-FAMILIES; UNWED MOTHERS.

John, D. W., and R. T. Johnson. "Peer Influences," In *Encyclopedia of Psychology,* vol. 2. edited by Raymond J. Corsini. New York: Wiley, 1984.

Leach, Penelope. *The Child Care Encyclopedia.* New York: Knopf, 1984.

peptides Fragments of protein consisting of two or more amino acids. Peptides result in the linkage of amino acids by chemical bonds between the amino and carboxyl groups of adjacent acids. There are peptides in the endocrine system and nervous system. Many hormones are peptides, such as some gastrointestinal hormones and several pituitary hormones. Examples are oxytocin and ACTH (adrenocorticotropic hormone). In the nervous system, there are peptides in nerve cells throughout the brain and spinal cord. Examples are endorphins and substances involved in the control of the pituitary gland.

Larger peptides, consisting of many linked amino acids, are referred to as polypeptides. Longer chains of amino acids, composed of linked polypeptides, are called proteins.

See also ENDOCRINE SYSTEM; ENDORPHINS; PITUITARY GLAND.

perception One's mental attitudes of sensations about the environment interpreted through the five senses of tasting, smelling, hearing, seeing and touching. False perceptions can occur when there is no sensory stimulation. These may take the form of hallucinations. Perception is usually based on an ability to organize information into some framework or pattern. For example, the individual must be able to recognize objects as separate from their background and as stationary or moving, such as a chair or a person. Such differentiation requires the use of memory. Finally, interpretation depends on one's attitudes, current mood and expectations. For example, a hungry person will pay attention to food sooner than a person who has just finished a meal.

Some mental health disorders, such as Alzheimer's disease and schizophrenia, involve distortions in perception.

Perception can also relate to one's feelings of fear or danger. What appears dangerous to one person may seem like a thrilling challenge to another. The individual who has a phobia of heights will react with sweaty palms, shaky knees and nausea when faced with climb to the top of a mountain, but another person may view the climb as exciting.

Perception also relates to one's attitudes. For example, a teenager's perception of appropriate behavior or wearing apparel may be what his or her peer group views as the current fad, but that perception may differ from the parents' idea of behavior or wearing apparel.

See also ALZHEIMER'S DISEASE; PEER GROUP; SCHIZOPHRENIA.

perfection The state of being expert, proficient, flawless, without fault or defect. It is an unrealistic goal, a drive toward the impossible and unattainable, and the desire to be perfect is a threat to good mental health for many people. Perfectionists are very achievement-oriented. They are unable to select what is important and have the faulty idea that perfectionism equals quality.

The perfectionist faces stresses and frustration with failure of any kind, imagined, real, large or small. The obsession with perfection ultimately results in fragmentation of self, loss of efficiency, sleep deprivation, less time for exercise, rest and quiet meals, increased use of alcohol and drugs and ultimately exhaustion. The perfectionist ideal leaves out the important fact that people are only human and have limitations of body, mind, and spirit.

Many people believe the myth that overachieving will bring recognition and perhaps even love. Today's society measures individuals in terms of productivity and accomplishment. However, there is a delicate balance between the amount of work the human body and mind can do and the amount of time required for rest and regeneration. That balance point differs for each person and is affected by feelings of stress, emotional overload, illness and fatigue.

Overcoming Perfectionism

People who are plagued by the need to be perfect and the incurred stresses should realize their own limitations and reevaluate personal priorities. They must decide what is important and what is not, as well as set realistic deadlines and short and long term goals and choose values that matter.

CONQUER PERFECTIONISM FOR BETTER MENTAL HEALTH

- Look for sources of satisfaction in simple pleasures.
- Pursue special interests such as painting, music, gardening, reading, handicrafts and other hobbies.
- Take better care of the personal self with improved diet, rest and exercise.
- Concentrate on the process of achieving a goal instead of the goal itself.
- Establish friendships outside work and family.
- Set personal priorities and stay with them.
- Find time to be alone and become better acquainted with yourself.

See also OBSESSIVE-COMPULSIVE DISORDER; SELF-ESTEEM.

Riess, Dorothy Young. "The Perils of Perfection." *Better Health Newsletter* (March 1989).

Shaw, Jean, ed. "Perfectionism: Internal Source of Stress Has High Emotional and Physical Costs." *Women's Health Advocate Newsletter* 4, no. 5 (July 1997).

performance anxiety   The extreme stress felt by many people before any kind of performance. They fear failure, criticism or not measuring up to real or imaginary standards. Issues of self-esteem are also involved. Time and energy spent thinking about these fears detracts from concentrating on preparation and the performance.

For some individuals, performance anxiety may cause loss of sleep, indigestion, dizziness or even faintness. However, if properly directed, the nervous energy generated by stress before a performance can become an advantage. When focused on the best possible outcome, that there will be a standing ovation, for example, the individual will be challenged to do a good job.

Performance anxiety is a common stressor to people who speak in public as well as musicians, actors and other performers. Anyone who is the central focus of other people's attention can experience performance anxiety.

Overcoming Performance Anxiety

Many individuals use meditation and deep breathing exercises to reduce stress before performances. Others carry a good luck charm, which provides their anxieties with a placebo-like effect. Some follow certain rituals before every performance; for example, a person might establish a routine way of getting dressed, avoid certain foods or beverages (caffeine and alcohol particularly) or take a walk. For severe cases of performance anxiety, physicians may prescribe medication.

See also BREATHING; CRITICISM; DIZZINESS; MEDITATION; PUBLIC SPEAKING; SELF-ESTEEM; SOCIAL PHOBIA; STAGE FRIGHT.

perphenazine   A phenothiazine-type antipsychotic drug used to relieve symptoms in certain psychiatric disorders, such as schizophrenia. Perphenazine is also sometimes used to relieve nausea and vomiting (antiemetic drug) caused by chemotherapy, radiation therapy or anesthesia.

Adverse effects may include abnormal movements of the face and limbs, blurred vision, drowsiness and headache. Parkinsonism may result from long-term use of the drug.

See also ANTIPSYCHOTIC MEDICATIONS; SCHIZOPHRENIA.

perseveration   A tendency to emit the same verbal response again and again to different questions or stimuli. This may involve constant repetition of one word or phrase or an inability to shift conversation away from a particular topic. It is a disorder of thought process, which refers to the way a person puts ideas together, the associations between ideas and the form and flow of thoughts in conversation.

See also SCHIZOPHRENIA.

personality   All of one's traits, habits, experiences, ways of emotionally responding (including temperament), and motivation. Personality development seems to depend on the interaction of many complex factors, including interaction of heredity and environment. While many theorists hold that genetics is more important than environment, many take the opposite view.

Personality tests are questionnaires designed to determine various traits, to assist in psychological research and at times to determine the suitability of an individual for a particular field of work or job assignment. Personality tests measure many aspects of an individual's being, such as how one relates to people and one's degree of extroversion or introversion.

See also EXTROVERSION; INTROVERSION; PERSONAL-ITY DISORDERS.

personality disorders A group of disorders involving behaviors or traits that are characteristic of a person's recent and long-term functioning. Patterns of perceiving and thinking are not usually limited to isolated episodes but are deeply ingrained, inflexible, maladaptive and severe enough to cause the individual mental stress or anxieties or to interfere with interpersonal relationships and normal functioning. Personality disorders are often recognizable by adolescence or earlier, continue through adulthood and become less obvious in middle or old age. An individual may have more than one personality disorder at a time.

The common factor among individuals who have personality disorders, despite a variety of character traits, is the way in which the disorder leads to pervasive problems in social and occupational adjustment. Some individuals with personality disorders are perceived by others as overdramatic, paranoid, obnoxious or even criminal, without an awareness of their behaviors. Such qualities may lead to trouble getting along with other people, as well as difficulties in other areas of life and often a tendency to blame others for their problems. Other individuals with personality disorders are not unpleasant or difficult to work with but tend to be lonely, isolated or dependent. Such traits can lead to interpersonal difficulties, reduced self-esteem and dissatisfaction with life.

Causes of Personality Disorders

Different mental health viewpoints propose a variety of causes of personality disorders. These include Freudian, genetic factors, neurobiologic theories and brain wave activity.

Freudian. Sigmund Freud believed that fixation at certain stages of development led to certain personality types. Thus, some disorders as described in the *Diagnostic and Statistical Manual of Mental Disorders* are derived from his oral, anal and phallic character types. Demanding and dependent behavior (dependent and passive-aggressive) was thought to derive from fixation at the oral stage. Characteristics of obsessionality, rigidity and emotional aloofness were thought to derive from fixation at the anal stage; fixation at the phallic stage was thought to lead to shallowness and an inability to engage in intimate relationships. However, later researchers have found little evidence that early childhood events or fixation at certain stages of development lead to specific personality patterns.

Genetic Factors. Researchers have found that there may be a genetic factor involved in the etiology of antisocial and borderline personality disorders; there is less evidence of inheritance of other personality disorders. Some family, adoption and twin studies suggest that schizotypal personality may be related to genetic factors.

Neurobiologic Theories. In individuals who have borderline personality, researchers have found that low cerebrospinal fluid 5-hydroxyindoleacetic acid (5-HIAA) negatively correlated with measures of aggression and a past history of suicide attempts. Schizotypal personality has been associated with low platelet monoamine oxidase (MAO) activity and impaired smooth pursuit eye movement.

Brain Wave Activity. Abnormalities in electroencephalograph (EEG) have been reported in antisocial personality for many years; slow wave is the most widely reported abnormality. A study of borderline patients reported that 38 percent had at least marginal EEG abnormalities, compared with 19 percent in a control group.

Types of Disorders

According to the American Psychiatric Association's *Diagnostic and Statistical Manual of Mental Disorders* (4th ed., rev., 1994), or DSM-IV, personality disorders are categorized into three major clusters:

Cluster A: Paranoid, schizoid and schizotypal personality disorders. Individuals who have these disorders often appear to have odd or eccentric habits and traits.

Cluster B: Antisocial, borderline, histrionic and narcissistic personality disorders. Individuals who have these disorders often appear overly emotional, erratic and dramatic.

Cluster C: Avoidant, dependent, obsessive-compulsive and passive-aggressive personality disorders. Individuals who have these disorders often appear anxious or fearful.

The DSM-IV also lists another category, "personality disorder not otherwise specified," that can be used for other specific personality disorders or for mixed conditions that do not qualify as any of the specific personality disorders.

Individuals with diagnosable personality disorders usually have long-term concerns, and thus therapy may be long-term.

See also AVOIDANT PERSONALITY DISORDER; BORDERLINE PERSONALITY DISORDER; DEPENDENT PERSONALITY DISORDER; OBSESSIVE-COMPULSIVE DISORDER; PARANOID; PASSIVE-AGGRESSIVE PERSONALITY DISORDER.

American Psychiatric Association. *Diagnostic and Statistical Manual of Mental Disorders,* 4th ed., rev. Washington, D.C.: APA, 1994.

Andreasen, Nancy C., and Donald W. Black. *Introductory Textbook of Psychiatry.* Washington, D.C.: American Psychiatric Association, 1991.

personal space   The invisible zone of privacy unconsciously put between an individual and other people. Personal space is something rarely noticed, unless it is invaded by someone approaching too closely, in which case people may feel stressed and become anxious, irritated and even hostile.

According to Lisa Davis, in *In Health* (Sept./Oct. 1990), "we invite others into our personal space by how closely we approach them, the angle at which we face them, and the speed with which we break a gaze. It's a subtle code, but one we use and interpret easily and automatically, having absorbed the vocabulary since infancy."

Anthropologists have reported that people follow fairly established rules regarding how far apart they stand, largely depending on their relationship to each other. For example, friends, spouses, lovers, parents and children tend to stand inside a "zone of intimacy," or within arm's reach, while a personal zone (about four feet) is comfortable for conversation with strangers and acquaintances.

The amount for personal space needed depends on many variables, including the individual's cultural background, gender and the nature of the occasion. Individuals from North European or British ancestry usually want about a square yard of space for conversation in uncrowded situations. However, people from more tropical climates choose a smaller personal area and are more likely to reach out and touch the occupant of another space. In Mediterranean and South American societies, social conversations include much eye contact, touching and smiling, typically while standing at a distance of about a foot. In the United States, however, people usually stand about 18 inches apart for a social conversation; they tend to talk at arm's length, moving closer only to shake hands.

Understanding cultural and gender differences in interpretations of personal space is becoming more important as intercultural trade and business transactions escalate. The observation of personal space leaves much room for misinterpretation. Consultants have developed businesses to interpret for people of all nationalities the meaning and use of personal space in order to relieve the possibilities for occurrences of stressful situations. It is possible that a culture's use of space is evidence of a reliance on one sense over another. For example, Middle Easterners get much of their information through their senses of smell and touch, which require a close approach, while Americans rely primarily on visual information, backing up in order to see an intelligible picture.

See also ACCULTURATION; CROWDING; MIGRATION.

Davis, Lisa. "Where Do We Stand?" *In Health* (Sept./Oct., 1990).

Freedman, Jonathan L. *Crowding and Behavior.* New York: Viking Press, 1975.

Padus, Emrika, ed. *The Complete Guide to Your Emotions and Your Health,* rev. ed. Emmaus, Pa.: Rodale Press, 1994.

Pertofrane   Trade name for the tricyclic antidepressant drug desipramine.

See also ANTIDEPRESSANT MEDICATIONS; PHARMACOLOGICAL APPROACH; TRICYCLIC ANTIDEPRESSANTS.

perversion, sexual   A psychiatric term for a culturally, morally or legally unacceptable form of sexual behavior. The term applies to practices that deviate widely from the norm, such as sadomasochism, exhibitionism, necrophilia, coprophilia, zoophilia and pedophilia. However, the preferred term is paraphilia, because it seems less judgmental.

See also PARAPHILIAS.

pets   Pets reduce loneliness, provide companionship and give the owner a sense of order to his or her life. No matter how the owner may feel about other events in his life, the routine of caring for a pet provides a distraction from life's stresses and problems and draws the owner out of himself. Dog owners often find that no matter how little they may feel like exercising, the dog's need for walks forces them out. They end up feeling better for it and possibly meet neighbors and other dog walkers along the way.

Pets have been found to be so important to mental health that nursing homes and other institutions may have pets in residence or programs through which pets visit residents or patients. It has been observed that simply stroking a dog or cat can reduce blood pressure.

The world may not really be divided into "dog people" and "cat people," but sometimes it seems that way. Cat owners admire their pets' independence, graceful shape and movements and wild instincts. Since cats tend to require less human companionship than dogs, they are ideal for busy people who must be away from home for long periods of time. However, their owners must be people who can enjoy providing food and other care to animals that may seem to be aloof. Dogs, on the other hand, have been called the "yes men of the animal world." With their affectionate, emotional nature and appetite for food (regardless of whether they are really hungry or it is really good for them), they offer unconditional love and act out human behavior that their more inhibited masters can enjoy vicariously.

The death of a pet can be a devastating experience for one's mental health. Although a child who has lost a pet may be inconsolable for a time, in the end it may be an experience that leads to the child's maturity, since it is frequently the child's first brush with genuine loss. Adults who lose pets are often reluctant to express themselves freely about their sorrow because they fear that others will think their behavior is childlike and self-indulgent. However, the fact that veterinary hospitals now frequently send a sympathy card or letter of condolence on the death of a pet is an indication of the increasing awareness of the effect of an animal's loss.

PET scan   See BRAIN IMAGING; POSITRON EMISSION TOMOGRAPHY.

peyote   The primary active ingredient of the peyote cactus is the hallucinogen mescaline. Peyote can be found in the fleshy parts of this cactus plant; it is ground into a powder and then taken orally. Mescaline can also be produced synthetically. A typical dose of mescaline will produce illusions and hallucinations that last from five to 12 hours.

See also HALLUCINATION AND HALLUCINOGENS; MESCALINE.

Media Resource Guide on Common Drugs of Abuse. Public Relations Society of America, National Capital Chapter, Fairfax, Va., September 1990.

Phaedra complex   Sexual love of a mother for her son. The term is derived from the Greek myth about Phaedra, daughter of Minos and wife of Theseus, who was in love with her stepson, Hippolytus; when he rejected her, she accused him of violating her and hanged herself.

See also OEDIPUS COMPLEX.

phallic stage   The third stage of psychosexual development (according to psychoanalytic thinking), which occurs between ages three and six. At this time the child first focuses sexual feeling on the genital organs; masturbation becomes a source of pleasure. According to Sigmund Freud, the penis becomes the center of attention, for both boys and girls. During the phallic phase or stage, boys experience sexual fantasies toward mothers and rivalry toward fathers; they eventually give up both because of fear of castration. Similarly, girls experience sexual fantasies toward fathers and hostility toward mothers, because of rivalry and blaming mothers for depriving them of penises. Girls usually give up these feelings out of fear of losing the love of both parents. The American psychoanalyst Erik H. Erikson (1902–   ) suggested that when a child does not advance beyond the phallic stage to the genital stage, he or she may experience later guilt, role fixation and inhibition, which may lead to anxieties about sexual activity and sexual dysfunction.

See also ELECTRA COMPLEX; OEDIPUS COMPLEX.

phallic symbol   According to psychoanalytic theory, any object that resembles or represents the penis may be considered a phallic symbol. In dreams or in everyday life, structures that are longer than they are wide may be phallic symbols. Examples include trees, sticks, cigars, pencils, snakes, flutes and other musical instruments, such as clarinets or trombones.

See also PHALLIC STAGE; SEXUAL FEARS.

phallic woman   Traditionally, in psychoanalytic terms, a woman who is fixated at the phallic stage of development, who consciously seeks to deny that she lacks a penis or unconsciously wishes to castrate all men so that they will also be deprived of a penis. Feminist theorists tend to discount the entire concept, viewing women who are angry at men as reacting to a male-dominated social structure rather than to an anatomical difference.

See also CASTRATION; FREUD, SIGMUND.

phantom limb pain; phantom pain   According to the American Cancer Society, individuals who have had a limb (or a breast) surgically removed may experience pain as if it were coming from the absent limb. While physicians are not sure why this occurs, phantom limb pain exists and is not imaginary. Individuals experiencing this kind of pain become anxious, irritable and nervous because they often do not understand what is happening to them. There is no single method of relieving phantom pain in individuals who experience it. However, relaxation techniques are effective for many people.

phantom lover syndrome   A type of schizophrenic delusion in which a woman believes that an unknown man is in love with her.

See also SCHIZOPHRENIA.

pharmacokinetics   A term relating to how the body deals with a medication, such as how the drug is absorbed into the bloodstream, distributed to different tissues, broken down and excreted from the body. This is important in determining appropriate dosage and anticipating side effects and possible adverse drug effects. Pharmacokinetics of medications used for mental health disorders are important considerations for the prescribing physician.

pharmacological approach   The treatment of mental health disorders with prescription medications. In many cases, the pharmacological approach is used in combination with psychotherapy, behavior therapy or some of many complementary therapies. Prescription medications are often helpful for individuals who have agoraphobia, anxiety disorders, bipolar disorder, depression, panic attacks and panic disorder, obsessive-compulsive disorder, post-traumatic stress disorder, as well as other disorders. In many cases, use of meditation, biofeedback, guided imagery and relaxation therapy continue to be helpful after prescription medication is stopped.

In some cases, the pharmacological approach may be helpful for the short term. However, chronic conditions may require long-term management, often with a combination of complementary therapies and pharmacological therapies.

The best principle with pharmacological therapy is to use the lowest effective dose for the shortest possible period of time. However, before any medication is taken, an individual should have a thorough medical and psychiatric examination.

Categories of Medications

There are several major classes of medications used for anxiety disorders and depression covered in this book: *benzodiazepines (BZDs), cyclic antidepressants* and *noncyclic antidepressants*. Additionally, a number of pharmacological agents are categorized as "other antianxiety medications."

Alcohol is the oldest antianxiety drug, and it remains the most frequently used (and misused) nonspecific tranquilizer. Barbiturate drugs have been available since 1903; they are respiratory depressants and are contraindicated in people with respiratory insufficiency. In 1957 the first BZD, chlordiazepoxide (Librium), was introduced for the management of anxiety. Since then most antianxiety medications and sleeping medications are now benzodiazepines because of their relatively decreased toxicity in overdose.

See also AGORAPHOBIA; ALPRAZOLAM; ANTIDEPRESSANT MEDICATIONS; ANTIMANIC MEDICATIONS; ANTIPSYCHOTIC MEDICATIONS; ANXIETY DISORDERS; BARBITURATE DRUGS, BENZODIAZEPINE DRUGS; BIOFEEDBACK; BIPOLAR DISORDER; COMPLEMENTARY THERAPIES; DEPRESSION; GUIDED IMAGERY; HERBAL MEDICINE; MANIC-DEPRESSIVE DISORDER; MEDITATION; MIND/BODY CONNECTIONS; OBSESSIVE-COMPULSIVE DISORDER; PANIC ATTACKS AND PANIC DISORDER; POST-TRAUMATIC STRESS SYNDROME; PSYCHOTHERAPIES; RELAXATION; VALIUM.

Appleton, William S. *Prozac and the New Antidepressants: What You Need to Know About Prozac, Zoloft, Paxil, Luvox, Wellbutrin, Effexor, Serzone, and More.* New York: Plume, 1997.
Carlin, Peter. "Treat the Body, Heal the Mind." *Health* (Jan./Feb., 1997).
Kahn, Ada P. *Stress A to Z: A Sourcebook for Facing Everyday Challenges.* New York: Facts On File, 2000.
Sachs, Judith. *Nature's Prozac: Natural Therapies and Techniques to Rid Yourself of Anxiety, Depression, Panic Attacks and Stress.* Englewood Cliffs, N.J.: Prentice Hall, 1997.
Turkington, Carol. *Making the Prozac Decision: A Guide to Antidepressants.* Los Angeles: Lowell House, 1994.
Wilkinson, Beth. *Drugs and Depression.* New York: Rosen, 1994.

phencyclidine   See PCP.

phenelzine   Generic name for the monoamine oxidase inhibitor antidepressant medication marketed as Nardil.

See also ANTIDEPRESSANT MEDICATIONS; MONOAMINE OXIDASE INHIBITORS; PHARMACOLOGICAL APPROACH.

phenobarbital   A medication known as a barbiturate drug used mainly as an anticonvulsant drug, although its usage has largely been replaced by newer anticonvulsant drugs. It is still used in children who have epilepsy along with phenytoin. In some cases, it is prescribed as a sedative and may be combined with antispasmodic drugs for treating irritable bowel syndrome.

See also EPILEPSY; IRRITABLE BOWEL SYNDROME.

phenothiazine drugs   The name of a group of drugs classed as antipsychotics; they are sometimes called major tranquilizers.

These medications, which became available in the mid-1950s, created a pharmacologic revolution because they suppressed delusions, hallucinations, regression, withdrawal and agitated behavior that resulted in the chronic hospitalization of schizophrenics.

Although phenothiazine drugs were once thought to be safe, permanent neurological symptoms (tardive dyskinesia) have been linked to their long-term use. Examples of such drugs include chlorpromazine, thioridazine and trifluoperazine.

phobia   A persistent and irrational fear of a specific object or situation. Usually the phobia causes the individual to avoid the object or situation. Commonly, the term "phobia" is misused to refer to people who merely have a distaste for certain things or situations, such as snakes or crowded rooms. In a true phobia, there are physiological reactions that occur, despite the individual's attempts at controlling them. Some individuals are actually incapacitated by their phobias; for example, those who will not ride elevators cannot work in high-rise buildings, and those who fear dust live in sealed environments.

Phobias are included in a group of disorders known as anxiety disorders. These also include generalized anxiety disorder, panic disorders, obsessive-compulsive disorders and post-traumatic stress disorder.

Phobias are defined by psychological as well as physiological reactions. Symptoms may include feeling irrational panic or terror when in a harmless situation, recognizing that the fear goes beyond normal boundaries and the real threat of danger and that others do not perceive a danger. The reaction is automatic, uncontrollable and pervasive. The individual suffers from many physical reactions associated with extreme fear and has an overwhelming desire to avoid or escape from the situation. Avoidance is a characteristic of the lives of phobic people.

According to a recent study by the National Institute of Mental Health (NIMH), people of all ages, at all income levels and in all geographic locations suffer from phobias. Estimates are that between 5 and 12 percent of Americans suffer from phobias. They are more common among women than men.

Phobias can be divided into three basic categories. Specific phobias are the most common and involve fear of particular things, such as one type of animal (dogs, cats, snakes), or of particular situations (such claustrophobia, fear of being in an enclosed place, or acrophobia, fear of heights).

Social phobias include a wide variety of situations most people encounter in everyday life. Most people become somewhat anxious in certain situations, such as interviewing for a new job, having dinner at the boss's home or meeting new in-laws. However, for some people, these situations cause more than simple nervousness. They become so upset that they eventually begin to avoid the kinds of situations that cause them distress. The most prevalent social phobia seems to be a fear of public speaking. Fears of meeting new people, of being seen while eating or writing or of using public toilets are also common social phobias. Social phobias seem to stem from a fear of being scrutinized and possibly criticized by others. Social phobias affect men and women equally. Often a person with one social phobia will also have other social phobias, as most social phobias relate to a fear of embarrassment.

Another type of phobia is agoraphobia. This condition is really a fear of fear, although technically the word comes from the Greek term meaning "fear of the market-place." Agoraphobia involves fear of having a panic attack and being far from a source of help or assistance. There are aspects of fears of embarrassment; many agoraphobics fear throwing up in public or fainting. Some agoraphobics will venture out with the company of a trusted companion, in some cases a child or a dog.

Agoraphobia seems to be more prevalent in individuals from families where other members also have the disorder. Agoraphobia is often accompanied by alcoholism. Most agoraphobics develop symptoms between the ages of 19 and 35. More women than men have agoraphobia.

Causes of Phobias

Some phobias may result from learned responses; for example, children brought up by parents who fear dogs may learn to fear dogs themselves. Others result from a traumatic experience. For example, if a young child receives a painful bite from a dog, he or she may fear all dogs. However, for many individuals, there is no learned component, and there may actually be an aspect of brain chemistry that makes one individual more susceptible to acquiring phobias than others.

Often phobic people are also depressed. It is difficult to generalize whether the depression comes first or the phobia, but it is understandable that the person who reacts with unwanted extreme fear to certain situations and feels helpless may also feel depressed.

According to the American Psychiatric Association, phobias may develop as result of panic attacks. After a panic attack, the individual may fear a situation associated with the attack and begin to avoid it. Not all phobic people experience panic attacks.

Treatment

Individuals with phobias should understand that greater knowledge of phobias has been gained during the last few decades and that help is available and seek treatment. Many forms of therapy are used to treat phobic individuals, ranging from behavioral therapy to psychoanalysis. In behavioral therapy, the therapist focuses on the symptoms and attempts to change the physiological reactions, enabling the sufferer to face the feared situation. Many phobic people have good results with exposure therapy and desensitization to the feared object or situation. In psychoanalysis, the analyst may delve into the individual's past to determine the roots of the current problem. Relaxation therapy and psychopharmacotherapy are used in conjunction with other therapies. In some individuals, antianxiety drugs help them reduce the panic they feel when even thinking about a feared situation. With medication, such individuals can learn to face their phobic situation and overcome it. A variety of medications are used to treat phobic individuals. Some help some people, while others are useful to others. Pharmacologic treatment for phobias is a very individual matter.

In many cases, those with social phobias can improve themselves by concentrating on improving their social skills. When they gain confidence, they will not think so much about their possible blushing, sweating or appearing nervous to others.

Phobias can be treated by a qualified psychiatrist, psychologist, social worker or other mental health professional.

Reading material in the form of pamphlets are available from several sources.

For further information, contact:

American Psychiatric Association
1400 K Street NW
Washington, D.C. 20005
Phone: (888) 357-7294
Web site: www.psych.org

Anxiety Disorders Association of America
11900 Parklawn Drive, Suite 100
Rockville, MD 20852
Phone: (301) 231-9350
Fax: (301) 231-7392
Web site: www.adaa.org

National Mental Health Association
1021 Prince Street
Alexandria, VA 22314-2971
Phone: (800) 969-6642
Fax: (703) 684-5968
Web site: www.nmha.org

See also AGORAPHOBIA; ANXIETY DISORDERS; BEHAVIORAL THERAPY; SCHOOL PHOBIA.

American Psychiatric Association. *Diagnostic and Statistical Manual of Mental Disorders* 4th ed., rev. Washington, D.C., 1994.

Bourne, Edmund J. *The Anxiety & Phobia Workbook.* Oakland, Calif.: New Harbinger Publications, 1995.

Doctor, Ronald M., and Ada P. Kahn. *The Encyclopedia of Phobias, Fears, and Anxieties. 2nd ed.* New York: Facts On File, 2000.

Kahn, Ada P. and Ronald M. Doctor. *Facing Fears: The Sourcebook for Phobias, Fears, and Anxieties.* New York: Facts On File, 2000.

Monroe, Judy. *Phobias: Everything You Wanted To Know, But Were Afraid to Ask.* Springfield, N.J.: Enslow Publishers, 1996.

Nardo, Don. *Anxieties and Phobias.* New York: Chelsea House, 1992.

physician assisted suicide   See END OF LIFE ISSUES.

Pick's disease   A rare brain disease that closely resembles Alzheimer's disease and is usually difficult to diagnose clinically. Disturbances in personality, behavior and orientation may precede and initially be more severe than memory defects. Like Alzheimer's disease, a definitive diagnosis is usually obtained at autopsy.

See also ALZHEIMER'S DISEASE.

pineal gland   A pea-sized endocrine organ. It is located in the brain at the entrance to an important canal for the circulation of spinal fluid and has a role in controlling the flow of cerebrospinal fluid. The gland secretes the hormone melatonin for a fixed period every 24 hours, during darkness. The period is set by a biological clock that is light-sensitive. If there are eight hours of darkness, it can produce its quota. If there are only six, if falls short. Some researchers have tied seasonal affective disorder to melatonin because of the way the hormone is produced in the dark, particularly during winter.

Pinel, Philippe (1745–1826)   French physician considered to be the most revolutionary psychiatrist of the 18th century. Shocked by the public belief that mentally ill persons were "wild beasts possessed by the devil," and even more by the practice of keeping them in chains and dungeons, he instituted more humane practices at the major medical institutions in Paris, such as talking between the physician and patient, showing empathy and kindness and providing occupational therapy.

See also SEASONAL AFFECTIVE DISORDER.

Goldenson, Robert M., ed. *Longman Dictionary of Psychology and Psychiatry.* New York: Longman, 1984.

pituitary gland   A pea-sized endocrine gland near the base of the brain known as the master gland of the endocrine system because it is a source of a number of hormones, including the gonadotropic hormones. The gonadotropins which stimulate the gonads (ovaries in women and testicles in men) are LH (luteinizing hormone) and FSH (follicle stimulating hormone). In women, LH and FSH regulate ovulation; in men they regulate production of testosterone. The pituitary is a fairly remarkable gland, as it also regulates thyroid function and adrenal function in addition to playing a role in regulation of nursing and fluid balance in the body. The pituitary is in turn regulated by the hypothalamus, a portion of the brain involved in primitive functions.

Pituitary problems, such as benign growths that produce prolactin, another pituitary hormone, are quite common and can cause menstrual irregularities or amenorrhea, abnormal breast secretions and infertility problems, which may lead to stress and anxieties.

See also BRAIN; ENDOCRINE SYSTEM; HORMONES; HYPOTHALAMUS.

placebo; placebo effect   A substance used as a treatment that has no pharmacologic medicinal effect but that superficially resembles an active drug and is administered either as a control in testing new drugs or as a psychotherapeutic agent. Sometimes placebos induce reactions because of the power of suggestion. Individuals in a "double-blind" study do not know if they are taking a placebo or the real drug. The "placebo effect" refers to the therapeutic benefit of the chemically inactive substance. The word is derived from the Latin word meaning "I shall please."

play therapy   Use of play activities and materials, such as dolls, puppets, clay and finger paint in child psychotherapy. Such activities mirror children's emotional life and fantasies, enabling them to play out their feelings and problems and to test out new approaches and relationships in action. Play ther-apy is also referred to as analytical play therapy and ludotherapy.

pleasure principle   A psychiatric term referring to the inner force that motivates individuals to seek immediate gratification of instinctual impulses such as hunger, thirst, elimination and sex. According to Sigmund Freud, when these needs are not satisfied, people are in a state of tension. When they are fulfilled, reduction in tension evokes the experience of pleasure. The pleasure principle dominates the early life of the child but is later modified by the reality principle. The development of maturity has a great deal to do with the capacity to delay instant gratification.

PMS   See PREMENSTRUAL SYNDROME.

polysubstance dependence   Repeated use of three or more compounds by an individual. Usually no single agent predominates. Use of one substance greatly increases the chance of that person using another. Some compounds are deliberately combined to produce a desired effect, such as cocaine, amphetamines and heroin.

See also SUBSTANCE ABUSE.

pornography   Writing or drawing that some individuals find sexually arousing. The term is derived from the Greek, meaning "writing of harlots." Pornography is also known as psychological aphrodisiacs.

Throughout history, there have been laws about printing and distributing pornography, but this has always been fraught with the subjectivity in deciding what is or what is not pornography. However, in a general way, pornography can be divided into erotica—which is generally graphic about "normal" heterosexual love—and exotica, which centers on sexual practices outside the cultural norm, such as sadism, masochism and fetishism.

Pornography appears in the Old Testament and in the plays of Aristophanes. The term "pornography" is probably derived from the name Porneius, a character in Greek legend.

See also VICTORIANISM.

Hendrickson, Robert. *Facts On File Encyclopedia of Word and Phrase Origins*. New York: Facts On File, 1987.

positive reinforcement A term used in behavioral therapy referring to rewards that strengthen responses. On the other hand, a negative reinforcer, such as a punishment, diminishes the response. Positive reinforcement is more effective in sustaining behavior than is negative reinforcement. Failure to provide reinforcements will usually extinguish a behavior, and variable and unpredictable schedules of reinforcement may be more effective in maintaining behavior than fixed regular reinforcements. An example is the pathological gambler who receives the positive reinforcement of winning only occasionally but continues to gamble and is rarely deterred by loss of financial assets.

positron emission tomography (PET) A brain imaging technique to measure blood flow in areas of the brain using radioactive tracers or isotopes. The technique became available in the middle to late 1970s. A major application of PET is to the study of the neurochemical systems within the brain. For example, PET is useful in assessing the amount of a psychoactive drug in various parts of the brain, as well as physiological abnormalities.

PET is used with Alzheimer's disease patients; 70 to 80 percent of such patients show a characteristic decrease in metabolic function or cerebral blood flow in posterior temporoparietal regions. Schizophrenia, major depression, manic-depression, anxiety disorders and obsessive-compulsive disorders have all been found to show decreases or increases in blood flow and sugar metabolism in various areas of the brain.

PET may be particularly useful in differentiating Alzheimer's disease from other disorders that are present with confusion and intellectual deterioration.

See also ALZHEIMER'S DISEASE; BRAIN IMAGING.

Andreasen, Nancy C., and Black, Donald W. *Introduction to Psychiatry*. Washington, D.C.: American Psychiatric Association, 1991.

postpartum depression Some women experience postpartum depression, sometimes referred to as "maternity blues," after childbirth. While the new mother may be elated with her new baby, some of the mild depression may be attributed to the letdown after months of eager anticipation. Hormonal changes after the birth of a baby may also affect a woman's mood. For example, rapidly plummeting estrogen and progesterone can lead to hot flashes and irritability, similar to the phenomena associated with menopause. Sleep deprivation caused by a crying baby can also lead to irritability and depression.

Some women become depressed after childbirth because they fear being a parent, fear being a failure as a parent, feel less loving toward the baby than they think they should and feel less sexually attractive to their mates because their bodies have not regained their normal shape. Women may also feel a loss of self-esteem if they go from careers outside the home into full-time motherhood. Because of demands of new babies, women may feel exhausted, overwhelmed with chores and chronically fatigued. In addition, any stresses within marriage that existed before the birth of a baby may worsen after the baby's arrival.

The extent to which women experience postpartum depression may also depend on their support systems, including husbands, families and additional helpers in the household. A significant number of persistent, severe postpartum depressions become recurrent major depression or bipolar (manic-depressive) disorders requiring psychiatric treatment.

See also ANTIDEPRESSANT MEDICATIONS; CHILDBIRTH; DEPRESSION; PREGNANCY.

Holt, Linda H., M.D., Skokie, Ill. (personal interview).

postpartum psychosis When postpartum depression expands from mild depression to severe thought disorders and complete dissociation, the situation is called postpartum psychosis; it is also referred to as puerperal psychosis. A psychotic episode during the month after childbirth may be schizophrenic or depressive, not uncommonly the beginning of a depressive disorder brought about by the stresses of the pregnancy and delivery. It may be caused or aggravated by factors such as pre-existing personality defects, marital instability and financial burdens.

See also POSTPARTUM DEPRESSION.

post-traumatic stress disorder (PTSD) Anxiety disorder produced by an unusual and extremely stressful event, such as assault, or an act of violence, rape, natural disaster or physical injury. PTSD has been referred to as battle fatigue or shell shock when caused by military combat.

Often PTSD surfaces several months or even years later, although its symptoms can occur soon after the event. Sufferers characteristically reexperience the trauma in painful recollections or recurrent dreams or nightmares. Some have diminished emotional responsiveness ("numbing"), feelings of estrangement from others, insomnia, disturbed sleep, difficulty in concentrating or remembering, guilt about surviving when others did not, avoidance of activities that cause recollection of the traumatic event and intensive thoughts related to the event. Avoidance behavior also affects sufferers' relationships because they often avoid close emotional ties with family, colleagues and friends.

Sometimes the reexperience comes as a sudden, painful rush of emotions that seem to have no cause. These emotions may be anger or intense fear; some PTSD sufferers endure anxiety and panic attacks. During panic attacks, their throats tighten, breathing and heart rate increase, and they may feel dizzy and nauseous.

Witnessing a Crime

People witnessing a crime may be faced with a decision whether to come to the aid of the victim. Once the decision for involvement has been made, they may face the stress of being questioned by the police, exposed to threats or harassment from the associates or family of the criminal and harried by postponement and rescheduling of the trial with no regard for their work schedule and other personal responsibilities.

A decision not to become involved is often made. These people may feel that there are other witnesses to the crime, and they want to avoid a difficult and personally dangerous situation. Some of them may later feel the guilt of doing nothing, and they will experience extreme stress.

Watching a violent crime may also result in PTSD with symptoms of anxiety, nightmares, insomnia and other fears. Recovery can be aided with a variety of psychotherapies administered by professionals. Victim/Witness Assistance Programs, whose services include psychological counseling, have been initiated in some areas of the United States. During the trial, program administrators may make arrangements for witnesses to get in and out of court buildings with minimum public and media exposure, as well as intervene to the court on behalf of the witness when he or she is a victim of stressful threats or intimidation.

Overcoming PTSD

Individuals who have PTSD can learn to work through the trauma and pain and to resolve their anxieties. Individual psychotherapy is one of many useful therapies. PTSD results, in part, from the difference between the individual's personal values and the reality of what he or she witnessed or experienced during the traumatic event. Psychotherapy helps the individual examine his or her values and behavior, with the goal of resolving the conscious and unconscious conflicts that were created. Additionally, the individual works to build self-esteem and self-control, develops a reasonable sense of personal accountability and renews a sense of integrity and personal pride.

In many cases, family therapy is recommended because members of the family may affect and be affected by the PTSD sufferer. Some spouses and children report that their loved one does not communicate, show affection or share in family life. The therapist can help members of the family recognize and cope with the range of emotions they feel, and when needed, help them improve their communication skills and learn techniques for parenting and stress management.

A newer technique for PTSD involves "rap" groups, in which survivors of similar traumatic events are encouraged to share their experiences and reactions. Group members help each other realize that many people have gone through and experienced similar events and emotions. Over time, the members gain an improved self-image and self-esteem. Antidepressant medications have also been reported to reverse symptoms of PTSD.

For further information:

Anxiety Disorders Association of America
11900 Parklawn Drive, Suite 100
Rockville, MD 20852
Phone: (301) 231-9350
Fax: (301) 231-7392
Web site: www.adaa.org

National Association of Veterans Administration Chiefs of Psychiatry
54th Street and 48th Avenue
Minneapolis, MN 55417
Phone: (612) 725-6767

National Institute of Mental Health
6001 Executive Boulevard
Bethesda, MD 20892
Phone: (800) 421-4211
Web site: www.nimh.nih.gov

U.S. Veterans Administration
Mental Health and Behavioral Sciences Services
810 Vermont Avenue NW, Room 915
Washington, D.C. 20410
Telephone: (202) 389-3416

See also ANXIETY DISORDERS; BREATHING; COMMUNICATION; CONTROL; COPING; DREAMS; EMOTIONS; GUILT; LISTENING; PANIC ATTACKS AND PANIC DISORDER; PSYCHOTHERAPIES, SELF-ESTEEM.

Cremniter, Didier et al. "Post-traumatic reactions of hostages after an aircraft hijacking." *Journal of Nervous and Mental Disease* 185, no. 5 (May 1997): 344–346.
Husain, Syed Arshad et al. "Stress Reactions of Children and Adolescents in War and Siege Conditions." *American Journal of Psychiatry* 155, no. 12 (Dec. 1998): 1718–1719.
Kahn, Ada P. *Stress A to Z: A Sourcebook for Facing Everyday Challenges.* New York: Facts On File, 2000.
Kahn, Ada P., and Ronald M. Doctor. *Facing Fears: The Sourcebook of Phobias, Fears, and Anxieties.* New York: Facts On File, 2000.
Porterfield, Kay Marie. *Straight Talk About Post-Traumatic Stress Disorder: Coping with the Aftermath of Trauma.* New York: Facts On File, 1996.

powerlessness The perception that one's own actions will not significantly affect an outcome. A person who feels powerless may be unable to set goals and unable to follow through on activities relating to school, work or family life. For some individuals, feelings of powerlessness may underlie depression, suspiciousness and aggressive behavior. Powerlessness is associated with withdrawal, passivity, submissiveness, apathy and, in some individuals, increasing frustration, agitation, anxiety, aggression, acting-out behavior and even violence.

Powerlessness can be induced by illness and hospitalization, because such events compromise one's sense of independence and control. Powerlessness also arises from interpersonal interactions and lifestyle. Strategies to help an individual who feels powerless include enabling him or her to have control of a situation, to increase knowledge and to promote a sense of well-being.

McFarland, Gertrude K., and Mary Durand Thomas. *Psychiatric Mental Health Nursing.* Philadelphia: J. B. Lippincott, 1991.

prayer An act of an individual speaking to God in adoration, confession, supplication or thanksgiving. According to researchers, repeating a prayer can help reduce anxieties and improve the physical condition by lowering the heart rate, breathing rate and brain wave activity.

At a national conference on faith in Boston, Massachusetts, in 1995, experts said that the importance of prayer is gaining support among cost-conscious health organizations. "The supposed gulf between science and spirituality in healing does not always exist," said Herbert Benson, M.D., a professor at Harvard Medical School. Benson explained that scientific studies have demonstrated that by repeating prayers, words or sounds and passively disregarding other thoughts, many people are able to trigger a specific set of beneficial physiological changes. Studies show that this relaxation response decreased visits to health maintenance organizations by 36 percent.

Another internationally known authority in the field of mind/body medicine, Larry Dossey, M.D., said that the power of prayer to heal should no longer be regarded as just a matter of faith. Dossey, a physician who has practiced medicine for more than 20 years, has become a believer, not in religion, but in a growing body of research suggesting that prayer is an important scientifically verifiable factor in healing. "I have come to regard it as one of the best-kept secrets in medical science," he says in his book, *Healing Words: The Power and the Practice of Medicine.*

See also BENSON, HERBERT; COMPLEMENTARY THERAPIES; DOSSEY, LARRY; RELAXATION; RELIGION.

Dossey, Larry. *Healing Words: The Power of Prayer and the Practice of Medicine.* San Francisco: Harper, 1993.
———. *Meaning and Medicine: Lessons from a Doctor's Tales of Breakthrough and Healing.* N.Y.: Bantam, Doubleday, 1991.

prazepam   Generic name for the benzodiazepine drug Centrax.

See also BENZODIAZEPINE DRUGS; PHARMACOLOGICAL APPROACH.

prefrontal system   One of the largest cortical subregions of the human brain, also known as the prefrontal cortex. It may constitute nearly a third of the human brain and receives connections from all over it.

The prefrontal areas have to do with motivation and initiative, as well as appreciation of the future consequences of behaviors or acts. Damage to the frontal lobes via head trauma, brain degeneration, tumors, strokes or chronic alcohol toxicity can cause marked behavioral changes and symptoms of apathy, with lack of spontaneous behavior. It can also cause a state of euphoria, with a deterioration of behavior including inappropriate sexual behavior or deterioration of personal habits.

See also BRAIN.

pregenital phase   A term for the stages of psychosexual development before the stages when the penis and clitoris become the central erogenous zones and when the sex organs begin to exert a dominant influence. The pregenital phase includes the first stages of sexuality, when the individual concentrates on the mouth, anus and urethra rather than the genital organs.

See also PSYCHOSEXUAL DEVELOPMENT.

pregnancy   Pregnancy evokes many mental health and physiological issues. Some women experience frequent mood swings, ranging from crying to euphoria, and many have exciting or frightening dreams, sometimes involving the unborn child. Emotional changes are due to hormonal as well as emotional adjustments involved in pregnancy.

Both parents as well as extended family make many psychological adaptations to pregnancy. An important influence on the progress of the pregnancy is the presence of a supportive emotional environment. For example, if there have been multiple previous pregnancies, the attitude toward the current pregnancy will be affected. The parents' attitude toward the pregnancy will also be influenced by factors such as whether the child was wanted or not, if an abortion had been attempted or considered or if there are hereditary disorders in the family. However, these anxieties usually are replaced by positive feelings as signs of life are experienced and the pregnancy progresses.

For many women, an early symptom of pregnancy is morning sickness, which is sometimes considered "imaginary" but is a very real problem for sufferers. Nausea during the first months of pregnancy may be due to a low level of vitamin B6 or may occur because of the natural slowing down of a pregnant woman's digestive process. When food remains undigested in the stomach for longer periods than normal, nausea and the urge to vomit occur. Morning sickness usually diminishes or disappears by the time the pregnancy is in the fourth month.

How a woman copes with pregnancy depends largely on the woman and her husband's attitude toward pregnancy. While most couples have a positive outlook, sometimes pregnancy occurs to please others, such as grandparents, or with the wish to be nurtured oneself. In some cases, conception occurs in an attempt to save a marriage that is dysfunctional or to deal with anxiety about sterility. At the time the new mother begins to feel the infant's movement, ambivalence about becoming pregnant may become apparent.

Many women cope with the psychological stresses of pregnancy better when they begin participating in "prepared childbirth" classes offered by many hospitals, which teach prospective parents about the physiological changes that occur during pregnancy and labor. Some classes provide exercises to help the new mothers learn to relax and reduce tension. For example, the Lamaze method, named for a French obstetrician, involves learning breathing, relaxing and massage routines for the mother and her coaching partner.

Men and Pregnancy

Couvade (from the French word for hatching) is the term applied to the range of sympathetic physical changes men go through during their wives' pregnancy. Some men actually experience symptoms such as nausea, fatigue, backache and weight gain as a result of the emotional conflicts of imminent fatherhood. Some cultures developed elaborate rituals to help men through these difficult times. In Western cultures, however, men have a role in pregnancy and often participate in prenatal education classes and the birth even itself.

Assisted Pregnancy

Pregnancy and motherhood without marriage has become more culturally acceptable in some Western countries. Couples who cannot conceive can now become parents with the use of "assisted reproductive" techniques, including in vitro fertilization and artificial insemination. Surrogate motherhood is also gaining some degree of acceptance, despite legal complications. Women who delay motherhood into their late thirties or early forties because of their own or their husbands' careers or because of the attraction of the single life face diminished fertility and greater anxiety about the possibility of birth defects that come with increased maternal age. However, amniocentesis (testing the amniotic fluid to detect abnormalities in the fetus) allays some fears of women who postpone motherhood.

Baby Blues

Subsequent endocrine changes after childbirth, as well as fatigue from being awakened during the night to feed the newborn, often lead to postpartum depression or "baby blues." Some women become weepy a few days after giving birth. Some who experience clinical depressive symptoms may feel withdrawn and partially reject the infant. This response may become evident in difficulties in feeding and patterns of mother-child interaction. In most cases, postpartum depression does not last more than two weeks. However, if it persists longer, professional help should be sought. A woman may develop irrational fears, despair and hopelessness and may have ideas involving violent anger toward the new baby.

Fears Involving Pregnancy

Fears of pregnancy stem from both psychological and physical sources. Some examples include unmarried women who fear conceiving and bearing a child out of wedlock; married women who do not want the burden of a child; women who fear the pain of childbirth or fear that they might die during pregnancy; and some who fear the interruption in their work and physical activity. Some women fear that their pregnant physical appearance will be unattractive to their husbands, and some fear that they will never return to their original physical appearance.

Many women become anxious and embarrassed by the physical symptoms associated with pregnancy. Morning sickness, food cravings, frequent urination, water retention, bloating and swollen breasts are frequent complaints. First-time mothers fear that they may not be able to recognize the first movements of the fetus and as a result may worry that the baby is abnormal or dead. While some mothers fear weight gain during pregnancy, others feel that they are not gaining enough. Recent findings about effects on the fetus of the mother's smoking and alcohol consumption have caused many pregnant women to abstain out of fear that they will have an unhealthy baby.

Pregnancy and Sexual Intercourse

Psychological stress arises for many couples during pregnancy when they become concerned about the advisability of continuing sexual intercourse during pregnancy. Although this is an individual matter for each couple, it causes stress in many relationships, as both partners may fear hurting the fetus, and the male may fear hurting the woman. However, depending on the course of the pregnancy, gynecologists usually allow women who have no unusual vaginal discharges, pain or other symptoms to continue sexual relations until the seventh month. In later months, modifications of coital position are suggested to assure that intercourse will not harm the baby or cause a miscarriage.

See also BONDING; CHILDBIRTH; COUVADE; POSTPARTUM DEPRESSION.

Davis, Kenneth; Howard Klar and Joseph T. Coyle. *Foundations of Psychiatry.* Philadelphia: W. B. Saunders, 1991.

Eisenberg, Arlene; Heidi Eisenberg Murkoff and Sandee Eisenberg Hathaway. *What to Expect When You're Expecting.* New York: Workman Publishing, 1984.

Rockwell, Beverly. "Expectant Fathers: Changes and Concerns." *Canadian Family Physician* 35 (May 1989).

premenstrual depression   Many women experience irritability and depressed feelings before menstrual periods. In recent years, researchers have been considering premenstrual depression as part of premenstrual syndrome (PMS) and are looking into causes and relationships to depressive disorders. Researchers at the National Institute of Mental Health have noted that in some women, premenstrual depression is a cyclical problem, as is seasonal affective disorder (SAD), which is more common among women than men. Both may be biologically linked. Symptoms of premenstrual syndrome (PMS) and SAD are similar, in that women feel lethargic and may oversleep or overeat. Some have more premenstrual symptoms seasonally, primarily during the winter, during which time they are depressed only when they are premenstrual. Light therapy that helps sufferers of SAD may also be helpful for premenstrual depression.

See also ANTIDEPRESSANT MEDICATIONS; DEPRESSION; PREMENSTRUAL SYNDROME; SEASONAL AFFECTIVE DISORDER.

premenstrual syndrome (PMS)   The recurrence of symptoms in the 14 days (or less) prior to menstruation with absence of symptoms after menstruation. Discomforts that may occur before a menstrual period include water retention, tender breasts, headaches, body aches, food cravings, lethargy and depression. Asthma, herpes, acne, baby battering, epilepsy and mood swings have little in common, but they all have a connection if they recur at the same time in each menstrual cycle. Until the 1970s or 1980s, many women experiencing these symptoms were told that they were imagining them. The medical profession did not recognize the constellation of symptoms as a "syndrome"; consequently, many women became even more stressed by lack of help from physicians and lack of understanding by family members.

There is no single definitive test to diagnose PMS, but there are ways to determine if it is present. Mainly, it is the perception of the woman and her family and a confirmation of the cyclical nature of the symptoms by "charting" them each month. The severity of symptoms may vary from one cycle to the next, but the main symptoms will remain the same.

Causes of premenstrual syndrome have not been determined and vary from woman to woman. Symptoms occurring several days before menstruation seem to be related to the interrelationships of hormones between ovulation and the beginning of menstruation.

The medical profession's attitude that the discomfort of PMS was "all in the mind" increased anxiety for many women. Attitudes are changing and PMS is now a recognized physical condition, but there is still some reluctance to take it seriously. Although there is no single successful treatment for PMS, many doctors now regard it as a challenging problem in need of solution. A variety of treatments, such as hormones, vitamins, analgesics and diuretics, have been tried with varying degrees of success.

During the 1980s and 1990s, many women suffering from PMS found practitioners within women's health centers sympathetic and interested in treating these problems. Women who once worried that they were "going crazy" before their menstrual period have now learned new ways of coping with their symptoms through a combination of diet, medication, exercise and counseling.

See also MENSTRUATION.

Lever, Judy, and Michael G. Brush. *Pre-menstrual Tension.* New York: McGraw-Hill, 1981.

primal anxiety A psychiatric term referring to the most basic form of anxiety that the infant first experiences during separation from the mother when he faces new stimuli in the real world.

primal fantasies Children often fantasize about conception, birth, sexual intercourse by their parents and castration. Children do this to fill the gaps in their knowledge. Many such unconscious fantasies are revealed in dreams and daydreams.

primal scene The sexual act between parents. Early psychoanalysts believed that witnessing the parent in a sex act would trigger a crisis in sexuality in the child. However, more recent theories have discounted the significance of this experience, pointing out that in most places in the world entire families share a room, with little evidence that children suffer sexual trauma or confusion resulting from this lack of privacy. Nonetheless, Western culture usually downplays parental sexuality in front of children.

See also PRIMAL THERAPY.

primal scream therapy See PRIMAL THERAPY.

primal therapy Primal therapy (also known as primal scream therapy) is used to treat some mental dysfunctions, including anxieties about sexuality, by encouraging the individual to relive basic or "primal" traumatic events and let go of associated painful emotions. Such events may have led to development of anxieties and frequently involve feelings of abandonment or rejection experienced in infancy or early childhood. The technique was developed by Arthur Janov (1924–), an American psychologist and author of *The Primal Scream* (1970). During therapy, the individual may scream or cry and afterward feel that the "primal pain" has been released.

See also PRIMAL SCENE.

primary depression Depression in which one's mood is unrelated to a preexisting mental disorder or to a physical condition, substance abuse disorder or a medication. Primary depressions occur in individuals with no previous history of any other mental illness. Primary depression is divided into unipolar and bipolar depressions. Some individuals with primary depression complain of a sad, blue, low mood; others also complain of hopelessness, helplessness, irritability, fearfulness and anxiety.

Sufferers complain of loss of interest in normal activities, diminished pleasurable experiences, withdrawal from other people and recurrent thoughts of death or suicide. Individuals who have primary depression may also have physical symptoms such as headache, fatigue, palpitations, gastrointestinal disturbances and weight loss.

procreation fantasy Imagined or fantasized participation in sexual reproduction, for example, by women who experience a false pregnancy. In men, a common procreation fantasy is playing the role of a father who begets a famous offspring.

See also FANTASY.

prodrome An early symptom of a mental or physical illness that serves as a warning sign that may lead to preventive measures. The word comes from the Greek word *prodromos,* which means "running before." An example of a prodrome, or prodromal sign, is the beginning of withdrawal from social activities by a depressed person. A prodromic dream is one that contains a warning of impending disorder.

prognosis Prediction of the future course, severity, duration and outcome of a disease or mental disorder. A prognostic test forecasts results of education or training for a specific skill.

progressive muscle relaxation A stress management technique in which individuals learn to make heightened observations of what goes on in their bodies. They learn to control all of the skeletal muscles so that any portion can be systematically relaxed or tensed by choice.

First, there is recognition of subtle states of tension. When a muscle contracts (tenses), waves of neural impulses are generated and carried to the brain along neural pathways. This muscle-neural phenomenon is an observable sign of tension.

Next, having learned to identify the tension sensation, the individual learns to relax it. Relaxation is the elongation (lengthening) of skeletal muscle fibers, which then eliminates the tension sensation. This general procedure of identifying a local state of tension, relaxing it away and making the contrast between the tension and ensuing relaxation is then applied to all of the major muscle groups.

As a stress management technique, progressive relaxation is only effective when individuals have the ability to selectively elongate their muscle fibers on command. They can then exercise the self-control required for progressive relaxation and more rationally deal with the stressful situation.

See also BIOFEEDBACK; COMPLEMENTARY THERAPIES; RELAXATION.

Jacobsen, E. *Progressive Relaxation,* 2nd ed. Chicago: University of Chicago Press, 1983.
———. "The Origins and Development of Progressive Relaxation." *Journal of Behavior Therapy and Experimental Psychiatry* 8 (1977): 119–123.
Lehrer, Paul M., and Robert L. Woolfolk, eds. *Principles and Practice of Stress Management,* 2nd ed. New York: The Guilford Press, 1993.

projection   A defense mechanism one uses unconsciously that involves blaming somebody else for one's own thoughts or actions. The individual unknowingly rejects emotionally unacceptable thoughts, attributing (projecting) them to others.

See also DEFENSE MECHANISMS.

prolactin   A substance secreted by the anterior pituitary, possibly with a circadian rhythm. It is released in response to suckling, physical and emotional stress, hypoglycemia and estrogen administration. Prolactin inhibitory factors (PIF) and prolactin releasing factors (PRF) are secreted at the hypothalamic level. Dopamine stimulates PRF secretion, whereas serotonin inhibits it. Studies of PRF secretion have been used to research the pathophysiology of affective disorders and schizophrenia.

Some women experience amenorrhea because of increased prolactin thought to be produced in the pituitary gland. This condition may also be caused by psychotropic medications such as neuroleptics. When occurring simultaneously, it can be diagnosed and treated by a general physician or specialist in endocrinology.

See also PITUITARY GLAND; SEROTONIN; PHARMACOLOGIC THERAPY; SCHIZOPHRENIA.

pro-life and pro-choice   Terms for individuals who oppose abortion (pro-life) and those who favor giving women the option of abortion (pro-choice). Pro-life advocates believe in a general set of values regarding the value of all human life. Pro-choice advocates believe their position supports a woman's civil rights. During the 2000s, controversy between these groups continues.

See also ABORTION; *ROE V. WADE.*

Prolixin   Trade name for fluphenazine, an antipsychotic drug.

See also PHENOTHIAZINE DRUGS.

promazine   An antipsychotic drug of the phenothiazine class used in some patients as a sedative. In some cases, after anesthesia, it is used to relieve nausea and vomiting (antiemetic).

See also PHENOTHIAZINE DRUGS.

promiscuity   The term given to certain sexual behavior of men or women; the term is somewhat judgmental, and the definition has changed over a period of years, particularly after the "sexual revolution" of the 1960s. In the United States today, however, the most commonly held attitude is that a person is generally considered promiscuous if he or she has sexual intercourse with several casual acquaintances over a short period of time. Premarital intercourse with one partner is not considered promiscuous. Promiscuous behavior has been discouraged to a great extent because of the increase in sexually transmitted diseases and AIDS. It appears that since the emergence of the AIDS epidemic, promiscuous sexual behavior among homosexual people has reduced.

See also ACQUIRED IMMUNODEFICIENCY SYNDROME; PEER GROUP; SAFE SEX; SEXUALLY TRANSMITTED DISEASES.

propranolol A medication in the family of beta blocking agents commonly used to treat high blood pressure, migraine headaches and some heart conditions. In some individuals, it is prescribed to reduce rapid heartbeat (tachycardia) and general nervousness associated with anxiety disorders. In other cases, it is prescribed to help control symptoms of stage fright and fears of public appearances. Many patients tolerate it well because it has few side effects. However, possible side effects include dizziness, slow pulse, sleep difficulties, diarrhea, coldness, numbness and/or tingling of fingers or toes. Individuals who have chronic lung disease, asthma, diabetes or certain heart diseases and those who are severely depressed should not take propranolol.

See also HEADACHES.

proprietary A medication for which one company holds a patent for production. This differs from a generic drug, which may be manufactured by other companies without a patent.

See also ETHICAL DRUG.

prostitution A service providing sexual activity based on payment of money or exchange of other property or valuables. The term can apply to male and female, heterosexuals and homosexuals. The service may be sexual intercourse or performance of acts that gratify sexual deviations, or paraphilias.

Fear of prostitutes is known as cyprianophobia. At the end of the 20th century, this fear has increased because of the risk of contracting a sexually transmitted disease or the AIDS virus. In many parts of the world, these diseases are found in epidemic proportions among prostitutes.

Kahn, Ada P., and Linda Hughey Holt. *The A to Z of Women's Sexuality.* Alameda, Calif.: Hunter House, 1992.

protriptyline Generic name for the tricyclic antidepressant medication marketed under the trade name Vivactil.

See also ANTIDEPRESSANT MEDICATIONS; PHARMACOLOGICAL APPROACH; TRICYCLIC ANTIDEPRESSANTS.

Prozac The trade name for an antidepressant drug (fluoxetine) that has been available since the late 1980s. It is part of a class of selective serotonin reuptake inhibitors (SSRIs) with low toxicity and free of many side effects attributed to tricyclic antidepressants. Fluoxetine is not a sedative, has no anticholinergic side effects and does not promote weight gain. Side effects may include possible nausea and weight loss—both usually time limited—insomnia and anxious agitation that occurs rarely and is dose-related. Most people adjust to these side effects.

See also SELECTIVE SEROTONIN REUPTAKE INHIBITORS (SSRIs).

Doctor, Ronald M., and Ada P. Kahn. *Encyclopedia of Phobias, Fears, and Anxieties.* New York: Facts On File, 2000.

pseudodementia A condition that sometimes accompanies depressive illness, which should be differentiated from dementia. In this disturbance, the depressed person seems to be demented. He or she is unable to remember correctly, cannot calculate well and complains of lost cognitive abilities and skills. The pseudodemented person has a treatable illness and is not truly demented. The "dementia" is usually caused by the depressive illness.

See also DEMENTIA; DEPRESSION.

psyche A term derived from the ancient Greek word for soul or spirit. It refers to the mind as opposed to the body. According to Sigmund Freud, the psyche could be divided into the conscious and the unconscious. The prefix "psych-" is derived from this word.

See also PSYCHIATRIST; PSYCHOLOGIST; PSYCHOLOGY.

psychedelic Drugs that are capable of producing altered states of awareness that may be marked by an unstable flow of ideas and moods, distorted perceptions, hallucinations or symptoms that mimic signs of mental disturbances observed in psychotic patients. Examples of psychedelic drugs are lysergic acid diethylamide (LSD) and mescaline.

The Multidisciplinary Association for Psychedelic Studies (MAPS) is a membership based nonprofit research and educational organization that assists scientists with designing, obtaining approval for, funding, conducting and reporting on research into the health and spiritual potentials of psychedelics and marijuana.

For information:

Multidisciplinary Association for Psychedelic
  Studies
2105 Robinson Avenue
Sarasota, FL 34232
Web site: maps.org
E-mail: info@maps.org

See also HALLUCINATIONS; LYSERGIC ACID DIETHYLAMIDE.

psychiatrist   A physician (medical doctor with an M.D. degree) who specializes in the diagnosis and treatment of mental health and emotional disorders. Psychiatrists can prescribe medications and can admit patients to hospitals.

In 1995, there were an estimated 33,486 psychiatrists in the United States, and the number has been increasing since then. Approximately 75 percent of psychiatrists in the American Psychiatric Association were men, yet psychiatry ranked high among medical specialties in the proportion of women and in the number of women practitioners. The number of women physicians choosing psychiatric careers has increased in recent years, as suggested by the greater proportion of women than men in psychiatry who are younger than 40 years of age.

The distribution of psychiatrists varies considerably within the United States, but averages 11.3 per 100,000 individuals ranging from 4.5 per 100,000 resident population in Mississippi to more than 25.8 per 100,000 in Massachusetts and 50.9 per 100,000 in the District of Columbia. Generally, the New England and the Middle Atlantic states have the most psychiatrists per population; the least are in the East South Central and the West South Central states. The Center for Mental Health Services calculated that 90.5 percent of the clinically trained psychiatrists in the United States are clinically active, though the percentage varies among the states. As of 1996 the American Psychiatric Association consisted of 76 percent of members who are

white, 7.6 percent who are a Asian, 4.4 percent who are Hispanic, 1.7 who are African American and .1 percent who are American Indian.

Psychiatrists practice within several theoretical frames of reference. Various approaches offer differing explanations of how symptoms or disorders develop, how they interfere with an individual's functioning and how and why they can be altered by interventions.

Today most psychiatrists are trained in a variety of diagnostic possibilities and treatments, including psychodynamic psychotherapy. There is also a stronger medical emphasis because of the rapid development of techniques of psychopharmacology, which require a knowledge of pharmacology, physiology, cardiology and endocrinology, all subjects taught in medical training. Recent advances in neuroscience as it relates to behavior have provided a strong medical as well as psychosocial focus for psychiatry, which now spans these areas of knowledge. According to data collected by the American Medical Association on the Physician's Professional Activities Census, approximately 6 percent of all U.S. physicians designate their specialty as psychiatry or child and adolescent psychiatry.

In addition to providing direct patient care, many psychiatrists devote some time to other professional activities such as administration, medical teaching and research. Many work in more than one setting during the week, according to data from the 1996 National Survey of Psychiatric Practice. Many psychiatrists are likely to devote at least part of their practice hours to salaried and managed care settings, including health maintenance organizations, preferred provider organizations and large hospital systems.

Cooperation and consultation between psychiatrists, primary care physicians and other providers continues to be important for the provision of comprehensive care to patients. Especially in rural areas, primary care providers are critical gatekeepers for the diagnosis and treatment of mental health problems. The detection of mental disorders and the treatment of the less severe disorders, including the prescription of medications, often take place in a primary medical setting. Primary care physicians, however, are less likely than psychiatrists to treat patients with serious or complex mental disorders, such as patients with dual diagnoses or coexistence of psychiatric and medical illnesses. Primary care physicians are more likely to prescribe medications for anxiety, while psychiatrists are more likely to prescribe drugs for depression.

psychic vaginismus   A painful vaginal spasm that prevents sexual intercourse, due to psychological rather than physiological causes.

See also DYSPAREUNIA; VAGINISMUS; SEXUAL DYSFUNCTION.

psychoactive drug   One of many chemical compounds that affect thought processes and mood. These drugs have been subject to both appropriate and inappropriate uses. Psychoactive drugs may make one more relaxed or more active. Antidepressant drugs and tranquilizers are two examples of psychoactive drugs. Alcohol is also considered a psychoactive drug. Psychoactive drugs are prescribed for a wide range of mental health disorders, including depression, anxieties and phobias.

It is possible to develop a dependency on one or more psychoactive substances prescribed by a physician. Close monitoring by a physician is necessary when taking psychoactive drugs.

See also ANTIDEPRESSANT MEDICATIONS.

psychoanalysis   The original mode of treatment for mental health disorders developed by Sigmund Freud and his followers. It aims to reorganize character structure, with an emphasis on self-understanding and a correction of developmental lags. Symptom relief usually occurs as a result of this understanding, but it is usually not the immediate goal of the treatment.

Psychoanalysis is practiced by clinicians who have undergone specialized training in this after residency training. Individuals who practice psychoanalysis are not necessarily medical doctors, but they must pass certain examinations given by many centers throughout the world. Analysts use features of free association, dream analysis and the development and working through of transference distortions in the relationship with the analyst. Sessions are usually held four or five times a week, and a completed analysis generally takes three to five years, but length of treatment varies considerably with the nature of the problems being treated.

The American Psychoanalytic Association has more than 3,400 members, and the International Psychoanalytical Association numbers over 10,100.

According to a report in *Psychiatric News* (Sept. 6, 1991), the nature of psychoanalysis is changing to include multiple theoretical viewpoints that work synergistically. There is a proliferation of psychoanalytic publications dealing with clinical and theoretical issues, as well as the application of psychoanalytic study to other fields such as history, literature, anthropology and art.

See also FREUD, SIGMUND; PSYCHOTHERAPIES.

psychobiology   An approach in which the individual is viewed as an integrated unit, and both normal and abnormal behavior are explained in terms of biological, sociological and psychological determinants. Symptoms are seen as real but distorted attempts at adjustment; these symptoms can be understood as such by observing the patient in everyday activity and by compiling a biographical report (anamnesis) based on all phases of his or her history—physical and mental, conscious and unconscious.

psychodrama   An adjunct to psychotherapy in which the patient acts out certain roles or incidents; this is sometimes useful for individuals trying to overcome the serious effects of stresses in their lives. The roles or incidents may or may not be related to people closely involved with the individual or situations that they find particularly stressful.

The purpose of psychodrama is to bring out hidden concerns and to allow expression of a person's disturbed feelings. Therapeutic value comes from the release of pent-up emotions and from insights into the way other people feel and behave. Psychodrama is often carried out with a partner or in a group. In many cases, use of music, dance and pantomine may be included.

The technique was developed by J.L. Moreno, a Viennese psychiatrist, in 1921. Psychodrama is considered an early form of group therapy or group psychotherapy.

See also COMPLEMENTARY THERAPIES; DANCE THERAPY; PSYCHOTHERAPIES.

psychogenic A disorder caused by a mental rather than a physical disturbance. For example, some sexual dysfunctions are of psychogenic origins.

See also SEX THERAPY.

psychogenic amnesia Memory loss from psychological causes. The disorder is defined as a single episode of sudden inability to recall important information, a loss too extensive to be explained by ordinary forgetfulness. This has been reported to occur after severe physical or psychosocial stressors, for example after war or a fire. In a study of combat veterans, 5 to 10 percent were amnestic for their combat experiences, and 5 to 14 percent of all military psychiatric casualties have amnestic syndromes.

See also AMNESIA; POST-TRAUMATIC STRESS DISORDER.

Andreasen, Nancy C., and Donald W. Black. *Introductory Textbook of Psychiatry.* Washington, D.C.: American Psychiatric Association, 1991.

psychogenic fugue A mental health disorder in which there is sudden unexpected travel away from home or customary workplace with the assumption of a new identity and an inability to recall the previous identity. The disturbance is not due to multiple personality disorder or to an organic mental disorder. The fugue may follow a severe psychosocial stress, is usually brief (hours or days) and involves only limited travel, but rarely it may extend for months and involve complex travel. Significant alcohol use seems to predispose to this disorder.

This disorder should be distinguished from multiple personality disorder, which more typically involves repeated shifts of identity—more than a single episode—and a history of identity disturbances since childhood. Psychogenic amnesia usually lacks purposeful travel or the assumption of a new identity.

See also PSYCHOGENIC AMNESIA.

Amchin, Jess. *Psychiatric Diagnosis: A Biopsychosocial Approach Using DSM-III-R.* Washington, D.C.: American Psychiatric Press, 1990.

psycho-imagination therapy (PIT) A process with major emphasis on subjective meaning through use of waking imagery and imagination to effect personality changes. The basic proposition of psycho-imagination therapy recognizes the individual's needs to become aware of how he defines himself in relation to others and how he thinks others define him. A person's imagery, more than any other mental function, indicates how he or she views the world. Use of systematically categorized imagery can open up the inner world to both patient and therapist. The technique was developed in 1965 by Joseph E. Shorr, an American psychologist, and is theoretically related to the interpersonal school of psychoanalysis that stems from the work of Harry Stack Sullivan (1892–1949), an American psychiatrist and dissenter of Sigmund Freud. Many psychotherapists use aspects from several different schools of thought.

See also PSYCHOTHERAPIES.

psychological tests There are many tests commonly used for diagnostic purposes. Some are used by therapists, while others are used by human resource departments as part of preemployment screening of applicants.

Usually devised by psychologists, such tests are designed to determine qualities of the applicant's or client's personality and the suitability of the individual for the assignment.

See also PSYCHOLOGIST; PSYCHOLOGY.

psychologist A nonmedical specialist in diagnosing and treating mental health concerns. In most states, a psychologist has a Ph.D. degree from a graduate program in psychology. Psychologists are licensed, receive insurance reimbursement, have hospital privileges and act as expert witnesses in court cases.

Prior to World War II, psychologists were primarily involved in academic institutions, with only a few individuals employed outside universities and actively engaged in mental health services. Not until 1977—with the passage of the Missouri psychology licensure act—did all 50 states and the District of Columbia grant statutory recognition to the profession. Since that time, the number of licensed psychologists has grown, rising from an estimated 20,000 in 1975 to almost 46,000 only 10 years later.

Along with this dramatic growth in the population of practitioners was a significant expansion in psychologists' role as direct mental health providers. Today, psychologists are involved in almost every type of mental health setting, including institutional or community-based, research- or treatment-oriented and general health- or mental health-focused. Within these environments, psychologists' roles have also expanded beyond traditional activities of diagnostic assessment and psychotherapy to include primary prevention, community-level intervention strategies, assessment of service delivery systems and client advocacy.

Within psychology, there are many sub-specialties. These include child, developmental, school, clinical, social and industrial. Many psychologists have private practices, are employed by a health care facility and teach in universities.

Psychologists cannot prescribe medications. They usually refer patients requiring medication to a physician.

See also PSYCHOLOGY.

psychology The study of all processes of the mind, such as memory, feelings, thought and perception, as well as intelligence, behavior and learning. Within the field, many different approaches are applied. For example, behavioral psychology studies the way people react to events and adapt accordingly; neuropsychology relates human behavior to brain and body functions; and psychoanalytic psychology emphasizes the role of the unconscious and experiences of childhood.

Subdivisions in the American Psychological Association's designated areas of specialization include medical, child, industrial, social and animal-experimental psychology.

See also BEHAVIORAL THERAPY.

psychometry The measurement of psychological functions, using devices such as intelligence tests, personality tests and specific aptitude tests. While such tests have been refined since the earlier versions, the validity of such tests is still questionable.

See also INTELLIGENCE; PERSONALITY.

psychoneuroimmunology (PNI) Psychoneuroimmunology is a relatively new branch of science that studies the interrelationships among the mind (psycho), the nervous system (neuro) and the immune system (immunology). The aim of this field is to investigate and document interrelationships between psychological factors and the immune and neuroendocrine systems. Research efforts include looking at the effects of emotional stress on the immune system and health. In a general way, PNI seeks to understand the scientific basis of the mind/body connection.

Steven Locke and Douglas Colligan, in *The Healer Within*, explain that a premise of PNI is that the immune system does not operate in a biological vacuum but is sensitive to outside influences. PNI researchers speculate that there is a line of communication between the mind and cells that compose the immune system. Tendrils of the brain's nerve tissues run through important sectors of the immune system, including the thymus gland, bone marrow, lymph nodes and spleen. Hormones and neurotransmitters secreted by the brain have an affinity for immune cells. Also, certain states of mind and feelings can have strong biochemical results.

The field began in 1981 with the publication, *Psychoneuroimmunology,* edited by Robert Ader. While most of the research presented was primarily based on animal models of stress and illness, the collection paved the way for clinical research with humans.

During the late 1980s and 1990s, researchers from various backgrounds were drawn to this new discipline. Social psychologists, experimental psychologists, psychiatrists, immunologists, neuroendocrinologists, neuroanatomists, biologists, oncologists and epidemiologists, among other specialists, have all made contributions to PNI research. Together, they seek to explain the way the brain and mind contribute to illness or keep people healthy.

See also COMPLEMENTARY THERAPIES; HUMOR; IMMUNE SYSTEM; LAUGHTER; MIND/BODY CONNECTION; NEUROTRANSMITTERS; PLACEBO EFFECT; RELAXATION; STRESS.

Kahn, Ada P. *Stress A to Z: A Sourcebook for Facing Everyday Challenges.* New York: Facts On File, 2000.

Locke, Steven, and Douglas Colligan. *The Healer Within.* New York: New American Library, 1984.

Moye, Lemuel A. "Research Methodology in Psychoneuroimmunology: Rationale and Design of the Images-P Clinical Trial." *Alternatives Therapies* 1, no. 2 (May 1995).

Padus, Emrika, ed. *The Complete Guide to Your Emotions and Your Health,* rev. ed. Emmaus Pa.: Rodale, 1994.

Schwartz, Carolyn E. "Introduction: Old Methodological Challenges and New Mind-Body Links in Psychoneuroimmunology." *Advances: The Journal of Mind-Body Health* 10, no. 4 (Fall 1994).

psychoneurosis   A term used interchangeably with neurosis, which relates to mental disorders associated with many psychological symptoms. In neurosis, the individual does not lose touch with reality but realizes that he or she is not mentally healthy. In psychosis, the individual loses touch with reality and believes that he or she does not have any illness.

See also NEUROSIS; PSYCHOSIS.

psychopathology   The study of abnormal mental processes. There are two major approaches, the descriptive and the psychoanalytic. In descriptive psychopathology, the clinician records symptoms that make up a diagnosis, such as delusions, hallucinations or mood disturbances. In the psychoanalytic approach, the clinician delves into the individual's unconscious motivations.

The terms "psychopathic personality" and "sociopathic personality" have been applied to the condition of antisocial personality disorder, which was first recognized during the 19th century as "moral insanity." It applied to immoral or guiltless behavior that was not accompanied by impairments in reasoning.

See also PSYCHOANALYSIS.

psychopharmacology   Treatment of mental disorders with medications. Generally, medications used to treat psychiatric illnesses are known as psychotropic medications. There are several major categories of these drugs, including neuroleptic (or antipsychotic) medications, antiparkinsonian medications, lithium, antidepressant drugs and antianxiety medications, as well as many other drugs that are known to be efficacious in some mental health conditions.

See also ANTIANXIETY MEDICATIONS; ANTICHOLINERGIC MEDICATIONS; ANTIDEPRESSANT MEDICATIONS; BENZODIAZEPINE MEDICATIONS; LITHIUM CARBONATE; NEUROLEPTIC.

psychosexual anxieties   Anxieties caused by mental attitudes about sexuality and physical conditions involving sexuality. Some anxieties are caused more by psychological attitudes, while others come from the physical aspects. Many psychosexual anxieties have arisen due to the new sexual freedoms that many individuals experienced in the latter decades of the 20th century. Sexual activity between men and women, unmarried as well as married, seemed to increase for a number of reasons. First, improved methods of contraception in the form of the birth control pill became available. Secondly, some sexually transmitted (venereal) diseases, most notably syphilis and gonorrhea, became curable with penicillin and other drugs.

During the last two decades of the 20th century, an increasing number of new sexually transmitted diseases (STDs) appeared, causing psychosexual anxieties that differed from previously recognized generalized sexual fears. For example, when an individual discovers, feels or suspects a genital lesion, he or she may lose interest in sexual intercourse or at least restrain himself/herself for fear of infecting the partner. Another situation is the concern faced by the innocently infected partner of an individual with a sexually transmitted disease who has had intercourse outside a stable relationship. The innocent partner may realize the implications of the STD but may not want to face the reality of the diagnosis.

Under the stress of having a sexually transmitted disease, a person may become angry, anxious or depressed. Anger may be directed at the physician consulted as well as the person who transmitted the infection. Professionals in clinics specializing in sexually transmitted disease deal with this kind of anxiety by letting the individual voice his or her feelings and later by offering reassurance. In some individuals, anxiety is so severe that a short course of antianxiolytic medication is given.

Guilt and depression over a sexually transmitted disease are not uncommon. In some cases, antidepressant medications are given. Many conditions, such as genital herpes, pelvic inflammatory disease, acute epididymitis and hepatitis B may also lead to anger, anxiety, guilt and depression.

Physical symptoms of gonococcal and nongonococal urethritis may be more easily and rapidly treated than the psychological symptoms. Resuming intercourse soon after tests indicate cure may help to heal the psychological wound that one or both partners in a stable relationship feel. Unfortunately, nongonococal urethritis may be recurrent, and the patient may be told not to resume intercourse until the inflammation clears. This advice may put an extra strain on a relationship.

Pelvic pain and pain during sexual intercourse (dyspareunia) usually interfere with satisfactory sexual intercourse. Pelvic inflammatory disease also causes pain during intercourse and may lead to infertility. Along with dealing with a women's feelings of loss of health and fertility, a physician may see the couple together to identify problems that have occurred because one or both partners has had sex with others and to discuss the anger and resentment the woman feels if it is the man who has not been monogamous (as is often the case).

Genital herpes may occur in one partner in a relationship when the other has never knowingly had the infection. Both may be confused about where the infection came from and may be angry, accusatory or resentful of the other partner. Discussion guided by a trained therapist enables the couple to face the facts together. Such a couple should discuss whether herpes, once healed, might disturb further sexual relationships (usually not).

Women and homosexual men who have had anorectal herpes may develop maladaptive behaviors after the primary attack. Vaginismus (tightening of the vaginal muscles) and anospasm (tightening of the anus muscles) may continue long after the ulcers have healed. Systematic desensitization (for example, using the partner's finger as a dilator) often is successful in overcoming this problem in a few sessions with an appropriately trained sex therapist.

Frequent recurrences of genital candidiasis (yeast infection) may leave both partners confused, frustrated and angry about the supposed source of the problem. If the relationship is unstable, symptoms may assume dimensions out of proportion to the signs. Trichomonas vaginalis and gardnerella vaginalis often involve offensive vaginal discharges, which may cause a loss of interest in the male partner. After treatment the odor may disappear, but the women may have lost confidence in herself, and the man may mistake the normal musky vaginal odor for the previous abnormal odor. The couple may need reassurance from a physician or sex therapist.

Syphilis, whether congenital or acquired, is feared by many people as "worse than cancer." Congenital syphilis that occurs in later life may devastate an individual when he or she realizes the implication of the disease with respect to his or her parents.

An individual who has a sexually transmitted disease or whose partner is unfaithful may lose interest in intercourse. Loss of libido may be due to anxiety, depression or a lack of interest in the partner. Individuals who are undergoing treatment for a sexually transmitted disease should discuss with their physician their attitudes about resuming sexual relations. Counseling with short-term psychotherapy may help the individual return to normal sexual function.

Some individuals may complain of symptoms of a sexually transmitted disease yet not have any illness. Some who have had an infection retain the symptoms after the infection has been cleared up with appropriate medication. Penile and urethral itching, penile and perineal pain, testicular pain and pelvic pain may either be psychosomatic or represent symptoms of reactive sexually transmitted diseases.

Many individuals visit sexually transmitted disease clinics for checkups because they fear having acquired an STD. Some continue to believe or fear that they have contracted an infection in spite of extensive and frequent reassurance. Some of these individuals may have delusions of venereal disease, which are fixed ideas that the individual cannot be talked out of (found in schizophrenic disorders, psychotic depression and monosymptomatic delusions), and phobias or obsessional fears. Individuals who have a fixed belief of venereal disease should be referred for psychotherapy.

See also DEPRESSION, DISEASES; GUILT; SEXUALLY TRANSMITTED DISEASES; SYPHILIS.

*Adapted with permission from *The Encyclopedia of Phobias, Fears, and Anxieties,* 2nd ed. by Ronald M. Doctor and Ada P. Kahn. New York: Facts On File, 2000.

psychosexual development   A psychoanalytical term for the effects of sexual maturation on the development of personality; also called libidinal development. Freud viewed this development as a stage-by-stage expression of the libido, or source of energy. In the first stage (oral), the mouth is the prime erotic zone, with sucking and biting the characteristic expressions. In the next stage (anal), the infant derives pleasure in expelling or retaining feces. In the phallic stage, the libido focuses on the genital organs, with masturbation the major source of pleasure. The Oedipus complex may develop at this time. Next is the latency stage, in which overt sexual interest is repressed and sublimated into peer activities. The genital stage is reached in puberty, when one focuses erotic interest and activity on a sexual partner.

See also PSYCHOSEXUAL DISORDERS.

psychosexual disorders   A group of sexual dysfunctions that arise from psychological rather than physical factors. These include gender identity disorders, paraphilias and psychosexual dysfunctions, such as disturbances in sexual desire or response.

See also PARAPHILIAS.

psychosexual dysfunctions   Disorders in which there is no known organic cause for an interference with the normal process of sexual response. Conditions termed "sexual dysfunctions" include lack of sexual desire, impotence, premature ejaculation, painful intercourse and lack of orgasm. These dysfunctions are common in men and women, often start in early adult life and, in many people, disappear with experience, increased confidence and personality maturation.

Many people respond well to sex therapy, which can be done with an individual or a couple.

See also DYSPAREUNIA; IMPOTENCE; SEXUAL RESPONSE CYCLE; VAGINISMUS.

psychosexual trauma   A frightening sexual experience in early life that may relate to a current psychologically induced sexual dysfunction. Examples include child abuse, incest or rape.

See also INCEST; RAPE, RAPE PREVENTION AND RAPE TRAUMA SYNDROME.

psychosis   A severe mental disorder in which the individual loses contact with reality. This differs from neurosis, which is a more mild group of mental disorders. Psychotic individuals have a distorted ability to think, perceive and judge clearly; they do not realize that they are ill. Neurotics, on the other hand, generally know they are ill.

A psychotic episode can involve hallucinations, delusions, disorientation and extremely aggressive behavior. Schizophrenic and manic-depressive psychoses are examples of functional psychosis. In toxic psychosis, psychoticlike behavior results from impairment of brain cell function. Medical and neurological illness such as Alzheimer's disease may also cause psychoses.

Many people recover from psychotic episodes with appropriate treatment, often involving use of psychotropic medications, carefully monitored by their physicians.

See also PSYCHOPHARMACOLOGY; PSYCHOTROPIC DRUGS.

psychosomatic (psychosomatic illness)   A term that refers to physical problems that may either be imagined or made worse by psychological factors. Some examples of conditions that sometimes have psychosomatic components include headache, nausea, asthma, irritable bowel syndrome, ulcers and certain types of eczema.

See also MUNCHAUSEN'S SYNDROME.

psychosurgery   Any operation on the brain as a treatment for symptoms of mental disorders, usually performed when all other treatments have been ineffective. Although psychosurgery has helped some people, successes with the operations have been inconsistent, with highly unpredictable results, and remain a controversial form of treatment for mental illness. Cingulotomy, a modified form of psychosurgery, has produced favorable results for a small number of patients with refractory mental disorders. At one time, prefrontal lobotomy was the most widely used form of psychosurgery but, as it often resulted in harmful side effects, has been replaced by other safer operations.

The term "neurosurgery" is preferred when referring to the relief of pain due to organic diseases.

See also BRAIN.

psychotherapies   Treatment of mental and emotional concerns by psychological methods. In psychotherapy, a therapeutic relationship between the patient and a therapist (psychotherapist) is established. The relationship is focused on the patient's symptoms. Patterns of behavior—mood swings, low self-esteem and not being able to deal with anxieties—can benefit from interaction between patient and therapist.

There are many types of psychotherapists who can be recommended by friends, family physicians or local community mental health centers. There are several rules to follow when choosing a therapist: Check out credentials. Know whether the therapist is a psychiatrist, psychologist or psychiatric social worker. Determine where the person received training, and check with that institution. Also, because there are professional societies for many specialties, check with the appropriate organization to see that the therapist has appropriate accreditation.

Choosing a Psychotherapist

People seeking help may be faced with the question of whom to choose. If they recognize what their problems are, and there are just occasional periods of feeling moody or low, a psychiatrist may not be needed. Guidelines for selecting a psychotherapist rather than a psychiatrist include:

The end of the anxiety-producing problem is in sight, but the individual just can't get there by himself or herself.

The individual realizes that symptoms are of short duration and that the stress that brought them on can be identified.

However, a person who has tried going to a therapist and has not found relief, may need a psychiatrist because of the following reasons:

M.D.s are the only mental health therapists who can prescribe medications. Some mental disorders, such as those caused by medical illnesses can be diagnosed by an M.D.

For certain emotional illnesses, medications may be helpful.

The individual has incapacitating or debilitating symptoms.

The individual has other concurrent medical problems for which care and medications are being received.

There is a history of mental illness in the family, if other family members have ever been hospitalized for mental illness or the individual requires hospitalization for a mental problem.

Group Therapy

Group therapy is treatment of emotional or psychological problems in groups of patients or in self-help support groups led by a mental health professional. These groups attract individuals with similar concerns. For example, such groups may be for recently widowed persons, divorced people, parents who have lost a child to sudden infant death syndrome, people suffering from depression or those concerned with obesity. Group therapy is also useful for people who have personality problems, alcoholism, drug dependency, eating disorders and anxiety disorders.

Therapy groups may include from three to 40 people, but they work best with 10 to 12 participants who meet for an hour or more, once or twice a week. There is therapeutic interaction among the individuals in the group; members find that others share their feelings and experiences, and this helps them feel less alone and less helpless.

Co-therapy

A form of psychotherapy in which more than one therapist works with an individual or group. Co-therapy is also known as combined therapy, cooperative therapy, dual leadership, multiple therapy and three-cornered therapy. Co-therapists work in various areas. For example, in sex therapy, one therapist is a male and the other is female to encourage understanding of both viewpoints in sexuality problems concerning a couple.

Geropsychiatry

This is a specialized form of mental health care that addresses the complexities involved between mental and physical illness in the elderly. For example, an elderly patient who appears to have psychotic symptoms may be experiencing symptoms of toxicity resulting from taking two or more incompatible drugs. Many psychosomatic disorders and chronic conditions manifest themselves with symptoms of depression. Physicians specializing in geropsychiatry are located in community hospitals where they can provide a safe and secure environment, offer psychological evaluation in conjunction with medical testing and provide liaison services for elderly patients being treated for medical or surgical conditions.

An increasing number of hospitals are adding this component to their mental health programs. Some hospitals contract with various managed care organizations who provide these services.

Family Therapy

Family therapy is a form of psychotherapy that focuses on the family unit, or at least the parent and child (in single-parent families), rather than separate treatment of one or more family members. It is based on the theory that an individual who is troubled or is mentally ill should not be seen in isolation from the family unit. Family members become aware of how they deal with each other and are encouraged to communicate more openly. The discussions and confrontations lead to understanding.

Family therapy usually focuses on here-and-now stresses and their practical solutions. It can be helpful when at least one member has a relatively serious problem, such as recurrent depression, or

needs ongoing assistance in coping with outbursts of anger and emotional withdrawal.

Family therapy has become increasingly popular for dealing with problems of children and adolescents. Typically, the therapy group will consist of both parents, a parent and stepparent, two separated parents or other parental pairings depending on the environment in which the child lives. In many cases, the child is brought to a mental health professional because of difficulties in school, such as exhibiting aggressive behavior or cutting classes.

See also ALCOHOLISM; ANXIETY DISORDERS; COMMUNICATION; DEPRESSION; EATING DISORDERS; GRIEF; LISTENING; MARITAL THERAPY; OBESITY; PSYCHIATRIST; PSYCHOLOGIST; SELF-ESTEEM; SEX THERAPY; SUDDEN INFANT DEATH SYNDROME; SUPPORT GROUPS.

psychotropic drugs Prescription medications that have effects on behavior, experience or other psychological functions. Psychotropic drugs include antidepressant drugs, sedatives, hypnotics, narcotics, stimulants, tranquilizer drugs and psychedelic drugs. Substances that have mind-altering effects that are not their primary function are not considered psychotropic drugs.

Psychotropic medications usually require highly individualized dosage schedules and are often prescribed to individuals who are receiving more than one drug at a time. Special attention should be given to the possibilities of drug interactions.

See also ANTIDEPRESSANT MEDICATIONS; PSYCHOPHARMACOLOGY.

PTSD See POST-TRAUMATIC STRESS DISORDER.

puberty and puberty rites The period during which adult sexual characteristics develop. Puberty normally occurs between age 10 and 14 in girls and one to two years later in boys, although precocious or delayed puberty can occur in both sexes. The onset of puberty is known as pubarche.

In females, puberty usually starts with breast budding and/or the appearance of pubic hair. Over the next year or so, the breast tissue underlying the initial "buds" enlarges, the hips widen and pubic and axillary hair thickens. Soon menarche, the first menstruation, occurs. When regular cyclic menses have been established, puberty is considered completed.

The high levels of estrogens that occur during puberty generally "seal" a girl's leg bones, so little additional height growth will occur after puberty. Occasionally, a girl can conceive if sexual intercourse predates full pubertal development and ovulation occurs at this time. Increasingly intense interest in the opposite sex occurs in young women and men, and though neither sex is ready for the responsibilities of parenthood, it is usually possible for a young man to impregnate a young woman and for a young woman to become pregnant and bear a child.

Puberty occurs earlier in well-nourished populations, and the average age of menarche has declined in the developed world over the past few generations to age 12. The occurrence of the normal adolescent tendency to try to establish independence; deteriorating social structures, such as church and family; and early sexual development have made adolescence a time of great turmoil for both children and their parents.

Precocious puberty is the premature development of functioning gonads in young women and young men; women ovulate and men produce mature spermatozoa. Precocious puberty may occur as early as the age of eight in girls and the age of 10 in boys; such young people also have adult levels of sex hormones and the secondary sex characteristics of their gender.

Sexual awakening is a term for the period of psychological change that accompanies puberty. During this time, young people undergo changes in attitudes, emotions and interests that are appropriate for approaching sexual maturity. Physical experimentation, including increased masturbation and petting, occurs during this phase.

In some societies, ceremonies are performed to mark the arrival of puberty and the beginning of adulthood; the rites are also known as initiation rites.

Formal rites may include teaching of legends and laws as well as sexual practices and responsibilities expected of an adult in the particular society.

quazepam   Generic name for the benzodiazepine medication marketed under the trade name Doral.

See also BENZODIAZEPINE MEDICATIONS; PHARMACOLOGICAL APPROACH.

racing thoughts   See THOUGHT DISORDERS.

random nuisances   Annoying or unpleasant situations with which individuals must cope. They may include difficult things, such as commuting in traffic, finding a parking spot and depending on public transportation when the weather is bad, or annoying things, such as construction noise outside your office window, phone calls from telemarketers at dinnertime, last minute dinner guests and zippers that get stuck at a critical moment. Such nuisances differ for each person, but if they produce anxieties, they affect one's mental health.

Successful people regard random nuisances as "small stuff." There is a saying, "Don't sweat the small stuff, and it's all small stuff," and random nuisances may seem small. However, the response to some of life's "small stressors" may escalate into physical responses, such as anger and rage, that are similar to responses to major stressors.

Hans Selye explained the concept of stress with two basic ideas: The body has a similar set of responses to many of life's stressors; this he called the general adaptation syndrome (G.A.S.). Also, stressors can make an individual ill. To prevent illness induced by stressors, keeping a positive perspective on life and everyday occurrences is essential. The individual should endeavor to cope with the small stressors and keep them from escalating into more serious consequences.

Many individuals find that meditation at the end of a day helps them meet challenges of home, children and paying bills. Others find that participating in regular exercise helps them forget about the random nuisances of each day.

See also ANGER; EXERCISE; GENERAL ADAPTATION SYNDROME; HARDINESS; MEDITATION; RELAXATION; SELYE, HANS; STRESS.

randomized clinical trial   An experiment designed to test the safety and/or efficacy of an intervention, such as a prescription drug, in which people are randomly allocated to experimental or control groups and outcomes are compared. Many new pharmaceutical products are extensively tested in this way.

rape, rape prevention and rape trauma syndrome   Rape is forcible sexual intercourse against the will of the partner. There is some variation among states as to the actual definition; in many states sexual assault need not involve either force, actual penetration or ejaculation. In some places genital contact under the heat of force or even implied threat of force meets the legal definition.

In the majority of cases the perpetrator is male and the victim female, but it is possible for the victim to be male. In many states, sexual contact between an adult and an underage child or adolescent is automatically considered rape.

Traditionally women have most feared violent sexual assault by a stranger. However, society has increasingly recognized that forced intercourse can occur with perpetrators known to the victim—even a husband. The incidence of "date rape" (rape by a person with whom one has had a social engagement) is increasingly reported.

Rape is now recognized as more a crime of violence than one of sexuality; rapists often have a history of other types of violent crime. As courts and law enforcement agencies have been more sympathetic toward victims, the number of reported rapes in the United States has increased dramatically.

Fear of rape, known as virgivitiphobia, underlies the entire female experience of sexuality. In early adolescence, girls are taught to be distrustful of men and fearful of being victimized. Adult women are often fearful of going out without a male escort out of fear of sexual harassment and possible assault.

Although public support and sympathy for rape victims have recently improved, society continues to hold a "blaming the victim" mentality toward rape victims. Often victims are blamed for being in the wrong place or dressed in a seductive fashion, and the role of the criminal is downplayed. In recent years, the efforts of rape victim advocacy groups have helped place rape in the violent context in which it belongs.

Immediate dangers of rape include direct injury, pregnancy and sexually transmitted disease (STD). Rape victims may be shot, knifed or beaten. The rape itself can cause perineal bruising or lacerations, particularly if the victim is very young, if anal penetration occurs or if dangerous objects are used in the assault. Cultures are taken for gonorrhea and other sexually transmitted diseases, and appropriate antibiotics may be recommended. For the victim exposed to herpes or AIDS, there is at present no effective way of preventing these diseases.

After the attack, the victim's body and clothing will be examined for traces of semen, hair or clothing of the rapist. Recent development of DNA "fingerprints" from semen and blood will allow for very accurate identification of the person responsible.

Women at risk for pregnancy may be offered "morning after" contraception. Unfortunately, many victims fail to press charges, either out of fear of having to relive the incident in court, out of fear of shame or other reprisal or actual fear of the assailant. In later years, many victims suffer depression and post-traumatic stress reactions, which can adversely affect their professional, personal and sexual lives.

Prevention of rape will depend on major restructuring of the way society views violence against women and prevention of the drug, alcohol and poverty problems that lead to violent crimes. To a lesser extent, self-defense and assertiveness training for women can decrease the risk to those women but fails to address the underlying psychopathology of the rapist.

Rape trauma syndrome is a term used to describe the results of sexual victimization against the victim's consent. The trauma that develops from this attack or attempted attack may include an acute phase of disorganization of the victim's lifestyle and, in some cases, a long-term traumatization with symptoms similar to post-traumatic stress disorder. Many factors influence the process of recovery from rape trauma syndrome, including the type of assault, the victim's coping style and level of self-esteem, the type of social support available, additional life stressors and additional history of victimization.

See also SEXUAL FEARS.

Becker, Judith V.; Linda J. Skinner; Gene G. Abel; and Joan Cichon. "Level of Postassault Sexual Functioning in Rape and Incest Victims." *Archives of Sexual Behavior* 15, no. 1 (1986).

Clark, Stephanie. "Perspectives on Sexual Assault." *Canadian Family Physician* 35 (Jan. 1989), pp. 77–80.

Edmonds, Ed M., and Delwin D. Cahoon. "Attitudes Concerning Crimes Related to Clothing Worn by Female Victims." *Bulletin of the Psychonomic Society* 24, no. 6 (1986).

Gordon, Margaret T., and Stephanie Riger. *The Female Fear.* New York: Free Press, 1989.

Harrison, Maureen, and Steve Gilbert, eds. *The Rape Reference: A Resource for People at Risk.* San Diego: Excellent Books, 1996.

Kahn, Ada P., and Linda Hughey Holt. *The A to Z of Women's Sexuality.* Alameda, Calif.: Hunter House, 1992.

Koss, Mary P.; Christine A. Gidycz and Nadine Wisniewski. "The Scope of Rape: Incidence and Prevalence of Sexual Aggression and Victimization in a National Sample of Higher Education Students." *Journal of Consulting and Clinical Psychology.* 55, no. 2 (1987).

Miller, Maryann. *Drugs and Date Rape.* New York: Rosen, 1995.

Rank, Otto (1884–1939) An Austrian psychoanalyst who broke away from Sigmund Freud and his teachings to emphasize short-term therapy and the birth trauma, which Rank believed was the root of anxiety disorders. He aimed his therapy at eliminating the effects of trauma, especially anxiety and dependence, and helping the individual achieve constructive independence and trusting relationships. Rank believed that once the individual's "primal anxiety" (known as "life fear") was uncovered, the analyst could concentrate on helping the individual look forward to the process of separation (the termination of the analyst-patient relationship) by gradually undoing the individual's reliance. The aim of this separation was to inspire the successive stages of what Rank called "the wills of life," which would enable the individual to become a fully integrated personality. The emphasis on "wills" led Rank's theory of neurosis to become known as "will therapy." This system directs attention to present functioning potential as opposed to the Freudian emphasis on the unconscious past.

See also ADLER, ALFRED; JUNG, CARL.

Doctor, Ronald M. and Ada P. Kahn. *Encyclopedia of Phobias, Fears, and Anxieties.* New York: Facts On File, 2000.

rapid cycling   A mood disorder in which episodes of mania or depression occur at least four times within a year.

See also DEPRESSION; MANIA; MANIC-DEPRESSIVE ILLNESS.

rationalization   One type of defense mechanism. The individual uses rationalization as an unconscious way to attempt to justify or make consciously tolerable by plausible means feelings, behavior or motives that otherwise would be intolerable, such as personal shortcomings. An example is an individual who cheats and explains the behavior by thinking "everybody cheats." Such an excuse is used to ward off feelings of guilt and maintain self-respect.

See also DEFENSE MECHANISMS; PROJECTION.

Doctor, Ronald M., and Ada P. Kahn. *Encyclopedia of Phobias, Fears, and Anxieties.* New York: Facts On File, 2000.

Rat Man, case of   A well-documented case, in which Sigmund Freud treated a young man tormented by anxieties and thoughts of harm to others and to himself. His most horrifying thoughts were of a form of torture involving rats eating at the anus of his father and the woman he loved.

Probing further, Freud found that the death of the man's father had occurred after he had imagined his death. Freud thought that the young man had developed a belief in what he termed "omnipotence of thought," a feeling that thinking about an occurrence could magically bring it about.

Schur, Max. *Freud: Living and Dying.* New York: International Universities Press, 1972.

Ray, Isaac (1807–81)   American physician and one of the most influential psychiatrists of his time. He helped create the Association of Medical Superintendents of American Institutions for the Insane, the forerunner of the American Psychiatric Association. He also contributed to the development of forensic psychiatry, and he collaborated with Thomas Kirkbride in developing policies and plans for well-built and well-managed mental hospitals, in which patients would have "abundant means for occupation and amusement," though he also advocated physical restraint.

Goldenson, Robert M., ed. *Longman Dictionary of Psychology and Psychiatry.* New York: Longman, 1984.

reflexology   A form of body therapy based on the theory that every part of the body has a direct line of communication to a reference point on the foot, hand and ear. By massaging these reference points, professional reflexologists say they can help the corresponding body parts to heal. Through improved circulation, elimination of toxic by-products and overall reduction of stress, the body responds and functions better because it is more relaxed.

USING REFLEXOLOGY TO IMPROVE MENTAL WELL-BEING

- Choose a quiet place.
- Apply a few drops of a light, absorbent, greaseless lotion to your feet and massage them, continuing until the lotion is totally absorbed.
- Grasp the ankle, heel or toes of one foot firmly in one hand, place the thumb of your other hand on the sole of your foot at the heel and apply steady, even pressure with the edge of your whole thumb.
- Keep your thumb slightly bent at the joint and use a forward, caterpillar-like motion. This is called thumbwalking; press one spot, move forward a little, press again, etc.

• When you reach the toes, start again at a new spot on the heel. Continue until the entire bottom of the foot has been worked. Then fingerwalk the top of the foot. Work your entire foot twice this way.

See also BODY THERAPIES; COMPLEMENTARY THERAPIES.

Feltman, John, ed. *Reflexology: Hands on Healing,* Emmaus, Pa.: Rodale Press, 1989.

regression   A defense mechanism involving reversion to immature behavior when one feels threatened or overwhelmed by internal conflicts. Some individuals may regress on an ongoing basis, and others do it on a temporary basis in specific situations. Examples of regression include crying or temper tantrums to gain attention. In psychoanalysis, individuals are sometimes encouraged to temporarily regress to help them remember some childhood events, their feelings and their methods of coping. In some alternative therapies, including primal therapy, individuals are also encourage to regress during therapy.

See also PSYCHOTHERAPIES.

Reich, Wilhelm (1897–1957)   Irish-American psychoanalyst and member of the psychoanalytic movement that broke with Sigmund Freud. Reich refused to accept the death instinct, and he developed his own theory that the achievement of "full orgiastic potency" is the single measure of psychological well-being.

See BIOENERGETICS.

Goldenson, Robert M., ed. *Longman Dictionary of Psychology and Psychiatry.* New York: Longman, 1984.

reinforcement   Strengthening of good habits (or bad habits such as addictions) or behaviors by positive rewards (positive reinforcement). For good mental health, individuals have a need for positive self-regard, much of which comes from approval (or disapproval) from significant others. When good habits are praised and rewarded, they are reinforced; when bad habits are ignored and rewards are withheld or punished (negative reinforcement), presumably they will diminish. In daily life as well as in therapy, individuals can be motivated to change behavior patterns to include more adaptive responses and more socially acceptable behaviors. Methods of reinforcement may include rewards such as privileges or increased social interactions. There is evidence suggesting that in humans positive reinforcement works better than negative reinforcement to change behavior.

relaxation   A feeling of freedom from anxiety and tension; mental conflicts and disturbing feelings of stress are absent. Relaxation also refers to the return of a muscle to its normal state after a period of contraction.

People who are very tense and anxious can learn to relax using relaxation training, a form of behavior therapy. Relaxation techniques are methods used to unconsciously release muscular tension and achieve a sense of mental calm. Historically, relaxation techniques have included meditation, t'ai chi, massage therapy, yoga, music and aromatherapy. More modern developments include autogenic training, progressive muscle relaxation, hypnosis, biofeedback and aerobic exercise.

Many of these techniques were developed to help people cope with stresses brought on by the challenges of life. They are different approaches with the same goal of relieving stress by bringing about generalized physical as well as mental relaxation. Relaxation techniques have in common the production of the relaxation response as one of their stress-relieving actions. Additionally, relaxation may counter some of the immunosuppressing effects of stress and may actually enhance the activity of the immune system.

Relaxation training programs are commonly used in conjunction with more standard forms of therapy for many chronic diseases. The mind/body connection between relaxation and ill health has been demonstrated in many conditions. Some of the physiological changes that occur during relaxation include decreased oxygen consumption, decreased heart and respiratory rates, diminished muscle tension and a shift toward slower brain wave patterns.

"The Relaxation Response"

In the 1970s, Herbert Benson, M.D., a cardiologist at Harvard Medical School, studied the relationship between stress and hypertension. In stressful situations, the body undergoes several changes, including rise in blood pressure and pulse and faster breathing. Dr. Benson reasoned that if stress could bring about this reaction, another factor might be able to turn it off. He studied practitioners of transcendental meditation (TM) and found that once into their meditative states, some individuals could willfully reduce their pulse, blood pressure and breathing rate. Dr. Benson named this "the relaxation response." He explained this procedure in his book, written with Miriam Z. Klipper, *The Relaxation Response* (1976).

Relaxation Applications

Relaxation training can be particularly useful for individuals who have "white coat hypertension," which means that their blood pressure is high only when facing certain specifically stressful situations, such as having a medical examination or visiting a dentist. It can also help reduce hostility and anger, which in turn affect the body and the individual's physical responses to stress. Anxieties can lead to panic attacks, nausea or gastrointestinal problems.

There are many applications of relaxation training to help individuals learn to control their mental state and body and to treat conditions as diverse as high blood pressure, cardiac arrhythmia, chronic pain, insomnia, premenstrual syndrome and side effects of cancer treatments. Relaxation training is an important part of childbirth classes to help women cope with the pain of labor.

In a training program, individuals are instructed to move through the muscle groups of the body, making them tense and then completely relaxed. Through repetitions of this procedure, individuals learn how to be in voluntary control of their feelings of tension and relaxation. Some therapists provide individuals with instructional audio tapes for use during practice, while other therapists go through the procedure repeatedly with their clients.

To determine the effectiveness of relaxation training, some therapists use biofeedback as an indicator of an individual's degree of relaxation and absence of anxiety.

See also AROMATHERAPY; AUTOGENIC TRAINING; BENSON, HERBERT; BEHAVIOR THERAPY; BIOFEEDBACK; GUIDED IMAGERY; HYPNOSIS; IMMUNE SYSTEM; KABAT-ZINN, JON; MASSAGE THERAPY; MEDITATION; MIND/BODY CONNECTIONS; MUSIC; PROGRESSIVE MUSCLE RELAXATION; STRESS; T'AI CHI; TRANSCENDENTAL MEDITATION; YOGA.

Benson, Herbert. *The Relaxation Response*. New York: Avon Books, 1975.
———. *Beyond the Relaxation Response*. New York: Berkeley Press, 1985.
Goleman, Daniel, and Joel Gurin, eds. *Mind Body Medicine: How To Use Your Mind For Better Health*. Yonkers, N.Y.: Consumer Reports Books, 1993.
Lehrer, Paul M., and Robert L. Woolfolk, eds. *Principles and Practice of Stress Management*, New York: The Guilford Press, 1993.
Locke, Steven, and Douglas Colligan. *The Healer Within*. New York: New American Library, 1984.

relationships   Relationship are formed between individuals connected by affinity. These relationships include the individual's family, spouse, lovers, friends and business or professional associates. Good relationships are healthy and nurturing and act as a buffer against stress on good mental health. However, even the most meaningful relationships can at times be nonsupportive and sources of anxiety.

HOW A HEALTHY RELATIONSHIP CAN CONTRIBUTE TO BETTER MENTAL HEALTH

- Realism: openness and honesty with each other
- Trust: allowing the individuals to share their feelings
- True friendship: having no hidden motives
- Forgiveness: accepting the individual as he or she is
- Security: knowing that individuals can count on one another
- Vulnerability: exposing weaknesses that allow the relationship to grow

---

Relationships and Health

Best friends are invaluable to good mental health. A best friend is on the same wavelength as you; understands your personal situations, such as dealing with a difficult boss or overbearing parent; appreciates and admires who you are, even if there isn't always agreement on what is being done or said; makes you feel important in his or her life; is very much like you and has the same values and belief systems.

People who lack outlets for anxiety release are susceptible to a list of anxiety-related illnesses. Having one or two close friends with whom they feel free to say anything is invaluable. When they are overwhelmed, they don't trust their own judgment, and an objective view from a friend can help.

Romantic Relationships

Romantic relationships are far riskier and potentially more anxiety producing to the individual's emotional and physical well-being than people realize. Not only are feelings likely to be hurt, self-esteem damaged and trust betrayed, but there can be physical and mental battery by an outraged spouse. America's high divorce rate suggests that intimacy has painful consequences.

According to Geraldine K. Piorkowski, author of *Too Close for Comfort: Exploring the Risks of Intimacy,* romantic relationships can produce anxiety because they are related to the process of getting close to another person. As we become more intimate (both emotionally and sexually), we reveal our deepest secrets, hopes, inadequacies and even fantasies. We become more vulnerable, and thus easily cut to the core by a hostile comment, act of betrayal or moment of rejection.

Furthermore, Piorkowski says, anxiety arises in relationships when our emotional needs and expectations are unrealistic. Also, we may lose our autonomy and wind up feeling suffocated by the other's demands; their neediness may drain energy needed to pursue our own desires and interests. We may be blamed for all the problems in the relationship and suffer guilt and loss of self-confidence as a result.

Relationships and Support Groups

A lack of connections with other people can be detrimental to good mental health, says Dr. Andrew Weil, author of *Spontaneous Healing.* "Surrounding yourself with supportive people is an important step for any healing you need to do. Whenever I take a family history from a patient, I always ask about people who are helping or hin-

dering someone's illness. For example, sometimes a friend or family member who means well only make matters worse, maybe by not wanting the patient to express sadness about being sick or show discomfort from pain."

In terms of building relationships through support groups, Dr. Weil urges patients to find and develop relationships with people who have the same conditions and have improved, rather than simply join a support group. "I find that some support groups can be counterproductive and cause more stress for the individual," he says. "For example, some patients with cancer are horrified and extremely stressed when they see another person with a more advanced form of the disease. There is a similar phenomenon with chronic fatigue syndrome."

Some people are more fatalistic about their illness while others tend to be positive thinkers. This should be factored into any relationships developed through a support group and especially with regard to the regular people in your life, suggests Dr. Weil.

See also AUTONOMY; DIVORCE; GUILT; INTIMACY; MARRIAGE; PARENTING; SELF-ESTEEM; SUPPORT GROUPS.

*Adapted with permission from *Encyclopedia of Phobias, Fears and Anxieties,* 2nd ed. by Ronald M. Doctor and Ada P. Kahn. New York: Facts On File, 2000.

Gilbert, Roberta M. *Extraordinary Relationships: A New Way of Thinking About Human Interactions.* Minneapolis: Chronimed Publishing, 1992.

Jaffe, Dennis T. *Healing From Within.* New York: Knopf, 1980.

Piorkowski, Geraldine K., *Too Close for Comfort: Exploring the Risks of Intimacy.* New York: Insight Books, 1994.

Weil, Andrew. *Spontaneous Healing: How to Discover and Enhance Your Body's Natural Ability to Maintain and Heal Itself.* New York: Knopf, 1995.

religion Systems of beliefs regarding oneself and the universe. Religion gives many people a sense of security, a feeling of meaning and order and an ethical pattern for living. Religious beliefs offer help, support and strength to those with both external and internal mental health concerns. Religious programs and rituals facilitate social interaction, which is important in an age when contact with lifelong friends and extended family is the exception rather than the rule and when urban anonymity has produced a sense of alienation for many.

Religious beliefs and practices satisfy mystical and illusory needs for many individuals. For example, the image of a divine being or beings meets a longing evident in many civilizations for a higher power in control of the universe. Prayer and meditation are comforting and helpful to many people. Modern psychotherapeutic discoveries have confirmed the benefits of breath control and mental centering practiced for centuries in Zen Buddhism and yoga. Religion has also focused the energies of important artists by giving them an outlet and inspiration for their creativity. Certain religions such as the Pentecostal movement in Christianity and Native American religions have fostered ecstatic, visionary states that satisfy a need for an experience that transcends reality.

Religious attitudes have been of concern to mental health professionals since the 1800s, but the relationship between the disciplines has not always been congenial, despite the fact that the meaning of the word "psychology" ("the science of the soul") implies a strong relationship between the fields. Members of the clergy, psychologists, psychiatrists and psychotherapists meet some overlapping needs in that they offer support, advice and wisdom and in many cases serve as confessors.

There is a sharp division in the mental health field regarding the role of religion in preserving a healthy state of mind. For example, Sigmund Freud (1856–1939) considered religion to be an "illusion" and an extension of childlike attitudes toward parents. Carl Jung (1875–1961) believed that proving or disproving the existence of God was not within the framework of psychology but that psychologists should accept thoughts and feelings related to religious beliefs as real and significant. In *Modern Man in Search of a Soul* (1933) Jung wrote, "Among all my patients in the second half of life, that is to say over 35, there has not been one whose problem in the last resort was not that of finding a religious outlook on life."

In the period from 1930 to 1960, theologian Paul Tillich (1886–1965), philosopher Martin Buber (1878–1965) and psychoanalyst Rollo May (1909–   ) published important works attempting to synthesize religion, psychology and modern philosophical movements. An interest in combining the mental health disciplines with the influence of religion has encouraged the development of training in pastoral counseling in recent years. In the early 1970s, priest-sociologist Andrew Greeley (1928–   ) in his book *Unsecular Man: The Persistence of Religion* (1974) described a conservative, religious social trend that recently has become more obvious in movements such as the creationist opposition to secular humanism in education, in the political influence of religious leaders and in celebrities publicizing their "born again" experiences.

Religion contains elements that are both supportive and damaging to good mental health. The Christian promise of reward in the afterlife has inspired and comforted many, but it has also been held responsible for making believers passive or accepting of hardships and inequities that they could overcome through their own efforts. Highly disturbed psychotic patients have been known to literally accept biblical passages as commands leading to self-mutilation. Others with obsessional disorders literally live a hellish life struggling with guilt and behaviors to undo what they feel are sinful (obsessive) thoughts. Many experience religion as being constraining and supportive of narrow-minded behavior. For example, Abraham Lincoln abandoned what he believed to be the pettiness of organized religion while adhering to the high aspirations of religious thoughts. Religious movements have brought about bloodshed and dissension, as in the Protestant-Catholic conflict in Northern Ireland in the latter part of the 20th century. Historically, religious visions and thoughts have been part of unstable behavior, particularly in such religious leaders as Martin Luther, John Wesley and Saint Ignatius. More recently, reports of fraud and sexual abuse by religious leaders have shown that the power that society gives religious leaders can corrupt.

Two surveys, one completed in 1991 for *Time* and one taken by the Gallup poll, indicate that while religion is a strong influence in the United States, there seems to be a lack of confidence or awareness of its importance. For example, the *Time* survey showed that 78 percent of those surveyed felt that children should be allowed to say prayers in public schools. Sixty-three percent said that they would not vote for a presidential candidate who did not believe in God. Fifty-five percent said that there was too little religious influence in American life, and 65 percent felt that religious influence was decreasing. The latter opinion can be both supported and contradicted by the Gallup poll, depending on one's point of reference. The percentage of those surveyed who felt that religion was "very important" or "fairly important" to them personally, about 85 percent, has remained fairly constant since the 1970s. Attendance at church or synagogue during the previous week had actually risen slightly from a low of 40 percent in the 1970s to 43 percent in 1989, while actual membership had dropped from 73 percent in 1965 to 68 percent in 1989.

The Gallup survey further defined the religious in the population. Female nonwhite adults over the age of 50, southerners and those with annual incomes under $20,000 are most likely to place importance on religion. On the other hand, the wealthy have a high rate of church attendance and membership.

An earlier survey of World War II veterans offered interesting insights into the religious state of mind of men who had experienced warfare. About 26 percent said that the war made them more religious; 19 percent that it made them less so. Fifty-eight percent of those surveyed said that even though their religious conviction may have increased, decreased or remained the same, their war experiences made them more interested in the subject of religion. The veterans exhibited an even stronger tendency when describing their religious attitudes during battle. Most were of the opinion that everyone prays in combat. The interesting variation was the comment "There were atheists in fox holes, but most of them were in love," implying that the thought of a loved one might carry a man through danger almost as well as an appeal to a higher power.

See also CULTS.

remarriage Although the divorced and widowed remarry at a high rate, the divorce rate for these unions is higher than for first marriages. Responses to a survey concerning the failure rate of second marriages consistently listed two leading causes:

children and money. Friction between stepparents and stepchildren is common. In remarriages, the husband is frequently several years older than the wife and may not want more children, while she may be eager for a family. The financial strains of a man called on to support two families are very often disruptive.

Other major obstacles are a reflection of the reasons for the second marriage. Some divorced men and women marry a person very similar to their first spouse and encounter similar difficulties; others try so hard to find a quality that was lacking in their first spouse that they may marry a person who has that particular quality and become blind to the fact that in other ways they are actually incompatible. Divorced or widowed persons may remarry out of emotional and financial need without fully establishing themselves or sifting through and resolving their feelings about their previous marriage. Some carry feelings of guilt about how the second marriage affects their children or previous spouse. The ex-wife or husband may interfere in the marriage, and family members may make it obvious that they preferred the previous spouse.

How well one is accepted by the extended remarriage family may relate to the circumstances of the courtship. For example, if a woman was the "other woman" while the new husband was still married, relatives may regard her as a "homewrecker." If she knew him before he was widowed and marries him soon after his wife's death, relatives may think the marriage was too hasty and disrespectful to the deceased. Many mid-life women grew up dependent on their families or their husbands. Until the 1950s, most women's mindset when entering marriage was "until death do us part." Having to seek a second, or third, husband weighs heavily on the self-esteem of divorced women.

In the 2000s, some individuals, after meeting a lovable other who loves them, choose not to marry for a variety of reasons ranging from not wanting to lose alimony payments, to waiting for vesting in a pension plan, to fear of making a mistake. Many older individuals who are past childbearing and child-rearing years opt for a "living together" arrangement instead of remarriage.

See also DIVORCE; MARRIAGE; STEPFAMILIES.

Belovitch, Jeanne. *Making Remarriage Work.* Lexington, Mass.: Lexington Books, 1987.

Kahn, Ada P., and Linda Hughey Holt. *Midlife Health: A Woman's Practical Guide to Feeling Good.* New York: Avon Books, 1989.

U.S. Department of Commerce. *Statistical Abstract of the United States, 1991.* Washington, D.C.: USGPO, 1991.

Wilson, Barbara Foley. "The Marry-Go-Round." *American Demographics* (Oct. 1991).

remembering   See MEMORY.

REM (rapid-eye-movement) sleep   A stage of sleep in which dreams occur. A sleep cycle consists of stages (known as Stages I, II, III and IV) in a cycle lasting about 90 minutes followed by the period of REM sleep for about 10 minutes. With each cycle, REM periods lengthen. During the last cycle, REM sleep may last for 30 to 60 minutes. REM sleep onset has been found to occur earlier in individuals with symptoms of depression and may be a biological marker for depression or vulnerability to depression.

See also DEPRESSION; DREAMING; SLEEP.

repression   In psychoanalysis, the basic defense mechanism, which excludes painful experiences and unacceptable impulses from consciousness. Repression operates on an unconscious level against anxiety often produced by objectionable sexual feelings and feelings of hostility.

resistance   The feelings, thoughts, attitudes and behaviors on the part of the patient that oppose therapeutic goals in a psychotherapeutic setting. Sigmund Freud viewed resistance as a defense mechanism, while behavioral therapists now explain resistance as part of avoidance learning; certain thoughts repeatedly associated with painful experiences, such as situations that produce anxieties or fears, become aversive. For best results, psychotherapists plan tactics to help overcome the patient's resistance to the therapist, to the process of treatment and to the loss of symptoms. An examination of resistance by the therapist may suggest certain diagnoses as well as whether the patient is amenable to certain modes of psychotherapy.

See also BEHAVIORAL THERAPY; DEFENSE MECHANISMS; FREUD, SIGMUND; PSYCHOANALYSIS.

Restoril   Trade name for the benzodiazepine medication known as temazepam.

See also BENZODIAZEPINE DRUGS; PHARMACOLOGICAL APPROACH.

retardation, mental   See MENTAL RETARDATION.

retirement   Withdrawing from the workforce, usually at an older age. Retirement is highly sought by some, but it produces mental health problems including anxieties, boredom and feelings of lack of productivity for others. Many retired people feel that they are not contributing members of society and become depressed and withdrawn. Some feel the lack of prestige they formerly received from their position.

Retired people who adjust the best to retirement seem to be those who enjoy getting into new activities and making new acquaintances. Most retired people enjoy having more time for family and friends, for travel and for pursuit of long-standing hobbies.

Those who enjoy their freedom from work usually have planned ahead by starting an interest or form of recreation before retirement that they pursue with additional vigor when additional time is available. For example, some individuals learn a musical instrument, while others pursue woodworking or sewing as a hobby. Others do volunteer work to help others in their previous profession. Some U.S. cities have "job corps" of senior citizens willing to use their knowledge in business and industry.

Many retired people enjoy going back to school and taking classes at local colleges and universities. Some participate in Elder-hostel activities, traveling to a distant college campus for a week or two to study a favorite topic.

Many people who retire actually go back to a paid position. According to researchers at the University of Southern California, retirement is no longer a once-in-a-lifetime happening. They tracked 2,816 American men who turned 55 between 1966 and 1976. Approximately one-third went back to work for an average of two or more years after they retired.

Other significant findings indicated that the average American male retires between age 61 and 62, that white-collar workers stay on the job about two years longer than blue-collar workers and that blue-collar workers spend an average of 10 years in retirement. White collar workers average 12 years of retirement.

Wives of retired men are sometimes affected by their mates' retirement. A research project reported in *Modern Maturity* (Dec. 1990–Jan. 1992) indicated that most women polled reported satisfaction with their husbands' retirement. Effects of retirement on 413 upper-middle-class women married to men retired an average of 16 years were examined. More than one-third of the women had no problems with their husbands' retirement, and two-thirds said they were fully prepared for it. Only 12 percent said they felt some loss of personal freedom, and 5 to 6 percent reported an increase in household chores. Among those who said they would have done things differently, the majority mentioned the need to be better prepared financially for retirement.

See also AGING.

Dennis, Helen, and John Migliaccio. "Redefining Retirement: The Baby Boomer Challenge." *Generations: Journal of the American Society on Aging* XXI, no. 2 (summer 1997): 45.

Godin, Seth. *If You're Clueless about Retirement and Want to Know More.* Chicago: Dearborn Financial, 1997.

Manchester, Joyce. "Aging Boomers and Retirement: Who is at Risk?" *Generations: Journal of the American Society on Aging* XXI, no. 2 (summer 1997): 19.

right to die   See LEGAL ISSUES.

Ritalin   A trade name for a drug (methylphenidate hydrochloride) sometimes used to treat hyperactivity in children. It is a mild stimulant to the central nervous system that may help some children increase their ability to concentrate in school and perform homework and other expected chores. Use of the drug has been controversial, because of concerns that it is too often prescribed for children. It is generally agreed that the diagnosis of Attention Deficit Hyperactivity Disorder (ADHD) should be carefully evaluated prior to its prescription for children. Newer medications have been developed and have replaced the use of Ritalin to some extent, although numerous studies support the beneficial effects of Ritalin in ADHD.

See also ATTENTION-DEFICIT/HYPERACTIVITY DISORDER.

rites of passage   See PUBERTY.

ritual   See OBSESSIVE-COMPULSIVE DISORDER.

Roe v. Wade   A 1973 ruling by the U.S. Supreme Court in which previous antiabortion laws enacted by individual states were struck down, making abortion legal in the United States and spelling out legal concerns about abortion during the three trimesters of pregnancy.

See also ABORTION; PREGNANCY; PRO-LIFE AND PRO-CHOICE.

Rogers, Carl R. (1902–1987)   An American psychologist and a major early contributor in the movement known as client-centered therapy (phenomenology). He identified critical features of the psychotherapy encounter; these features, which apply to all therapies, include consequence on the therapist's part, unconditional positive regard ("prizing" of the client), "empathetic understanding" (being in the frame of mind of the client) and communication of these qualities to the client.

Rogers considered clients as unique persons with unique perceptions, and he took psychotherapeutic techniques out of the area of disease and extended their use to normally functioning persons. His work has influenced all therapies.

See also CLIENT-CENTERED THERAPY.

role playing   A technique used in psychotherapy in which the client acts according to a role that is not his or her own. It can be useful in a variety of ways. For example, it can help a therapist determine how socially phobic people react to certain social roles and how they see themselves in social situations. Role playing can also help the individual gain insight into the conduct of others as well as catharsis, or release from their anxiety symptoms.

See also CATHARSIS.

Rolfing   One of many contemporary body therapies used to relieve stress and improve mental and physical health. It is a form of deep tissue massage and is a combination of the disciplines of Eastern philosophical systems and practices and medical knowledge of muscular and skeletal structure.

The technique, which is often combined with other body therapy techniques, was developed by Ida Rolf (1896–1979), an American biochemist. As a young woman, she had an accident and was successfully treated by both an osteopathic physician and a yoga instructor. She combined these two techniques with the medical system of homeopathy, a practice which calls upon the patient's own healing powers rather than merely treating symptoms. The therapy gained recognition through Rolf's work at the Esalen Institute in California during the 1960s. From what had been considered fringe or one of many complementary therapies, Rolfing and other body therapies entered the mainstream of mental and physical treatments in the mid-1900s.

Rolfing focuses on the network of connective tissue—fascia, tendons and ligaments—that contains the muscles and links them to the bones. Whenever connective tissue fails to work effectively, pain results. For many, Rolfing helps to heal the body by bringing it into proper alignment and proper relationship to the forces of gravity. A Rolfing practitioner puts pressure on certain areas of the patient's connective tissue to improve the structure of the body. Certified Rolfers have had training in human anatomy, physiology, kinesiology and various massage techniques.

Finding a Rolfing Therapist

The Rolf Institute, headquartered in Boulder, Colorado, has produced Rolfers since 1972. There are more than 600 practitioners across the United States and in 23 other countries. The Institute provides a complete listing of its graduates, their addresses and telephone numbers. The Institute also has a free pamphlet that lists books, videotapes and audio-visual information currently available about Rolfing.

For information:

The Rolf Institute
P.O. Box 1868
Boulder, Colorado 80306
Phone: (303) 449-5903

See also BODY THERAPIES; MASSAGE THERAPY.

Rolf, Ida P. *Rolfing: Reestablishing the Natural Alignment and Structural Integration of the Human Body for Vitality and Well Being.* Rochester, Vt.: Healing Arts Press, 1989.

Rorschach test (inkblot test)   A standardized test in which an individual responds to a set of inkblot pictures. Presumably, the individual reveals his or her attitudes, emotions and feelings by interpreting the pictures. The test was developed by Hermann Rorschach (1884–1922), a Swiss psychiatrist and psychoanalyst.

See also PSYCHOLOGICAL TESTS.

rumination   The act of being excessively anxious about, worrying about, thinking about and pondering one concern for an inordinate period of time. Rumination is a common symptom of obsessive-compulsive disorder. Ruminations are repetitive, intrusive thoughts or obsessions about some aspect of one's life, such as fear of contamination, fear of harming others or fear of not doing certain tasks correctly. The thoughts may be evoked by external cues or come out of the blue. Ruminations impair concentration and are hard to drive out of one's mind.

See also OBSESSIVE-COMPULSIVE DISORDER.

runner's high   A feeling of physical and mental well-being, which may occur during or after a period of exercise that makes the cardiovascular system work harder for longer than it usually does. For example, about 30 to 40 minutes of jogging may produce the feeling in many individuals. There is a common misconception that runner's high is caused exclusively by the release of endorphins, brain chemicals that can reduce pain and elevate mood in a manner similar to that of opiate drugs. In addition to release of endorphins, exercise causes the body to release many neurochemicals that in turn trigger physiological reactions. For example, stimulation of the sympathetic nervous system, along with activation of the endocrine system's adrenal medulla, causes the heart rate to increase and more oxygen to be delivered to the brain, all of which contribute to "runner's high."

See also ENDORPHINS.

Rush, Benjamin (1745–1813) An American physician who was physician general during the Revolutionary War. He later turned his attention to psychiatry, establishing a separate wing of the Pennsylvania Hospital for the active treatment and intensive study of mental patients, on the theory that insanity is a disease and essentially treatable. His treatment methods, however, included not only calming patients through kindness but also bloodletting, purging, keeping them awake and on foot for 24 hours and intimidation.

S

SAD See SEASONAL AFFECTIVE DISORDER.

sadism A sexual deviation (paraphilia) in which an individual needs to inflict pain on another in order to achieve sexual satisfaction. The term "sadism" is named for the Marquis de Sade (1740–1814), a French novelist whose works described his own bizarre sexual activities. Works such as *The Story of Juliette* (1797) and *The Bedroom Philosophers* (1795) were long banned for obscenity; de Sade spent many years in prison for his views.

Sadistic acts may include physical cruelty, such as beating or tying up the victim, or mental cruelty, as in humiliating the partner. Such acts may be inflicted on either a consenting or a nonconsenting person and may range from mild injury to raping, torturing or even killing the victim. Masochism is the term applied to instances in which an individual must be subjected to pain in order to achieve such satisfaction.

The term "sadism" was first used by Baron Richard von Krafft-Ebing (1840–1902), a German author and neurologist, in his classic work *Psychopathia Sexualis* in 1882. He described the forms that sadism might take following unsatisfying intercourse, sadistic acts that increase desire and acts that brought about orgasm without intercourse in cases of impotence.

Mental health professionals say that sadism as a psychological syndrome alone is rare. Most cases of sadism have been reported by prostitutes. Sadism is most frequently combined with masochistic behavior, a tendency to derive sexual pleasure from being dominated or injured by the sexual partner. A study of individuals who showed some type of sadomasochistic behavior showed that while men tended toward sadism and women toward masochism, both sexes derived pleasure from some behavior patterns of each type.

See also MASOCHISM; PARAPHILIAS; SADOMASOCHISM; SEXUAL DYSFUNCTION.

sadomasochism Two forms of sexual preference, one in which a person derives pleasure and sexual gratification from inflicting pain (sadism), and the other being when one becomes sexually aroused by experiencing pain (masochism). This practice is abbreviated as SM. Many sadomasochistically oriented people center their activities around reading magazines featuring photographs of women dressed in leather and spike-heeled shoes while they chain, whip and torture their victims; others actually practice this behavior. Some normal couples enjoy acting out sadomasochistic fantasies during lovemaking; the behavior becomes aberrant when it crosses into inflicting pain or humiliation on either individual.

See also PARAPHILIAS; SADISM; SEXUAL DYSFUNCTION in BIBLIOGRAPHY.

Katchadourian, Herant A., and Donald T. Lunde. *Fundamentals of Human Sexuality.* New York: Holt, Rinehart and Winston, 1972.

SADS See SCHEDULE FOR AFFECTIVE DISORDERS AND SCHIZOPHRENIA.

"safe sex" A term coined during the 1980s as the AIDS (Acquired Immunodeficiency syndrome) epidemic heightened and was known to involve the heterosexual population of men and women. The term "safe sex" means avoiding behaviors in which the AIDS virus can be transmitted. Anal intercourse seems to carry the highest risk for infection of all sexual techniques.

Safe sex practices involve avoiding sexual intercourse with known drug users and those who test positive for the HIV virus (known to cause AIDS), knowing about one's partner's sexual background, using condoms as well as a spermicide and becoming involved in a monogamous relationship. Safe sex practices can also help avoid transmission of many sexually transmitted diseases.

See also ACQUIRED IMMUNODEFICIENCY SYNDROME; SEXUALLY TRANSMITTED DISEASES; SEXUALLY TRANS-MITTED DISEASES in BIBLIOGRAPHY.

Kahn, Ada P., and Linda Hughey Holt. *Midlife Health: A Woman's Practical Guide to Feeling Good.* New York: Avon Books, 1989.
Paalman, M. E. M. "Safer Sex." *World Health* (Nov. 1988).

"sandwich" generation   The generation of midlife adults who are involved in their adult children's (and in some cases grandchildren's) lives while still caring for aging parents. Estimates are that women in particular will spend more time caring for aging parents than they did in raising their own children.

"Sandwich" generation adults have many stresses in their lives because of their multiple roles. For many, financial considerations are important, as they begin to face the possibility of requiring nursing home care for aging parents when they have just finished paying off college tuitions. Many find that just as their children have left home, parents' needs increase, and an increasing amount of time and energy is spent in caring for them.

In many homes during the 2000s, adult children have returned to what parents thought would be an empty nest. With two (and sometimes three) generations in the home, as well as an elderly parent either in the home or elsewhere, adults find that they need to stretch their adaptive skills in family dynamics. Their children are no longer children, but in returning home they seem to have put themselves in that role.

Those who adapt well in this new dimension of parenting become good listeners, but not critics, helpers and supporters in emotional and financial ways (to the extent possible) without becoming domineering. Just as when the children were younger, the goal of most parents is to encourage personal growth and independence in their children. In most cases, the younger generation wants to be on their own as soon as possible, and successful parents patiently encourage that goal.

See also ELDERLY PARENTS; EMPTY NEST SYNDROME; PARENTING.

Zal, H. Michael. *The Sandwich Generation.* New York: Plenum Press, 1992.

schedule for affective disorders and schizophrenia (SADS)   A structured interview to aid in the diagnostic process as well as for use in research projects. Available since the 1970s, it covers symptoms and past history. The first section evaluates the current condition; the second evaluates symptoms occurring during the patient's lifetime. It differs from other such standard research diagnostic interview formats in that it records the severity of each symptom (on a 1–6 scale).

schizoaffective disorder   A category of illness used when a differential diagnosis between affective disorders and schizophrenia or schizophreniform disorder cannot be made. Elements of mood swings associated with bipolar disorder as well as psychotic symptoms associated with schizophrenia occur. Patients with the manic form of schizoaffective disorder have been found to have increased likelihood of relatives with bipolar disorder.

See also AFFECTIVE DISORDERS; SCHIZOPHRENIA; SCHIZOPHRENIFORM DISORDER.

schizoid personality disorder   A personality characterized by social withdrawal, hypersensitivity, absence of tender feelings for others, indifference to praise or criticism, close friendships with only one or two persons and sometimes unusual thoughts or beliefs. Usually eccentricities of behavior, thought and speech are not present.

See also SCHIZOPHRENIA; SCHIZOPHRENIFORM DISORDER.

schizophasia   Jumbled speech characteristic of advanced schizophrenia. It is also known as word salad.

See also SCHIZOPHRENIA.

schizophrenia A group of mental illnesses or related disorders characterized in a general way by distortions of perception, speech and thoughts. Although symptoms vary among individuals, common symptoms include disturbances in affect, inappropriate affect, withdrawal from reality, hallucinations and delusions. Schizophrenia causes pervasive dysfunction in many areas of behavior and is one of the most catastrophic mental illnesses because of its chronicity and the devastating effects it has on family members.

Individuals whose symptoms involve feelings of persecution and fixed delusions are said to have paranoid schizophrenia, despite the capacity to function socially and occupationally at some level; those who have incoherent thought and speech but do not have delusions are said to have disorganized schizophrenia. Approximately 150 out of every 100,000 persons in the United States have schizophrenia; men and women of all races are affected equally. The U.S. government estimates the cost of schizophrenia at more than $40 billion annually in direct medical costs and lost productivity. It is the fourth most costly diagnosis for Medicaid nationally.

Historical Background

In the late 1800s, Emil Kraepelin (1856–1926), a German psychiatrist, combined "hebrephrenia" and "catatonia" with certain paranoid states and called the condition "dementia praecox." Kraepelin said the condition consisted of large irreversible intellectual deterioration that began around or shortly after adolescence. Eugene Bleuler (1857–1939), a Swiss psychiatrist, modified Kraepelin's conception in the early 1900s to include cases with better outlook and in 1911 renamed the condition schizophrenia. The word "schizophrenia" is derived from the New Latin terms for "split mind" (*schizo* and *phrenia*).

Diagnostic criteria in the *Diagnostic and Statistical Manual of Mental Disorders* (4th ed., rev.) may include: (1) delusions, prominent hallucinations, incoherence/loosening of associations, catatonic behavior, inappropriate/flat affect (at least two); or (2) bizarre delusions; or (3) prominent hallucinations, for at least one week.

Gradual Onset of Symptoms

Schizophrenia usually begins gradually during adolescence or young adulthood, except for the paranoid variety, which may develop in the late twenties or after. Early symptoms may not be detected by family and friends for a while. Initially, the sufferer may feel tense, is unable to sleep or concentrate and may become socially withdrawn, and there is general deterioration of job performance and self-appearance. Symptoms become increasingly bizarre as the disease progresses. Some individuals talk in nonsensical terms, and others have unusual perceptions. The condition improves (remission or residual stage) and worsens (relapses) in cycles. Sometimes sufferers may appear relatively normal, while other patients in remission may appear strange because they speak in a monotone, have old speech habits, appear to have no emotional feelings and are prone to have "ideas of reference" (the idea that random social behaviors are directed at them). During an acute phase, schizophrenics suffer from hallucinations, delusions or thought disorders.

The most commonly noted hallucination is hearing voices that give commands, comment on behavior or insult the patient. Hallucinations also occur in visual or tactile form. Visual hallucinations may include having nonexistent perceptions, such as walls bending in and out as they breathe. Tactile hallucinations may include itching or burning sensations or a sense that "unhealthy" processes are affecting the body.

Delusions are bizarre thoughts that have no basis in reality. Some sufferers believe that someone can hear their thoughts, put thoughts into their heads or control their feelings. Some believe that others are spying on or planning to harm them, while others have delusions that they are a famous person from history or that they are part of some religious process.

Thought disorders involve loosely associated thoughts, shifting from one topic to other, unrelated topics with no logical connection. Some substitute rhymes or make up their own words that mean nothing to others.

Because of their illness, schizophrenics have a distorted ability to determine whether a situation or event they perceive is real, because while they are doing one activity, they may hear a voice talking about something totally unrelated. For example, while trying to read, they may hear a voice they attribute to Martians telling them to do something else.

Diagnosis and Causes

Psychiatrists diagnose schizophrenia when the condition has lasted at least six months and has included a psychotic phase. Although there are no accepted laboratory tests for schizophrenia, studies of brain metabolism during a task requiring mental concentration have shown lack of normal increases in the frontal lobes of the brain.

Some scientists believe that there may be an inherited susceptibility to schizophrenia, because the illness does run in families. According to the American Psychiatric Association, if one identical twin has the disease, there is a 50 to 60 percent chance that the sibling (identical genetic makeup) also has schizophrenia. With one parent suffering from schizophrenia, a child has an 8 to 18 percent chance of developing the illness. If both parents have the disease, the child has a risk of between 15 and 50 percent.

There are many theories regarding schizophrenia. The onset of schizophrenia in most cases seems to be during puberty, as the body undergoes structural and biochemical changes. It may be that a schizophrenic's brain is more sensitive to certain biochemicals or that it produces excessive or inadequate biochemicals necessary for good mental health, that the brain does not develop normally or that the brain may not effectively screen stimuli when processing information that healthy people easily handle.

Some researchers have suggested that schizophrenia may have similarities to some "autoimmune" diseases, which are disorders caused when the body's immune system attacks itself. Another theory is that the mother of a schizophrenic suffered with a viral infection while he or she was in the uterus. A recent finding of MRI (magnetic resonance imaging) abnormalities in non-concordant identical twins with schizophrenia not present in the normal twin supports the possibility of intrauterine influence. The virus could have infected the baby in such a way that changes occurred many years after birth. Several factors put together, such as the genetic predisposition, the immune system and the virus, may interact to cause an individual to develop the disease.

Treatment

Treatment involves use of medication, hospitalization in some cases and psychotherapy for the individual as well as the sufferer's family members. Treatment plans are individualized according to the patient's condition and the needs of the families involved.

New medical technology enables researchers to use several tools to diagnose or confirm diagnosis of schizophrenia and plan a treatment approach. One such technique is computerized axial tomography (CAT scan), which shows subtle abnormalities in the brains of some sufferers; ventricles (fluid-filled spaces within the brain) are larger in some schizophrenics' brains. Enlarged ventricles are also seen in bipolar disorder, and CAT findings are therefore not diagnostic.

In some schizophrenics, the prefrontal cortex in the brain appears to have either atrophied (shrunk, dried out) or developed abnormally.

Medications that interfere with the brain's production of dopamine (a biochemical) are successful with schizophrenics because their brains are either extraordinarily sensitive to dopamine or produce too much dopamine.

A number of antipsychotic medications help bring biochemical imbalances closer to normal in a schizophrenic. Medications reduce delusions, hallucinations and incoherent thoughts and reduce or eliminate chances of relapse.

According to the American Psychiatric Association, 60 to 80 percent of those who did not take medication as part of their treatment had a relapse the first year after leaving the hospital, while only 20 to 50 percent of those who took medication were rehospitalized the first year. When patients continued taking medication beyond the first year, relapse rates were reduced to 10 percent.

Antipsychotic drugs have some side effects, including dry mouth, blurred vision, drowsiness, constipation and dizziness upon standing up; in a few weeks, these side effects usually disappear. A more serious possible side effect is tardive dyskinesia (TD), a condition that affects 20 to 30 percent of people taking antipsychotic drugs. TD involves small tongue tremors, facial tics and abnormal jaw movements, and spasmodic movements of the hands, feet, arms, legs, neck and shoulders. TD symptoms are relieved in many cases when medication is stopped. A new "atypical antipsychotic" group of medications including clozapine, risperidone, olanzapine, quetiapine, and ziprasidone have been shown to be more effective with so-called negative symptoms (social withdrawal, lack of initiative and motivation) than the older antipsychotic drugs. These newer medications do not depend solely on blockage of dopamine as do the older antipsychotic medications. These medications also have a much lower incidence of extrapyramidal side effects and tardive dyskinesia. A proportion of patients who have shown limited progress while treated with older medications have shown much improved responses with the use of "atypical antipsychotic" medications.

Psychotherapy for the individual as well as family members helps all involved cope with the disease and its processes. Family members need reassurance and suggestions for handling the emotional aspects of the disorder. Suggestions may also be made regarding changes in the patient's living and working environment that will reduce stress and anxieties.

A variety of other therapies are useful for many schizophrenics, including dance therapy, art therapy, psychodrama and occupational therapy.

The following are some resources for information on schizophrenia:

American Mental Health Fund
2735 Hartland Road (#302)
Falls Church, VA 22043
Phone: (703) 573-2200

American Psychiatric Association
1400 K Street NW
Washington, D.C. 20005
Phone: (888) 357-7924
Web site: www.psych.org

National Alliance for the Mentally Ill
2107 Wilson Boulevard
Arlington, VA 22201
Phone: (703) 524-7600 or (800) 950-6264

Fax: (703) 524-9094
Web site: www.nami.org

National Alliance for Research on
  Schizophrenia and Depression
60 Cutter Mill Road, Suite 404
Great Neck, NY 11021
Phone: (516) 829-0091
Fax: (516) 487-6930
Web site: www.narsad.org

National Mental Health Association
1021 Prince Street
Alexandria, VA 22314-2971
Phone: (703) 684-7722
Fax: (703) 684-5968
Web site: www.nmha.org

See also AFFECTIVE FLATTENING; ANTIPSYCHOTIC MEDICATIONS; CLOZAPINE; PSYCHOSIS; TARDIVE DYSKINESIA; THOUGHT DISORDERS.

Facts About Schizophrenia. Washington, D.C.: American Psychiatric Association, 1988.

schizophrenic depression The term applied to a mental illness that is characterized by the combined symptoms of schizophrenia and depression.

See also DEPRESSION; SCHIZOPHRENIA.

schizophreniform disorder A disorder that meets the criteria of schizophrenia but is of shorter duration, generally lasting two weeks to six months. Although the onset is acute rather than gradual, there is a greater chance of recovery from schizophreniform disorder than from schizophrenia. The term was first used in 1939 to describe an acute disorder that occurred in persons with normal personalities.

See also SCHIZOPHRENIA.

schizotypal personality disorder A pattern of peculiar behavior, odd speech and thinking and unusual perceptual experiences; a mild form of schizophrenia without psychotic symptoms. Treatment often centers on issues that disturb the patient, such as mild feelings of paranoia or ideas of reference. A supportive approach and training in social skills help many individuals feel more comfortable in social situations.

See also PERSONALITY DISORDERS; SCHIZOPHRENIA.

school phobia In children, one of the most common anxiety disorders; also known as school refusal or school absenteeism. There is some controversy whether refusal to go to school is related to separation anxiety, truancy secondary to conduct disorder or a fear of failure. Fear of going to school may begin as early as kindergarten, but it usually develops during grade or junior high school. In many cases, the child begins to devise reasons for staying home from school. Some develop symptoms, such as nausea, stomachache or headache. Others leave home for school but then return without their parents knowing that they are absent from school, or spend their day elsewhere.

School avoidance should be evaluated and treated as soon as it is detected to prevent future personal, academic and social consequences. A therapist, along with teachers, parents and the child, should try to determine the underlying reasons for the school avoidance. Reasons may include low self-esteem, being teased or bullied by others, being criticized by others or feeling inferior to others. Situations surrounding actual school issues should be considered, such as riding on the school bus, eating in the school lunchroom, using the public washrooms and undressing in the gym locker rooms. Issues of body image may be involved. Often the child's mother covertly remembers her own phobic behavior or has anxieties about the child and needs supportive help to not convey her anxieties to the child.

Treatment of a child who avoids school should be regarded as a crisis intervention. The goal should be to get the child back in school as soon as possible and attending regularly with less fear and more confidence to meet the daily challenges, whether in the classroom, the playground or the gym.

With appropriate counseling and conferences with teachers or other school officials, children and parents can develop a new understanding of the anxieties regarding school attendance. There is some evidence linking early history of school phobia with later occurrences of panic disorder and agoraphobia.

Fear of school, or school phobia, is known as didaskaleinophobia.

See also ANXIETY DISORDERS; PHOBIA.

Andreasen, Nancy C., and Donald W. Black. *Introductory Textbook of Psychiatry.* Washington, D.C.: American Psychiatric Association, 1991.

screen memory The memory of an unacceptable experience, often of a trivial or harmless nature, which unconsciously serves the purpose of concealing or screening out an associated experience of a more significant nature. Screen memory (also known as cover memory) is a form of resistance frequently encountered in psychotherapy.

seasonal affective disorder (SAD) Seasonal affective disorder (SAD) seems to result from the stress of not seeing much sunshine or daylight. It affects an estimated 35 million Americans. It is characterized by severe mood swings that correspond to the change of seasons. Depression usually becomes more prevalent during the winter months, while the mood switches to mania with the coming of spring.

The incidence of SAD rises with geographic latitude, affecting 1.4 percent of Floridians but almost 10 percent of the population of New Hampshire.

Therapy for SAD includes use of specially made bright lights that extend the hours of illumination during short winter days. In some cases, medications and psychotherapy are useful.

Role of Genetics

People who eat more, sleep more and are more depressed during the winter months probably have family members experiencing similar changes, according to an article in the *Archives of General Psychiatry* (January 1996). Researchers from Washington University School of Medicine in St. Louis, Missouri, surveyed 4,639 adult twins from Australia to determine if there is a biological predisposition to seasonal rhythms in mood and behavior (seasonality). Two types of seasonality have been clinically described: one characterized by a winter pattern and a second by a summer pattern of depressive mood disturbance. Other surveys, cited by the researchers, have shown that one in four adults suffers from some type of seasonality disorder.

Many of the twins surveyed for this study (40 percent) lived in the Australian state of Victoria.

The region has seasonal changes in sunlight exposure similar to Montgomery County, Maryland, where research on SAD was pioneered, according to the article.

The researchers found that winter was much more likely than summer to lead to changes in mood, energy, social activity, sleep, appetite and weight. They also found a "significant genetic influence" on those changes. The researchers wrote: "Thirteen percent of our sample complained that seasonality was a personal problem, 17 percent reported that they felt worse during the winter and eight percent reported that they experienced a summer pattern of worsening in mood. Only 2 percent of our sample reported a degree of seasonality that resembled the response of patients who were clinically diagnosed as having seasonal affective disorder (SAD)," which is the most extreme form of seasonality.

The researchers concluded that "There is a tendency for seasonality to run in families, and this is largely owing to a biological predisposition." These findings support continuing efforts to understand the role of seasonality in the development of mood disorders.

See also DEPRESSION; PHARMACOLOGICAL APPROACH; PSYCHOTHERAPIES.

Madden, Pamela A. F. "Seasonal Changes in Mood and Behavior." *Archives of General Psychiatry* (Jan. 1996).

secondary depression A depression occurring in an individual who has another illness—either mental or physical—that precedes the depression. Depression may accompany psychiatric disorders, such as obsessive-compulsive disorder, alcohol abuse or alcoholism (most common), and it may occur after or along with a medical illness. Careful evaluation of secondary depression is essential to determining the cause and course of treatment.

See also ANTIDEPRESSANT MEDICATIONS; DEPRESSION.

secondary gain Advantages derived from an anxiety disorder, other than the primary gain of relieving the internal conflict or anxiety. Examples of such gains include attention, sympathy, avoidance of work and domination of others. These gains are reactions to the illness instead of causal factors. They often prolong the anxiety disorder and may create resistance to therapy.

secrets The word "secret" is derived from the Latin word "secretus," meaning separate, or out of the way. The current definition, according to the *American Heritage Dictionary of the English Language,* includes the following:

- Something kept hidden from others or known only to oneself or to a few
- Concealed from general knowledge or view
- Dependably close-mouthed; discreet
- Not visibly expressed; private; inward

Most of us know something that fits into the above definitions that we don't tell others. What the definition doesn't say, however, is that many of us are uncomfortable and stressed by the secrets we keep. Many of us have a lifelong struggle with the keeping of secrets. Some of us think that there is something wrong in having a secret, but we don't know what to do about it. Some of us even think there is something wrong with us.

Some of us have serious secrets, such as having committed a crime, while others have less serious secrets, such as having had orthodontia as a teenager. We use energy worrying about keeping the secret. We feel scared, threatened and held back from letting our real selves emerge. Some secrets become all-consuming.

There are those whose sexual orientation may be unknown to their friends and families, adults who have never had a sexual experience, secret alcoholics, agoraphobics afraid to venture out of their homes without a trusted person, women who have had abortions or gave babies away, people who know they are adopted and choose not to tell their spouses. Some people were married once and never told their second spouse. Some are currently victims of abuse by their husbands or wives. Others may have a history of mental illness in their family, once attempted suicide or struggled with mental health issues.

An increasing number of individuals undergo cosmetic surgery. Then there are those who never tell their wartime secrets, or those who undergo rigorous religious training for the priesthood or rabbinate but later perform more secular jobs, or those in professional capacities, such as doctors or lawyers who hide just as many secrets about themselves (e.g., psychiatrists who are drug addicts) as the rest of us. Hiding a non-visible handicap, such as vision or hearing impairment, diabetes or cancer, produces stresses that can lead to anxiety disorders. Just as the size of ears and noses vary among individuals, so do the sizes and shapes of secrets vary among individuals. But the common factor among them is the indecision, anxiety and stress they produce.

As we continue to worry about hiding our secret, the stress produced by the hiding leads to body tension, thereby producing psychophysiological illnesses, such as headaches and stomachaches, and behavioral symptoms, such as irritability, short temper and difficulty concentrating, and psychological reactions, such as anxieties, depression and frustration.

Telling Secrets

Some secrets should be kept. Divulging some secrets at the wrong time to the wrong people can be embarrassing, shameful and may interfere with one's life and lifestyle. On the other hand, telling a secret at an appropriate time to an appropriate person may help you feel freer, unburdened and able to let go of the fears that you have faced. Telling can be a positive force and work to your benefit.

Secrets to Share

Secrets can be divided into those to keep, those to let go of and those to share; the person with the secret must decide which category pertains to his or her particular knowledge. Many couples share secrets—the intimacies of their relationship is one example. Business associates share secrets. Mothers and daughters, fathers and sons share secrets. Many admit to shared secrets, and for many their sharing has helped bond their loving and supportive relationship. Fortunately for them, their shared secrets are "constructive" secrets.

Kahn, Ada P. *Stress A to Z: The Sourcebook for Facing Everyday Challenges.* New York: Facts On File, 2000.

security object   A special object, such as a blanket or a favorite toy, that gives a young child reassurance and comfort. Many children sleep with their security object or take it with them wherever they go. If the item is lost or taken away, the child will become extremely distressed until it is returned.

sedative drug   One of many substances that tend to moderate or tranquilize (sedate) a person's state of mind and help induce sleep. Many drugs have sedative side effects; examples include antianxiety drugs, antipsychotic drugs, some antidepressant drugs and some sleeping medications. Many sedative side effects decrease as the patient takes the medication over time, and the patient accommodates to the side effects. Many people receive sedative drugs before surgery.

See also BARBITURATE DRUGS; CENTRAL NERVOUS SYSTEM; HYPNOTIC DRUGS.

seizures   A sudden episode of uncontrolled electrical activity in the brain. Symptoms may be as subtle as a twitching of a small area of the body—such as the face or an arm or leg—or more severe, causing a convulsion of the body. Consciousness is almost always lost during a seizure. Recurrent seizures are known as epilepsy. Seizures can occur because of infection, head injury, brain tumor or stroke (cerebrovascular accident) or may be alcohol-related.

See also ANTICONVULSANT MEDICATIONS; CONVULSIONS; EPILEPSY.

selective serotonin reuptake inhibitors   (SSRIs)   A class of antidepressant medications introduced in the 1980s. Popular medications in this category are fluoxetine (trade name: Prozac), sertraline (Zoloft), paroxetine (Paxil), fluvoxamine (Luvox), venlafaxine (Effexor) and nefazodone (Serzone). The SSRIs lack the cardiac toxicity of tricyclic antidepressants and most also lack anticholinergic adverse effects. Although they are generally well-tolerated, adverse effects common to this group include nausea, headache, insomnia, dry mouth and restlessness, especially at the beginning of treatment.

The SSRIs appear to be effective in various anxiety states, particularly panic disorder and obsessive-compulsive disorder, as well as in anxious depression. There is also circumstantial evidence for their efficacy in social phobia.

See also ANTIDEPRESSANTS.

Boer, J.A. Den, and H.G.M. Westenberg. "Serotonergic Compounds in Panic Disorder, Obsessive-Compulsive Disorder and Anxious Depression: A Concise Review." *Human Psychopharmacology* 10 (1995): pp. S173–S183.

selegiline A medication (trade name: Deprenyl) that slows the progress of Parkinson's disease. It was approved for use in the United States in 1989. It is a monoamine oxidase (MAO) Type B inhibitor at low doses that increases brain dopamine level; at higher doses it inhibits MAO Type A and may be useful for depression.

See also PARKINSON'S DISEASE.

self-esteem Liking, respecting and accepting oneself and appreciating one's self-worth. In the 1990s, self-esteem has been targeted as a major characteristic of good mental health. Low self-esteem can lead to mental and physical disorders, such as depression, poor appetite, sleeplessness and headaches.

People tend to compare themselves with others, their own standards and standards set for them by others. If they think they do not measure up, they have low self-esteem. Such individuals may feel inferior, either intellectually or physically, while individuals with high self-esteem feel confident and capable. People with low self-esteem often depend on approval from others. Some become workaholics, and some become totally dependent on outside approval.

Lack of self-esteem can be life threatening, particularly in young people when it is a major factor in suicide. Lack of self-esteem has been pointed to as a cause for many social ills, including juvenile delinquency, crime and substance abuse. While it may not be the most important causative factor, it usually plays a role.

Causes of low self-esteem vary among individuals, but there are many common themes. For example, many people have low self-esteem because of physical appearance. Obesity is a common situation; this can be overcome by seeking counseling regarding a diet and exercise program. Some adults have lifelong low self-esteem because of a prominent facial feature, such as a misshapen nose or ear; with counseling and possibly cosmetic surgery, improvements can be made in both outlook and appearance. But some people have obsessional ideas about unattractive body features (dysmorphophobia), which seems to be a subtype of obsessive-compulsive disorder; this should be understood and treated.

There are other common physical causes of low self-esteem. Child abuse, whether sexually or psychological, can be a major factor. Abused spouses and lovers also suffer from low self-esteem. Being bullied or criticized in school can also harm a child's confidence and self-worth.

Some children lose their self-esteem on the athletic fields because they do not compete well or do not have the physical ability to keep up with others. Other children lose self-esteem in the classroom when they find doing math or science difficult and are advised to pursue other avenues of career choice. Simple comments by teachers can ruin a child's self-esteem; for example, when a child is told that he cannot sing well and should just mouth the words, he may lose his confidence in ever trying to sing again. A high school student criticized because of lack of public speaking ability may become afraid of standing up in front of a crowd. In such cases, lack of self-esteem can lead to social fears and phobias.

In a Gallup poll in early 1992, 612 adults were interviewed by telephone. Respondents were asked about situations that would make them feel very bad about themselves. Situations included not being able to pay bills, being tempted into doing something immoral, having an abortion, getting a divorce, losing a job, feeling they had disobeyed God, being noticeably overweight, doing something embarrassing in public and being criticized by someone they admire. People over 50 years of age were more likely to feel bad about these situations than younger people. However, overall, 63 percent said that time and effort spent on self-esteem is worthwhile; only 34 percent said that time and effort could be better spent on work.

Extreme over-inflation of self-esteem is a characteristic of manic behavior. An individual may feel extremely powerful and influential and may even experience delusions. Narcissistic individuals act as if they feel very important, but in fact they rely constantly on external support for money, clothes, important friends and success to counteract their inner emptiness and low self-esteem.

See also BODY IMAGE; CODEPENDENCY; CRITICISM; DEPRESSION; INFERIORITY COMPLEX; SCHOOL PHOBIA; SUICIDE.

Kahn, Ada P., and Sheila Kimmel. *Empower Yourself: Every Woman's Guide to Self-Esteem.* New York: Avon Books, 1994.

self-help groups   These consist of people who share a common experience and wish to assist one another with or without the use of a trained mental health professional. Such groups became popular during the 1970s and continue to be so. Central to a self-help group is the idea of sharing feelings, perceptions and problems with others who have had the same experience. The group can pass on practical advice to new members, such as what life is like after divorce or how to cope with aging parents.

The National Self-Help Clearinghouse can provide information about groups throughout the United States, as well as books and pamphlets on how to start a group and what to look for in an existing group.

For information, contact:

National Self-Help Clearinghouse
33 West 42nd Street
New York, NY 10036
Phone: (212) 642-2944

self-help techniques   During the 1990s, American society has been offered self-help in the form of magazine articles, radio call-in shows, television talk shows, speakers, support groups, audio and video tapes. Self-help can work if the individual is motivated to make it work. In fact, even with psychotherapy under the guidance of a mental health professional, much of the improvement in a person's mental health actually comes from self-help.

Self-help techniques include meditation and progressive relaxation. Both are skills that can be learned and applied to relieve many mental health concerns, such as stress, anxiety and phobias.

Many individuals join self-help groups or support groups to learn various techniques for particular situations.

See also ANXIETY; MEDITATION; STRESS.

"Special Focus on Self-Help." *Anxiety Disorders Association of America Reporter* VI, no. 3 (summer/fall 1995).

self-hypnosis   See HYPNOSIS.

self psychology   A term for the psychological system propounded by Heinz Kohut (1913–1981), an Austrian-born American psychoanalyst. This theory holds that all behavior can be interpreted in reference to the self. He proposed that the young child has tendencies toward assertiveness and ambition as well as tendencies toward idealization of parents and the beginnings of ideals and values. Both groups of tendencies contribute to strong ties between the infant and parent. He believed that the real mover of psychic development is the self, rather than sexual and aggressive drives, as Sigmund Freud suggested. Kohut used the term "selfobject" to describe an object in an infant's surrounding that the infant regards as part of him- or herself. People with narcissistic personality disorder cannot separate adequately from the selfobject and thus cannot perceive or respond to the individuality of others. Kohut believed that lack of emphatic response between parent and infant is the cause of later psychological disorders in the growing child.

Kohut developed his major theories in several publications, including *The Analysis of the Self* (1971), *The Restoration of the Self* (1977) and *The Search for the Self* (1978).

self-talk   See AFFIRMATION.

Selye, Hans (1907–1982)   An Austrian-born Canadian endocrinologist and psychologist well known for his work in stress research. He introduced the concept of stress to the psychological world during the early 1940s. He is the author of *The Stress of Life* (1956) and *Stress without Distress* (1974).

He received his medical training in Europe, but he did most of his innovative research on the effects of stress in Montreal at McGill University and the Institute de Medicine et de Chirugie Experimentales de l'Universite de Montreal. He received his medical degree and his Ph.D. from the German University in Prague. He held earned doctorates in medicine, philosophy and science, as well as at least 19 honorary degrees from universities around the world. He authored more than 32 books and more than 1,500 technical articles. For many years he was professor and director of the Institute of Experimental Medicine and Surgery at the University of Montreal.

In 1950, Selye coined the term "general adaptation (or stress) syndrome." Selye borrowed the term "stress" from physics and applied it to the mutual actions of forces that take place across any section of the body and threaten homeostasis. Although not all states of stress were noxious, according to Selye, he held that the more severe, protracted and uncontrollable situations of psychological and physical distress led to disease states. His concept of GAS focused on the reaction of the body to illness or foreign substances as opposed to concentrating on specific illnesses and their treatment. Although his work was medical and in some ways controversial, the mental health disciplines profited from his groundbreaking stress research.

He defined stress as "the nonspecific response of the body to any demand made upon it." It is more than "merely nervous tension," and he ultimately categorized well over 1,000 physiological things that occur in stress and adaptation. His theory is a description of what one may expect in the body's attempts to adapt and return to "normality" during chronic exposure to stressors.

Selye believed that "stress is the spice of life. Without it you would be a vegetable—or dead."

His famous and revolutionary concept of stress opened countless new avenues of treatment through the discovery that hormones participate in the development of many degenerative diseases, including coronary thrombosis, hardening of the arteries, high blood pressure, arthritis, peptic ulcers and even cancer.

See also DIS-STRESS; EUSTRESS; GENERAL ADAPTATION SYNDROME; HOMEOSTASIS; STRESS.

Selye, Hans *The Stress of Life* New York: McGraw-Hill, 1956.

———. *Stress without Distress.* Philadelphia: J. B. Lippincott, 1974.

senile dementia   See DEMENTIA; SENILITY.

senility   Changes in mental ability brought on by old age, including impaired memory and reduced ability to concentrate. Dementia affects about one in five individuals over age 80.

See also DEMENTIA; MEMORY.

sensate-focus-oriented therapy   The approach developed by Masters and Johnson to overcome sexual difficulties involving training sessions in which both partners learn to think and feel sensually by progressively touching, stroking, fondling, kissing and massaging all parts of their mate's body. The therapy also includes a complete history of each partner's attitudes, steps toward improvement in communication between the partners and at-home practice.

See also SEX THERAPY; SEXUAL DYSFUNCTION.

sense of humor   See LAUGHTER.

separation anxiety   A distressed feeling one experiences when separated from parents or individuals with whom one has an attachment. Infants and toddlers normally experience anxiety about separation from parents or caregivers, but the intensity usually diminishes by the time the child is four to five years old. Children who fear separation cry, cling to the parent and demand to be held and cuddled.

In childhood, symptoms of separation may be headaches, stomachaches and other vague complaints in an effort to keep the parent from leaving or to keep the child from going off to school. School phobia, or school refusal, is sometimes a case of separation anxiety rather than a fear of being bullied or a fear of failure. What some children fear is that something dreadful will happen to their parent(s) if they are away or that the parent will not be there when the child returns.

Sometimes the parent (usually the mother) has fears of danger when her child is away from her, which get transmitted to the child and augments the child's fears. This means that often the mother of a child with separation anxiety may need supportive psychotherapy to help the child. There is some evidence that a child who has a history of separation anxiety is associated with panic attacks and agoraphobia as an adult.

See also AGORAPHOBIA; SCHOOL PHOBIA; SECURITY OBJECT.

Serax   Trade name for the benzodiazepine medication oxazepam.

See also BENZODIAZEPINE DRUGS; PHARMACOLOGICAL APPROACH.

Seroquel   The trade name for quetiapine, an "atypical antipsychotic" medication used in the treatment of schizophrenia.

serotonin   A neurotransmitter (also known as hydroxytryptamine, 5-hydroxytryptamine or 5-HT) found in the central nervous system, in many tissues, in the lining of the digestive tract and in the brain. Serotonin influences sleep and emotional arousal and is indirectly involved in the psychobiology of depression and impulsive behavior. It may be that low levels of serotonin are a factor in the development of depression and impulsive, sometimes violent behavior. Some antidepressant drugs increase the levels of serotonin and norepinephrine, another neurotransmitter. Serotonin is derived from tryptophan, an essential amino acid found throughout the body and in the brain. Serotonin stimulates smooth muscles (involuntary muscles such as in the intestinal wall) and constricts blood vessels. Serotonin was identified in the 1950s.

See also ANTIDEPRESSANT MEDICATIONS; DEPRESSION; NEUROTRANSMITTERS.

sertraline hydrochloride   An antidepressant drug (trade name: Zoloft). This medication is indicated for the symptomatic relief of depressive illness. It should not be taken along with monoamine oxidase inhibitors.

See also ANTIDEPRESSANT MEDICATIONS; DEPRESSION; SEROTONIN.

Serzone   Trade name for nefazodone, an antidepressant medication which increases brain serotonin function but may have fewer sexual side effects because of its capacity to block out the serotonin receptor (5HT receptor).

sex addiction   According to Joel Z. Spike, D.D., associate professor and director of Education and Drug Prevention, Southeastern College of Osteopathic Medicine, North Miami Beach, Florida, sex addiction meets the criteria of addiction that we tend to use, including compulsive behavior, loss of control and continuing behavior despite knowing the negative consequences.

Men are more affected with sexual addictions than women; Dr. Spike reports the ratio as being about eight to one. Sexual addictions occur in all socioeconomic groups; concurrent psychopathology may or may not be present. About 90 percent of sex addicts have other types of addictions. In a study from the Sexual Dependency Unit of Golden Valley Health Care Center, Golden Valley, Minnesota, in which 85 percent of patients were male, 42 percent of whom had incomes above $30,000, 58 percent were college graduates, and half were married. According to Dr. Spike, "These people are totally preoccupied with sex. They feel a compulsion to have sexual activity, which while not pleasurable for them, is a way of relieving stress and anxiety. They repeatedly have sexual activity followed by guilt, shame and depression. It is not unusual for these men to have literally thousands of partners in a year."

About 87 percent of male sex addicts come from dysfunctional families in which some addictions or substance abuse occurred. Many male sex addicts have backgrounds of childhood physical, sexual or emotional abuse. Many were victims of sexual trauma, such as seductions or incest.

Lives of sex addicts revolve around compulsivity, having experiences and recovering from the experiences. Addicts spend large amounts of time every day with their activity; many have financial problems, spending thousands of dollars on massage parlors, prostitutes, phone sex and pornography. Very often there are also major family issues, causing these men to seek relationship counseling.

Recognizing Sex Addiction in Men

The most notable signs are presence of a sexually transmitted disease, urinary tract symptoms and depression. Sex addicts want help, even though they show excessive reliance on denial. Sex addicts express cognitive distortions including denial, minimization, rationalization, suspicion, paranoia and self-delusion. Addicts work hard to maintain their secret and believe that they are the only one who feels such severe pain.

Most sex addicts have feelings of low self-esteem and isolation, and some may come in for treatment with ideas of suicide. They have basic beliefs about themselves that they are bad and unworthy people and feel unlovable as they are. They suffer from "stroke hunger" and want attention. They feel a major conflict with their own role system, values and morals.

Sex addiction involves a continuum of compulsive behavior and loss of control. Behavioral abnormalities may include reduced community involvement and social interactions, as well as family, employment and legal problems. Risking increasing consequences to achieve more exciting highs indicates an escalation of a sexual addiction. Individuals often escalate within their own levels. Level I addiction involves exaggeration of behaviors considered normal, acceptable or tolerable. Such behaviors, however, are carried out compulsively; there is anonymous sexual behavior.

Level II addictions involve even greater risks of social, moral and legal sanctions. The addict may be a "nuisance" offender, such as a voyeur or "flasher;" he may be perceived by others as pathetic. Escalation may place him at risk of inflicting damage to others and of legal consequences for himself in committing incest, rape or pedophilia.

Treatment

To treat a sex addiction, the patient must be drug-free. According to Dr. Spike, "Any substance abuse or dependency must be treated before beginning active treatment of the sex addiction." Sexual addiction is more difficult to treat than drug dependency or alcoholism. One must help the patient develop communication skills, deal with the issues of truth and improve cognitive distortions. Behavioral therapy may help in treating sexually dys-functional individuals as they come out of other addictions.

Treatment for sex addiction may consist of abstinence, education, medication and group, co-joined and individual therapy. Group therapy helps because it breaks down denial more than can be done in individual therapy. In some programs, addicts enter into an eight-week celibacy contract, avoiding all forms of sexual expression, including masturbation and fantasy, that may act as a bridge between their past and future.

See also SEXUAL DYSFUNCTION IN BIBLIOGRAPHY.

sex anxiety inventory (SAI) A questionnaire used by therapists with individuals in counseling for sexual anxieties. Responses to the SAI give some indications of the individual's sexual attitudes, experiences and possible basis for anxieties. Developed in 1974, the 25-item questionnaire permits the respondent to select alternative answers.

See also SEX THERAPY; SEXUAL FEARS.

Janda, L. H., and K. E. O'Grady. "Development of a Sex Anxiety Inventory." *Journal of Consulting and Clinical Psychology* 48 (1980).
Kleinknecht, Ronald A. *The Anxious Self.* New York: Human Sciences Press, 1986.

sex drive The desire to have sexual activity. This drive varies in strength in different women and men and at different ages and stages of life in the same individual. Differences may be due to inhibitions about sexual activity produced by parental attitudes toward sex and those of peer groups. One's expression of sex drive may differ also, according to whether or not one has a partner. For example, sex researchers have found that some widowed postmenopausal women who have no partner do not believe that their sex drive is very strong, while women in the same peer group who date and have regular, attractive male companions feel a strong sex drive.

Although some researchers believe that sex drive decreases with age, many senior adults will attest to the fact that sex drive can persist throughout all stages of life. Good health, freedom from chronic disease and companionship with others of the opposite sex stimulate the sex drive to continue until older age.

See also LIBIDO; SEX THERAPY.

Trudel, Gilles, Lyne Landry, and Yvette Larose. "Low Sexual Desire: The Role of Anxiety, Depression and Marital Adjustment." *Sexual and Marital Therapy* 12, no. 1 (Feb. 1997): 95–99.

sex therapy Counseling and treatment of sexual difficulties that are not due to physical causes. Many people are helped by a combination of sex therapy and marital counseling. The purpose of sex therapy is to reduce anxieties the couple has about sexual activity and increase their enjoyment of their relationship. In sex therapy, couples learn about normal sexual behavior and to reduce their anxieties about sex by gradually engaging in increasingly intimate activities. Couples learn to communicate better with each other regarding sexual matters and preferences and to retrain their approaches and response patterns.

Sex therapists use several techniques. One is sensate-focus therapy, in which the couple explores pleasurable activities in a relaxed manner without sexual sensations. The couple might start with massage of nonerogenous areas of the body. Gradually, as anxieties diminish, the couple progresses to stimulation of sexual areas and finally to sexual intercourse.

Other techniques sex therapists use are directed toward reducing premature ejaculation, relieving vaginismus (muscle spasm of the vagina) and helping both partners reach orgasm.

For sexual problems related to physical causes or illness, individuals should consult a physician, particularly specialists in gynecology or urology.

See also ANORGASMIA; DYSPAREUNIA; EJACULATION; ORGASM; SENSATE-FOCUS-ORIENTED THERAPY; SEXUAL FEARS; SEXUAL FULFILLMENT.

Kahn, Ada P., and Linda Hughey Holt. *The A to Z of Women's Sexuality.* Alameda, Calif.: Hunter House, 1992.

sexual abuse The forced participation of an unwilling individual in sexual activity by use of direct or implied threats. Abuse may involve actual physical contact, acts of exhibitionism or indecent exposure between adults and children. Fear of sexual abuse is known as agraphobia or contrectophobia. Sexual abuse occurs at all ages, from infants through older-age adults.

See also ABUSE; DISSOCIATION; DOMESTIC VIOLENCE; INCEST; RAPE.

Matas, M., and A. Marriott. "The Girl Who Cried Wolf: Pseudologia Phantastica and Sexual Abuse." *Canadian Journal of Psychiatry* 32 (May 1987).
Walker, Edward et al. "Relationship of Chronic Pelvic Pain to Psychiatric Diagnoses and Childhood Sexual Abuse." *American Journal of Psychiatry* 145, no. 1 (Jan. 1988).

sexual dysfunction Any condition that interferes with the process leading to and including coitus. Masters and Johnson estimated that 50 percent of American marriages were affected by some form of sexual dysfunction. Individuals may have temporary dysfunctions or situations that persist throughout life. Use of some prescription drugs may cause sexual dysfunction for some individuals; in some cases, other similar drugs may be substituted by a physician that do not have these unpleasant side effects.

To some extent, sexual dysfunction is culturally defined; for example, anorgasmia in women was considered proper and even desirable in the Victorian era but is considered a dysfunction at present. Homosexuality and masturbation have at different times been considered abnormal and at other times normal behavior. Present forms of female sexual dysfunction include anorgasmia, painful sexual intercourse (dyspareunia) and vaginismus. Example of male sexual dysfunctions include impotence, difficulty in maintaining erection, premature ejaculation and retarded ejaculation.

See also ANORGASMIA; DYSPAREUNIA; IMPOTENCE; ORGASM; SEX THERAPY; SEXUAL RESPONSE CYCLE; VAGINISMUS.

Avery-Clark, Constance. "Sexual Dysfunction and Disorder Patterns of Working and Non-working Wives." *Journal of Sex and Marital Therapy* 12, no. 2 (summer 1986).
Brown, Pamela. "Sexual Dysfunction in Women." *Canadian Family Physician* 35 (June 1989).
De Amicis, Lyn A. et al. "Clinical Follow-up of Couples Treated for Sexual Dysfunction." *Archives of Sexual Behavior* 14, no. 6 (1985).

Pinhas, Valerie. "Sexual Dysfunction in Women Alcoholics." *Medical Aspects of Human Sexuality* (June 1987).

sexual fears   Many people have fears that impair or weaken their sexual responses to partners. For example, some women are afraid of experiencing pain during intercourse or that they will not experience orgasm. Some men fear that they will not be able to achieve or maintain an erection long enough for a satisfactory experience.

Ill health can cause people to fear that they will not be able to enjoy sexually fulfilling experiences. For example, some people after surgery fear being hurt by their partner or hurting their partner during sexual activity.

The threat of acquiring a sexually transmitted disease (STD) or the HIV virus (known as the cause of AIDS) is a contemporary fear of many people who are not in monogamous relationships. These fears can largely be overcome by the use of "safe sex" practices.

See also BEHAVIORAL THERAPY; DYSPAREUNIA; SAFE SEX; SEX THERAPY; SEXUAL DYSFUNCTIONS.

sexual fulfillment   A feeling of contentment after a pleasurable and satisfying sexual encounter. An individual has a feeling of intense fulfillment in the orgasmic and resolution phases of the sexual response cycle. This is accompanied by a feeling of extreme relaxation, sometimes a "high" feeling and emotional closeness with the partner.

See also ORGASM.

sexual harassment   Unwanted and uninvited sexual attentions whether from men toward women, women toward men or toward same-sex individuals. Such attentions may include jokes and remarks, questions about the other's sexual behavior, "accidental" touching and repeated and unwanted invitations for a date or for a sexual relationship.

In 1980, a U.S. Supreme Court decision (*Meritor v. Vinson*) declared that sexual harassment is a form of sex discrimination and therefore a violation of Title VII of the 1964 Civil Rights Act.

sexual identity   An individual's biologically determined sex orientation.

See also GENDER IDENTITY.

sexuality   The ability to think and behave as a sexual being; also, any aspect of human thought or behavior that has sexual meaning. Sexuality implies a self-concept of oneself as a sexual being as well as having the capacity to respond to erotic stimuli and sexual activity. Sexuality encompasses being comfortable with sexual fantasies and erotic zones of the body as well as with one's own gender identity, although no specific set of behaviors or sexual preference is necessary to have a good sense of one's own sexuality. There are social, psychological and biologic dimensions to human sexuality.

sexually transmitted diseases (STDs)   Sexually transmitted diseases is the term given to a group of diseases that affect both men and women and are generally transmitted during sexual intercourse. These diseases cause discomfort, may lead to infertility and may be life threatening. They cause psychological distress for many reasons, including a need to communicate one's problem to one's partner and a need to disclose information about past sexual activities. The term "safe sex" relates to prevention of STDs as well as AIDS.

Historically, syphilis and gonorrhea were referred to as venereal diseases long before the term STD was coined during the latter part of the 20th century. Several STDs became notably widespread during the 1980s. These include herpes, chlamydia, hepatitis B, pubic lice, genital warts and other vaginal infections. Syphilis and gonorrhea are still prevalent, and some sources say they are on the increase owing to the upswing in other concurrent STDs.

Concerns about STDs are prevalent among individuals who are widowed or divorced and who begin seeking new partners after their loss, as well as among never-married individuals. Fears of acquiring STDs have led many formerly sexually active people to seek fewer sexual partners. Such concerns have also increased the use of condoms, as they are thought to reduce the likelihood of spreading most STDs (as well as AIDS).

Herpes

Herpes (technically known as Herpes simplex or herpes virus hominus) outbreaks cause either single or multiple blisters that occur on mucous membranes such as lips or the vagina. Herpes simplex I causes most oral "cold sores." Herpes simplex II causes most genital herpes. Transmission can occur when a herpes blister comes in contact with any mucous membrane or open cut or sore. Herpes is most often transmitted through sexual intercourse and can also be transmitted during mouth-genital contact or with manual contact during heterosexual or homosexual relations.

Herpes can be debilitating in an active stage. Herpes recurs and often attacks when the previously infected individual is under stress, fatigued or has another illness. Women who know that they have the herpes infection are concerned about giving birth to a baby who may also have herpes, as the infection can be transmitted to the baby during the birth process. Women who have active vaginal herpes blisters are routinely given cesarean sections.

Many individuals who have herpes take drugs to relieve the pain of the blisters and prophylactically (as a preventive) to reduce the severity of future attacks. A medication in the form of a cream is also available.

Chlamydia

Chlamydia is two or three times more common than gonorrhea but less well known. It is only in the latter quarter of the 20th century that information about this disease has appeared in the medical and popular press. Chlamydia is feared because untreated infections in women can lead to infections in the fallopian tubes and uterus (pelvic inflammatory disease). The disease affects men and women, but women are less likely to notice symptoms in early stages. The signs in women are unusual vaginal discharge, irregular bleeding, bleeding after intercourse or deep pain during and after intercourse. Men may notice clear, mucus-like discharge from the penis and burning during urination. Chlamydia is treated with antibiotics, and sexual partners must be treated to avoid a ping-pong effect of reinfection. Thus, when one individual discovers that he or she has it, psychological concerns arise regarding telling the partner(s) and encouraging treatment for both.

Hepatitis B

This infection may develop about two months after sexual activity. It is usually acquired during sexual intercourse with an infected individual. Hepatitis B is common in underdeveloped countries and among intravenous drug users in the United States. People who are concerned about getting Hepatitis B can obtain an immunization against it; the immunization is recommended for health care workers and for household and sexual contacts of infected individuals.

Pubic Lice

These are tiny bugs, also known as "crab lice" or "crabs," that burrow into the skin and suck blood. They thrive on hairy parts of the body, including the pubic mound, outer lips of the vulva, underarms, the head and even eyebrows and eyelashes. Eggs take from seven to nine days to hatch; persons infected may notice itching one to three weeks after exposure. The most direct way of acquiring pubic lice is through sexual or close physical contact with an infected person's body. However, pubic lice can also be transmitted by shared towels or bedsheets. Pubic lice is commonly treated with a standard pesticide (known in the United States as Kwell) that is also used for head lice. Those who have pubic lice (or live in the same household with someone who has them) can reduce risks of spread by washing towels and bedding with disinfectant, such as household bleach, in boiling water and drying the items in a hot dryer to be sure of killing off the unhatched eggs of the lice.

Genital Warts

Warts, or small bumps, on the mucous membrane of the vulva, the clitoral hood, in the perineum, inside the vagina, in the anus, on the penis or in the urinary tract may be genital warts. They cause discomfort and anxiety to the sufferer and may be particularly painful during sexual intercourse or when the sufferer wears tight clothing. Genital warts are caused by a sexually transmitted virus and can be removed by a physician. Certain strains of the wart virus have been implicated as a cause of cervical cancer. If either partner has a history of genital warts, a condom should be used during sexual intercourse to reduce transmission of the wart virus.

Gonorrhea and Syphilis

Gonorrhea is caused by a bacterium that can infect the genital organs and spread to other parts of the body. Gonorrhea can cause complications including pelvic inflammatory disease, joint pains, heart disease, liver disease, meningitis and blindness. Gonorrhea has been referred to as the "dose," "clap" or "drip." Gonorrhea is treated with large doses of penicillin, usually injected, often with follow-up doses of oral antibiotics. During the latter part of the 20th century, many cases of penicillin-resistant gonorrhea have appeared, making the disease more fearsome than during the years when penicillin was hailed as the "magic bullet" against the disease. Because there are fewer symptoms in women than men, gonorrhea is usually detected later in women. In a woman, the gonorrhea germs travel to the uterus, fallopian tubes and ovaries. As the disease advances, she may notice abdominal pain. Males may notice painful urination and pus discharging from the penis.

Syphilis, though less common than gonorrhea, can result in serious complications when untreated. Syphilis—also known as "lues," "syph," "pox" and "bad blood"—is caused by a microorganism from the spirochete family. An initial outbreak (primary syphilis) causes a large punched-out lesion called a chancre. After this initial outbreak, symptoms may not recur for several months, when a skin rash, or secondary syphilis, occurs. Years later, central nervous system symptoms in the form of mental aberrations and a stumbling gait may occur (tertiary syphilis). Treatment with penicillin or other antibiotics is usually effective during the early stages of the disease and will prevent complications. Treatment is difficult in the later stages of the disease.

Acquired Immunodeficiency Syndrome (AIDS)

This has become a widely known disease during the latter part of the 20th century. The AIDS virus is known to be transmitted by direct exchange of body fluid, such as semen or blood.

Other Diseases

One commonly known infection is trichomonas, which is caused by microscopic parasitic organisms that live in small numbers in the vagina. The organisms, known as trichomonads, also live under the foreskin of a man's penis or in the urethra, usually without producing any symptoms. Medications are available to combat this infection. However, a treated individual must inform his or her sexual partner so that the partner can also be treated.

Yeast infections (monilia) are not necessarily sexually transmitted diseases, but the organisms also live in the vagina and under the foreskin of the penis and can be transmitted during sexual intercourse. Many women, however, have yeast infections without having had sexual intercourse. Taking antibiotics can trigger a yeast infection by destroying the balance of organisms in the vagina.

Bacterial infections can also be transmitted during sexual intercourse; these are treatable with sulfa creams or oral antibiotics.

Reducing Risks of Acquiring an STD

Although some STDs seem to be increasing in prevalence, people can reduce their risk of these diseases by taking certain precautions:

1. Have a monogamous relationship. Have sexual contact with only one partner who limits contact to you only.
2. Look your partner over. Ask about any suspicious-looking discharges, sores or rashes.
3. Be clean. Partners should bathe before and after sexual intercourse. Wash with soap and water.
4. Use condoms. Condoms provide some (though not complete) protection against STDs. However, the condom must be put on before sexual activity begins and not removed until the end of the activity.
5. Use foam, a diaphragm with spermicides, or sponge spermicides, which kill many infectious agents; these should be used in addition to the condom.
6. Avoid the ping-pong effect of infection. If one partner has an STD, the other partner must be informed and treated at the same time to avoid reinfection.

See also ACQUIRED IMMUNODEFICIENCY SYNDROME.

Kahn, Ada P., and Linda Hughey Holt. *The A to Z of Women's Sexuality.* Alameda, Calif.: Hunter House, 1992.

sexual response   Physiological reaction to sexual stimulation and arousal. In women, vaginal lubrication is an early sign in the sexual response cycle. In men, erection of the penis occurs. Responsiveness is a highly individual matter, largely determined by mutual feelings of love and affection between the partners and a wide variety of emotional and physical circumstances. Levels of responsiveness vary among individuals and vary within the same individual at different times. Many people become anxious about their responses, not realizing that a wide range of differences, are considered normal.

See also SEX THERAPY.

sexual revolution   Changes in sexual attitudes and behaviors during the 1960s, 1970s and early 1980s. These included more liberal attitudes toward premarital sexual activity, changes in the sexual double standard in which sexual activity is seen as more acceptable for men than for women and more open discussion of women's sexual needs. Changes in the double standard and increases in premarital activity evolved in part as a result of development of better and easier means of birth control, including oral contraceptives during the late 1950s.

For many young people, dating habits during the sexual revolution included sexual intercourse early in the relationship. However, with the recognition of the increase of sexually transmitted diseases and acquired immunodeficiency syndrome (AIDS) in the heterosexual population in the 1980s, many people became more cautious and selective about their choice of sexual partners and monogamy regained favor.

The sexual revolution was closely tied with the Women's Liberation Movement. Many college dormitories became coeducational, offering women more options regarding housing. There was wider acceptance of unmarried adults "living together."

Movies and plays during the sexual revolution included more sexually explicit scenes, and sexuality was discussed more openly in the media.

See also ACQUIRED IMMUNODEFICIENCY SYNDROME; WOMEN'S LIBERATION MOVEMENT.

shell shock   A term that referred to mental disorders that occurred as a result of battle. This term, as well as "combat fatigue," was used during World War I. A newer term for the same syndrome or effects is post-traumatic stress disorder (PTSD). There are still some elderly veterans in Veterans Administration hospitals who are there because of lifelong mental difficulties ensuing after shell shock.

See also POST-TRAUMATIC STRESS DISORDER.

shiatsu   A specific method for manipulating *tsubos* (the points along the meridians where the flow of energy may become blocked). There are many forms of shiatsu. The manipulation may occur through pressing with the fingers and hands, or through the use of elbows, knees and feet.

Shiatsu is considered a complementary therapy and may be useful for some individuals to prevent or relieve the effects of stress, thus improving their mental health. Manipulation of the body's approximately 360 tsubos, also known as acupressure or acupuncture points, is thought to release the flow of energy (*chi*).

See also BODY THERAPIES; COMPLEMENTARY THERAPIES; MASSAGE THERAPY.

shift work   Many psychological factors related to adaptation to night-shift work are based on how well the individual handles the interruption of the circadian rhythm. The break in circadian rhythm can affect mental ability, alertness and temperament. Some night-shift workers experience anxiety and lapses in memory as a result of sleep deprivation. Coping mechanisms to combat fatigue, and later to induce sleep, may include overeating, alcohol consumption and use of sedatives and stimulants.

Social needs of night-shift workers are a consideration. For example, the rest of the world operates on a 9 to 5 schedule, with most socialization occurring after work and on weekends. For night-shift people to have a family or social life, they must schedule creatively.

Hurley, Margaret, and Elizabeth A. Neidlinger. *Schumpert Medical Quarterly,* Schumpert Medical Center, Shreveport, La., vol. 9, no. 2 (Oct. 1991).

shock therapy   See ELECTROCONVULSIVE THERAPY.

shopaholism   Stress reduction by shopping that can create a compulsive syndrome. Excessive shopping shares some characteristics with obsessive-compulsive disorder, in which people perform certain rituals to relieve tension. In this way, compulsive shopping is similar to the problems of alcoholics or compulsive gamblers.

Compulsive shoppers buy things in order to make themselves forget the pressures of their lives and make themselves feel good. However, what happens is that it takes more and more spending and buying to improve their moods.

According to Thomas C. O'Guinn of the University of Illinois, probably 2 percent of Americans can be described as compulsive buyers, and another 2 or 3 percent are on the verge. Advertising suggests that shopping is a good way to relieve anxiety.

In a symposium on compulsive buying during a conference of the American Psychological Association in San Francisco in September 1991, advertisers and store owners drew some blame for encouraging irresponsible spending, as did credit card companies. Stores that are most tempting to compulsive buyers feature soft lights and music, in which reality is shut out and the customers can indulge in fantasy; some gambling casinos have similar characteristics. After studying hundreds of compulsive buyers, O'Guinn concluded that such buyers have a knack for deluding themselves when they want to buy something. They believe that they will have the money to pay for the items when the bills come, but they really will not.

Many people who are normally good about balancing their budget overbuy around holidays. According to Dr. James Jefferson, director of the Center for Affective Disorders, University of Wisconsin Hospital and Clinics and professor of psychiatry at the University of Wisconsin Medical School, for people who are compulsive shoppers, the problem can be magnified during holidays. Excessive shopping can be attributed in part to an attempt to promote a better self-image through buying multiple or expensive gifts. For others, gift giving is seen as a way to change people's perceptions about the giver, to make an economic statement or to serve as a substitute for other, weaker aspects of the relationship.

Evan Steffans, consulting therapist for Shopper Stoppers, a support group for addictive spenders in Dayton, Ohio, has some tips for shopaholics:

Work Out Your Stress   Most people with addictive illnesses do not know how to cope with stress. Learn alternatives to blotting out the stress, which is what the shopping does.

Develop Social Outlets   Cultivate groups of friends with whom you can share activities as a healthful alternative to shopping.

Exercise   Physical exercise is a good stress reliever and will clear the mind for better concentration later on.

While it is impossible to give up shopping entirely, compulsive shoppers who understand their addiction can help themselves by following a few reminders:

- Shop with a list and buy only what is on the list.
- Shop with a partner who will help you resist temptations.
- Do not browse.
- Avoid sales. The excitement can trigger a shopping spree.
- Avoid use of credit cards. Use them only for business, if you need to.

Debtors Anonymous is a Chicago-area support group for overspenders based on the 12-step recovery program of Alcoholics Anonymous. DA members work toward financial solvency the way AA members work toward abstinence. Experienced DA members review new members' finances and help them formulate an action plan for resolving debts and a spending plan for the future. DA members look to one another for support, hope and strength in dealing with the stresses of indebtedness.

For information, contact:

Debtors Anonymous
P.O. Box 20322
New York, NY 10025–9992
Phone: (312) 274-DEBT

See also OBSESSIVE-COMPULSIVE DISORDER; OBSESSIVE-COMPULSIVE DISORDER in bibliography.

Moore, Judy Kay. "Holiday Shopping Can Be Compulsive For Some: UW Expert." *Feature Story,* Center for Health Sciences, University of Wisconsin—Madison (Nov. 1991).

Nilsson, Pam. "No, It Won't Kill You . . . But Shopaholism Will Murder Your Bank Account." *Today's Chicago Woman,* November 1991.

shyness Generally refers to avoidance of other people, or excessive discomfort, embarrassment and inhibition in the presence of others; it is a source of anxiety for many individuals who would like to become more dynamic and outspoken.

Many people would like to be more outgoing, meet new people and learn new activities. Their reluctance to facing possible criticism or even being watched holds them back from pursuing advancements and goals in life. Shyness is fairly common in children and adolescents. However, as the young person develops an increasing sense of self-esteem, shyness often disappears.

See also PHOBIAS; PUBERTY AND PUBERTY RITES; SELF-ESTEEM.

sibling rivalry Competition between brothers and/or sisters is normal. The first situation occurs after the birth of a new baby, when an older sibling feels "displaced" and constantly seeks to command the parents' attention. Feelings of rivalry may persist throughout life. One child may be continuously compared with another in the family, and the parents may influence the feeling of rivalry by showing one child as the better example. Throughout school, brothers and sisters may feel competitive with one another in order to gain more affection from their parents.

Personality differences may account for sibling rivalry. For example, while one child may be extroverted, have an outgoing personality and make friends easily, another child in the family may be more introspective and find it difficult to mingle in new groups of children. The quieter child may be jealous of the other child, even though he excels in academic skills, while the child with many friends may be jealous of her sibling's academic achievements.

Sibling rivalry may persist even after the death of parents, when brothers and sisters become jealous over uneven distribution of their parents' possessions.

See also JEALOUSY.

sick building syndrome A contemporary personal and societal threat to mental health once known as building-related illness. People who work in office buildings may experience symptoms such as headaches, itchy eyes, itchy nose and throat, dry cough, diminished mental acuity, sensitivity to odor and tiredness. These symptoms may be caused by air conditioning systems, fluorescent lighting systems and poor ventilation. Modern buildings are tighter in construction and depend on air-circulators, as opposed to outside air, for ventilation.

Additionally, the sources of stressful symptoms may be caused by the frustration of feeling closed in and unable to control the amount of heat or light in the immediate environment. Thus the stress of the syndrome is also related to feelings of lack of personal control.

A ripple effect sometimes occurs when one employee in such a building starts complaining. Soon others believe that they too have headaches as a result of the workplace. The notion of becoming ill from the building in which one works is not entirely farfetched when one considers the outbreak of Legionnaire's disease, a form of pneumonia, which was first identified among American Legion conventioneers in a Philadelphia hotel during the 1970s and was caused by bacteria in the air conditioning system; similar outbreaks have occurred as recently as 1995. Tests identified the organisms responsible for the disease as a contaminant of water systems that had been responsible for earlier epidemics of pneumonia, although the cause had not been understood earlier.

The influence of sick building syndrome as a source of employee stress was recognized on a fairly large scale when complaints characteristic of sick building syndrome made to the U.S. Department of Occupational Safety and Health (OSHA) doubled between 1980 and 1981. Recognized by the insurance industry under the name "tight building syndrome," Fireman's Fund Insurance Company established a "tight building syndrome" laboratory in late 1983, after investigating 48 buildings in the

U.S. and discovering that about one-third presented health hazards from indoor air pollution.

Relieving Anxieties Caused by Sick Building Syndrome

Individuals who believe that they are being made ill by their building should consult their company psychologist, if there is one, or the department of human resources. Reports should be filed in a timely way so that investigations can be made. Removal of the pollutant, if possible, is essential. There may be possibilities for improvement of air balance and adjustment, including circulating a percentage of outside air. All humidifiers, filters and drip pans must be checked. Overall maintenance of the building should be evaluated and care should be taken regarding selection of cleaning materials, air fresheners and moth repellents. New carpeting should be installed on a Friday, so as to allow ventilation of the building over the weekend.

Additionally, individuals should determine if there are any steps they can take to relieve their personal stress. These may include being moved to another part of the building, or bringing a small electric fan or heater to work with them. If necessary, a short vacation away from the pollutants may be helpful.

See also ENVIRONMENT; WORKPLACE.

Crawford, Joanne O., and Sean M. Bolas. "Sick Building Syndrome, Work Factors and Occupational Stress." *Scandinavian Journal of Work, Environment and Health* 1996 22, no. 4 (Aug. 1996): 243–250.

sick role A protective role given to a person who is mentally ill, physically ill or injured. Often many people with illnesses begin to enjoy the attention and achieve what is known as secondary gain.

See also SECONDARY GAIN.

side effects of drugs Results that occur after taking medications that are unrelated to the hoped-for effect. Not all individuals experience the same side effects. Usually individuals are warned about possible side effects of medications, such as dry mouth as a common side effect of some antidepressant drugs. Other common side effects of some drugs include dizziness, nausea and constipation. Sometimes side effects occur because of synergism between drugs (additive effects) or an individual's allergies.

When an individual experiences side effects of a prescription medication, this situation should be discussed with the prescribing physician. Some people choose to stop taking their medication because of a side effect, and when this occurs, they are putting themselves at risk for the more severe consequences of their unmedicated condition.

SIDS See SUDDEN INFANT DEATH SYNDROME.

Siegel, Bernie S(hepard) (1921–) Surgeon, lecturer and author of the best-selling book, *Love, Medicine and Miracles* (Harper, 1986). He completed his surgical training at Yale New Haven Hospital and the Childrens' Hospital of Pittsburgh. He received his M.D. degree from Cornell University and his B.A. from Colgate University. He has been a practitioner of pediatric and general surgery.

Siegel is the founder of Exceptional Cancer Patients (ECP), a support group whose members try to help heal themselves. By sharing their fear and anger with each other, ECP members undergo a form of alternative therapy which, according to Siegel, aids in the healing process. They utilize the concept of "carefrontation," a loving, safe, therapeutic confrontation, which facilitates personal change and healing.

Siegel believes that getting well is not the only goal; more important is learning to live without fear and to be at peace with life and ultimately death. He utilizes group therapy involving patients' dreams, drawings and images. Siegel travels extensively to speak and run workshops sharing his techniques and experiences.

See also CANCER; SUPPORT GROUPS.

Siegel, Bernie S. *Love, Medicine and Miracles,* New York: Harper & Row, 1986.

sign An objective indication of a disorder that is observed or detected by a physician or another person as opposed to indications reported by the individual, which are known as symptoms. For example, repeated bruises on a child may be a sign to a physician that the child is a victim of child abuse. On the other hand, headaches, which the physician cannot see, may be reported by a patient and may be a symptom of underlying disease.

See also SYMPTOM.

Sinequan Trade name for doxepin hydrochloride, a tricyclic antidepressant drug.

See also ANTIDEPRESSANT MEDICATIONS.

Skinner, Burrhus Frederic (1904–1990) An American psychologist and pioneer in operant behavior-modification techniques of psychotherapy. Skinner's work affected approaches to treatment of anxieties, phobias and other areas of mental health. He constructed a major learning theory and was an influential spokesman for radical behaviorism. His theory of behavior was based on a deterministic philosophy that included the notion that individuals' behavior and personality are determined by both past and present events, as well as genetic makeup, and not by internal influences. He believed that psychologists should focus on observable and verifiable behavior and also that behavior can be best understood and modified by manipulating its consequences.

See also BEHAVIOR THERAPY.

Doctor, Ronald M. and Ada P. Kahn. *Encyclopedia of Phobias, Fears, and Anxieties.* New York: Facts On File, 2000.

SK-Pramine See IMIPRAMINE HYDROCHLORIDE.

sleep Recurring periods of relative physical and psychological disengagement from one's environment. Sleep-related problems are among the most common complaints individuals have when they visit physicians or other therapists. Depression seems to be a major factor that interferes with sleep, causing some individuals to sleep too much and preventing others from getting to sleep or sleeping through the night. Sleep in individuals with a chronic illness or pain is often interrupted.

Sleep patterns vary with age, state of health, medication and psychological state. Sleeping habits affect most people's moods. Many feel somewhat

irritable and short-tempered without adequate sleep. According to Rosalind Cartwright, Ph.D., director of the Sleep Disorder Service at Rush-Presbyterian-St. Luke's Medical Center, Chicago, people who can't fall asleep are usually the complainers and worriers, those who don't learn how to relax before sleeping and those whose minds don't stop to let them relax.

The old adage "early to bed and early to rise" is too generalized a plan for most people, says Dr. Cartwright. There are many individual patterns of sleep that work well. Some elderly people don't go to bed until 4:00 A.M. They stay awake until then, reading, knitting or doing some creative work. They wake up at 8:00 A.M. when everyone else does and they feel good. Such individuals once went to bed at midnight and worried about staying awake four hours; now they turn those hours into doing something constructive.

Stages of sleep differ in proportion to how we spend our time during the day. People who do hard physical work do not necessarily need more sleep than sedentary office workers, but their sleep is deeper. According to Dr. Cartwright, they have more prolonged stage 4 sleep at the beginning of the night.

There are some sleep differences between men and women. One difference is that men lose their ability for deep sleep (delta sleep) as they age sooner than women, even though more women complain about insomnia and light sleeping. Men begin to lose their deep sleep in their late forties and fifties, while women continue to have deep sleep later in life.

Sleep Disorders

There are two basic categories of sleep disorders. One is known as DIMS, or disorders of initiating or maintaining sleep. These include difficulty getting to sleep or staying asleep or waking too early. The second category is known as DOES, or disorders of excessive sleep. Characteristics may include falling asleep inappropriately and difficulty in awakening. Such individuals are known as hypersomniacs.

Another common and more serious disorder of sleep is sleep apnea. This consists of brief periods of ceasing to breathe. There may be at least 250,000 people in the United States who cease breathing so often or for such long periods of time at night that they are tired all day and are likely to drift off into sleep at any moment. They must walk around often to fight off sleep. Such individuals can't drive safely.

Signs of sleep apnea are loud snoring, prolonged periods between breaths (apnea), weight gain and elevated blood pressure. Diagnosis of sleep apnea can be made from a tape recording at the bedside of the snorer. If there are repeated pauses of more than 10 seconds between snores, it may mean that the oxygen level in the brain is going down. The person must wake himself to restart the brain. There is treatment for sleep apnea, and it is important that such people be treated because this disorder causes a strain on the heart.

Repetitive Nocturnal Myoclonus

This involves involuntary jerky motions of the legs, episodes of muscle spasms and twitching that disturb sleep. This is an uncomfortable sensation that occurs just before falling asleep. The individual feels an urge to get up and walk around. This sensation may increase with age and, according to some researchers, frequently runs in families. It is more common in individuals age 50 to 60 than in younger people.

Sleep Difficulties of Menopausal Women

Many women experience changes in their sleep patterns around menopause. Some changes may be due to hot flashes or to many other factors involving other individual psychosocial stresses. According to Dudley Dinner, M.D., director of the Sleep Disorders Center, the Cleveland Clinic Foundation, while women may have slept seven to eight hours at age 20, they may decrease up to six or six and a half hours between age 55 and 60. In addition, sleep tends to become more "fragmented." Women in this age group may awaken more often and spend more time awake during the night, although the total time in bed may increase.

Sleep Disturbance Related to Medication

Because many medications can cause sleepiness in some individuals, all such medications should be taken only under a physician's supervision. Some medications may make sleep apnea worse.

Medications Used for Inducing Sleep

Many individuals have sleeping medications prescribed for them at some time during their life. Often at a time of great bereavement, such as after the death of a spouse or parent, an individual will have difficulty sleeping and can be helped with the assistance of an appropriately prescribed medication for short-term use.

Dreaming

Most dreaming takes place during the REM (rapid-eye-movement) stage. Nightmares of being unable to move have a real basis during this phase of sleep because of the limpness of the muscles. Most people forget dreams unless they awaken during a REM period or within 10 minutes afterward.

According to Dr. Cartwright, dreaming has a role in our mental health. This is indicated by the fact that people in poor mental health are distinctly different. "Dreaming doesn't cause mental illness, but when dreams work well, they help process our emotions of the day. We put our emotions to rest during sleep. When we are upset, our dreaming does not serve us well," Dr. Cartwright said.

Research

Evaluation of individuals' problems as well as sleep research is carried out in many sleep laboratories across the United States. Sessions for a troubled sleeper in a sleep laboratory depend on the diagnosis and how complex the problem is. Some tests, such as those for narcolepsy—a disorder of excessive daytime sleepiness—are done during the day, with a series of five short naps. However, most sleep lab evaluations are done during the night. Patients are monitored for many things, including naso-oral air flow and heart rate. Insomniacs are tested to determine how much they really sleep. Typically, many physiological parameters are measured on a 16-channel machine. One person can be measured on 16 channels, or two people on eight channels. There is an intercom from the control room, and researchers can talk to any sleeper in a room or tape-record from any room.

With use of an electroencephalogram (EEG), a graphic depiction of the brain's electrical potentials recorded by scalp electrodes, sleep is divisible into two categories: nonrapid-eye-movement sleep (NREM) and rapid-eye-movement (REM) sleep. Dreaming sleep is another term for REM sleep. There are four stage of NREM sleep. Stage I occurs immediately after sleep begins with a pattern of low amplitude and fast frequency. Stage II has characteristic waves of 12 to 16 cycles per second known as sleep spindles. Stages III and IV have progressive further slowing of frequency and increase in amplitude of the wave forms. After the beginning of sleep, over a period of 90 minutes, a person goes through the four stages of NREM sleep and goes from them into the first period of REM sleep. Dreaming usually occurs during REM sleep, and short cycles (20 to 30 minutes) of REM sleep recur about every 90 minutes throughout the night. This type of sleep is so named because of the coordinated rapid eye movements that occur.

Sleep and Sex Research

Sex researchers test individuals' capabilities for sexual arousal while they are asleep to determine if sexual dysfunctions are caused by physiological problems. In males, a penile plethysmograph indicates changes in blood flow and size of the penis as it undergoes erection. In females, a vaginal plethysmograph records vaginal blood flow during sexual arousal. When individuals show indications of high sexual arousal during sleep, psychotherapy often helps them achieve improved sexual function during waking hours.

Snoring

Snoring is a serious problem for more than 10 million Americans. It is a problem for the snorer as well as their bed partner or roommate, often causing the other to awaken tired and irritable after many awakenings throughout the night. Snoring is the cause of many marital arguments.

Heavy snoring accompanied by slowed breathing patterns may indicate the presence of sleep apnea.

See also DREAMING; JET LAG; REM SLEEP; SNORING.

Kahn, Ada P., and Linda Hughey Holt. *Midlife Health: A Woman's Practical Guide to Feeling Good.* New York: Avon Books, 1989.

HOW TO GET A GOOD NIGHT'S SLEEP

It takes most people about 15 minutes or less to fall asleep. If you have trouble getting to sleep and staying asleep long enough to feel good throughout the day, try some of these suggestions:

- Drink a cup of warm milk before bedtime. Eat a light snack. Avoid stimulating beverages that contain caffeine, such as coffee, cola beverages and chocolate.
- Take a warm, relaxing bath.
- Relax in bed and read something you enjoy. As your mind becomes engrossed, your muscles will relax. When your body is relaxed, you are likelier to become sleepy and ready for sleep. Watching television may have the same effect.
- Read something you find very dull. When your mind cannot handle what you present, your internal coping mechanism of falling asleep may take over. Watching television may have the same effect.
- Experiment by changing your environment. Make the room warmer or colder. Use different combinations of covers. Some people like the feeling of the "weight" of blankets, while others do not. If you like warmth without weight, use an electric blanket. Some have dual controls so that each bed partner can have individual arrangements.
- Avoid stressful situations before bedtime. Postpone discussions of problems until morning when possible. Avoid lengthy telephone conversations that may upset you before bedtime.
- If you have an argument or tension-filled discussion late at night, don't go to bed mad.
- If you are alone and feel hostile, call a friend and talk. Venting may help you unload and you will sleep better.
- Avoid using sleeping pills. People build up a tolerance to them, and some have daytime hypnotic effects. Some pills induce sleep apnea.
- If you must take a sleeping pill during times of extreme stress, such as after the death of a loved one, after surgery or during extreme jet lag, take short-acting sleeping medications.
- Nightly use of sleeping medications may not be effective after a while. If you have to use them at all, use them only every other night, or every third night.
- Avoid taking naps during the day; go to bed a little later each night.

sleep apnea   See SLEEP; SNORING.

sleep disorders   See SLEEP.

sleep paralysis   A sensation of being unable to move at the moment of waking up or going to sleep. This feeling may last for only a few seconds and be accompanied by frightening hallucinations.

This occurs in some people who have narcolepsy but also occasionally happens in normally healthy people as well.

See also NARCOLEPSY; SLEEP.

sleep therapy   A treatment sometimes used for depression in which the individual is monitored in a sleep laboratory and the sleep-wake cycle is altered. For example, the individual might be kept awake during one full night or during specific hours of several nights. This is termed sleep deprivation therapy. Russian psychiatrists have used sedative drugs to promote sleep for several days as a form of therapy. This type of sleep therapy is not used in the United States as a standard treatment.

See also DEPRESSION; PSYCHOTHERAPY; SLEEP.

sleepwalking (somnambulism)   Walking while asleep during NREM (nonrapid eye movement) sleep; this affects about 5 percent of adults and many more children. For unknown reasons, boys are more likely to sleepwalk than girls. A child may sleepwalk after awakening from a nightmare or night terror and may scream, talk or even urinate in an inappropriate place.

It is difficult to awaken a sleepwalker; the best approach is to calmly lead him or her back to bed. However, in a household where an individual is known to sleepwalk, it is best to close off stairwells and remove loose objects in the possible pathway to prevent injury.

Since somnambulism occurs during stage IV sleep, it frequently responds to benzodiazepine medications, such as flurazepam (Dalmane) or temazepam (Restoril).

slips of the tongue   Also known as "lapsus lingae," slips of the tongue occur when one says one thing but means another. Most people do this at times, and doing so does not mean that one is losing one's memory. These are mistakes that grouped together with other errors such as mislaying objects, memory lapses and writing errors are known as symptomatic acts. Sigmund Freud theorized that these acts have a subconscious basis with some motivation that is not recognized by the person who commits them. This type of behavior is temporary and correctable. Although undesirable, it tends to fall within normal limits and is not considered pathological.

Campbell, Robert Jean. *Psychiatric Dictionary.* New York, Oxford University Press, 1981.

smoking   The actual physiological effects of smoking are somewhat at odds with the sensations that smokers report. When nicotine enters the bloodstream, it raises the heart rate, blood pressure and blood flow and dilates the arteries. It also raises the level of glucose in the blood. However, smokers report a sense of tranquility, despite the stimulating effects of nicotine.

Smoking is generally experienced as an uncomfortable, negative experience the first time it is attempted, but it soon becomes a habit that is difficult to break despite its link with cancer and heart disease.

The habit of smoking is usually started in adolescence and seems to be a function of a desire to conform to peer pressure. Rebellious attitudes, lower socioeconomic status, desire for tension relief and patterns of family smoking also seem to be factors that contribute to teenage smoking.

According to a 1989 Gallup poll, 63 percent of smokers would like to quit the habit and many of those have made a serious but unsuccessful effort to stop. Although the survey showed a decline in smoking, down to a low of 27 percent from a peak of 45 percent in 1954, smoking is still prevalent among adolescents and has actually increased slightly to 13 percent of 13- to 17-year-olds, up from 10 percent in previous years.

Possibly a reflection of the importance of athletics to teenagers is the fact that more teenage girls (14 percent) smoke than teenage boys (11 percent). In the general population, men have traditionally smoked more than women, although these figures are now somewhat even at 28 percent of men and 26 percent of women. Although their numbers have decreased, men are still heavier smokers than women. One-fourth of men smoke more than a pack of cigarettes a day, while only 14 percent of the women surveyed exceed a pack a day. Light smoking of less than a pack a day is common among the population in the 18- to 29-year-old age bracket.

Smoking is now regarded as an addiction. Many stop-smoking programs exist to help cigarette addicts. However, for the programs to be helpful, the individual must attend regularly and follow the rules set forth. For many, unfortunately, this is easier said than done. Dr. Alexander Gussman of the Psychiatric Institute, Columbia Medical School, has shown that smokers have a significantly higher past history of depression and may reexperience depression when trying to withdraw from smoking, requiring antidepressant treatment.

Since antismoking laws have been passed in the United States during the 1980s and 1990s, there are frequent incidents of anger and hostility between smokers and nonsmokers. Although scientists have documented harmful effects of smoking to smokers as well as those who are forced to breathe secondhand smoke, many smokers still believe that it is their "right" to smoke when and where they want to. Nonsmokers maintain the same "right" to clean air. Increasingly, workplaces are adopting non-smoking policies and setting up outdoor smoking areas for smokers. Most restaurants have non-smoking areas, but there are some that do not. For those that do not, ventilation systems are not always effective, and non-smokers are frequently offended by smoke in the air. For many non-smokers, smoke in the air is more than an annoyance; for asthmatics and those with other respiratory disorders, being forced to breathe in secondhand smoke can bring on an attack and cause them to be ill.

Because of the known health effects of smoking (credited as a factor in 500,000 deaths per year), the United States may eventually become a smokeless society. However, in Third World countries, numbers of smokers are increasing and cigarette consumption is increasing, especially as American tobacco manufacturers have turned elsewhere in the world to market their products.

STRESS RELIEVERS FOR THOSE WHO ARE QUITTING SMOKING

- List your reasons for wanting to stop smoking
- Note when and where you smoke the most
- Set a date for quitting; tell your family and friends
- Remove cigarettes, ashtrays and matches from your home, car and office
- Minimize stressful situations and other occasions where you previously craved a cigarette
- Spend time where smoking is prohibited
- Reach for high-fiber, low-calorie snacks, such as vegetables or fruits when you have the urge to smoke
- Talk to someone who is supportive until the urge to smoke passes
- Increase aerobic exercise (walking, biking)
- Use relaxation techniques (meditation, guided imagery)
- Reward yourself for quitting smoking

For information:

American Heart Association
7320 Greenville Avenue
Dallas, TX 75231
Telephone: (214) 373-6300

American Lung Association
1740 Broadway
New York, NY 10019
Telephone: (212) 315-8700

Centers for Disease Control
Office of Smoking and Health
1600 Clifton Road NE
Atlanta, GA 30333
Telephone: (404) 639-3311

National Cancer Institute
9000 Rockville Pike
Building 31, 4A-21
Bethesda, MD 20892
Telephone: (800) 4-CANCER

See also ADDICTIONS; HABITS.

Hammond, S. Katharine, "Environmental Tobacco Smoke Presents Substantial Risk in Workplaces." *The Journal of the American Medical Association* (Sept. 26, 1995.)

Spitzer, Joel, "Medical Implications of Smoking." Skokie, Ill. The Good Health Program, Rush North Shore Medical Center, 1995.

snoring An annoying condition that results when the soft palate vibrates because an air passage is blocked during sleep. Snoring frequently results when one sleeps on his or her back; the tongue slides back into a position that partially blocks the nasal passage, forcing one to breathe through the mouth, particularly in a deep sleep. Snoring may deprive both the snorer and the bed partner of necessary sleep, possibly resulting in irritability and tension the next day.

Snoring is more common in overweight people, in part because they are more likely to sleep on their backs and because fatty tissue in their throat may cause blockage. Snoring may also be caused by enlarged tonsils and nasal problems. Heavy drinking, smoking or eating just before sleep may also cause snoring.

Snoring is more common in men than in women and tends to increase with age. A significant number of snorers can be heard in the next room. Measurements of snoring volume have recorded decibel levels as high as the sound of a jack hammer or pneumatic drill. Robert W. Hart, M.D., writing about snoring in *Chicago Medicine* (Dec. 21, 1991), characterized it as "mild, moderate, severe or heroic." According to Hart, the incidence of habitual snoring in an unselected population has been estimated near 20 percent. However, in overweight males between the ages of 30 and 59, that incidence reaches 60 percent. Some sources estimate that 40 million Americans snore.

Snoring and Sleep Apnea

Many individuals who report chronic fatigue and irritability are victims of sleep apnea, known as obstructive sleep apnea syndrome (OSAS). If untreated, OSAS can have lethal consequences when daytime sleepiness leads to automobile and industrial accidents, as well as consequences for interpersonal relationships because of short tempers due to tiredness.

OSAS is characterized by repetitive episodes of complete (apnea) or incomplete (hypopnea) obstruction of the upper airways during sleep. OSAS is more common in males and post-menopausal females, with its frequency increasing with age and weight. The OSAS sufferer may complain of feelings of choking or suffocating during the night or feel panicky because of an inability to take in enough air.

TIPS FOR SNORERS

- Learn to sleep on your side or stomach.
- Attach something to the back of your pajamas or night-gown to awaken yourself when you lie on your back.
- Avoid having an alcoholic nightcap, because it aggravates snoring; alcohol causes too much relaxation in the oral-

pharynx region. The same thing happens after taking tranquilizers and sleeping pills.
- Elevate the head of your bed several inches. This may alleviate the tendency to snore.
- Devices are available that help. One is a vinyl molded tooth guard, much like an athletic mouth guard, that captures and holds the tongue so that it doesn't fall to the back of the throat. It makes the airway stay open.
- Masks are available for really heavy snorers. These prevent snoring by supplying positive air pressure and keeping the throat open.
- Surgical techniques may be a last resort for an individual with severe and serious snoring problems. One procedure involves tightening up the tissues in the back of the throat. Another procedure involves making a permanent hole in the breathing system before the voice box. The hole bypasses the throat area when open and prevents the movement of the tissues that lead to snoring.

Treatment options for OSAS include general measures, such as weight loss, abstinence from alcohol and other offending substances, pharmacologic approaches for limited periods of time, devices (such as oral and orthodontic devices) and surgical procedures (such as nasal surgery or uvulopalatopharyngoplasty).

OSAS syndrome is linked to hypertension, ischemic heart disease and cerebrovascular disease and may have consequences for an individual's physical as well as mental health.

See also CHRONIC FATIGUE SYNDROME; SLEEP.

Borbely, Alexander. *Secrets of Sleep.* New York: Basic Books, 1984.
Hales, Dianne. *The Complete Book of Sleep.* Reading, Mass.: Addison-Wesley, 1981.
Hart, Robert W. "Snoring and Sleep Apnea: A Clinical Approach." *Chicago Medicine* 94, no. 24 (Dec. 21, 1991).

social anxiety   See ANXIETY DISORDERS; PHOBIA.

social phobia   See PHOBIA.

Social Security disability   Individuals incapacitated by a mental health disability may be entitled to a monthly stipend under the provisions of the Social Security Administration disability program. For example, some people with schizophrenia, chronic depression and chronic fatigue syndrome meet standards for such benefits. Eligibility standards are strict, however.

A person is considered disabled when she has a severe physical or mental impairment or combination of impairments that prevents her from working for a year or more or that is expected to result in death. The work does not necessarily have to be the kind of work done before disability; it can be any gainful work found in the national economy. This definition requires total disability.

To be eligible for this benefit, a person must have worked long enough and recently enough to be insured under the system that is funded by Social Security taxes paid by employers, employees and self-employed persons. To apply, an individual should begin by contacting the local office of the Social Security Administration. Documentation must be complete, including letters from physicians and mental health professionals, possibly laboratory test results and test results of various psychometric tests, which measure psychological or cognitive damage. Letters from previous employers, friends and relatives can be helpful, as can letters from congressional representatives and attorneys. Social Security will want to know how one's impairment limits function.

Following written application, the process will include personal interviews with a case worker. If the first application is rejected, there is a process of appeal, and many cases are granted disability status after one or more appeals.

The Clearinghouse on Disability Information is a centralized source of information about federal, state and local programs. It also follows related legislations and can make referrals on a local basis. The clearinghouse publishes a newsletter on federal activities affecting people with mental as well as physical disabilities and several small guidebooks.

Clearinghouse on Disability Information Office
    of Special Education and Rehabilitative
    Services
U.S. Department of Education
Switzer Building, Room 312
Washington, D.C. 20202
Phone: (202) 732-1723

The National Organization of Social Security Claimants' Representatives (NOSSCR) is a membership organization of attorneys who represent individuals applying for Social Security disability. They can answer questions about the process of application and appeal and can make referrals to local attorneys.

NOSSCR
6 Prospect Street
Midland Park, NJ 07432
Phone: (800) 431-2804 or
    (201) 444–1415

See also MEDICARE.

social support system   An individual's relationships with others and with the environment. This includes significant others, job, community, church and material resources. An individual with a mental health problem may have inadequate social support because family members do not understand why certain regimens are important and thus may not offer the assistance or encouragement that would help the person comply. An inadequate support system may encourage noncompliance and interfere with the individual's improvement.

See also NONCOMPLIANCE.

social workers   Social workers have been major providers of mental health services since the early 1920s, when they were an integral part of the beginning of the child guidance movement. Social workers are trained to have expertise concerning community resources available for various types of support and therapy, as well as to intervene when the individual and the environment do not mesh smoothly, causing discomfort or disruption for the individual or family.

Social workers are found in the public and private sectors. Many work in publicly funded health and mental health clinics, public schools, family agencies, clinics, hospitals and private practices. Some work in employee assistance programs (EAP), alcohol and chemical dependency programs and in religious settings.

Social workers early identified the importance of the family as a central focus rather than an individual in isolation. Much early professional literature emphasized the importance of the family and identified it as the unit for treatment. This had an impact on the early child guidance movement, as well as other mental health efforts, and influenced the development of family therapy.

In the 1960s and 1970s, with the establishment and development of comprehensive community mental health centers, clinical social workers were heavily utilized and provided a major proportion of outpatient mental health treatment services. In the 1980s, an increasing number of clinical social workers moved into full- or part-time private practice. In the 1990s, private practice was the fastest-growing setting for clinical social workers.

As of August 2001, there were more than 150,000 members of the National Association of Social Workers (NASW), an organization limited to those persons who have a bachelor's, master's or doctoral degree from a university program accredited by the Council on Social Work Education.

National Institute of Mental Health. *Mental Health, United States, 1990.* Manderscheid, R. W., and Sonnenschein, M. A., eds. DHHS Pub. No. (ADM) 90–1708. Washington, D.C.: USGPO, 1990.

sodium lactate infusions Intravenous infusions of sodium lactate will provoke a panic attack in most patients with panic disorder but not in normal subjects. The mechanism by which this occurs is not clear, and researchers hope that future test results may provide keys to biochemical factors in the causes of panic attacks.

The mechanism for sodium lactate precipitation of panic attacks is not clear, but it is also known that increased carbon dioxide (CO_2) accumulation can precipitate panic attacks, leading to a theory that the change in acid-base balance may also be affected by carbon dioxide levels.

See also PANIC DISORDER.

solvent abuse Glue sniffing or inhaling fumes of industrial solvents and aerosol sprays containing hydrocarbons, which can produce feelings of intoxication. These substances can produce a state of euphoria followed by depression of the central nervous system. Results of this habit can damage the brain, liver and kidneys. Occasionally death occurs as the result of a direct toxic effect on the heart or asphyxiation.

See also SUBSTANCE ABUSE.

somatic A term that means related to the body (soma) or related to body cells, as opposed to germ cells (eggs and sperm). The term "somatic" also relates to the body wall as opposed to the viscera (internal organs). The psyche relates to the mind. Somatic treatments in psychiatry include the use of medications and electroconvulsive therapy (ECT).

See also SOMATIC FIXATION; SOMATIZATION.

somatic fixation A process whereby a physician or patient or family focuses exclusively and inappropriately on physical or biomedical aspects of a complex problem. This can occur in any illness, especially chronic illness, when there is a one-sided emphasis on the biomedical aspects of a multifaceted problem. Somatically fixated patients tend to have anxiety, depression, trouble coping and numerous physical symptoms.

Some individuals have been raised in an environment in which they receive considerable attention for physical pain and little, if any, attention for emotional pain. Families operate on a continuum from full encouragement of emotional and physical experience to complete lack of acceptance of emotional experience. Emotionally repressed families condition children to experience any need or problem as physical. Thus physical symptoms may become their language for a range of experiences, from physical to emotional

According to Susan McDaniel, M.D., and colleagues from the University of Rochester School of Medicine, Rochester, New York, physicians should evaluate both the biomedical and psychosocial elements of a patient's problem, elicit the patient's and family's understanding of the problem and learn about any recent stressful events or unresolved crises in the lives of family members.

Treatment of a patient with a somatic fixation should involve medical treatment as well as extensive emotional support for the patient and family members.

Somatization disorder (Briquet's syndrome) is seen in people who have numerous physical symptoms without abnormal tests or medical findings who have repeated medical evaluations and increased amounts of surgery compared with others. Studies have shown that such people live long lives but persist in having numerous physical symptoms and medical treatment.

See also HYPOCHONDRIASIS; SOMATIZATION.

McDaniel, Susan; Thomas Campbell; and David Sea-burn. "Treating Somatic Fixation: A Biopsychosocial Approach." *Canadian Family Physician* 37 (Feb. 1991).

somatization The term for a feeling of physical symptoms in the absence of disease or out of proportion to a given ailment. From a public health point of view, somatization is important. According to the *Harvard Health Letter* (Apr. 1992), in any given week almost 80 percent of basically healthy people have symptoms that are not caused by physical disease. About one in five health care dollars is spent on patients with somatization. Nearly half of the patients seen in physicians' offices are the "worried well."

People who have ongoing somatic complaints may undergo uncomfortable invasive procedures that may cause complications. For example, it is possible that a person who repeatedly reports chest pains could eventually undergo coronary angiography to rule out serious arterial narrowing. These individuals may also be taking many medications needlessly, some with serious side effects.

Individuals who "somatize" are said to have somatoform disorders.

somatoform disorders See SOMATIC; SOMATIC FIXATION; SOMATIZATION.

somnambulism See SLEEPWALKING.

soteria Possessions or other objects, including collections, that are acquired for a feeling of security. An example of a soteria is a child's "security" blanket that is carried around at all times.

specific phobias See PHOBIA.

spectator role A term referring to a behavior pattern in which one's natural sexual responses are blocked by observing oneself closely and worrying about how well or poorly one is performing rather than participating freely. The term was introduced by William H. Masters (1915–), an American physician and sex researcher, and Virginia Johnson (1925–), an American psychologist and sex researcher.

See also SEX THERAPY.

spinal tap See BRAIN.

split personality An inappropriate term for dissociative identity disorder. It is sometimes also erroneously used to refer to schizophrenia; Bleuler used the term "split personality" to refer to the separation of thought and emotion in this disorder.

See also DISSOCIATION; DISSOCIATIVE DISORDERS; SCHIZOPHRENIA.

SSRIs See SELECTIVE SEROTONIN REUPTAKE INHIBITORS.

stage fright A feeling of nervous anticipation that individuals experience before giving a public speech, making an appearance on a stage (as in a theatrical production), playing a musical instrument or singing publicly, being on a radio or television program or being videotaped.

Those who go out of their way to avoid public speaking and public appearances may actually have a phobia about public appearances. Symptoms of stage fright and public speaking phobia may include becoming dizzy and nauseated when getting near the stage, having sweaty palms, weak knees and difficulty breathing and feeling a rapid heartbeat. While most people feel these symptoms in a very mild manner, phobic people will suffer so much that they momentarily fear they will die because of their rapid heartbeat and difficulty in getting enough air to breathe comfortably. (They may be overbreathing but not realize it.)

Some people have these symptoms for a few moments before going on stage, and as soon as they walk onto the stage, their fears disappear as they focus all of their attention and energy on their performance.

Those who do not lose their fears hold on to them for many reasons, including fear of criticism, fear of making a mistake, fear of being a failure or believing that they are not adequate for the task.

Behavioral therapy techniques can help people overcome stage fright. By systematically becoming accustomed to being in front of people, many individuals learn to lose their fear and become successful public figures.

See also ANXIETY DISORDERS; PHOBIA.

state anxiety A term used to differentiate types of anxiety. State anxiety, also called A-state, is a temporary and changing emotional state involving feelings of tension and apprehension and increased autonomic nervous system activity. It is a response to a specific situation that the individual perceives as threatening, but the response changes as the situation changes. An example of state anxiety is the unpleasant feelings one experiences when taking an examination or facing a new and strange situation. When the situation is over or one has become accustomed to it, the anxiety disappears. State anxiety may be contrasted with trait anxiety, a part of the personality that causes consistent anxiety in some people.

See also ANXIETY; AUTONOMIC NERVOUS SYSTEM; TRAIT ANXIETY.

Doctor, Ronald M., and Ada P. Kahn. *The Encyclopedia of Phobias, Fears, and Anxieties.* New York: Facts On File, 2000.

state-trait anxiety inventory (STAI) A psychological test developed about 1970 to research anxiety. Use of the test has led to advances in understanding anxiety. The test differentiates between state anxiety, also known as A-state, in which the anxiety is a temporary and changing response to a situation, and trait anxiety, which is an ongoing personality trait.

The STAI A-Trait portion includes 20 statements relating to anxiety, tension and their opposites. Respondents indicate on a scale ranging from 1 to 4 how often each statement generally pertains to them. The STAI is considered reliable and valid. There is also a version of the STAI for children known as the STAIC.

See also ANXIETY; STATE ANXIETY; TRAIT ANXIETY.

Doctor, Ronald M., and Ada P. Kahn. *The Encyclopedia of Phobias, Fears, and Anxieties.* New York: Facts On File, 2000.

Spielberger, C.D. et al. *The State-Trait Anxiety Inventory.* Riverside, Calif.: Consulting Psychologists Press, 1970.

STDs See SEXUALLY TRANSMITTED DISEASES.

stepfamilies Relationships in stepfamilies are far more complex than in traditional nuclear families. Stresses and challenges arise partly from the fact that society does not define the role of the stepparent as well as that of the natural parent. As a result, everyone may have a different set of ideas regarding how stepparent and stepchild get along. Frequently, a stepparent may feel that he or she should assume the role of an actual parent, but this may be very uncomfortable and objectionable to the child, especially as he may continue to have a strong relationship with his own natural parent. Children who live with a single parent may have had a partial sense of being the center of attention in the household and may have difficulty giving up that role when the stepparent arrives.

When two families merge, the living arrangements may cause stresses and challenges to the mental health of all involved. For example, some children may be in residence, and others may visit. Living arrangements may change during the course of the marriage in some anticipated way. A child who had been living with the other parent may suddenly decide he wishes to leave that parent, possibly because of a stepparent in that household, and move in. If conflicts erupt between stepsiblings, parents usually side with their own child rather than being peacemakers as in the traditional marriage. Children may also feel that their inheritance rights are threatened by the arrival of a stepfather or -mother, especially in cases involving older couples and adult children.

There may be a highly charged sexual atmosphere in the home because the couple are actually newlyweds but with children present. This may arouse real or potential relationships between stepsiblings that are technically, although not biologically, incestuous. There is also a potential for technical incest between stepparent and stepchild, particularly if the stepparent is young, even close to the age of the child. Stepparents sometimes even encourage these feelings in children by their attempts to be warm and friendly.

See also DIVORCE; REMARRIAGE.

Belovitch, Jeanne. *Making Re-marriage Work*. Lexington, Mass.: Lexington Books, 1987.
Wald, Esther. *The Remarried Family*. New York: Family Service Association of America, 1981.

steroids   A group of chemical compounds with similar structure that act as chemical activators and regulators. They are secreted by various glands and activate various body functions. An example of a steroid is cortisol, which is higher in individuals who have depression and lessens as they are recovering. Anabolic steroids (synthetic compounds) are misused by some athletic trainers to stimulate muscle development. Anabolic steroids can be legally obtained in the United States only with a physician's prescription.

See also ANABOLIC STEROIDS; BRAIN CHEMISTRY; CORTISOL.

stillbirth   The death of a fetus between the 20th week of gestation and delivery. The major cause of stillbirth appears to be loss of oxygen to the baby, because of either a problem with the placenta or an umbilical cord accident before or during labor. However, there is no known cause for more than half of stillbirths. A stillbirth causes a special kind of grief for the parents. Although they have never seen their child, they have imagined how he or she would look, what they would use for a name and how the child would interact with others in the family. After the stillbirth, there are no "real" memories, such as photographs or items the child actually used or touched. Friends and others in the family do not share the grief with the parents in the way that they might with an older infant who died, making grief even more difficult for the parents.

Even though another child may arrive a year or more later, most parents of a stillborn never fully recover from their loss. Some remember the "due date" for years and observe it with sadness and revival of the feeling of loss.

See also GRIEF; MISCARRIAGE; PREGNANCY.

stimulant drugs (stimulants)   Drugs that stimulate the central nervous system and increase the activity of the brain or the spinal cord. Examples of stimulant drugs include amphetamines, cocaine, caffeine and nicotine. As these agents produce a feeling of euphoria and may temporarily increase alertness, they are often overused and abused; this occurs particularly with amphetamines and cocaine. Stimulants do have some legitimate uses in medicine. Children with ADHD (Attention Deficit Hyperactivity Disorder) may benefit from stimulant treatment. Stimulants are used with success for the augmentation of antidepressant medications in patients with treatment resistant or refractory depression. Stimulants are also helpful in treating some cases of post-stroke depression as well as cognitive dysfunction and loss of motivation resulting from traumatic brain damage.

See also AMPHETAMINE DRUGS; COCAINE; METHAMPHETAMINES; SUBSTANCE ABUSE.

stimulus properties   In differentiating between fear and anxiety, some therapists describe the two feelings in terms of stimulus properties—the *identifiability, specificity* and *predictability*—of the source that brings on a response. Fear is considered a response to a clearly identifiable and circumscribed stimulus; whereas with anxiety, although it is a similar response, the stimulus to which the individual is responding is unclear, ambiguous and/or pervasive. If a response occurs to a stimulus that is a *realistic* threat and therefore useful, it is said to be fear. Conversely, a response is called anxiety if it is elicited by a stimulus that is not seen as a realistic or consensual threat, and is therefore irrational and not useful.

Another factor that differentiates fear from anxiety is the predictability of the source of the threat to which the individual responds. When an object or situation provides a signal of danger or threat, and is therefore predictable, the state experienced is called fear. For example, the response of a person in the middle of a thunderstorm who worries about being struck by a lightning bolt would be considered fear because the stimulus is clearly identifiable and predictable and the threat is realistic.

See also PHOBIA.

Doctor, Ronald M., and Ada P. Kahn. *The Encyclopedia of Phobias, Fears and Anxieties.* New York: Facts On File, 2000.

St. John's Wort (Hypericum perforatum) Widely prescribed by physicians for depression in Germany and other European countries. Researchers reviewing and meta-analyzing data representing 1,757 outpatients with depressive disorders concluded that "extracts of hypericum are more effective than placebo for mild to moderately severe depressive disorders." Another researcher found the St. John's extract to be as efficacious as amitriptyline for mild to moderate depression, with fewer side effects. In a six-week multicenter study, the same hypericum extract was tested against imipramine for severe depressive episodes. It was found equivalent in efficacy and superior in adverse effects. However promising these results may be, interpretation is limited by the relatively short duration of the studies when compared with the longer-term nature of major depression, as well as by dosage and standardization considerations.

Barrett, Bruce, David Kiefer, and David Rabago. "Assessing the Risks and Benefits of Herbal Medicine: An Overview of Scientific Evidence." *Alternative Therapies* 5, no. 4 (July 1999): 40–49.

stress A major factor in achieving a feeling of well-being and ongoing mental wellness. Stress is an everyday part of life and can be a source of energy or a source of impaired mental health. Everyone feels a sense of emotional strain, tension and anxiety at times. Different individuals can cope with differing levels of stress. Sometimes individuals feel completely overloaded by what is going on in their lives. Because each individual experiences life in unique ways, circumstances that one enjoys may be stressful to others.

Events that cause stress for different individuals vary. Some find happy events, such as starting a new job or planning a trip, sources of stress. Others find that trouble at home or on the job causes stress. Major life changes, such as the death of a loved one, divorce, loss of a job or moving to a new city, cause stress. At all stages of life, individuals sometimes find their personal agenda too full for comfort and feel overwhelmed. Stress increases when they feel a lack of support from those around them.

Stress is an internal response to circumstances known as "stressors." These include difficulty in getting along with people, feeling trapped or inadequate, finding little pleasure in life and feeling distrustful. Stress can lead to depression, frustration and anxiety.

When an individual feels stressed, chemical changes take place in the body. The adrenaline starts flowing and the nervous system is activated, which causes a fight or flight response. During extreme stress, some people notice that they have a faster heartbeat and a sick feeling in their stomach; it is hard to work or function efficiently at such times.

Stress affects all aspects of life. Some individuals find that stress actually raises their energy level and helps them focus their mind better on their work or on a sports activity. Some thrive on many kinds of stressors. People who do are often attracted to high-stress occupations and professions.

Stress that starts at work can affect home life, and the reverse is also true for many people. Stress within a family causes tension and difficulty in communicating with one another. In some cases, interpersonal stresses develop when an individual has two feelings at the same time, such as wanting to be an independent adolescent yet feeling dependent on parents. As life is a series of progressions through emotional stages, it is helpful to remember that change and growth always involve some degree of stress. In a family, several people are trying to cope with their own stress and the stress of others about whom they care.

Diet and exercise can help relieve stress. Normal eating of three meals a day reduces effects of stress for some people. "Crash diets" and "fad diets" can lead to anxiety, depression and an inability to maintain a good weight. Well-balanced meals provide a slow release of necessary nutrients throughout the day. For some people, too much caffeine causes additional stress by bringing on symptoms of anxiety.

Many people find that regular physical workouts involving running, walking or exercising in a gym, health club or on exercise equipment at home help them relieve stress and get ready to effectively face challenges of the day ahead. Using muscles is a way to use up some of the fight or flight readiness in the body.

Some people use massage or soothing music as stress relievers. Sources of relaxation are very individual matters. What allows one person to relax may actually cause stress for another. An example is noise level in the workplace or at home. Each individual should try to create an environment in which to work and live that is the least stressful and concentrate on reaching peak performance and feeling of well-being.

Individuals who have been exposed to sudden and unexpected events, such as seeing someone attacked or beaten, seeing a suicide or death or surviving a natural disaster (such as an earthquake of flood), may have a pattern of stress known as post-traumatic stress disorder. Over a period of weeks, months or even years, the mind and body may continue to react in many ways. The individual may have bad dreams, flashbacks and feelings that the event is recurring. With support from family, friends and mental health professionals, these individuals can find help.

General Adaptation Syndrome

Stressors represent significant changes. How one adjusts to change influences the extent of stress one feels. Hans Selye used the phrase "general adaptation syndrome" to explain how individuals coped with the stressors in their lives. Individuals experience events in different ways. What results in emotional strain and anxiety for one person may not bring about those reactions in others.

Stress affects all aspects of life. Some individuals find that stress actually raises their energy level and helps them focus their mind better on their work or on a sports activity. Some thrive on many kinds of stressors. People who do are often attracted to high stress occupations and professions.

Learning to Manage Stress

"Stressors cannot be eliminated, so our goals should be to control and manage stress," says Elaine Shepp, LCSW, a psychotherapist in private practice and on the staff at Rush North Shore Medical Center, Skokie, Illinois. "It is possible to 'neu-tralize' the toxic effects of unrelenting stress," she explains. "People I know who win the battle against stress put their personal and professional lives into perspective. They may experience a constantly high level of pressure and unrealistic performance objectives at work. However, they have enough moral courage to become somewhat 'inner directed.' They develop their own ideals of conduct and objectives and test themselves by their own standards." "Some report that they have made a conscious decision not to continue having a 'non-life life.' They are able to prioritize their work and enjoy some diversions."

Professional Help in Coping with Stress

There are times when individuals find that their mental outlook detracts from the energy required for productive work and effective personal functioning. At these times, talking to a friend just isn't enough; fortunately, psychological help is available to help deal with stress. "People who seek professional help to overcome extreme stress should not consider themselves 'weak' or 'losers,'" says Elaine Shepp. "Seeking psychological help is an intelligent way of using tools that are available to increase one's level of functioning. Counseling can help prevent 'burnout' or assist in dealing with life situations that require the input of a non-involved, knowledgeable person."

If you find yourself feeling totally overwhelmed by your stressors and decide to get professional help, how should you choose a psychotherapist? You may want to talk with a close colleague or friend who has experienced psychotherapy. However, the issue of confidentiality is just as important as the need to find a mental health professional who is nonjudgmental. The psychotherapist should be one with whom you have a sense of comfort, who understands your particular stressors and who can suggest practical ways for you to handle these stressors. Find a therapist who is multifaceted in his or her approach to problems and knowledgeable about the many options available to treat particular problems. Look for one who is open to consulting with other professionals who have additional expertise.

Finding Relief From Stress

Sources of relaxation are very individual matters. Many people find that regular physical workouts help them relieve stress and get ready to effectively face challenges of the day ahead. Using muscles is a way to use up some of the "fight or flight" readiness in the body.

Some people use massage or soothing music as stress relievers. What allows one person to relax may actually cause stress for another; an example is the noise level in the workplace or at home. Each individual should try to create an environment in which to work and live that is the least stressful and that allows him or her to concentrate on reaching peak performance and achieving feelings of well-being.

Many complementary therapies are used to relieve stress; they include acupuncture, biofeedback, guided imagery, hypnosis, meditation, progressive muscle relaxation and yoga. Also, hobbies help many people relieve stress. When they participate in an activity simply for enjoyment, their stress level goes down; such hobbies may include dancing, art and painting, sewing, building model trains or plane, bird watching or playing a musical instrument. Choices of hobbies are as diverse as human nature.

Diet and exercise are basics of wellness and can also help relieve stress. Normal eating of three meals a day reduces effects of stress for some people. "Crash diets" and "fad diets" can lead to anxiety, depression and an inability to maintain a good weight. Well-balanced meals provide a slow release of necessary nutrients throughout the day. For some people, too much caffeine causes additional stress by bringing on symptoms of anxiety.

REDUCE STRESS TO IMPROVE MENTAL HEALTH

- Develop a sense of humor and increase your ability to see humor in sometimes intolerable situations.
- Learn to recognize your own signs of stress:
  Increased irritability with "difficult" clients or family members
  Headaches
  Overeating
  Increased alcohol consumption
  Sleeplessness
  Depression
  Chronic fatigue
- Identify external and internal stress-producing factors over which you have little or no control. Internal factors include perfectionism and unrealistic expectations.
- Be realistic in your daily outlook. Don't expect too much of yourself or others.

- Prioritize your responsibilities. Learn to occasionally say "no" to requests you consider unreasonable or undoable. Focus your energy on other needed areas.
- Pay attention to the basics of living, such as eating a well-balanced diet.
- If you consume a large quantity of caffeinated beverages, cut down. Coffee, tea and cola can increase your heart rate and your irritability level.
- Develop a regular habit of exercising. A twenty-minute walk each day can be effective in fighting muscle tension.
- Keep your job stress separate from stress related to your home life.
- Learn some relaxation techniques that work for you, such as deep breathing or listening to music you like.
- Recognize that you may need professional help if you feel so overwhelmed that you just cannot cope.
- Understand that getting professional help to deal with major stressful events, such as death, divorce, illness or job loss, is a sign of good self-care, not weakness.

STRESS MANAGEMENT

Learn to recognize your own signs of stress, common stressors and ineffective coping methods. If you experience any of the symptoms below, consider that stress may be a possible cause.

Stress Signals

Nervous tic
Muscular aches
Inability to sleep
Increased sweating
Stuttering
Nausea or stomach pain
Grinding teeth
Headache, dizziness
Low-grade infections
Rash or acne
Desire to cry or crying
Constipation or diarrhea
Frigidity or impotence
High blood pressure
Dry mouth or throat
Irritability or bad temper
Lethargy or inability to work
Cold, clammy or clenched hands
Sudden bursts of energy
Finger-tapping
Depression
Fear, panic or anxiety
Hives
Coughing
Nagging
Fatigue
Pacing
Frowning
Restlessness
Accident prone

STRESS MANAGEMENT *(continued)*

Common Thoughts and Feelings

Impulsive
Freeze up
Become rigid
Falling apart
Thoughts "jumble up"
Feeling tense
Constant worrying
Feeling time pressure
World is caving in

Stressors (in your family)

Holidays, vacations
Marital difficulties
Injury or illness
Problems with children
Giving a party
Child is leaving home
Spouse has a new job
Not enough time
Sexual difficulties

Stressors (as an individual)

Aging
Pressure on the job
Feeling unattractive
New job
Great achievement
Change in habits
Success problems

Finances

Inability to pay bills
Mortgage
Major purchase

As a Member of Society

Leading a group
Starting a relationship
Lack of freedom
Feeling insecure
Being popular

As a Family Member

Problems with others
Lack of Privacy
Leaving home
Death in the family
Divorce or remarriage

Ineffective Methods of Coping with Stress

Increased smoking
Overeating
Increased consumption of any drug
Denial
Sedentary life
Sleeping all the time

See also ANXIETIES; BEHAVIOR THERAPIES; BENSON, HERBERT; CAFFEINE; COMPLEMENTARY THERAPIES; GENERAL ADAPTATION SYNDROME; HEADACHES; HIGH BLOOD PRESSURE; HOBBIES; HOMEOSTASIS; KABAT-ZINN, JON; MEDITATION; MIND/BODY CONNECTIONS; POST-TRAUMATIC STRESS DISORDER; RELAXATION; SELYE, HANS

*Adapted with permission from Kahn, Ada P. *Stress* (booklet), Mental Health Association of Greater Chicago, 1989.

Kahn, Ada P. *Stress A to Z: The Sourcebook for Facing Everyday Challenges.* New York: Facts On File, 2000.

Selye, Hans. *Stress Without Distress.* Philadelphia: J. B. Lippincott Company, 1974.

———. *The Stress of Life,* rev. ed. New York: McGraw-Hill, 1978.

stroke A unit of positive recognition or love, which may take the form of a kind word, compliment, reinforcing feedback or a physical "pat on the back." Individuals need frequent doses of good strokes to maintain their good mental health.

Stroke also refers to damage to the brain caused by interruption to its blood supply. Movement, sensation or function controlled by the damaged area is often impaired. Intellectual impairment is often permanent.

According to Robert W. Teasell, M.D., assistant professor of Medicine, University of Western Ontario, and chief of Physical Medicine and Rehabilitation, University Hospital, London, Ontario, clinically significant depression occurs in more than 30 percent of stroke patients. This depression reduces motivation and, with an adverse effect on activities of daily living and socialization, often adds to family problems and stresses.

Treatment should include positive feedback, emotional support and psychological counseling. Some antidepressant drugs can be appropriately used under careful supervision following a stroke.

One person's stroke affects the well-being of others in the family. Those providing care to a stroke victim face their own adjustment problems, as their personal needs are often sacrificed to meet the needs of the stroke patient. With limited opportunities for rest, caregivers are often under great stress and themselves suffer a higher rate of depression and deterioration of health.

See also CAREGIVERS; CHRONIC ILLNESS; REINFORCEMENT.

Teasell, Robert W. "Long Term Sequelae of Stroke." *Canadian Family Physician* 38 (Feb. 1992).

stupor   A mental state in which there is marked decrease in reactivity to the environment and reduction of spontaneous movements and activity. The individual may be totally unresponsive to any stimulus. Stupor may occur as a result of epilepsy, brain disease, serious depression or many other causes such as catatonia. In catatonic stupor the patient may seem totally unresponsive but later show awareness of everything that happened around her during the catatonic stupor.

See also BRAIN; EPILEPSY.

stuttering   A speech disorder involving repeated hesitation and delay in saying words or in which certain sounds are unusually prolonged. Also known as stammering, it usually starts in early childhood and may be a temporary situation. About half of the children whose stuttering persists after age five continue to do so throughout adulthood.

Some people who have a stammer find it more pronounced when they become anxious or fearful. For example, some individuals who are fearful of public speaking (a common social phobia) have difficulty getting words out if they have to stand up in crowd and say something. These same individuals have no difficulty in reading or singing in unison.

For many, stuttering is a source of embarrassment. Some stutterers become socially withdrawn because they fear ridicule from others. Some individuals improve their speech pattern through speech therapy, which may include learning to give equal weight to each syllable.

Causes of stuttering are not understood; theories suggest that it may be due to a subtle form of brain damage or may be related to a psychological problem.

subconscious   According to psychoanalytic theory, the subconscious is the part of the mind through which information passes on its way from the unconscious to the conscious mind. The subconscious contains thoughts, feelings or ideas that one is temporarily unaware of but that can be recalled under certain circumstances.

sublimation   A process by which individuals redirect impulses into socially acceptable forms of behavior. For example, aggressive urges may be channeled into sports activities. Sublimation is also regarded as a defense mechanism.

See also FREUD, SIGMUND; PSYCHOANALYSIS.

substance abuse   An addiction or a problem with alcohol or other drugs. Many people look to alcohol and drugs to help them cope with stress, anxiety or depression. Other people misuse substances they obtain with a physician's prescription. Some people develop a dependence on drugs, which means that they have a compulsion to continue using the substance because it gives them a feeling of well-being. One can be psychologically dependent on a drug and not physically dependent; the reverse is also true. Dependence can occur after periodic or prolonged use of a drug, and the characteristics of dependence vary according to the drug involved.

The toll exacted on society, health and the economy by substance abuse remains staggering in the early 2000s. In the inner cities in the United States, the drug problem appears to be worsening, with a concomitant increase in violent crime. For example, in 1989, the number of murders in Washington, D.C. averaged more than one a day, and more than 70 percent were drug related.

In a comprehensive economic analysis conducted in 1983, costs of alcohol problems in the United States were estimated to exceed $70 billion per year, with the majority of these costs attributed to reduced productivity. An additional $44 billion in economic costs were attributed to drug problems. Alcohol is implicated in nearly half of all deaths caused by motor vehicle crashes and fatal intentional injuries such as suicides and homicides; victims are intoxicated in approximately one-third of all homicides, drownings and boating deaths.

Adolescents who use alcohol and other drugs are much more likely than their non-using peers to experience other serious problems. An estimated one in four adolescents is at very high risk of alcohol and other drug problems, school failure, early unwanted pregnancy and/or delinquency.

An estimated 21.2 million Americans have tried cocaine at least once. Use of crack cocaine, which appears to be even more addictive than the powdered form, has become increasingly widespread, especially in some urban centers. Among serious consequences of cocaine use is the incidence of developmental disabilities among infants of crack-addicted mothers.

Substance abuse significantly increases the risk of transmitting the human immunodeficiency virus (HIV). This can occur directly through the sharing of contaminated needles, sexual contact with intravenous drug abusers or other drug injectors or via in utero infection and indirectly through adverse effects on immune system functioning and the increased risk of unsafe sexual practices.

Recognition of the gravity of the substance abuse problem in the United States is evidenced on almost every national opinion poll that places substance abuse as a priority concern. The national effort to prevent these problems has mobilized government, schools, communities, businesses and families.

The combination of increased public resolve, advanced scientific understanding and treatments available for those who seek help gives some small degree of optimism for overcoming the national substance abuse problem in the United States.

See also ADDICTIONS; ALCOHOLISM: EMPLOYEE ASSISTANCE PROGRAMS.

success A threat to good mental health both when it happens and when it does not happen. Some who view success as a source of stress fear that they will not be able to compete at a higher plateau or that they will not be able to fulfill further expectations. Those reaching for success may fear that with achievement they will have to move to a better neighborhood, bigger house or send children to a better school. All these expectations may lead to worries and stressful feelings about finances.

While success can be a source of satisfaction, it can also be stressful because some individuals may fear that achievement will place them in another social or academic class and they will then lose friendships. Some individuals actually avoid success because they want to continue conforming to their group.

Expectations for success are stressful because fears of failure are associated with the striving process. An inability to reach what the individual regards as success may reflect unfavorably on one's self-image and self-esteem.

Certain personality types are driven toward success. The "type A" personality, for example is associated with intense drives for success. Such individuals have competitive feelings, are extremely goal oriented, take on multiple commitments and become preoccupied with meeting deadlines. Often, after serious illness, such individuals learn to relax more and redirect their drives away from success, instead placing more value on family and friendships.

See also SELF-ESTEEM; TYPE A PERSONALITY.

sudden infant death syndrome (SIDS) SIDS, or "crib death," is the sudden death of an infant that cannot be explained by prior medical history or postmortem examination. Victims of SIDS are infants, usually between the ages of two and four months, who stop breathing during a normal sleeping period. Ninety percent of all victims die within the first four months, but it may strike children as old as one year. Although causes of SIDS are unknown, it is not caused by childhood vaccines, suffocation, vomiting and choking. Many research projects are under way to determine predictive factors that may prevent some deaths in the future.

A SIDS death can affect as many as a hundred people, among them parents, siblings, grandparents, extended family, coworkers, neighbors, babysitters and daycare workers. A SIDS death produces an intense reaction for many of these people. After the initial shock wears off, many parents find themselves experiencing feelings of guilt and depression. Support groups can be helpful for parents who have lost a child to SIDS.

For information on SIDS, contact:

Sudden Infant Death Syndrome Alliance
1314 Bedford Avenue, Suite 210
Baltimore, MD 21208

Phone: (410) 653-8226
Fax: (410) 653-8709
Website: www.sidsalliance.org

suicide Killing oneself voluntarily and intentionally. Many people do not like to talk about suicide or acknowledge its existence. A diagnosis of suicide is usually not one that the family wants to hear. When a high possibility of suicide exists within a family, certain measures should be taken. Suicidal tendencies should be explained to family members as a manifestation of depression that can be successfully treated. In an acute suicidal crisis, the family should be instructed to remove all weapons and all lethal means from the home, including prescription drugs. They should be told not to leave the individual alone at any time. Friends or loved ones who show signs of depression or express hopelessness or suicidal impulses should be helped to get immediate professional help before a suicidal crisis develops.

Associated with the word "suicide" are the terms suicidal ideation (having thoughts of committing suicide or thoughts of methods by which to commit suicide), suicide attempt (self-destructive behavior that could be lethal), suicidal gesture (self-destructive behavior that is usually not lethal and is often viewed by others as manipulative behavior) and self-destructiveness (behavior by which one damages himself immediately, impulsively or chronically).

Suicide is the eighth leading cause of death in the United States and the second most frequent cause of death for young people in the 15 to 25 age bracket. About 12 percent of those who threaten or attempt suicide actually kill themselves. Current statistics may understate the actual occurrence of suicide. Many auto and other accidents may have suicidal intention. Because of social stigma, insurance coverage issues and legal criteria for classifying cause of death, suicide may not be recorded as the cause in many cases.

Prevention of Suicide

One of the most difficult challenges clinicians face is the prevention of suicide by their patients. Such psychiatric clinicians routinely deal with patients whose diagnoses are associated with a high risk for

suicide; assessment and intervention always make such cases a high priority.

SUICIDE POTENTIAL: RISK FACTORS AND CHARACTERISTICS

The possibility that the individual will kill him- or herself voluntarily and intentionally is referred to as suicide potential.

Risk Factors	Characteristics
Depression	Ambivalence
Other mood disorders	Withdrawn, isolative
Schizophrenia	behavior
Other psychoses	Impaired concentration
Neurological disorders	Constricted thought
Delirium	processes, tunnel vision
Use or withdrawal of	Psychomotor agitation
alcohol or other	Psychomotor retardation
substances	Anxious
Organic brain disorders	Attentive to internal
Hallucinations, delusions	stimuli
Stress, acute or chronic	Verbalizes suicidal
Isolation	thoughts, feelings,
Loss of significant other	plan
Loss of self-esteem	Verbalized references
Loss of physical health,	to death, dying
function	Gives away possessions
Cultural factors	Anger, hostility
Spiritual anxiety	Impulsive behaviors
Personality disorders	Depressed mood
Impulse control disorders	Appetite disturbances
Internal conflicts, guilt	Hopeless-helpless
Family dysfunction, crisis	Disturbed sleep
Loss of resources, social	patterns
and economic	
Unmet needs	

The physician, psychotherapist or mental health worker is sometimes the only person with the opportunity of recognizing suicidal intent. Studies have shown that from 40 to 75 percent of suicidal individuals will see physicians within six months to a year preceding their self-destructive acts. A number of studies have pointed out that even while receiving psychiatric treatment, psychiatric hospitalization or treatment with psychotropic drugs, patients do commit suicide.

Although suicide rarely can be a logical, rational decision based on an individual's situation, evidence seems to support the contention that most suicides occur in the context of psychiatric illness. However, the absence of psychiatric treatment at the time of suicide does not necessarily preclude the existence of a serious mental disturbance. It has been observed that severely depressed patients may appear symptom-free just prior to suicide. This may lead to an erroneous assumption that the individual is "normal" at the time of suicide. While suicidal behavior may manifest itself in patients fitting any psychiatric diagnostic category, it has been found most prevalent in depression, especially manic-depression and psychotic depression, as well as in alcoholism, substance abuse and schizophrenia, especially in younger age groups.

Typically, the high-risk patient is one with symptoms of a serious depressive syndrome manifesting signs such as sleep disturbance, weight loss, dry mouth, loss of sexual drive, gastrointestinal discomfort, complete loss of interest, impairment of function, delusional guilt, neglect of personal appearance and cleanliness, inability to make decisions, a feeling of emptiness, psychomotor retardation or agitation in a depressed mood, feelings of hopelessness and helplessness and severe anxiety or panic attacks. Generally, the risk of suicide appears to be greatest in the early course of depressive illness (first three episodes) and decreases as drive and affect are "burned out" and life becomes a kind of partial death, without ambition and seemingly without purpose.

The Chronically Suicidal Individual

Repeated communication of a wish to die or suicidal thoughts is a characteristic of the chronically suicidal person. However, this in itself is not sufficient to distinguish the high- from the low-risk individual, since it has also been observed that the majority of the much larger group of patients who attempt but do not complete suicide also convey intent in advance.

Intense dependency is often an underlying dynamic in the suicidal individual. This dependency has been observed throughout all spheres of the suicidal individual's lifestyle, where inordinately excessive demands are made on others for constant attention, affection and approval. The individual also feels unable to cope by himself, thereby needing continual supervision and guidance. Others have independently observed this basic feeling of helplessness in patients who commit suicide.

CHRONIC PRE-LETHAL FEATURES*

1. Suicidal communications
2. Symbiotic dependency and reliance on external controls
3. Rigid thinking
4. Paranoid traits
5. Externalized anger
6. Intermittent loss of control
7. Chronic stimulus seeking
8. Impaired personal coping

Tendencies toward rigid thinking that does not allow for alternatives in a crisis—and thinking in opposites—have been observed in the personalities of many suicidal individuals. Perfectionism as a personality trait is carried to a pathological state, and this finds expression in the form of an anxious striving toward perfection in all undertakings.

A less commonly recognized characteristic repeatedly associated with a high risk of suicide is paranoia. While paranoia can serve as a temporary defense against depression, unrecognized suicidal impulses may result when this defense fails.

Sigmund Freud viewed suicide and depression as unconscious rage toward a lost loved object turned back on oneself; however, cases have suggested a high frequency of externalized anger and even violent tantrums in the histories of patients who commit suicide or make serious attempts.

Perhaps the most important characteristic of the chronically high-risk individual is that of impaired capacity for interpersonal relating. One study showed that 91 percent of those who completed suicide made no attempt to communicate their intent just prior to their suicide, but the suicide-gesture group contacted a significant other 73 percent of the time.

Assessing Acute Pre-lethal Factors

Mental health professionals are often placed in a difficult position regarding a patient's family or friends when they believe that suicide is a strong imminent possibility. However, there are a number of acute behavioral and situational factors found with the greatest frequency in seriously attempted and completed suicides.

Suicide in Major Affective Disorder

A study reported during 1990 indicated that among 954 patients with major affective disorders, nine clinical features were associated with suicide. Six of these—panic attacks, severe psychic anxiety, diminished concentration, global insomnia, moderate alcohol abuse and severe loss of interest or pleasure—were associated with suicide within one year. Three others—severe hopelessness, suicidal ideation and history of previous suicide attempts— were associated with suicide occurring after one year. These findings drew attention to the importance of: (1) standardized prospective data for studies of suicide; (2) assessment of short-term suicide risk factors; and (3) anxiety symptoms as modifiable suicide risk factors within a clinically relevant period.****

Situational Precursors of Suicide

The most commonly understood instances of increased suicidal risk in the depressed individual are situations associated with separation or loss. The loss does not necessarily have to be the final loss or death of a loved one as Freud emphasized, but it may be simply a temporary loss to the individual who is in a depressive crisis. For example, losses may be spouse, home, job, hospital discharge, temporary separation from therapist, money, love, and so on.

ACUTE PRE-LETHAL FEATURES*

1. Specific suicidal plan
2. Abrupt clinical change
3. Decreasing fear of death concomitant with an increasingly positive attitude toward death
4. Failure of psychological defenses (severe anxiety or panic attacks)
5. Mental regression
6. Delusional hopelessness
7. Loss of future perspective
8. Sudden decline of interpersonal relating, with help negation
9. Dreams of symbolic peaceful scenes of dying in which death is looked upon as exciting or euphoric.

SITUATIONAL PRECURSORS OF SUICIDE*

1. Threatened or actual loss of relationship
2. Failure situation
3. Real or perceived physical illness

The "failure situation" ranks high as a precursor of suicide. This situation may occur after a hospital discharge when a patient is trying to regain or attain higher levels of function, such as successfully starting a job or returning to college. This factor also ranks high when individuals try to meet higher expectations of themselves or others.

Additionally, the presence of real or perceived physical illness may be significant in the assessment of suicidal risk. In malignant or incurable illness, two critical suicidal periods seem to be those of: (1) uncertainty while diagnosis and prognosis are still at issue, and (2) shock following the first realization of the upheavals and suffering, actual or fantasized, that are to follow.*

Suicide in Youth*

There are some clues to predicting suicide among youngsters or adolescents. They are more likely to communicate with those in their peer group than their parents. They may give away a prized possession with the comment that they will not be needing it any more. They may be more morose and isolated than usual. Although there may be signs of insomnia, worry and anorexia, the youngster may not have all the classical signs of depression.

One study listed symptoms occurring in 25 college-age suicides in order of their frequency: despondency, futility, lack of interest in schoolwork, a feeling of tenseness around people, insomnia, suicidal communications, fatigue and malaise without apparent organic cause, feelings of inadequacy or unworthiness and brooding over the death of a loved one.

According to an article published in December 1991 in the *Journal of the American Medical Association*, having a gun at home may increase the risk that a psychologically troubled teen will commit suicide.*** David A. Brent, M.D., Western Psychiatric Institute and Clinic, Pittsburgh, Pennsylvania, and colleagues noted that the odds that potentially suicidal adolescents will kill themselves are up 75-fold when a gun is kept in the house. They commented on the differences between teen suicides and that of adults. For teens, they said, a suicide attempt may be an attempt to communicate that they are in great pain, although they may be ambivalent about wanting to die. For such adolescents, ready access to a firearm may guarantee that their plea for help will not be heard.

In a study, the authors matched 47 adolescents who had committed suicide in Pennsylvania from

July 1986 through February 1988 with 47 adolescents who had attempted suicide and 47 never-suicidal psychiatric controls. All three groups were similar with respect to age, gender, race and socioeconomic status. (The study population was predominantly white, male and 15 to 17 years of age.)

Researchers found that guns (handguns and long guns) were twice as likely to be found in the homes of suicide victims as in the homes of attempters or psychiatric controls. There was no difference in the methods of storage of firearms among the three groups, so that even guns stored locked or separated from ammunition were associated with suicide by firearms.

The authors commented that it is clear the firearms have no place in the homes of psychiatrically troubled youngsters. Physicians who care for psychiatrically disturbed adolescents with any indicators of suicidal risk, such as depression, conduct problems, substance abuse or suicidal thoughts, have a responsibility to make clear and firm recommendations that firearms be removed from the homes of these at-risk youths.

Assisted Suicide

In 1991, *Final Exit,* a "how-to" book by Derek Humphry, executive director of the Hemlock Society—a group aimed at promoting death with dignity—was published. His premise was that his book, for the terminally ill, is not meant to be a book for unhappy or depressed people.

Many mental health professionals worried that this book and others might legitimize suicide for troubled people with undiagnosed depression who could be treated if their illnesses were diagnosed correctly. Many expressed fear that such books could push up suicide rates, particularly among the elderly who are not terminally ill. However, according to David Clark, president of the American Society of Suicidology—an organization dedicated to preventing suicide—many people are extraordinarily glad when they recover from an attempt that someone did not help them die.**

In March 1990, a group of physicians writing in the *New England Journal of Medicine,* in an article entitled "The Physician's Responsibility Toward Hopelessly Ill Patients," held that "it is not immoral for a physician to assist in the rational suicide of a terminally ill person."**** Two of the 12 authors of the paper dissented from this statement.

Later in 1990, Dr. Jack Kevorkian assisted in the suicide of Janet Adkins, an Oregon woman said to have Alzheimer's disease. He provided her with a device that she activated to administer a lethal dose of drugs. Questions were raised about Dr. Kevorkian's ability to confirm the patient's diagnosis, about the patient's ability to make an informed decision and about the circumstances. The event took place in a van parked on a side road in Michigan, far from the patient's family and outside any institution.****

Suicide Rates Among the Aging Population

A federal study published during 1991 showed that from 1980 to 1986, suicides by Americans aged 65 and older jumped 23 percent for the men, and 42 percent for black men. The rate for white women rose 17 percent, while there were too few suicides among black women to show a meaningful trend. A study in Illinois using a grant from the American Association of Retired People Andrus Foundation showed that the great majority of the elderly who committed suicide were physically healthy. However, 79 percent had shown symptoms of a major treatable psychiatric illness, usually depression or alcoholism.**

For further information:

American Psychiatric Association
1400 K Street NW
Washington, D.C. 20005
Phone: (888) 357-7924
Web site: www.psych.org

American Association of Child and Adolescent
    Psychiatry
3615 Wisconsin Avenue NW
Washington, D.C. 20016
Phone: (202) 966-7300
Web site: www.aacap.org

American Association of Suicidology
4201 Connecticut Avenue NW, Suite 408
Washington, D.C. 20008
Phone: (202) 237-2280
Fax: (202) 237-2282
Web site: www.suicidology.org

National Alliance for the Mentally Ill
2107 Wilson Boulevard, Suite 300
Arlington, VA 22201
Phone: (800) 950-6264 or (703) 524-7600
Fax: (703) 524-9094
Web site: www.nami.org

National Depressive and Manic-Depressive
 Association
730 North Franklin Street, Suite 501
Chicago, IL 60610
Phone: (800) 826-3632
Fax: (312) 642-7243
Web site: www.ndmda.org

See also DEPRESSION.

***Brent, David A. et al. "The Presence and Accessibility of Firearms in the Homes of Adolescent Suicides." *Journal of the American Medical Association* 266, no. 21 (Dec. 4, 1991).

Fawcett, Jan et al. "Time-Related Predictors of Suicide in Major Affective Disorder." *American Journal of Psychiatry* 147, no. 9 (Sept. 1990).

*Fawcett, Jan, and Paul Susman. "A Clinical Assessment of Acute Suicidal Potential: A Review." *Rush-Presbyterian—St. Luke's Medical Bulletin* 14, no. 2 (Apr. 1975).

**Katz, Marvin. "Critics Fear Misuse of Suicide Books." *Bulletin, American Association of Retired Persons* 32, no. 11 (Dec. 1991).

****"Should the Doctor Ever Help?" *Harvard Health Letter* 16, no. 10 (Aug. 1991).

Sullivan, Harry Stack (1892–1949) An American psychiatrist and a dissenter from Sigmund Freud. Sullivan defined personality as "the relatively enduring pattern of a recurrent interpersonal situation which characterizes a human life." He noticed that individuals sometimes used language as a defense mechanism or form of "distortion" rather than as a common ground for communication. He said this "verbal shield" was caused by low self-esteem, which results in anxiety. Sullivan defined anxiety as a physiological and psychological reaction learned in early childhood. He was instrumental in setting up the World Federation of Mental Health and the United Nations Education, Scientific and Cultural Organization committee on investigating the causes of tension among a variety of cultures.

Doctor, Ronald M., and Ada P. Kahn. *The Encyclopedia of Phobias, Fears, and Anxieties.* New York: Facts On File, 2000.

sundowning (sundown syndrome) Increased symptoms of confusion during the late afternoon or evening hours, as exhibited by patients with dementia usually in nursing homes or long-term care institutions. Manifestations of sundowning include increased confusion, disorientation, agitated behavior and an increase in verbal behavior. Such spells can extend into the night, resulting in restlessness and sleeplessness.

See also AGING; ALZHEIMER'S DISEASE; AGING, ALZHEIMER'S DISEASE in BIBLIOGRAPHY.

superego A psychoanalytic term for the aspect of personality that represents the standards of parents and society and determines the individual's own sense of right and wrong as well as aspirations and goals. The more common term for superego is conscience.

See also CONSCIENCE.

superiority complex The unrealistic and exaggerated belief that one is better than others. In some people, this develops as a way to compensate for unconscious feelings of low self-esteem or inadequacy. For example, bullies who push other children around act like they are stronger and smarter than others their age. The reality is that they have low self-esteem. In adults, even business executives may put on a tough facade and try to make others think well of them, but inside they feel inadequate and do not respect themselves.

See also BULLIES; SELF-ESTEEM.

superstition Beliefs that have survived since ancient times among cultures around the world. Mental health may be affected in many people who still hold superstitious beliefs.

Many notions and customs persist; some are odd, amusing, harmless, and others are harmful. Scientific thinking helps destroy superstitious thinking because modern science believes that everything in nature has a natural cause, and it emphasizes the laws of nature that explain cause and effect.

Superstitious beliefs are more common among people with little education, but there is a tendency in many well-educated people to cling to superstitious beliefs. For example, hotels, cruise ships and other commercial enterprises sometimes skip the number thirteen because many persons believe it is unlucky. Other common American superstitions include: Fridays that fall on the 13th day of the month are considered unlucky. If your ears burn, it means someone is talking about you. Bad luck follows walking under a ladder, breaking a mirror or having a black cat cross your path. It is supposed to be good luck if one finds a penny or a four-leaf clover.

Stressful interactions may arise between family members or friends when one clings to an old superstition and another counters it with a more practical explanation.

See also TABOO.

Kahn, Ada P. *Stress A to Z: The Sourcebook for Facing Everyday Challenges.* New York: Facts On File, 2000.

support groups   Also known as self-help groups, support groups consist of individuals with the same mental health disorder or concern for the disorder who join together to help one another by sharing experiences and advice and providing emotional support for one another.

Support groups exist for patients themselves, as well as for spouses and family members. For example, individuals with manic-depressive illness began an organization that has now become nationwide, with chapters in many cities. Individuals with chronic fatigue syndrome (CFS) have done the same, with the result that sufferers no longer need feel alone and that they are the only individuals with the problems. Another example is Y-ME, a national organization of women who have had breast cancer.

There are support groups for parents of children with specific mental health concerns, as well as groups for middle-aged people who care for aging parents.

Many physicians recommend that patients join support groups because they realize that help with the anger and confusion can augment any therapies provided by medical means.

An additional benefit of belonging to a support group for a particular concern is than one can stay up to date on research progress being made as researchers work toward cures and better treatments. Many groups circulate articles from popular and scientific publications and bring in experts to discuss their latest findings.

According to Karyn Feiden, author of *Hope and Help for Chronic Fatigue Syndrome,* the work of support groups generally falls into three interlinked areas:

• Informing and educating the general public, and particularly patients, their families and the medical community.

• Counseling and consoling those who have been diagnosed with the particular disorder.

• Organizing and advocating for the cause at both the local and the national level.

See also BEHAVIORAL THERAPY; CHRONIC FATIGUE SYNDROME; DEPRESSION; EXPOSURE THERAPY; SELF-HELP GROUPS.

supra-additive effect   See SYNERGY.

Surmontil   Trade name for the tricyclic antidepressant medication generically known as trimipramine.

See also ANTIDEPRESSANT MEDICATIONS; PHARMACOLOGICAL APPROACH; TRICYCLIC ANTIDEPRESSANTS.

surrogacy   Any person who substitutes or takes the place of another. The term "surrogacy" may be used by mental health professionals for purely emotional or social family relationships. A child who lacks a parent may develop a relationship with a friend, teacher or relative and make that person his surrogate mother or father. An only child may adopt a surrogate brother or sister from her extended family or circle of friends.

Surrogacy gained a more physical, clinical meaning in recent years as science developed techniques whereby a woman could carry and give birth to a child for a woman who was incapable of normal pregnancy and childbirth. This technique has aroused religious opposition and seems to some unnatural or the first step toward a futuristic society that might take an overly clinical, calculating attitude toward reproduction.

Emotional as well as legal problems have arisen from the fact that the surrogate mother may become attached to the child she is carrying and be reluctant to give it up. Surrogate mothers at first were women who agreed to be artificially inseminated with the sperm of the prospective father. Advances in in vitro fertilization later offered the possibility of natural parenthood for both wife and husband for cases in which the wife produced normal eggs but had some other physical problem that made pregnancy difficult, dangerous or impossible. The egg and sperm are brought together outside the parents' bodies and then implanted in a surrogate mother for a normal pregnancy.

An unusual 1991 case of surrogate motherhood involved a woman who agreed to give birth to her own grandchildren. The grandmother was of childbearing age and in good health. Her daughter, who was born without a uterus, was capable of producing normal eggs but not of carrying a child. Eggs from the daughter fertilized with her husband's sperm were successfully implanted in her mother and resulted in twins.

Sex surrogates have also become a controversial issue in recent years. Surrogate sexual partners have been known to act as therapists by engaging in sex with people who have severe sexual dysfunctions. Rape victims, nonorgasmic men and women and people who have remained virgins well into adult life are thought to be appropriate candidates for this type of therapy. Because of a lack of trained therapists and a lack of standards or licensing for the field, it is vulnerable to quacks and practitioners whose motives are dubious. A serious problem in treatment by a sex surrogate is that an attraction may develop that makes the relationship unprofessional or that the patient may become emotionally dependent on the surrogate.

See also INFERTILITY; SEX THERAPY; SURROGATE ACT.

Goldenson, Robert M. "Surrogate." In *The Encyclopedia of Human Behavior,* vol. 2. Garden City, N.Y.: Doubleday and Co., 1970.

"How Safe Are Surrogates?" *Cosmopolitan* (Nov. 1990).
Singer, Peter, and Deane Wells. *Making Babies.* New York: Scribner's, 1985.

Surrogate Act In 1991, the Health Care Surrogate Act was signed into law in the state of Illinois. Typical of acts in other states, the law in some instances permits a surrogate to make decisions concerning medical care, including such life-sustaining treatment as artificial nutrition and hydration, for a person unable to make such decisions. For example, in some instances the act authorizes surrogates, including a person's spouse or adult children, to make certain health care decisions when the person has a terminal condition, is in a state of permanent unconsciousness or has an incurable or irreversible condition as defined by the act. The act does not apply if a person has a valid living will or durable power or attorney for health care.

See also LEGAL ISSUES; SURROGACY.

survivor guilt See HOSTAGES; POST-TRAUMATIC STRESS DISORDER.

switching Swings of mood from high energy, increased confidence, increased assertiveness and decreased need for sleep to periods of lethargy, fatigue, loss of confidence and increased need for sleep. Symptoms of switching are diagnosed as cyclothymia, a mild form of bipolar depression. In bipolar disorder, mania with exaggerated confidence, grandiosity and sometimes psychosis is alternated with severe depression. Sudden changes from one arousal state to the other can occur dramatically and rapidly, without necessary environmental stresses.

See also BIPOLAR DISORDER; DEPRESSION; MANIA; MANIC-DEPRESSIVE ILLNESS.

symbolism In dreams, phobias and the unconscious mind, an object or idea that may signify something else, based on a resemblance between the original and its substitute.

See also DREAMING; FREUD, SIGMUND; PHALLIC SYMBOL.

symbiosis A relationship between two people characterized by excessive dependence and mutual exploitation for needs. The term is also used to denote the stage in infantile development when the infant's dependence is total and he or she is neither biologically nor psychologically separate from the mother; this is a normal phase followed by further development.

A "symbiotic marriage" occurs when one or both members of a couple depends upon the other for the gratification of certain psychological needs. Both partners may have neurotic or otherwise unusual needs that could not be satisfied easily outside the marriage.

sympathetic nervous system (SNS) One of two divisions of the autonomic nervous system. The SNS controls many involuntary activities of the glands, organs and other parts of the body. For example, the SNS is responsible for preparing people for fighting, fleeing, action or sexual climax. Among many effects, the SNS speeds up contractions of blood vessels, slows those of the intestines and increases heartbeat.

See also AUTONOMIC NERVOUS SYSTEM.

sympatholytic drugs Drugs that block actions of the sympathetic nervous system. These include beta blocker drugs, guanethidine, hydralazine and prazosin. They work either by reducing the release of the stimulatory neurotransmitter norepinephrine from nerve endings or by occupying the receptors that the neurotransmitters normally bind to, thus preventing their normal actions.

See also NEUROTRANSMITTERS; NOREPINEPHRINE.

symptom An indication of a disease or disorder that is noticed by the sufferer, such as a headache. A symptom is different from a sign, which is an indication of a disorder noticed on an objective basis by another person, such as a physician. A group of symptoms as well as signs are sometimes referred to as a syndrome. An example is post-traumatic stress disorder, in which the individual may experience a wide range of symptoms, such as nightmares, feelings of claustrophobia and an inability to concentrate. The physician may notice increased heartbeat, rapid breathing and other signs during examination.

See also SIGN; SYNDROME.

synapse A microscopic gap between the neurons in the chemical network of the brain. Billions of neurons send and receive electrical messages across synapses through specific amounts of neurotransmitters.

See also BRAIN; NEUROTRANSMITTERS.

syndrome A group of symptoms or signs occurring together that make up a particular mental or physical disorder. For example, the syndrome that leads a physician to diagnose depression in an individual may include difficulty sleeping, loss of weight, lack of interest in previously enjoyed activities, inability to concentrate, lack of interest in sexual activity and other factors. Another example is post-traumatic stress disorder, a syndrome with many different symptoms experienced by different individuals.

See also SIGN; SYMPTOM.

synergy The cooperation or joint action of two drugs that when taken together are more effective than when used individually. Because of this phenomenon, an amount of a drug that might be safe under normal circumstances can have a harmful effect if taken with a drug that acts synergistically. An example is a small amount of alcohol combined with a small dose of a barbiturate drug, which can have a much greater effect than either alcohol or a barbiturate taken alone.

O'Brien, Robert, and Sidney Cohn. *The Encyclopedia of Drug Abuse.* New York: Facts On File, 1984.

syphilis See SEXUALLY TRANSMITTED DISEASES.

systematic desensitization A behavioral therapy procedure that is highly effective in the treatment of some anxiety disorders and anger. It originated with Joseph Wolpe (1915–1997), who used in vivo and imaginal desensitization with his patients and reported greater than 80 percent recovery rates for a variety of anxiety, phobic and emotional reactions. The essence of systematic desensitization is the gradual exposure of an individual to components of a feared situation while he or she is relaxed. Systematic desensitization is the major treatment procedure for phobias and agoraphobia. Exposure may occur in imagination (self-visualization) or in actuality (in vivo). Systematic desensitization is best used with the help of a skilled therapist. Once relaxation skills are mastered (a process which takes five to six weeks), a hierarchy involving gradually more intimate (and reactive) triggering stimuli is developed, and imaginal or in vivo exposure is started.

Systemic desensitization is a highly effective treatment method for simple phobias. The cure rate for simple phobias is about 80 percent to 85 percent after 12 to 15 sessions. Social phobias, agoraphobia and panic require more patience, time and skill in using systematic desensitization; they also usually require in vivo exposure rather than imaginal to be effective.

See also AGORAPHOBIA; BEHAVIOR THERAPY; WOLPE, JOSEPH.

Doctor, Ronald M., and Ada P. Kahn. *The Encyclopedia of Phobias, Fears, and Anxieties.* New York: Facts On File, 2000.

taboo An idea, concept or practice that is not discussed or carried out openly by a given culture. Some taboos are so specific to the culture that they are difficult for outsiders to understand. The source or reason for a taboo may be unknown or forgotten; taboos may once have given groups of people moral and ethical codes by which they lived.

Certain taboos that are common to many cultures may be a source of anxiety and a threat to good mental health. For example, references to the dead and death are frequently avoided, made in hushed tones or accompanied by a ritual gesture or phrase; suicide is not discussed in many cultures, nor is incest. In fact, references to the behavior and act of incest have been suppressed. During the 1990s in the United States there were revelations that incest had a higher incidence than previously thought. As a consequence, the taboo to speak out and protest about it was, to a large extent, lifted.

The word "taboo" is derived from the language of the Polynesian people meaning "forbidden" or "dangerous." It is the term used for behavior related to their king. He was thought to be so full of power, or *mana,* that his shadow, parts of his body and even objects he touched, were considered dangerous.

See also SUPERSTITION.

Douglas, Mary. "Taboo." In *Man, Myth and Magic,* edited by Richard Cavendish. New York: Marshall Cavendish, 1983.
Gregory, W.E. "Taboos." In *The Encyclopedia of Psychology,* edited by Raymond J. Corsini. New York: Wiley, 1984.

tachycardia Rapid beating of the heart. A rapid heartbeat is often associated with anxiety and panic attacks. Individuals who are already feeling anxious or fearful may become even more so when they realize that their heart is beating rapidly. Under such circumstances they may fear that they are having a heart attack. Individuals who are experiencing a panic attack with physical symptoms of rapid heartbeat, difficulty breathing and dizziness may fear that they are going to die. Rapid heartbeat is normal under some conditions, such as exercise or sexual activity.

See also ANXIETY; ANXIETY DISORDERS; PANIC ATTACK; PANIC DISORDER; PHARMACOLOGIC THERAPY in BIBLIOGRAPHY.

t'ai chi A physical, mental and spiritual practice that uses movement to balance energy and helps achieve and maintain harmony within oneself. Those who practice t'ai chi say that it helps them to develop more mental and spiritual energy, feel more overall vitality and obtain relief from anxieties.

T'ai chi is an outgrowth of Chinese martial arts, spirituality and medicine, and has been practiced for more than 2,000 years. As a martial art and a popular meditative practice, it is often called meditation in motion. According to Chinese philosophy, to do t'ai chi is to connect the individual with nature through movement. It is considered "great shadow boxing," which draws on Taoist beliefs in the interdependence of the body and the mind. In the open spaces and parks of China today, millions of young and old people practice t'ai chi, gently swaying, gliding and stepping.

Mental Health Benefits of T'ai Chi

Practitioners of t'ai chi usually experience deep and restful sleep. Their nervous system is soothed and calmed. The gentleness of t'ai chi ensures that they do not suffer strains and other muscular injuries but instead develop greater strength, flexibility and suppleness. Some athletes use t'ai chi as a way of warming up.

People who perform t'ai chi move all of their joints and exert more energy than it appears. Through the use of slow breathing, individuals can pace some of the systems of their body. They can stabilize their heartbeat, the exchange of oxygen and carbon dioxide and the secretion and absorption of endocrine fluids. The movements also improve health by assisting the flow of blood, creating tranquillity for the entire nervous system and fostering deep peace of mind through deep concentration.

United States researchers have been studying the physical and mental benefits of t'ai chi, particularly for older people, many of whom suffer from a lack of balance and frequent falls. In an article in the *Journal of the American Geriatrics Society* (May 1996), an evaluation of a 15-week course taken by 72 men and women over age 70, showed that t'ai chi not only improved their balance, but helped these people abort falls by teaching them to cope with missteps and precarious positions. Another study reported in the *Harvard Health Letter* (July 1997) said that older adults who practiced t'ai chi had significantly lower blood pressure readings after the exercise and a decreased fear of falling.

T'ai Chi Classes

Books and videos on t'ai chi are available, but the best way to learn is in classes held in t'ai chi studios, adult education courses at high schools and colleges, YMCAs and YWCAs and senior adult centers. Many people combine t'ai chi with other forms of exercise.

See also BREATHING; COMPLEMENTARY THERAPIES; MEDITATION.

Chen, W. William, and Wei Yue Sun. "Tai Chi Chuan: Alternative Form of Exercise for Health Promotion and Disease Prevention for Older Adults in the Community. *International Quarterly of Community Health Education* 16, no. 4 (1997): 333–339.

"talking" treatment Psychotherapy by means other than medication. A wide variety of therapies involve the troubled individual talking to the psychotherapist and the therapist listening attentively with empathy and understanding and available to make constructive suggestions. When modern anti-depressant drugs became available in the latter half of the 20th century, some feared that the "old-fashioned" talking treatment would be abandoned. However, when medications are given, they are usually given in combination with psychotherapy and some verbal contact.

More recently, studies comparing short term therapy (interpersonal or cognitive psychotherapy) with medication treatment or the combination have shown that this combined means of therapy can be successful in treating outpatients with mild to moderate depression.

See also PSYCHOTHERAPY.

Talwin The trade name for pentazocine, a purely synthetic opioid used as a strong painkiller. It is useful for medical purposes but also has a strong potential for the development of tolerance, as well as psychological and physiological dependence. Many addicts seek treatment for their addiction but also sometimes turn to hospital emergency rooms if they are experiencing acute symptoms of overdose or withdrawal.

See also SUBSTANCE ABUSE.

tangentiality See THOUGHT DISORDERS.

tantrums Angry physical outbursts may occur at any time in life, but they are most common in childhood and are thought to be a normal part of a child's developmental process. Tantrums may take many forms, usually involving some combination of screaming, rushing around madly, writhing on the floor and breaking available objects or using them as a weapon. Small children's tantrums are usually triggered by frustration and are beyond the child's control. Mental health professionals feel that the emotional flood that constitutes a tantrum may be just as terrifying for the child as for the adult, because the child fears his own loss of control.

A child may be angered by a new experience or obstacle that she cannot successfully master. Toys or other objects that the child wishes to handle that are either too large or too complex or intricate can trigger an outburst but may also provide a learning experience. There is some evidence that brighter children who are more eager to learn and explore may actually have more tantrums. Tantrums may also be started by the child's inability to understand that the adult world does not always revolve around him as he has come to expect. Most children grow out of their tantrums as they develop a better understanding of their role in the family and learn how people interact on a more mature level.

Leach, Penelope. "Tantrums." In *The Child Care Encyclopedia,* New York: Knopf, 1984.

tardive dyskinesia Uncontrolled, involuntary facial tremors and grimacing and jerky movements of the arms and legs caused as a side effect of the use of some neuroleptic drugs. This syndrome develops late in treatment (after six months to 20 years) and is estimated to occur in about 20 percent of chronic schizophrenic patients. It is most likely to occur in postmenopausal females with depressive features. This condition may continue after withdrawal of the medications and may become worse after treatment.

It is believed that tardive dyskinesia is caused by chronic blockage of dopamine receptors, resulting in a prolonged supersensitivity of dopamine receptors to normal levels of dopamine. However, this theory does not explain why some patients get tardive dyskinesia and others who must take chronic neuroleptic medications do not.

The best prevention for tardive dyskinesia is using antipsychotics only when indicated and in the lowest effective doses. Patients taking them should be monitored frequently with trials off medication to assess their ongoing need for the medication.

See also SCHIZOPHRENIA; THORAZINE; PHARMACOLOGIC THERAPY.

Tay-Sachs disease A genetic disorder that leads to progressive central nervous system damage. Approximately one in 3,600 infants among eastern European Jewish populations in born with Tay-Sachs disease, while only one in 360,000 non-Jewish infants is affected. The frequency of the abnormal gene for Tay-Sachs disease in the former populations is quite high. There is normal development for three to six months, followed by severe neurological deterioration, blindness, deafness and seizures. Individuals who believe they carry an abnormal gene should obtain genetic counseling before they have children. Tay-Sachs disease is considered a form of mental retardation.

See also MENTAL RETARDATION.

teeth grinding Known medically as bruxism, teeth grinding is a habit many people practice when stressed or anxious. Some people grind their teeth during the day, and some only do it at night.

For about 5 percent of the population, teeth grinding causes serious consequences. For example, it is possible to grind the enamel off the teeth, making them more susceptible to cavities and very sensitive to heat and cold. Years of grinding can cause facial and jaw pain from fatigued muscles. Grinding may also damage the joint between the jaw and the cranium (temporomandibular joint). When a person eats, the muscles responsible for chewing exert just enough pressure to hold in place the disk of cartilage that cushions the joint. When the person grinds his or her teeth, however, this disk gradually becomes displaced, causing soreness, inflammation and even arthritis.

Dentists can prepare plastic retainer-like appliances, called mouth guards or night guards, to prevent grinding. Many people find that relaxation therapy, guided imagery, hypnosis and biofeedback also help to relieve this unwanted habit.

See also ARTHRITIS; BIOFEEDBACK; GUIDED IMAGERY; HABITS; HYPNOSIS; RELAXATION; TEMPOROMANDIBULAR JOINT SYNDROME.

Kahn, Ada P. *Stress A to Z: The Sourcebook for Facing Everyday Challenges.* New York: Facts On File, 2000.

Tegretol The trade name for carbamazepine, a commonly used antiepileptic drug, especially for temporal lobe epilepsy. Carbamazepine is chemically related to tricyclic antidepressant drugs.

See also EPILEPSY.

temperament One's usual manner of reacting to things. For example, some people are usually calm and passive, and others are active and excitable. Traits of temperament are often noticeable in newborns and become obvious within a few days. Temperament traits may be inherited and become a part of personality, and they usually follow a lifelong pattern.

See also PERSONALITY.

temporal lobe epilepsy (TLE) Also known as psychomotor epilepsy, this disorder manifests itself with personality changes such as extreme and excessive interest in religion, hypergraphia (writing prolifically), hyposexuality, temper outbursts and, occasionally, mood disorders. It is due to an electrical and functional disturbance in the brain and is best evaluated by laboratory tests using neurophysiology and functional neuroimaging, as well as the electroencephalogram (EEG). Individuals with this condition may experience temporal lobe illusions (temporal lobe hallucinations, temporal hallucinations).

See also EPILEPSY.

temporomandibular joint (TMJ) syndrome Symptoms, including pain, that affect the jaw, face and head. TMJ occurs when the ligaments and muscles that control and support these areas do not work together properly. A spasm of the chewing muscles can bring on the disorder. In some individuals, this occurs because of bruxism (teeth grinding) or clenching of the teeth as a response to stress and tension. Treatment may include relieving pain by applying moist heat to the face, taking muscle-relaxant drugs and using a bite splint at night to prevent teeth clenching and grinding. Some individuals resort to surgery on their jaw; others undergo orthodontia to correct their bite. Psychological counseling is often recommended to help the individual overcome the underlying causes of tension that may have led to the disorder.

See also BRUXISM; STRESS.

TENS (transcutaneous nerve stimulation) See PAIN; TRANSCUTANEOUS NERVE STIMULATION.

tension headache See HEADACHES.

terminal illness An illness from which medical experts have agreed there will be no recovery. Since modern medicine has prolonged the final stages of illnesses, the mental and physical state of dying patients has received increased attention. In 1969, Elisabeth Kubler-Ross (1926–   ) described the final stages of terminal illness as denial, anger, bargaining, depression and acceptance. These attitudes and feelings may take different forms and may overlap, but they do seem to form a common experience among dying patients. Kubler-Ross observed that most patients find their death incomprehensible and the product of some intentional, destructive force, no matter what the actual cause. Terminally ill patients, in addition to fearing their own annihilation, fear the withdrawal of loved ones, real or imagined, and their own growing dependence and inability to cope with daily life. Patients frequently suffer from a loss of self-esteem and may express fears that they are being abandoned or persecuted. On the other hand, elderly patients approaching death may seem to experience it as a sort of summing up and end, a natural part of life.

A frequent problem in dealing with dying patients is that while they may wish to talk about their situation, listeners are hard to find because of the common resistance among those in good health to be confronted with the possibility of their own eventual annihilation.

Mental health professionals have found certain techniques and attitudes useful in dealing with dying patients. For example, it has been helpful to imagine the person without his illness, so that the illness does not become the most important thing about him, and to dwell on the patient's traits and talents in normal life. It is also important for the professional to be aware of her own fears and to maintain a balanced attitude between gloom and unrealistic optimism.

Professionals in health care have also found it helpful to combat the patient's fears about the potential pain and suffering as his illness reaches its final stages by informing him that those approaching death usually do not experience suffering.

See also ACQUIRED IMMUNODEFICIENCY SYNDROME; CAREGIVERS; CHRONIC ILLNESS; DEATH; HOSPICE.

Felner, R. D. "Terminally Ill People." In *Encyclopedia of Psychology,* vol. 3, ed. Raymond J. Corsini. New York: Wiley, 1984.

Zimmerman, Jack McKay. *Hospice.* Baltimore: Urban & Schwarzenberg, 1986.

terrorism   In a 1986 public report issued by then Vice President George Bush's Task Force on Combating Terrorism, terrorism was defined as: "The unlawful use or threat of violence against persons or property to further political or social objectives. It is usually intended to intimidate or coerce a government, individuals or groups to modify their behavior or politics."

Worldwide terrorism interferes with many people's feeling of mental well-being, as it makes them fearful and apprehensive about traveling and trusting strangers.

Terrorists are usually young men who are fanatical about their cause to the extent that they have no concern for their victims or for their own lives. Boys as young as 14 or 15 have been used for dangerous missions. Some terrorist groups are self-supporting through activities such as bank robbery or selling drugs, but most are supported by governments who find terrorism and hostage taking effective and inexpensive in comparison with the costs of conventional military force. Terrorism aimed at U.S. diplomats increased dramatically in the 20 years before the Bush report.

See also HOSTAGES; POST-TRAUMATIC STRESS DISORDER.

testosterone   A male androgenic sex hormone that stimulates muscles, bones and sexual development. During puberty it leads to deepening of the voice and growth of facial hair. The most important of the androgen hormones, testosterone is produced in the testes (and in very small amounts in a woman's ovaries). Testosterone in medicinal form is sometimes used to treat infertility in males who have disorders of the testes or pituitary gland. Since related androgenic hormones promote muscle development and strength, they have been self-administered by athletes to improve their function. Not only may this promote the development of cardiac disease, but increases in aggression and impulsive behavior (including homicide) have also

occurred. Androgenic drugs are outlawed by all athletic leagues and organizations.

See also INFERTILITY; PITUITARY GLAND.

thalamus   See BRAIN.

therapeutic alliance   The trusting rapport and understanding between the psychotherapist and the patient. In order to derive benefit from the psychotherapeutic consultations, the patient must trust the therapist and believe the therapist can help. The therapist, in turn, must communicate respect, interest and empathic understanding in order to facilitate the patient's trust.

See also PSYCHOTHERAPY.

thematic apperception test (TAT)   A personality diagnostic test. The TAT may be useful in giving therapists information about an anxious or phobic individual, because in doing the test, the individual displays attitudes, feelings, conflicts and personality characteristics. Individuals are asked to make up stories with a beginning, middle and end about a series of pictures; the therapist looks for common themes in the stories, and scores the test in a primarily subjective manner.

See also PERSONALITY TYPES.

Doctor, Ronald M., and Ada P. Kahn. *The Encyclopedia of Phobias, Fears, and Anxieties.* New York: Facts On File, 2000

therapeutic touch   A nontraditional therapy (also called alternative or complementary) developed by Dr. Dolores Krieger, professor of nursing at New York University, in which she relieves the pain and distress of illness by passing her hands over the patient. It is also known as the healing touch and is derived from the laying on of hands. Her method is described in her book, *The Therapeutic Touch: How to Use Your Hands to Help or to Heal.*

Since the mid-1970s, Dr. Krieger has conducted courses in therapeutic touch and taught thousands of people. New York University offers a fully accredited graduate course at the master's level, designed to formally teach the process of therapeutic touch and to investigate how and why it works. In addition, more than 50 universities offer formal instruction in therapeutic touch, usually as part of the nursing curriculum.

How Therapeutic Touch Works

The healer eases into an altered state of consciousness while focusing energy on the patient, then slowly passes his or her hands about four to six inches above the patient's body in an effort to sense a transfer of energy. The healer scans the body for an area of temperature change as an indication that part of the body is troubled, then lays his or her hands on the affected area, while the patient senses a change in temperature, perhaps a feeling of deep heat, in the area being touched.

According to Dr. Krieger, at the very least, the method produces a relaxation response in the patient and works well for inflammation, musculoskeletal problems and psychosomatic disorders. Explanation by healers whose patients have been helped say that energy passes between themselves and their patients. Skeptics believe that this healing has a placebo effect, but it seems to work for some individuals.

Historically, physicians touched their patients far more than they do today a fact due, in part, to the advent of so many highly technical diagnostic machines. Until the invention of the stethoscope in the mid-1800s, physicians pressed their naked ears to the bodies of patients to listen for heartbeats and other internal sounds. This intimate gesture probably had a soothing effect on the patient, much as therapeutic touch has today. As author Lewis Thomas wrote in *The Youngest Science*, "it is hard to imagine a friendlier human gesture, a more intimate signal of personal concern and affection, than the close-bowed head affixed to the skin."

Now many nurses and other health care practitioners, including body therapists, realize the need for human touch; they practice healing touch either knowledgeably or unconsciously along with massage and other techniques.

See also BODY THERAPIES; COMPLEMENTARY THERAPIES; MASSAGE THERAPY; PLACEBO EFFECT.

Engebretson, Joan. "Urban Healers: An Experiential Description of American Healing Touch Groups." *Qualitative Health Research* 6, no. 4 (Nov. 1996): 526–541.

Kahn, Ada P. *Stress A to Z: The Sourcebook for Facing Everyday Challenges.* New York: Facts On File, 2000.

Locke, Steven, and Douglas Colligan. *The Healer Within.* New York: New American Library, 1986.

Macrae, J. *Therapeutic Touch: A Practical Guide.* New York: Alfred A. Knopf, 1988.

therapy See PSYCHOTHERAPIES: PHARMACOLOGICAL APPROACH.

thiamine deficiency Thiamine deficiency may lead to Wernicke-Korsakoff syndrome (also known as alcohol amnestic disorder) and Korsakoff's psychosis (usually caused by alcohol abuse), an amnestic disorder (inability to remember recent events). In some cases, malabsorption or dietary inadequacy can lead to these disorders. Individuals with Korsakoff's syndrome often fabricate answers to questions in an attempt to fill in details they do not recall (confabulation). The most common memory impairment involves difficulty in learning new information. Korsakoff's syndrome improve in about 75 percent of people who stop alcohol abuse and who maintain an adequate diet for more than six months.

See also ALCOHOLISM.

thioridazine An antipsychotic medication (trade name: Mellaril) used primarily to treat schizophrenia and other psychoses. The use of thioridazine has also been suggested to relieve anxiety, agitation and depression associated with mood disorders. The drug is used in conjunction with psychotherapy, but its use for anxiety alone is limited because it carries with it the risk of tardive dyskinesia.

See also ANTIPSYCHOTIC MEDICATIONS; ANXIETY DISORDERS; DEPRESSION; SCHIZOPHRENIA; TARDIVE DYSKINESIA.

Thorazine Trade name for chlorpromazine hydrochloride, the first antipsychotic agent marketed; it is a phenothiazine derivative also referred to as a neuroleptic medication. It was used primarily to treat schizophrenia, other psychoses or mania. For a while during the 1950s it was used to treat anxiety disorders, but it has been replaced with newer anxiolytic agents because of its serious side effects and limited efficacy in anxiety. The primary indication for chlorpromazine and related medications is the treatment of psychosis.

Prior to the introduction of chlorpromazine around the mid-1950s, the population of state mental hospitals was increasing at a rate of 10 percent per year. After the introduction of chlorpromazine, the population decreased at the rate of 10 percent per year.

Psychiatrists, pharmacologists and neuroscientists have not solved the problem of schizophrenia, but the neuroleptics which have been developed do suppress hallucinations, delusions and symptoms of withdrawal seen in schizophrenia, organic psychoses, psychotic depression and other psychotic disorders. They do not by themselves restore schizophrenic patients to normal function and cause a range of side effects that limit compliance and their use. Related drugs (Prolixin and thioridazine) are examples of other phenothiazines. Side effects include extrapyramidal effects, Parkinsonian symptoms such as muscle rigidity, akathisias (a state of physical agitation often producing anxiety) and sedation. Acute administration may cause neuroleptic malignant syndrome, associated with rigidity, disorientation and high fever with possible chronic neurological damage. Long-term use carries a 4 percent per year risk of tardive dyskinesia. For these reasons, chlorpromazine and related medications are used in severe psychotic disorders.

See also ANTIPSYCHOTIC MEDICATIONS; TRANQUILIZER DRUGS.

thought disorders   Disturbance of thought processes or thought content. Thought process refers to the way an individual puts ideas together, to the associations between ideas and to the form and flow of thoughts in conversation. Thought content refers to the ideas the person communicates.

Disorders of thought processes include racing thoughts, a situation in which they individual is flooded with ideas and is unable to keep up with them. This is seen in some people who have schizophrenia and also in manic states. Another is circumstantiality, which involves thinking that is indirect in reaching a goal or getting to the point. People who are obsessional sometimes have this characteristic. Blocking is a sudden interruption or obstruction in the spontaneous flow of thoughts, considered by the individual as an absence of thought. This occurs in severe anxiety states and schizophrenia. Perseveration is a tendency for an individual to respond with the same sound or words to varied stimuli, and also an inability to shift the trend of conversation away from one specific topic.

Other thought process disorders include flight of ideas, verbally skipping from one related idea to another; tangentiality, in which the person replies to questions in irrelevant ways; clanging, which involves using the sound of a word, instead of its meaning (such as rhymes) to communicate; word salad, which is a jumble of words and phrases lacking comprehensive meaning or logical coherence; and echolalia, parrotlike repetition of another's speech (seen in organic brain syndrome and in mania). Loose associations involve transitions from one idea to another, unrelated idea.

Disorders of thought content include delusions, false beliefs firmly held despite incontrovertible and obvious proof to the contrary. There may be delusions of grandeur or delusions of persecution. Some individuals who have delusions of control believe that one's feelings and actions are imposed by some external source. Somatic delusions are beliefs about body image or body function. Thought broadcasting is the belief that other people can read one's thoughts. Ideas of reference involve incorrectly interpreting casual incidents and external events as having direct personal reference. These ideas are usually delusions. Depersonalization is a sense of unreality or strangeness concerning oneself and feeling detached from and being an outside observer of one's mental processes or body. Derealization refers to feeling detached from one's environment so that a sense of reality of the external world is lost. Depersonalization and derealization are fairly common in severe anxiety states and also in borderline personality disorder.

Another thought disorder is preoccupation (persistent ideas), which includes obsessions, compulsions and phobias. Some depressed people have morbid preoccupations about guilt or death.

See also ANXIETY DISORDERS; DELUSION; DEPRESSION; OBSESSIVE-COMPULSIVE DISORDER; PHOBIA; SCHIZOPHRENIA.

thought field therapy (TFT) A form of therapy based on body meridians and the restoration of energy balance in the body used to help some people deal with certain anxiety disorders. It is based on a Chinese medical principle that energy flows along meridians and can be balanced and released by contact on acupressure points. The therapy is aimed at breaking up negative emotions and beliefs. Clients learn to press certain pressure points on glands and energy pathways in particular patterns based on the type of energy blockage involved.

The therapy is said to have no adverse side effects. TFT does not require the individual to talk about their problem, something that often causes considerable distress or embarrassment and which discourages many from seeking treatment. The technique was developed in the 1980s by Roger D. Callahan, Ph.D., an American psychologist.

Doctor, Ronald M., and Ada P. Kahn *Encyclopedia of Phobias, Fears, and Anxieties.* New York: Facts On File, 2000.

thought stopping A behavioral therapy technique in which the individual imagines hearing the word "stop" whenever an undesirable thought occurs. Developed by Joseph Wolpe (1915–1997), an American psychiatrist, this technique is sometimes useful in treating anxieties, phobias, smoking and sexual deviations.

See also BEHAVIORAL THERAPY; REINFORCEMENT.

3-methoxy-4-hydroxyphenylglycol (MHPG) The major metabolite of norepinephrine in the central nervous system. Urinary excretion of MHPG is usually decreased in individuals with bipolar disorder while they are in the depressed mode as compared with the manic state. Levels of this substance are also increased during episodes of extreme anxiety or fear. Levels of MHPG diminish after use of imipramine or clonidine or after anxiety episodes diminish. Measurements of the substance help determine effectiveness of some antianxiety medications.

See also ANXIETY; LABORATORY TESTS.

thyroid gland A gland located at the back of the neck, which may have a biologic link to depression.

Normally the pituitary gland generates a hormone at night that stimulates the thyroid, but sleep suppresses this action. In individuals who cycle to mania or in depressed persons deprived of sleep, levels of the thyroid-stimulating hormone fluctuate between highs and lows. Increased levels of thyroid disease occurs in some manic-depressive individuals, especially those with rapid cycles of the highs and lows.

See also THYROTROPIN-RELEASING HORMONE TEST.

thyrotropin-releasing hormone test A test used as an aid in diagnosing depressions and assessing the status of the thyroid gland. Some clinicians and researchers believe that some individuals who suffer from a subclinical form of hypothyroidism should be monitored for thyroid function as a diagnostic tool. The thyroid-stimulating hormone (TSH) is measured after infusion of protirelin (thyrotropin-releasing hormone, TRH). Manics seem to have a blunted response compared with that of normal controls. Thus the thyroid-stimulating hormone (TSH) response to the thyrotropin-releasing hormone (TRH) infusion has indicated that the TRH test can be useful for both diagnosis and treatment.

Studies suggest that a significant proportion of individuals with depression may have early hypothyroidism. Many researchers also believe that both depressed inpatients and outpatients may be appropriate candidates for a comprehensive thyroid evaluation, including the TSH test. This evaluation is especially important if the patient is taking, or being considered for treatment with, lithium carbonate, which is known to cause hypothyroidism in some individuals.

See also BIOLOGICAL MARKERS.

Roesch, Roberta. *The Encyclopedia of Depression.* New York: Facts On File, 1991.

tic Rapid, repetitive movements of individual muscle groups. Most noticeable tics involve the facial muscles, such as the lips or eyelids. Tics may also be vocal. In some cases, tics are associated with anxiety and stress. Tics are also a characteristic of Tourette syndrome, a disorder of the nervous system.

See also BEHAVIORAL THERAPY; TOURETTE SYNDROME.

tiredness See CHRONIC FATIGUE SYNDROME.

titration A technique physicians use to determine the optimum dose of a drug required to produce a desired effect in a particular individual. Dosage may be gradually increased until the patient notices an improvement or decreased from a level that is excessive because of side effects. For example, antidepressant drugs are titrated for each individual. Certain blood tests of serum drug concentration levels are also used for this purpose. Because titration of many medications is essential, it is important for people who start drug therapy to be closely supervised by their physician.

See also ANTIDEPRESSANT MEDICATIONS; ANTIPSYCHOTIC MEDICATIONS.

TM See TRANSCENDENTAL MEDITATION.

TMJ See TEMPOROMANDIBULAR JOINT (TMJ) SYNDROME.

tobacco The active ingredient in tobacco is nicotine, which is addictive. It affects the central nervous system through routes that differ from other drugs, but it produces very similar results, such as pleasurable euphoria, dependency and withdrawal symptoms when stopped suddenly.

Nicotine acts as both a stimulant and a depressant. Shallow puffs seem to increase alertness, but deep ones are relaxing. Smokers sense their nicotine levels and tend to self-regulate them by varying inhalation patterns, as well as their frequency of smoking. In regular smokers, nicotine improves short-term memory, intellectual performance and concentration. Although smoking speeds up the heart rate and raises blood pressure, it also seems to relieve stressful feelings for some smokers. Nicotine consumption also appears to control weight to some extent, probably by lowering circulating insulin levels and thus decreasing smokers' craving for sweets and tendency to store fat. This particular aspect of nicotine makes smoking appeal to those who are afraid of gaining weight.

Smokers who quit may experience genuine physical discomfort and cravings. Withdrawal symptoms from nicotine include headaches, irritability, upset stomach, breathing and circulation problems, trouble sleeping, dizziness and numbness.

During pregnancy, smoking increases the risk of miscarriage, fetal death, premature delivery and low birth weight. Infants of mothers who smoked during pregnancy also have a 50 percent greater chance of sudden infant death syndrome (SIDS) than infants whose mothers did not smoke.

See also ADDICTION; SMOKING.

Media Resource Guide on Common Drugs of Abuse. Public Relations Society of America, National Capital Chapter, Fairfax, Va., September 1990.

Tofranil Trade name for imipramine hydrochloride, a tricyclic antidepressant drug, used in treatment of depressive episodes of major depression and bipolar, dysthymic panic and phobic disorders.

See also ANTIDEPRESSANT MEDICATIONS.

toilet training Learning to use the toilet presents the first great potential conflict between mother and child. Some mental health professionals connect toilet training that is too early or too harsh with later behavior that is obedient but resentful. On the other hand, a child whose toilet training was delayed may develop a self-indulgent, narcissistic personality. A strong atmosphere of conflict surrounding toilet training may cause feelings of guilt, self-doubt and rage.

Modern child development professionals say that toilet training can best be accomplished when a child is ready for it and has some sense of assuming responsibility for the functions of his own body that will make him like the adult world. Parents are usually most successful in presenting toilet training as an interesting idea and avoiding an authoritarian manner. One difficulty that must be surmounted in toilet training is that small children have little or no ability to connect the bodily sensation from the bladder or the intestines with the necessity of heading for the bathroom. Some awareness of the function does begin to develop between the 12th and 18th month, but usually at this point the child exhibits some interest but does not anticipate. Even children who are trained have so little ability to anticipate that their need to use the toilet is usually instantaneous. Once children are partly trained, parents can begin to rely on the child's own resistance to soiling himself rather than constantly reminding him, which may actually delay the time when he is fully trained.

Freeman, Lucy, and Kerstin Kupfermann. *The Power of Fantasy.* New York: Continuum, 1988.

Leach, Penelope. "Toilet Training," *The Child Care Encyclopedia.* New York: Knopf, 1984.

Tourette syndrome   A neurological syndrome characterized by rapid, repeated and purposeless involuntary movements of various muscle groups (motor tics) and by grunts, barks and sniffing sounds (vocal tics). It is the most debilitating of several tic disorders. It often begins before age 21 with one or more vocal tics. Behavioral difficulties such as attentional problems, compulsions and obsessions are commonly observed in TS patients.

Until the 1970s, TS was frequently misdiagnosed as schizophrenia, obsessive-compulsive disorder, epilepsy or nervous habits. Once thought to be rare, TS is now considered a relatively common disorder affecting up to one person in every 2,500 in its complete form and three times that number in its partial expressions that include chronic motor tics and some forms of obsessive-compulsive disorder.

TS was first described in 1885 by Georges Gilles de la Tourette, a French physician. The cause of the disorder is unknown; however, there is recognition that TS is familial and genetic. Researchers are actively engaged in searching for the chromosomal location of the TS gene of affected individuals. There is not yet a genetic or biochemical test to determine if a person with TS or an unaffected individual carries the gene; there is no prenatal test for the vulnerability to TS.

An inability to control one's own body and even one's own thoughts is taken for granted by most people and is often a source of anxiety, guilt, helplessness and depression. TS patients react in individual ways; some become withdrawn, others become overly aggressive and still others become perfectionists. Self-esteem problems are common.

Psychotherapy can be helpful to the individual as well as to the family involved. There is evidence that Tourette syndrome may be associated with symptoms of obsessive-compulsive disorder.

Medications help some individuals who have TS. Among those used are haloperidol (trade name: Haldol), pimozide (trade name: Orap), phenothiazine drugs (particularly fluphenazine) and clonidine (trade name: Catapres).

For additional information, contact:

Tourette Syndrome Association
42-40 Bell Boulevard
Bayside, NY 11361
Phone: (718) 224-2999

See also CHRONIC ILLNESS; FAMILY THERAPY; OBSESSIVE-COMPULSIVE DISORDER; TIC.

toxic shock syndrome   See MENSTRUATION.

trait   A long-lasting aspect of one's personality, such as dependence, independence, introversion or extroversion, that helps to predict how a person will respond in a variety of situations.

See also PERSONALITY.

trait anxiety   A general, persistent pattern of responding to situations with anxiety. Trait anxiety (also known as A-trait) resembles timidity, but it is really a habitual tendency to be anxious over a long period of time in many situations. The person with a high A-trait perceives more situations as threatening than a person who is low in A-trait. Phobic individuals are high in A-trait. The term "A-trait" is used in research projects to differentiate between types of anxieties. For example, American psychologist Charles Spielberger (1927–   ) developed an instrument to measure A-trait vs. A-state anxiety, the latter being more situational and varied over time.

See also STATE ANXIETY; STATE-TRAIT ANXIETY INVENTORY (STAI).

Doctor, Ronald M., and Ada P. Kahn. *The Encyclopedia of Phobias, Fears, and Anxieties.* New York: Facts On File, 2000.

Spielberger, C. D. et al. *The State-Trait Anxiety Inventory.* Riverside, Calif.: Consulting Psychologists Press, 1970.

tranquilizer medications Anxiety-reducing medications that act on the brain and nervous system and may have sedative side effects. Tranquilizer medications are generally divided into two categories: major tranquilizers (or antipsychotic drugs) and minor tranquilizers (known as antianxiety drugs). The sedative effect may promote tranquilizing effects but is not necessary for the later effect.

See also ANTIANXIETY MEDICATIONS; ANTIPSYCHOTIC MEDICATIONS.

transactional analysis (TA) A type of group or individual therapy in which the goal is to develop one's identity and independence and to better one's means of coping with interactions with others. TA was developed by Eric Berne, a Canadian-born American psychologist (1910–1970), and described in 1967 by Thomas A. Harris in the book *I'm OK, You're OK*. In TA, all behavior, thinking, feeling and experience is categorized into three ego states: parent (critical and/or loving); adult (practical and evaluative); and child (feelings, such as dependency, or fun-loving and caring). These ego states can be identified by nonverbal changes, changes in voice tone, expressions and words. All three states are considered to serve a valuable purpose. Individuals can learn to identify which ego state is in control.

TA analyzes transactions to gain insight into the dynamics of interpersonal problems. When the lines of the transaction are parallel, the transaction is complementary. When the lines of the transaction cross, communication stops.

transcendental meditation (TM) A technique for meditation based on ancient Hindu writings, developed by Maharishi Mahesh Yogi and introduced in the United States in the early 1960s. Typically, the meditator spends two 20-minute periods a day sitting quietly with eyes closed and attention focused totally on the verbal repetition of a special sound or "mantra." Repetition of the mantra blocks distracting thoughts. The effect achieved is better relaxation and relief from stress. TM has also been referred to as mystic union.

See also COMPLEMENTARY THERAPIES; MEDITATION.

transcutaneous nerve stimulation (TENS) A method for relieving pain using tiny electrical impulses to nerve endings under the skin. TENS seems to work by blocking pain messages to the brain by providing alternative stimuli. TENS is usually recommended for individuals who do not respond to analgesic medications. Careful monitoring by a physician is required when an individual uses this type of therapy.

See also PAIN.

transference The unconscious process during psychotherapy in which a person displaces emotional feelings and attributes of a significant attachment figure from the past—usually a parent—to the therapist. During psychoanalytic therapy, an understanding and resolution of this process must be achieved to understand how old conflicts could be resolved more satisfactorily.

Transference often occurs between patient and physician, worker and boss, student and teacher, but is not often recognized. Transference may be positive (trusting, feelings of strength and support) and negative (distrust, anger, anticipation of criticism, etc.), often depending on the individual's experience with parent figures. The process is often unconscious and unrecognized except in psychotherapy with a well-trained therapist. It can lead to very intense pervasive feelings.

See also COUNTERTRANSFERENCE; FREUD, SIGMUND; PSYCHOANALYSIS.

transsexualism A feeling that exists when a person feels that she or he is a member of one gender trapped in a body that has sexual characteristics associated with the other gender, usually evident to that person since childhood. The term "transsexualism" was coined by Harry Benjamin in 1966. The first well-known case of transsexualism was Christine Jorgensen, who had a sex change operation from male to female in 1952.

See also GENDER IDENTITY.

transvestitism Individuals who wear the clothing of the other sex, a practice known as cross-dressing. Transvestitism takes many forms. For example, pseudotransvestites try cross-dressing for fun and not to fulfill any need. The fetishistic transvestite cross-dresses episodically because women's clothes are fetish objects and create sexual arousal.

Tranxene Trade name for the benzodiazepine drug clorazepate.

See also BENZODIAZEPINE DRUGS; PHARMACOLOGICAL APPROACH.

tranylcypromine Generic name for the monoamine oxidase inhibitor medication marketed as Parnate.

See also ANTIDEPRESSANT MEDICATIONS; MONOAMINE OXIDASE INHIBITORS (MAOIs).

trazodone The generic name for the drug Desyrel, an antidepressant medication.

See also ANTIDEPRESSANT MEDICATIONS; DESYREL; PHARMACOLOGICAL APPROACH.

tremor An involuntary movement of muscles (shaking) in part of the body, most commonly the hands. Individuals who are extremely anxious may experience tremors at times of excitement or fear. Many elderly people have a slight tremor not related to any disease. Essential tremor is a disorder that sometimes runs in families but seems to have no known cause.

Some tremors are associated with neurological diseases such as Parkinson's disease. Other disorders in which tremor is a characteristic include multiple sclerosis, mercury poisoning and hepatic encephalopathy. Some drugs may cause tremors in some individuals; among them are amphetamine drugs, antidepressant drugs and lithium. Alcohol withdrawal may produce tremors.

See also ALCOHOLISM; PARKINSON'S DISEASE.

triazolam A benzodiazepine medication marketed under the trade name Halcion.

See also BENZODIAZEPINE MEDICATIONS; PHARMACOLOGICAL APPROACH.

trichtillomania See HAIR PULLING; OBSESSIVE-COMPULSIVE DISORDER.

tricyclic antidepressant medications A group of antidepressant drugs. Tricyclic drugs are so named because their molecular structure is characterized by three fused rings.

See also ANTIDEPRESSANT MEDICATIONS; DEPRESSION.

trimipramine Generic name for the tricyclic antidepressant medication marketed as Surmontil.

See also ANTIDEPRESSANT MEDICATIONS; PHARMACOLOGICAL APPROACH.

trisomy 21 See DOWN'S SYNDROME.

Type A personality A designation that usually relates to a lifestyle, and style of work and performance, characterized by competitive feelings, drive, ambition, impatience, goal orientation, anxiety, worry or hostility. Such individuals may tend to emphasize speed and quantity over quality of work. They may take on multiple commitments and become preoccupied with meeting deadlines. Their behavior may be characterized by abrupt gestures, and they may express themselves explosively. They tend to feel guilty if not working and take little pleasure in other activities. Many of these individuals neglect family responsibilities in favor of working and tending to business interests.

Some researchers believe that Type A people have individualistic traits that set them apart from others and that they tend to be suspicious people who lack the emotional support that comes from close relationships.

Type A personalities have sometimes been associated with high incidence of coronary heart disease. Many individuals make efforts to change their personality traits after a serious illness and, as a result, relax more and learn to spend their leisure time in enjoyable ways instead of working or competing. Studies involving Type A individuals have shown that this kind of behavior can be changed through learning relaxation techniques, development of a sense of humor and other lifestyle changes. They thus become a combination of Type A and Type B personalities. A study reported by psychologist Ariel Kerman, Ph.D., in her book, *The H-A-R-T Program: Lower Your Blood*

Pressure Without Drugs, indicated that researchers at Duke University found that when Type A personalities participated in a walking/jogging program (three miles per day, three days a week), their Type A characteristics became less dominant in their lives.

See also ANGER; HIGH BLOOD PRESSURE; HOSTILITY; RELAXATION; TYPE B PERSONALITY.

Kerman, D. Ariel. *The H.A.R.T. Program: Lower Your Blood Pressure Without Drugs,* New York: HarperCollins, 1992.

Pelletier, Kenneth. *Healthy People in Unhealthy Places.* New York: Delacorte Press, 1984.

Type B personality   Personality traits that enable an individual to enjoy activities that are not competitive. These individuals usually work without agitation or a sense of urgency and are not particularly goal-oriented, as are Type A personalities.

At one time A and B personality traits were thought to be strongly related to achievement and health and were also seen as being more rigid. However, more recent research indicates that the single trait of hostility is more strongly related to heart disease than the whole spectrum of traits known as Type A. It has also been found that Type A behavior is not as strong a predictor of achievement as once thought. Successful executives have actually been found to be people who can move back and forth between the Type A and Type B characteristics, depending on appropriateness to the situation. A and B personality types have been found to be scattered fairly evenly among top and middle management. For optimal mental health, it seems that a combination of the A and B traits may be best, so that an individual can enjoy a balanced life, with aspects of work, family, love, friends, recreation and fun.

See also FRIENDS.

Type C personality   Individuals who have Type C personalities refuse to let any negative feeling show. They usually seem in control and do not express emotions, especially those regarding anger, fear, sadness or even joy.

Type Cs tend to be patient, cooperative and highly focused on meeting other people's needs while showing little or no concern for their own. Usually, Type Cs tend to stay in stressful situations, such as bad marriages or frustrating jobs, longer than other people. They don't recognize their emotions and may not even realize when they are under stress. However, their bodies produce stress hormones, including cortisol, which has been known to suppress the immune system.

Because they don't express their emotions, Type C people do not produce natural opiates, the brain chemicals that have a pain-killing effect similar to artificial drugs such as morphine. This, too, reduces the overall effectiveness of their immune system.

According to psychologist Lydia Temoshok, Ph.D., author of *The Type C Connection: The Behavioral Link to Cancer and Your Health,* Type C personalities often are in the relapse group when compared with recoveries by individuals in other personality categories.

BETTER MENTAL HEALTH FOR TYPE C PERSONALITIES

- Be aware of your emotions; get psychotherapeutic help if necessary.
- Be able to express your anger in a constructive way.
- Become more assertive; learn how to say "no" when you want to.
- Develop relaxation techniques that work best for you.

See also ASSERTIVENESS TRAINING; CODEPENDENCY; DEPRESSION; RELAXATION; SELF-ESTEEM; STRESS.

Temoshok, Lydia. *The Type C Connection: The Behavioral Links to Cancer and Your Health.* New York: Random House, 1992.

tyramine   A substance found in some foods that may interfere with the effectiveness of certain antidepressant drugs because it affects constriction and expansion of bloods vessels. It is generally recommended that individuals who take MAO (monoamine oxidase) inhibitors as mood elevators for depression avoid ripe cheeses, anything fermented, pickled or marinated foods (such as herring), sour cream, yogurt, nuts, peanut butter, seeds, pods of broad beans (lima, navy, pinto, garbanzo and pea), chocolate, vinegar (except white vinegar) and any foods containing large amounts of monosodium glutamate (such as some Asian foods).

Individuals who suffer from migraine headaches are also advised to avoid foods containing tyramine.

See also ANTIDEPRESSANT MEDICATIONS; HEADACHES; MONOAMINE OXIDASE INHIBITORS.

unconscious The area of the mind in which memories, perceptions or feelings are stored; the individual is not aware of this store and cannot willfully recollect them.

See also FREUD, SIGMUND; PSYCHOANALYSIS.

underachiever A student or other individual who is of average or superior ability but performs poorly in school. Underachievement may be applied to specific areas such as arithmetic or reading ability if the child has shown potential beyond his achievement in that area. Underachievement affects the student's mental health as well as that of his parents.

Educational factors may contribute to underachievement. Teachers who have personality conflicts with certain students can contribute to poor performance by ignoring or contributing to their difficulties. Large class size or school systems that lack the personnel and techniques to delve into the causes of poor performance may cause or exacerbate a child's learning problems. Underachievement, particularly in very bright students, may result from boredom when classroom activities do not stimulate them or challenge their abilities. Average or bright students with short attention spans can also appear to be below normal.

A child's relationship with her parents may also cause underachievement. Parents who are high achievers themselves may have unrealistic expectations of their children, which causes a child who already has low self-esteem to suffer from an ever poorer performance. Parents with average abilities who produce a child with exceptional intelligence or other ability may not understand and even discourage their child's superior performance. Family problems such as divorce, conflict, death or serious illness of a parent may also hold a child back.

Children may also become underachievers because they are perceived as different and are not socially well-adjusted to their peer group. Factors such as exceptionally high intelligence, ethnic or religious difference, a financial status that is far above or below classmates or very mature or immature behavior patterns may set a child apart, limit her friendships and lower her school performance. Achievement is also reduced when a child desires to become a member of a gang so badly that he associates with troublemakers or other students who perform poorly in school.

Sex role expectations also influence a child's performance. For example, girls may respond to social conditioning that they are not supposed to be as bright as boys, particularly in subjects such as math or science. These expectations may adversely affect some boys as well. If their families expect consistently superior performance from them, they may become so frustrated that the results are the opposite.

See also PEER GROUP; SELF-ESTEEM.

Thiel, Ann; Richard Thiel and Penelope B. Grenoble. *When Your Child Isn't Doing Well in School.* Chicago: Contemporary Books, 1988. "Underachievement," In *American Educator's Encyclopedia,* Edward Dejnozka, Westport, Conn.: Greenwood Press, 1982.

unemployment Unemployment relates to all people who want to work but have been unable to find jobs—those who have worked but were laid off, recent high school and college graduates, people with disabilities, the poor and uneducated, women returning to the workplace after child-rearing and retirees who need additional income and/or stimulation. Because unemployment often means financial hardship, it can challenge the mental health not only of the people directly involved, but that of their spouses, children, and parents as well.

Unemployment is also a source of stress for those who have jobs but are constantly threatened with losing them. However, in a 1995 poll conducted by Towers Perrin, a management consulting firm, most workers are "amazingly stress hardy and pragmatic when coping with the uncertainties of corporate America." The poll also showed that one measure of a worker's adjustment to today's climate of job instability is that less than half of the workers surveyed expect to spend their entire careers with one company. Among those under age 34, only one-third counted on retiring from their present employer.

According to Carrie Leana and Daniel Feldman in their book, *Coping with Job Loss,* "unemployment as a fact of life will continue, if not worsen. Current statistics on unemployment and layoffs underestimate the dimensions of the problem. Even with unemployment at 6 percent, there would still be 7 million people out of work. Because government statistics do not include the discouraged job seekers (individuals who have stopped applying for new positions) and those who have joined the expanding ranks of the permanently unemployed, these figures vastly underrepresented the number of people actually out of work."

Leana and Feldman also reported that among the many situational factors influencing how a person reacts to a stressful life event such as losing a job, perception of unemployment levels has a "substantial influence." They explained: "The higher workers perceive the unemployment rates in their communities and/or professions to be, the more pessimistic they will be about the prospects for finding new jobs, especially ones at equal pay."

Fran Lowry, writing in *Canadian Family Physician* (February 1995), said, "Now when unemployment is still an important problem in many parts of the country [Canada], idle hands are making more work for physicians. People who are out of work make more visits to their physicians for a variety of complaints. Areas of high unemployment also report a higher incidence of alcohol use, and more marital and family abuse and violence."

See also GENERAL ADAPTATION SYNDROME; LIFE CHANGE SELF-RATING SCALE; STRESS.

Kahn, Ada P. *Stress A to Z: The Sourcebook for Facing Everyday Challenges.* New York: Facts On File, 2000.
Leana, Carrie R., and Daniel C. Feldman. *Coping with Job Loss: How Individuals, Organizations and Communities Respond to Layoffs.* New York: Lexington Books, 1992.
Lowry, Fran. "Larger Private Sector Role in Health Care Needed Now, Think Tank Warns." *Canadian Medical Association Journal* 154, no. 4: 549–51.

unipolar disorder (unipolar depression)   An affective illness (mood disorder) in which only depressive episodes occur. This is contrasted with bipolar disorder, in which episodes of depression as well as mania occur.

See also BIPOLAR DISORDER; DEPRESSION; RAPID CYCLING.

unwed mothers   A woman who becomes pregnant out of wedlock faces many psychological stresses in making many decisions. In most cases, there are several options to consider. She may either choose to terminate the pregnancy with a legal abortion or have the child and choose between single parenthood and giving the child up for adoption. Depending on her relationship with the father, she may also choose marriage. Research on the latter option has shown various results. It was once believed that a "shotgun" marriage was a poor choice, both because of the failure rate of such marriages and because the wife frequently dropped out of school. Some studies of this type of marriage in the 1980s showed a fairly high success rate, often dependent on the father being older than the mother and having finished school. A study of such marriages involving low-income black teenagers in Baltimore showed that one-third were still married 17 years later. Some researchers believe that these marriages may be of some benefit even if they do not last. In another study, women who had married under these circumstances and had stayed married for five years were found to be better off financially.

Changing social standards and even the examples of celebrities have encouraged unwed mothers to keep and raise their babies, but they still must face problems of providing financial support, coping with illness and other childhood disasters while working, and taking the responsibility for child rearing alone.

Often grandparents participate very actively in decision making about an out-of-wedlock pregnancy and also in rearing the child, with more or less favorable results depending on the flexibility of their attitudes. However, having one's child reared by one's parents brings several stressors into the picture. The young woman and her parents may have different ideas of appropriate behavior with the result of giving mixed messages to the child. In addition, the grandparents may be at an age and lifestyle at which having a young child around interferes with their long-planned activities.

In addition to women who unintentionally become pregnant out of wedlock, an increasing number of single women choose unwed motherhood. Some single women "feel the biological time clock ticking," meaning that they are in their late thirties and want to have children, although they have not yet found a man to marry. Some single women choose adoption; others choose to become impregnated by a man whom they know they will not marry, sometimes even retaining a friendly relationship with the man. Still others choose artificial insemination.

See also ABORTION; ADOPTION.

Chance, Paul. "Return of the Shotgun Wedding." *Psychology Today* 21 (Sept. 1987).
Kantrowitz, Barbara. "Mothers on Their Own." *Newsweek* (Dec. 23, 1985).

upper   The street name for amphetamine drugs. These are central nervous system stimulants with actions that resemble those of the naturally occurring substance adrenaline. Until recent years, physicians prescribed amphetamines for obesity, depression and narcolepsy. Amphetamines have also been widely misused by students studying for examinations and truck drivers on long trips in an attempt to stay alert for long periods of time.

Amphetamines are commercially produced but are limited by the Controlled Substances Act of 1972.

See also AMPHETAMINE DRUGS; SUBSTANCE ABUSE.

urethral phrase   A stage of psychosexual development representing transition from the anal to the phallic stage, involving conflicts about urethral control, resolution of which leads to self-competence and gender identity.

See also GENDER IDENTITY.

urolagnia   A paraphilia (sexual aberration) in which the woman or man has a morbid attraction for urine or the urinary processes of the sex partner or someone else. Such individuals may obtain sexual stimulation by watching the partner urinate, by sniffing garments smelling of urine during intercourse or masturbation, by drinking the partner's urine or by yielding to one's desire or the partner's desire to be urinated upon.

See also PARAPHILIAS; UROPHILIA.

urophilia   A psychosexual disorder marked by interest in urine and urination as a source of sexual excitement.

See also UROLAGNIA.

vacations According to Emrika Padus in *The Complete Guide to Your Emotions and Your Health* (Rodale Press, 1992), "getting away from it all—breaking free from routine—can bring a new perspective to old dilemmas and put a positive charge in your mental outlook. You'll get to know yourself a little better. And when you come home, you'll be happier, healthier and much more effective in coping with stress."

The book offers many healthy reasons for taking a vacation; Edward Heath, Ph.D., professor in the department of Recreation and Parks, Texas A&M University, and Richard I. Curtis, author of *Taking Off* (Harmony Books, 1981) concur. These reasons include:

Getting away from the daily routine
Relaxing
Seeing new sights
Opening up to different experiences
Making new friends
Sharing an event
Learning new skills
Participating in an adventure
Enjoying beauty
Anticipating pleasure
Remembering the joy

Said Dr. Heath, "The major goal of a vacation is happiness. You leave your troubles behind you . . . return refreshed and renewed. You should like your life a little better after a vacation."

However, vacations do not always result in better mental health. Vacations themselves can add to one's stress load. First there is the choice of how to travel—by car, train, ship or plane. Dealing with reservations can produce anxious feelings. Packing and preparing those left behind, in the case of families, can be difficult, especially when parents leave young children. When grandparents take on the responsibilities of caring for the children, intergenerational conflicts may result.

Delays of trains and planes, missed connections, and accommodations not up to one's expectations can be stressful. Bad weather can do more than dampen one's spirits; weather affects the enjoyment level of many sites. Additionally, interpersonal relationships are really put to the test on vacations, as friends, couples or other groupings are in close quarters and together every day.

See also HOBBIES; RECREATION.

Kahn P. Ada. *Stress A to Z: A Sourcebook for Facing Everyday Challenges.* New York: Facts On File, 2000.

vaginismus An involuntary muscle spasm of the vaginal opening that makes vaginal penetration and hence sexual intercourse painful. Vaginismus is one of the more common sexual dysfunctions that women experience. It is often triggered by a distasteful or painful early sexual problem such as rape or being the victim of sexual molestation. It can also be caused by physical problems such as chronic vaginitis or an imperforate hymen. At times vaginismus treatment requires intensive psychotherapy to search into its causes; in other cases, simply correcting a physical problem will alleviate vaginismus. Behavioral modification techniques have proven highly successful in treatment, based on a woman and her partner practicing stretching the vaginal opening, often with vaginal dilators.

See also BEHAVIORAL THERAPY; SEXUAL DYSFUNCTION.

Valium An antianxiety drug. Chemically known as diazepam, Valium is in a class of drugs called benzodiazepines. It has been used more extensively and for more conditions than any of the other benzodiazepines.

Valium is effective in the management of generalized anxiety disorder and panic disorder in selected patients. It is also used for skeletal muscle relaxation, for seizure disorders, for preanesthetic medication or intravenous anesthetic induction and for alleviating abstinence symptoms during alcohol withdrawal.

Valium is subject to abuse and may produce physical dependence after prolonged administration.

See also ANTIDEPRESSANT MEDICATIONS; BENZODIAZEPINE MEDICATIONS; DEPRESSION.

venereal disease See SEXUALLY TRANSMITTED DISEASES.

verbal slips See SLIPS OF THE TONGUE.

vertigo An illusion that one is spinning around or that one's surroundings are spinning around. The term is incorrectly used to describe dizziness or faintness. Some people who have agoraphobia or other phobias experience vertigo.

Healthy people experience vertigo when in boats, on amusement park rides or even when watching certain types of movies. Vertigo is caused by a disturbance of the semi-circular canals in the inner ear or the nerve tracts leading from them. Severe vertigo may be an indicator of several medical disorders, such as ear infections, influenza or Meniere's disease. Severe vertigo may be accompanied by ringing in the ears (tinnitus), jerky eye movements (nystagmus) and unsteadiness.

If symptoms of vertigo persist, the individual should seek medical treatment; pharmacologic therapies are available that help many people.

See also ANXIETY DISORDERS; DIZZINESS.

Viagra (sildenafil) A medication useful in helping men with impotence attain penile erections. The medication does not increase sexual desire but increases capacity for erections. It has been tried with variable results in females for achieving orgasm, especially to counter the sexual side effects of SSRI (selective serotonin reuptake inhibitor) antidepressant medications.

See also IMPOTENCE.

Victorianism In the United States, habits practiced during the years 1865 to 1918. The term comes from the name of Queen Victoria, who reigned in England from 1819 to 1901. Victorian attitudes held that women were weak and without sexual feeling and that female sexual activity was primarily to serve male needs for gratification. Married women were considered the guardians of children. Prostitutes, not wives or mothers, were considered the ideal "bad women." A proper middle-class woman did not dress in a provocative or revealing manner. Skirts were an inch off the ground, with many petticoats; a bustle extended up to three feet from the back of the dress, and her body was firmly held by a corset outfitted with tight strings and metal stays.

Although strict public standards of purity and decency were enforced, there was considerable prostitution and pornography. Laws relating to sexual interests included the Comstock Law (1873), regarding the mailing of obscene matter within the United States.

Sigmund Freud's view that sexuality affected every aspect of life had an effect on Victorianism. Freud said that repression of sexual instincts in men could lead to neuroticism and other harmful results. Freud also allowed that women were also sexual, but they were simply imperfect men because they lacked a penis. Freud put forth his theory of two types of female orgasm, the vaginal and clitoral (dual-orgasm theory), which tied in with his theory of developmental stages, which held that female development moved away from the clitoris to the vagina as the center of sexual pleasure. He considered failure to transfer the focus from the clitoris to the vagina as immature. Freud's theory indirectly argued that the male is not only sexually superior, but that women are dependent on a male penis inserted into the vagina for a "mature" sexual response. Freud viewed female masturbation as a sign of immaturity and ill health. Many agreed with Freud's views, including the dual-orgasm theory, until the 1960s when sex researchers, including Kinsey, debunked these notions.

During the Victorian era, female masturbation was generally thought to result in many ailments, including a harmful effect on reproduction. To cure adolescent female masturbation, vaginal mutilation and removal of the clitoris was at times carried out.

In public places, genitals on statues were covered with fig leaves. It was considered improper to talk about sexuality publicly. Books and plays (including those of Shakespeare) were censored.

Dissenters from Victorian views saw sexuality as healthy and natural. Writers such as Emerson and Thoreau advocated a return to nature and appreciation of human relationships, including sexuality. Many women's leaders attacked the sexual repression of women. Victorian outlooks and habits changed around the time the United States entered World War I.

See also FREUD, SIGMUND.

Kahn, Ada P., and Linda Hughey Holt. *The A to Z of Women's Sexuality.* Alameda, Calif.: Hunter House, 1992.

Masson, Jeffrey Moussaieff. *A Dark Science: Women, Sexuality and Psychiatry in the Nineteenth Century.* New York: Farrar, Straus and Giroux, 1986.

violence   See DOMESTIC VIOLENCE; FAMILY VIOLENCE.

Vivactil   Trade name for the tricyclic antidepressant medication known generically as protriptyline.

See also ANTIDEPRESSANT MEDICATIONS; PHARMACOLOGICAL APPROACH.

volunteerism   There are more people giving their time and energy without direct compensation to improve the quality of life in the United States than ever before. Estimates are that there are 80 million volunteers in the United States, contributing more than 19.5 billion hours of voluntary effort worth $150 billion in 1987 alone (according to the 1987 Gallup survey "Giving and Volunteering in the U.S.").

Deciding to volunteer is a personal commitment and covers the vast range of causes, concerns, beliefs, attitudes and needs of the diverse American population. A wide variety of options are open to volunteers, making it possible for people to find something to do that meets a real need and at the same time fits what they like to do or want to learn. This "right match" is what most often brings real fulfillment and joy to the volunteer.

It is often during life's major transitions, such as loss of a loved one, moving to a new community, loss of a job or divorce, that individuals experience great loneliness. According to Marlene Wilson's book *You Can Make a Difference!* volunteering can be a very helpful and healing experience during these times, because it is in the reaching out to others that people "get out" of themselves.

For information on volunteerism, contact:

Volunteer Management Associates
320 South Cedar Brook Road
Boulder, CO 80304
Phone: (303) 447-0558 or (800) 944-1470

Wilson, Marlene. *You Can Make a Difference!* Boulder: Volunteer Management Associates, 1990.

voyeurism   A sexual disorder in which an individual (male: voyeur, female: voyeuse) derives sexual satisfaction from secretly observing people's nude bodies in the act of undressing or during sexual activity. When this is the person's preferred or exclusive method of sexual excitement, the practice is considered a paraphilia. Voyeurism is also known as inspectionalism and "peeping Tomism." Voyeurism is considered a crime in many states in the United States.

war neurosis   A term largely replaced with posttraumatic stress disorder. War neurosis referred to a traumatic neurosis caused by wartime experiences, including bombings, exposure to combat conditions and internal conflicts over killing. Symptoms included anxiety, nightmares, irritability, depression and fears.

See also POST-TRAUMATIC STRESS DISORDER.

Watson, John B. (1878–1958)   An American psychologist and founder of behaviorism. Watson wrote, "Psychology as the behaviorist views it is a purely objective branch of natural science. Its theoretical goal is the prediction and control of behavior. Introspection forms no essential part of its methods, nor is the scientific value of its data dependent upon the readiness with which they lend themselves to interpretation in terms of consciousness." Watson emphasized learned behavior, stimulus-response connections and conditioning, and he regarded behavior as the product of both heredity and the environment. He believed that the task of psychology is to determine what is instinctive and what is learned. Watson is best known for his article "Psychology as the Behaviorist Views It" (1913). After leaving psychology he had a successful career in advertising.

See also BEHAVIORISM; RESPONSE; STIMULUS.

Harre, Rom and Roger Lamb. *The Encyclopedic Dictionary of Psychology.* Cambridge, Mass.: The MIT Press, 1984.

weekend depression   A type of depression that some individuals experience when away from their work. Particularly for some individuals who live alone, facing solitude creates emotional difficulties. To overcome the dislike and fear of being alone, as well as the change in mood from the workweek when one is surrounded by people, individuals may schedule pleasurable activities with friends or like-minded others so that they will not spend the entire weekend alone. Weekend depression should be distinguished from chronic depression.

See also DEPRESSION.

weight gain and loss   Concern about one's weight is often related to one's mental perception of body image and self-esteem. Weight gain and loss are also sometimes related to eating disorders such as anorexia nervosa or bulimia. Some individuals who fear gaining weight practice bulimia, the "bingeing and purging" syndrome, in which they gorge themselves and then induce vomiting. Many individuals become worried and impose stress on themselves because of their weight. Acceptance of oneself and one's body shape contributes to better mental health.

See also EATING DISORDERS.

Weil, Andrew (1942–)   American physician and author, known for his work in promoting complementary therapies and his books dealing with mind/body connections. Among his best-selling books that include tips for improving mental and physical health are *Eight Weeks to Optimum Health* and *Spontaneous Healing.* He advocates self-administered, common sense cures such as eating less fat, getting more exercise and reducing stress. He also suggests herbalism, acupuncture, naturopathy, osteopathy, chiropractic and hypnotism.

See also COMPLEMENTARY MEDICINE; MIND/BODY CONNECTIONS.

Wellbutrin   A trade name for an antidepressant drug, known generically as bupropion hydrochloride.

See also ANTIDEPRESSANT MEDICATIONS.

weltanschauung   A German word literally meaning "world outlook." The term refers to the totality of an individual's conception of reality, or philosophy of human life, society and the world at large.

Weltanschauung is a broader concept but roughly similar to the cognitive triad of negative view of the self, the future and the world, believed to underlie depression according to cognitive behavior theory.

Western blot test   A blood test for HIV (human immunodeficiency virus). The first-line serum test used to detect HIV is known as the enzyme-linked immunosorbent assay (ELISA). If the result is positive, the serum is then subjected to the more accurate Western blot test, because false positives may occur with ELISA. Persons should not be notified of a positive result until the Western blot test has been performed. In some states, all positive results are reported to public health authorities.

See also ACQUIRED IMMUNODEFICIENCY SYNDROME; ENZYME-LINKED IMMUNOSORBENT ASSAY.

wet dream   In the adult male, a sleep period in which ejaculation occurs (often characterized by dreams with sexual content). Wet dreams are common during adolescence and are considered normal even in adult males with regular sexual partners. Wet dreams sometimes cause embarrassment for young men.

See also EJACULATION; NOCTURNAL EMISSION.

will to survive   The mental fortitude and determination to live despite an adverse state such as a severe illness, disabling disorder or extreme environmental conditions, such as lack of water and food. Will to survive, or will to live, is often mentioned when survivors are found in mine shafts. Will to survive is credited with prolonging some terminal patients' lives.

See also HOSTAGES.

wish fulfillment   According to Sigmund Freud's wish-fulfillment theory of dreams, dreams express fulfilled wishes. The theory assumed that dreams have psychological meaning, that the hallucinatory quality of dreams enables the dreamer to represent as fulfilled wishes those that would otherwise have awakened him and that the wishes expressed are usually ones unacceptable to the sleeper's waking self. Only a small proportion of one's dreams are manifestly wish-fulfilling. The wish-fulfillment theory has been challenged by later psychiatrists and psychologists.

See also DREAMING; FREUD, SIGMUND.

withdrawal effects   Symptoms may appear when a drug on which the user is physically dependent is abruptly stopped or severely reduced. Withdrawal symptoms occur most consistently in cases of addiction to central nervous system depressants or narcotics.

Intensity and duration of withdrawal symptoms usually depends on the susceptibility of the individual, properties of the particular drug, and the degree of addiction. Usually, shorter-acting substances, such as heroin, cause more severe withdrawal symptoms than longer-lasting, more slowly eliminated drugs, such as methadone. If administered during heroin withdrawal, methadone can ease the intensity of the withdrawal experience.

Many people experience withdrawal symptoms after taking tranquilizers and other sedatives on a prescription basis. Withdrawal symptoms from depressants (barbiturates, sedatives, and tranquilizers) may occur within a few hours after the drug is stopped. Physical weakness, anxiety, nausea and vomiting, dizziness, sleeplessness, hallucinations, delirium, delusions, and convulsions may occur as soon as three days to a week following withdrawal and may last for many days. Withdrawal from the minor tranquilizers is similar but may take longer to develop. Not all symptoms that emerge after taking tranquilizers are withdrawal effects. Some may be anxiety that was repressed by the medications.

While certain substances, such as stimulant drugs (amphetamine and caffeine), are considered more psychologically than physically addictive, sudden abstinence may produce withdrawal effects. These may include headache, stomach cramps, lethargy, chronic fatigue, and possibly severe emotional depression. Individuals taking tricyclic antidepressants or MAO inhibitors should be aware that use of these drugs should be tapered off to avoid withdrawal reactions. If symptoms of withdrawal occur, the drugs may be reinstated temporarily and then tapered off even more gradually. The longer the period of use, the likelier there are to be withdrawal effects.

*Adapted with permission from Doctor, Ronald M., and Ada P. Kahn. *The Encyclopedia of Phobias, Fears, and Anxieties,* 2nd ed. New York: Facts On File, 2000.

Wolpe, Joseph (1915–1997)   An American psychiatrist who discovered that phobic people could be desensitized if they were trained to relax and gradually confront the phobia in their imaginations. He developed a theory of "reciprocal inhibition" (two opposing emotions cannot be experienced at the same time) and designed such contemporary therapies as assertiveness training, sexual therapies and aversive conditioning from this idea.

Dr. Wolpe was a professor of psychiatry at Temple University's medical school in Philadelphia from 1965 to 1988. Concurrently, he was director of the behavior therapy unit at the Eastern Pennsylvania Psychiatric Institute, also in Philadelphia. He was the second president of the Association for Advancement of Behavior Therapy.

In an obituary for Dr. Wolpe, Dr. Roger Poppen, a psychologist at Southern Illinois University at Carbondale and author of *Joseph Wolpe,* a 1995 biography, said that Dr. Wolpe was a major force in steering psychotherapy in the direction of empirical science. "He inspired and encouraged the direct comparison of carefully specified psychotherapy procedures by means of clear measurements of the therapy's outcome."

women's health movement   As part of the women's liberation movement of the 1970s, women in many parts of the United States started their own health centers and hired their own physicians. The aim of these centers is to increase knowledge about feminine anatomy and physiol-ogy, with strong emphasis on preventive health care and better patient-practitioner communications.

When possible, women's health centers have hired women physicians. Proponents of the women's health movement advocate more self-help groups and women helping women. During the 1980s, many hospitals reorganized their facilities to include "women's centers," in which women can obtain necessary health care in one place. Incorporated into the philosophy of such centers is better understanding of women's needs and health concerns and respect for women's rights to information about their health care.

See also WOMEN'S LIBERATION MOVEMENT.

women's liberation movement   Activities undertaken during the 1960s, 1970s, and early 1980s with intent to elevate women from total responsibility for child rearing and homemaking and from inferior positions in business, the professions and social clubs; to gain equal pay as men in the same work; and to gain freedom from the sexual double standard. In general, the movement worked toward less overall dominance by men and against the traditional stereotype of women as dependent, passive and fragile. The movement has enabled a generation of women to follow career paths not open to their mothers or grandmothers, to enjoy motherhood at the same time and to participate in previously male-dominated professional and social organizations. The "sexual revolution," during which women began to express sexuality with an increase in premarital and extramarital relationships, was an outgrowth of the women's liberation movement.

Significant steps in the women's liberation movement include publication of *The Feminine Mystique* (1963) by Betty Friedan, which exploded the myth of the happy housewife; the passage of the Equal Pay Act by the U.S. Congress in 1963; the founding of the National Organization for Women (1966); the first accredited women's studies course at Cornell University (1969); publication of *Sexual Politics* (1970) by Kate Millett; the founding of the National Women's Political Caucus (1971); the historic *Roe v. Wade* decision by the U.S. Supreme Court legalizing abortion (1973); the election of the first woman governor in her own right (Ella Grasso, Connecticut, 1974); the declaration of 1975 as the International Year of the Woman by the United Nations; the First National Women's Conference in Houston (1977); the march in 1978 of nearly 100,000 women in Washington to support extension of the Equal Rights Amendment; the appointment of Sandra Day O'Connor as the first woman to become an associate justice of the U.S. Supreme Court; and the candidacy of Geraldine Ferraro as the U.S. Democratic candidate for vice president in 1984.

See also SEXUAL HARASSMENT; WOMEN'S HEALTH MOVEMENT; WORKING MOTHERS.

Cott, Nancy F. *The Grounding of Modern Feminism.* New Haven: Yale University Press, 1989.

women's roles   The functions of women in society that traditionally were homemaking and child rearing were expanded in the later 20th century to include increasing participation in business, the military, government and other fields previously considered "men's fields." The change in women's roles has led in many cases to stress for women and the men in their lives; as competition between the sexes increases, jealousies over being the provider in the family occur, and males feel an increasing loss of power and control over women in their personal and professional lives.

Women with College Degrees

According to Challenger, Gray & Christmas Inc., an international outplacement firm that tracks workplace trends, the job outlook for women in highly skilled positions is improving. According to the firm's report, *21st Century Workplace Trends* (2000), the number of women earning four-year college degrees has surged 44 percent over the last two decades, from 444,045 in 1979 to approximately 640,000, or 56 percent of the estimated 1,140,000 college graduates, in 1999, according to the Department of Education.

In recent years, the number of men earning four-year degrees has actually fallen 6 percent from 532,881 in 1993 to 500,000 in 2000. As fewer and fewer men obtain bachelor's degrees, women will make further inroads into the managerial and

executive ranks as the job candidates of choice.

See also WOMEN'S LIBERATION MOVEMENT.

word blindness   See LEARNING DISABILITIES.

work addiction (workaholism)   A compulsive dependence on work as the most important means of maintaining one's self-esteem; the term "workaholic" refers to a person addicted to his or her work and who works excessively long hours, even when not necessary.

See also ADDICTION.

workaholism   See WORK ADDICTION.

working through   Exploration of a problem by an individual and therapist until a satisfactory solution is found or until a symptom has been traced to its unconscious sources. During the working-through process, the individual learns to understand the full implications of some interpretation or insight. Working through involves getting used to a new stage in life or getting over a loss or painful experience. As an example, the state of mourning requires some working through, as it involves the recognition that the deceased person is no longer available in many contexts in which he or she previously was a central figure.

workplace   The workplace affects the mental health of most people to varying degrees and for many varied reasons. Some people are stressed because they have too much work, while others are stressed because they are bored due to not enough work. Interactions with coworkers and bosses can lead to stress. Additional sources of stress include environmental situations, such as noise, poor lighting or lack of fresh air, as well as the frustration of being underpaid and overworked.

Contemporary technological stressors at the workplace range from back strain due to sitting at a computer terminal or to standing on a manufacturing assembly line to repetitive stress syndrome (carpal tunnel syndrome) from the use of computers.

Each occupation carries with it particular stresses, many of which are hidden by the employees. For example, many secretaries may resent doing the same chores over and over. Data processors may be bored with their work. Physicians find regulations imposed on them by managed care companies and insurance companies stressful. Accountants find the tax preparation season particularly stressful, while air controllers are under constant pressure every minute while at work. Lawyers must meet the demands of their clients as well as the superiors in their law firms.

The issue of control is an important one in determining the level of workplace anxiety. Those who feel they have more control over their situations, such as flexibility with work schedule or decision-making abilities in setting their own deadlines, may experience less stress than those who have no sense of control. Personal space is another issue. Workers who feel they have no privacy may feel more stressed than those who have offices or spaces with doors.

Jobs with fairly controllable situations include computer programmers, writers, artists, appliance repair persons and truck drivers. While these jobs can be very demanding, the minute-to-minute pace may be unhurried. Certain positions may be slow paced but with uncontrollable factors. These include janitors, security guards and bus drivers. Fast-paced and controllable professions include some physicians in private practice, business executives and city administrators. Fast-paced and uncontrollable professions include waiters, cashiers, firefighters and nurses.

Job mismatches can lead to mental health concerns. For some individuals, leaving the job is the solution. However, for many, that solution is not practical. Most people cannot walk away from their professions or businesses. The more realistic solution is to learn to cope better with current pressures.

Better Mental Health in the Workplace

Some of the stresses of workplace relationships can be eased by taking certain actions. Listen carefully when someone is speaking to you instead of planning your response as they are speaking. Careful listening can help prevent misunderstandings that might make you angry. Additionally, ask for feedback, which is another person's perception of what

you are doing or saying. Feedback is not evaluative or judgmental. Speak with your coworkers or superiors at an appropriate place and time. Do not initiate a difficult conversation without appropriate privacy. Finally, always ask for a clear statement of performance expectations. Confront a superior with questions about job role and expected outcomes.

In the early 2000s, workers have been faced with additional stresses of possible and actual downsizing of corporations during which many employees are laid off, necessitating early retirement for many and finding new jobs for others. The term "right-sizing" has come to mean scaling down the number of employees to an efficient and profitable level.

See also AUTONOMY; BOREDOM; CONTROL; COPING; FRUSTRATION; LISTENING; PERSONAL SPACE; STRESS.

Adams, Scott. *The Dilbert Principle: A Cubicle's-Eye View of Bosses, Meetings, Management Fads and Other Workplace Afflictions.* New York: HarperBusiness, 1997.

Field, Tiffany et al. "Job Stress Reduction Therapies." *Alternative Therapies* 3, no. 4 (July 1997).

Kahn, Ada P. *Stress A to Z: The Sourcebook for Facing Everyday Challenges.* New York: Facts On File, 2000.

Murphy, Lawrence R. "Stress Management in Work Settings: A Critical Review of the Health Effects." *American Journal of Health Promotion* 11, no. 2 (Nov./Dec. 1996): 112–135.

Peterson, Michael. "Work, Corporate Culture, and Stress: Implications for Worksite Health Promotion." *American Journal of Health Behavior* 21, no. 4 (1997): 243–252.

Rosch, Paul J. "Measuring Job Stress: Some Comments on Potential Pitfalls." *American Journal of Health Promotion* 11, no. 6 (July/Aug. 1997): 400–401.

Zeitlin, Lawrence R. "Organizational Downsizing and Stress-Related Illness." *International Journal of Stress Management* 2, no. 4 (Oct. 1995): 207–219.

worry A state of mental uneasiness, distress or agitation due to concern for a past, impending or anticipated event, threat or danger. Some degree of worrying is a common, everyday occurrence for most people. For some people, however, excessive worry interferes with mental health. Individuals who have anxiety disorders tend to worry more than others; for example, one with agoraphobia may worry about what will happen if he or she goes out, or one with a phobia may worry about what will happen if the phobic object or situation is encountered. Various forms of psychotherapy and self-helps relieve excessive worrying for many people.

Worrying may be called negative imagery because the worrier focuses on negative images or worst case scenarios (catastrophizes). Worrying to excess can be an unhealthy stressor because it causes the body to react; the heart pounds, breathing quickens and sweating may occur. For some individuals, guided imagery techniques, through which they imagine themselves in a given situation with a pleasant outcome, may be useful. Additionally, relaxation techniques, such as meditation and biofeedback, may be helpful. In a relaxed state, individuals can think more constructively and in a more organized manner.

WORRY LESS FOR BETTER MENTAL HEALTH

- When you try not to worry about something, it is likely that you will worry about it more. It may be advantageous to stay with the worry and really concentrate on it because you may stop worrying and begin solving your problem.
- Make a distinction between matters you can do something about and those you cannot.
- Instead of asking yourself repeatedly, "what if . . .," write down a number of possible solutions to a specific problem and then list the advantages and disadvantages of each idea.
- Use a diversionary technique, such as going for a walk, doing some other form of exercise, playing a musical instrument or listening to music. Doing so will help you organize your thoughts and come up with possible solutions. The best solutions may occur when you are not thinking about the immediate problem.
- Various forms of psychotherapy and self-help can relieve the stresses of excessive worrying for many people.

See also AGORAPHOBIA; ANXIETY; BIOFEEDBACK; CATASTROPHIZE; COPING; GENERAL ADAPTATION SYNDROME; GUIDED IMAGERY; MEDITATION; PHOBIA; RELAXATION; STRESS MANAGEMENT.

Diamond, David. "Bound to Worry." *Health* (July/Aug. 1992).
Padus, Emrika, ed. *The Complete Guide to Your Emotions and Your Health.* rev. Emmaus, Pa: Rodale, 1992.

worry beads Along with other types of beads, worry beads became the stylish way to relieve anxiety in the 1960s. Initially, the term "worry" was more nearly equivalent to the sense of the term meaning to shake or manipulate, but through usage it began to be associated with anxiety relief.

The modern source for worry beads is a peasant custom in Greece. Greeks customarily fingered sets of beads called *komboloi*. The habit is associated with the inclinations to use beads such as rosaries for religious purposes in other cultures, but in Greece it was simply a secular custom satisfying the tendency to want to do something with one's hands. A flood of tourism to Greece aroused an interest in Greek folk art, including *komboloi*. The beads became an international fad, were produced in ever more expensive and attractive styles and materials and ultimately were used by members of the Greek upper class who had looked down upon them.

See also ANXIETY; ANXIETY DISORDERS; WORRY.

Kulukundis, Elias. "Worry, Worry, Worry, the Greeks Have a Cure for it." *Holiday* (Apr. 1969).

writer's block An obstacle to the free expression of ideas on paper; occurs when there is an interruption in the flow between the thought and the recording of it. When a block occurs, the writer may feel frustrated and stuck. Unable to go on while waiting for an inspiration, the writer may have self-doubts about his or her capabilities, hopes and even future.

Many writers suffer from writer's block at some time. The block may involve an inability to get started with a writing project or to set words down on paper; it may occur in the middle of a project and the writer feels unable to go on. Writers may be concerned about the validity of the topic, ability to communicate on paper and acceptance by teachers, readers or publishers.

Too much stress can paralyze the writer, and too little stress can lead to apathy. The ideal state of mind, the one that unblocks, was called "eustress," or good stress, by Hans Selye, the Canadian author of *The Stress of Life* (1956) and *Stress Without Distress* (1974). The middle point in the stress spectrum is the state of relaxed concentration accompanied by energy. Because writing can be hard work, one must be in the right mental framework to take risks and have confidence and self-esteem regarding one's own abilities.

Overcome Writer's Block for Better Mental Health

Writing usually involves several steps: incubation, planning, research, organization, first draft, revision and final draft. Before starting, the writer unconsciously develops ideas and insights for the written material; this is the important incubation process. To bring these ideas out of the mind and onto paper and to break writer's block, he or she must reach a state of relaxed, energized concentration, in which self-criticism is set aside and there is room for creative thoughts.

There are a number of exercises one can perform to help reach the state of energized relaxation. Physical exercise energizes and is conducive to a relaxed state of mind. Meditation and imagery exercises are also very useful in reducing stress and minimizing the self-doubt that obstructs expression. Proper nutrition and enough sleep are similarly important to the writer.

Another way to avoid writer's block is to avoid people who are critical of the writer's work or ideas in the early stage of the project. While their criticisms may be helpful later, early in the project, criticism may be stifling.

See also CREATIVITY; FRUSTRATION; MEDITATION; SELF-ESTEEM; SLEEP; STRESS.

Kahn, Ada P. *Stress A to Z: The Sourcebook for Facing Everyday Challenges.* New York, Facts On File, 2000.
Sloane, Beverly LeBov. "Creativity." *Town Hall of California Reporter* (Mar./Apr. 1987): 6–7.

Wundt, Wilhelm Max (1832–1920) German psychologist and physiologist who founded experimental psychology with the establishment of the first official psychological laboratory in Leipzig. He applied introspective and psychophysical methods to a wide range of subjects, including reaction time, word associations, attention, judgment and emotions. He published monumental works on the history and foundations of psychology and also on logic, ethics and the psychological interpretation of history and anthropology.

See also PSYCHOLOGY.

Xanax Trade name for alprazolam, a triazolobenzodiazepine compound with antianxiety and sedative-hypnotic actions. It is efficacious in agoraphobia, has approval by the U.S. Food and Drug Administration for use in panic disorders and is also used to treat generalized anxiety disorder. Studies suggest that alprazolam also has antidepressant activity in moderate depression.

See also AGORAPHOBIA; ANTIDEPRESSANT MEDICATIONS; ANXIETY DISORDERS; DEPRESSION; PANIC DISORDER.

X-linked disorders Genetic disorders in which the abnormal gene or genes are located on the X chromosome and in which almost all those affected are males. Examples of this type of disorder are color vision deficiency and hemophilia.

See also CHROMOSOME; GENE.

X-linked mental retardation (XLMR) X-linked mental retardation (XLMR) accounts for approximately 20 to 25 percent of all known mental retardation. XLMR is also thought to cause the male excess observed in the mentally retarded population. The most well known XLMR is the fragile X syndrome, which is identified by the presence of a cytogenetic abnormality seen on chromosome analysis.

Males with fragile X syndrome frequently demonstrate behavioral problems, including hyperactivity and autistic behavior. Fragile X syndrome is the most common transmissible form of mental retardation. Approximately one-quarter to one-third of females who carry the fragile x genetic abnormality are also mentally retarded, generally in the mild range of severity.

XYY syndrome Down's syndrome in most cases is due to chromosomal defects resulting in three copies of chromosome number 21. Down's syndrome produces a variety of physical abnormalities and various degrees of mental retardation from relatively mild to quite severe. Among normal males, only 0.13 percent have two Y chromosomes. Compared with other males, XYY individuals are taller, often have severe acne and generally have low intelligence, although rarely in the retarded range.

See also CHROMOSOME; DOWN'S SYNDROME; MENTAL RETARDATION.

Davis, Kenneth; Howard Klar and Joseph T. Coyle. *Foundations of Psychiatry*. Philadelphia: W. B. Saunders, 1991.

yoga   A method of attaining a higher level of consciousness that eliminates anxiety-producing thought patterns. Yoga is a mental and physical discipline intended to help one get in touch with one's true nature and mystical feelings outside everyday existence and improve mental health.

There are several types of yoga practice and varying emphasis on physical, mental and social activity. Some yoga disciplines are more spiritual and metaphysical. The most commonly practiced yoga in the West is Hatha Yoga; it concentrates on spiritual improvement through the practice of physical exercise, which consists of postures called asanas. Mantras, or sacred sounds, are used in Mantra yoga. Still another branch of yoga practice concentrates on the kundalini or serpent power, which is thought to lie at the base of the spine and which can be released through postures, mantras and meditation. In some yoga practice, various forms are combined.

Yoga is an ancient practice that influenced and was in turn influenced by Brahminism, Jainism, Buddhism and Hinduism. Yoga practice started to move westward as a result of the Muslim invasions of India, but only the colonial expansion of the British brought Europeans in contact with yoga.

Critics of yoga say that it can be physically dangerous if practiced without supervision and that it may lead to introversion or a hedonistic philosophy. The degree to which adherents depend on their teacher or guru may decrease a sense of independence in the student and may give the teacher too strong a sense of his own power.

"Kundalini" and "Yoga," In *Harper's Encyclopedia of Mystical and Paranormal Experience,* Rosemary Ellen Guiley. San Francisco: Harper, 1991.

yohimbine   A substance considered by some as an aphrodisiac, or an erotic potion to increase capacity for and interest in lovemaking. Yohimbine is an alkaloid chemical derived from the bark of the African yohimbe tree. Its use was first observed by Europeans among natives in the 19th century; samples were brought back to Germany for study. The drug stimulates the nervous system and can cause anxiety. It is dangerous in large doses. It is sold under the trade name Yocon in the United States for sexual performance disorders. There is controversy concerning its effectiveness.

Z

Zen A form of Buddhism used as a basis for relaxation and stress management and concerned with the individual meaning of a person's life, rather than just the removal of symptoms or improvement of his or her adjustment to life. The goal of Zen is pursued through contemplation about the nature of humankind. During this process, individuals release tensions and experience oneness with the universe.

See also COMPLEMENTARY THERAPIES; MEDITATION; RELAXATION; STRESS; TRANSCENDENTAL MEDITATION.

zidovudine (AZT) A drug currently approved for use in patients with AIDS that has been shown to improve longevity and quality of life and may delay progression from ARC (AIDS-related complex) to the full-blown disease. AZT has also been demonstrated to ameliorate cognitive impairment in some individuals.

See also ACQUIRED IMMUNODEFICIENCY SYNDROME.

Vella, Stefano. "Zidovudine May Improve Survival for AIDS Patients." *Journal of the American Medical Association* (Mar. 3, 1992).

Zoloft An antidepressant drug (generic name: sertraline hydrochloride) indicated for the symptomatic relief of depressive illness. It is one of a category of medications known as selective serotonin reuptake inhibitors (SSRIs).

See also ANTIDEPRESSANT MEDICATIONS; DEPRESSION, SEROTONIN.

Zyprexa Zyprexa (olanzapine) is an "atypical antipsychotic" medication approved for use in schizophrenia and acute bipolar disorder. This medication has a low incidence of extrapyramidal side effects and tardive dyskinesia than traditional antipsychotic medications.

See also SCHIZOPHRENIA, BIPOLAR DISORDER.

RESOURCES

RESOURCES

ADDICTIONS

American Society of Addiction Medicine
4601 N. Park Avenue Arcade, Suite 101
Chevy Chase, MD 20815
Phone: (301) 656-3920
E-mail: usamoffice@aol.com

Center for Substance Abuse Prevention
5600 Fishers Lane, Rockwall II
Rockville, MD 20857
Phone: (301) 443-0365
Web site: www.samhsa.gov

Cocaine Anonymous
3740 Overland Avenue, Suite H
Los Angeles, CA 90034-6337
Phone: (310) 559-5833
Web site: www.ca.org

Debtors Anonymous
P.O. Box 400
Grand Central Station
New York, NY 10163-0400
Phone: (212) 642-8220

Gamblers Anonymous-International
Service Office
P.O. Box 17173
Los Angeles, CA 90017
Phone: (213) 386-8789
Web site: www.gamblersanonymous.org

Marijuana Anonymous
P.O. Box 2912
Van Nuys, CA 91404
Phone: (800) 766-8779
Web site: www.marijuana-anonymous.org

Narcotics Anonymous
P.O. Box 9999
Van Nuys, CA 91409
Phone: (818) 773-9999
Web site: www.wsoinc.com

National Clearinghouse for Alcohol and Drug
Information
11426 Rockville Pike
Rockville, MD 20852
Phone: (800) 729-6686
Web site: www.health.org
E-mail: info @health.org

National Council on Problem Gambling
P.O. Box 9419
Washington, D.C. 20016
Phone: (410) 730-8008
Web site: www.ncpgambling.org

National Institute on Drug Abuse
6001 Executive Boulevard
Bethesda, MD 20891
Phone: (800) 644-6432
Web site: www.nida.nih.gov

Substance Abuse and Mental Health Services
Administration
Center for Mental Health Services
5600 Fishers Lane
Rockville, MD 20857
Phone: (800) 789-2647 or (301) 443-2792
Web site: www.samhsa.gov/cmhs/cmhs.html

AGING AND ELDER CARE

Administration on Aging
330 Independence Avenue SW
Washington, D.C. 20201
Phone: (202 401-4511 or (202) 619-0724
Web site: www.aoa.dhhs.gov

Aging Network Services
4400 East-West Highway, Suite 907
Bethesda, MD 20814
Phone: (301) 657-4329
Web site: www.agingnets.com

Alliance for Aging Research
2021 K Street NW, Suite 305
Washington, D.C. 20006
Phone: (202) 293-2856
Web site: www.agingresearch.org

American Association for Geriatric Psychiatry
7910 Woodmont Avenue, Suite 11050
Bethesda, MD 20815
Phone: (301) 654-7850
Web site: www.aagpgpa.org

American Association of Retired Persons
601 E Street NW
Washington, D.C. 20049
Phone: (800) 424-3410
Web site: www://www.aarp.org

Care Options (Elder Care Management)
2012 Business Center Dr., Suite 130
Irvine, CA 92715
Phone: (714) 254-4140

National Aging Information Center
330 Independence Avenue SW
Room 4656
Washington, D.C. 20201
Phone: (202) 619-7501
Fax: (202) 401-7620
Web site: www.aoa.gov/naic

National Institute on Aging
31 Center Drive, Building 31
Room 5C27
MSC 2292
Bethesda, MD 20892-2292
Phone: (301) 496-1752
Web site: www.nih.gov/nia/

Social Security Administration
Office of Public Inquiries
6401 Security Boulevard
Room 4-C-5 Annex
Baltimore, MD 21235-6401
Phone: (800) 772-1213
Fax: (410) 965-0696
Web site: www.ssa.gov

AGORAPHOBIA

Anxiety and Phobic Program
P.O. Box 43082
Upper Montclair, NJ 07043
Phone: (973) 783-0007

Agoraphobics Building Independent
Lives, Inc. (ABIL)
3805 Cutshaw Avenue, Suite 415
Richmond, VA 23240
Phone: (804) 353-3964
E-mail: abill996@aol.com

Agoraphobics in Motion (AIM)
1719 Crooks Street
Royal Oak, MI 48067
Phone: (248) 547-0400
E-mail: anny@ameritech.net

Anxiety Disorders Association of America
11920 Parklawn Drive, Suite 100
Rockville, MD 20852
Phone: (301) 231-9350
Web site: www.adaa.org

AIDS (ACQUIRED IMMUNE DEFICIENCY SYNDROME) AND HIV

AIDS Clinical Trials Information Service
P.O. Box 6421
Rockville, MD 20849-6421
Phone: (800) TRIALS-A
Web site: www.actis.org

AIDS Health Project
1930 Market Street
San Francisco, CA 94102
Phone: (415) 476-6430
Web site: www.ucsf-ahp.org

National AIDS Clearinghouse (Information
and Publication orders)
Centers for Disease Control and Prevention
Box 6003
Rockville, MD 20850
Phone: (800) 458-5231

National AIDS Hot line: (800) 342-2437
TTY/TDD: (800) 243-7889
English Hot line: (800) 342-AIDS
Spanish Hot line: (800) 344-SIDA

National Association of People with AIDS
Hot line and TTY/TDD
Phone: (202) 898-0414

Project Inform
National HIV Treatment Line
Phone: (800) 922-7422

ALCOHOLISM

Al-Anon/Alateen Family Group Headquarters,
Inc.
1600 Corporate Landing Parkway
Virginia Beach, VA 23454-5617
Phone: (800) 344-2666
Web site: www.al-anon.alateen.org

Alcoholics Anonymous
A.A. World Services, Inc.
P.O. Box 459
New York, NY 10163
Phone: (212) 870-3400
Web site: www.alcoholics-anonymous.org

National Council on Alcoholism and Drug Dependence
12 West 21st Street
New York, NY 10010-6902
Phone: (212) 206-6770
Web site: www.ncadd.org

National Institute on Alcohol Abuse and
  Alcoholism
6000 Executive Boulevard, Wilco Building
Bethesda, MD 20892-7003
Phone: (301) 496-4452
Web site: www.niaaa.nih.gov

ALZHEIMER'S DISEASE

Alzheimer's Association
919 N. Michigan Ave., Suite 1000
Chicago, IL 60611-1676
Phone: (800) 272-3900
Fax: (312) 335-1110
Web site: www.alz.org
E-mail: info@alz.org

Alzheimer's Disease Education and
  Referral Center
P.O. Box 8250
Silver Spring, MD 10898-8507
Phone: (301) 495-3311 or (800) 438-4380
Web site: www.alzheimers.org/adear
E-mail: adear@alzheimer's.org

ANXIETY DISORDERS

Anxiety Disorders Association of America
11920 Parklawn Drive, Suite 100
Rockville, MD 20852
Phone: (301) 231-9350
Fax: (301) 231-7392
Web site: www.adaa.org

Anxiety Disorders Institute
1 Dunwoody Park, Suite 112
Atlanta, GA 30338
Phone: (770) 395-6845

Anxiety & Phobia Clinic
Davis Avenue at Port Road
White Plains, NY 10601
Phone: (914) 681-1038
Web site: www.phobia-anxiety.com

Council on Anxiety Disorders
79 Oconee Lane
Clarkesville, GA 30523
Phone: (706) 947-3854
Fax: (706) 947-1265
Web site: slvau@stc.net

Freedom From Fear
308 Seaview Avenue
Staten Island, NY 10305

Phone: (718) 351-1717
Fax: (718) 667-8893
Web site: www.freedomfromfear.org
E-mail: ffnadsd@aol.com

National Anxiety Foundation
3135 Custer Drive
Lexington, KY 40517
Phone: (606) 272-7166
Web site: www.lexington-on-line.com/naf.html

National Center for Post-Traumatic
  Stress Disorder
215 N. Main Street
White River Junction, VT 05009
Phone: (802) 296-5132
Web site: www.ncptsd.org

TERRAP Programs
932 Evelyn Street
Menlo Park, CA
Phone: (415) 327-1312 or (800) 2-PHOBIA
Fax: (415) 364-4703
Web site: www.terrap.com

ATTENTION DEFICIT DISORDERS

Attention Deficit Information Network (AD-IN)
475 Hillside Avenue
Needham, MA 02194
Phone: (781) 455-9895
Fax: (781) 444-5466
Web site: addinfonetwork.com
E-mail: adin@gis.net

Children and Adults with Attention
  Deficit Disorders
8181 Professional Place, Suite 201
Landover, MD 20785
Phone: (800) 233-4050 or (301) 306-7070
Fax: (301) 306-7090
Web site: www.chadd.org
E-mail: national@chadd.org

National Attention Deficit Disorders Association
  (ADAA)
P.O. Box 972
Mentor, OH 44061
Phone: (800) 487-2282
Web site: www.add.org

BODY THERAPIES

American Massage Therapy Association
820 Davis Street, Suite 100

Evanston, IL 60201-4444
Phone: (847) 864-0123
Web site: www.amtamassage.org

Feldenkrais Guild of North America (FGNA)
P.O. Box 489
Albany, OR 97321
Phone: (800) 775-2118
Web site: www.feldenkrais.com

North American Society of Teachers of the
    Alexander Technique (NASTAT)
P.O. Box 517
Urbana, IL 61801
Phone: (217) 367-6956

The Rolf Institute
P.O. Box 1868
Boulder, CO 80306
Phone: (303) 449-5903
Web site: www.rolf.org

CHRONIC FATIGUE SYNDROME

American Association for CFS (AAFCFS)
c/o Harborview Medical Center
325 9th Avenue
Box 359780
Seattle, WA 98104
Phone: (206) 521-1932
Fax: (206) 521-1930
E-mail: debrap@washington.edu

Chronic Fatigue Immune Dysfunction Syndrome
    Association of America Inc.
P.O. Box 2203398
Charlotte, NC 29222-0398
Phone: (800) 442-3437
Fax: (704) 365-9755
Web site: www.cfids.org

Chronic Fatigue Immune Dysfunction Syndrome
    Activation Network
P.O. Box 345
Larchmont, NY 10538
Phone: (212) 280-4266
Fax: (914) 636-6515
E-mail: cfidsnet@aol.com

National Chronic Fatigue Syndrome and
    Fibromyalgia Association
P.O. Box 18426
Kansas City, KS 64133
Phone: (816) 313-2000
E-mail: keal55A@prodigy.com

COMPLEMENTARY THERAPIES

American Art Therapy Association
1202 Allanson Road
Mundelein, IL 60060
Phone: (847) 949-6064
Web site: www.arttherapy.org

American Association of Naturopathic Physicians
P.O. Box 20386
Seattle, WA 98102
Phone: (206) 323-7610
Web site: www.naturopathic.org

American Association of Oriental Medicine
433 Front Street
Catasauqua, PA 18032
Phone: (610) 266-1433
Web site: www.aaom.org

American Chiropractic Association
1701 Clarendon Boulevard
Arlington, VA 22209
Phone: (703) 276-8800
Web site: www.amerchiro.org

Association of Applied Psychophysiology and
    Biofeedback
12267 W. 44th Avenue, #304
Wheat Ridge, CO 80303
Phone: (303) 422-8436
Fax: (303) 422-8894
Web site: www.aapb.org

Ayurvedic Institute
P.O. Box 23445
Albuquerque, NM 97192-1445
Phone: (505) 291-9698

Center for Dance Medicine
41 East 42nd Street, Room 200
New York, NY 10017
Phone: (212) 661-8401

Chopra Center for Well Being
7590 Fay Avenue, #403
La Jolla, CA 92037
Phone: (619) 551-7788

The Herb Research Foundation
1007 Pearl Street, Suite 200
Boulder, CO 80302
Phone: (303) 449-2265
Web site: www.herbs.org/herbs/

International Foundation for Homeopathy
2366 Eastlake Avenue E, #301
Edmonds, WA 98020

Phone: (206) 776-4147
Web site: www.healthy.net/ifh

National Academy of Acupuncture & Oriental
Medicine
P.O. Box 62
Tarrytown, NY 10591
Phone: (914) 332-4576

Mind-Body Medical Institute
New Deaconess Hospital
Harvard Medical School
185 Pilgrim Road
Cambridge, MA 02215
Phone: (617) 632-9530

National Center for Complementary and
Alternative Medicine
National Institutes of Health
6120 Executive Boulevard, Suite 450
Rockville, MD 20892-9904
Phone: (301) 402-4741
Web site: www.nccam.nih.gov

National Center for Homeopathy (NCH)
801 North Fairfax Street, Suite 306
Alexandria, VA 22314
Phone: (703) 548-7790
Fax: (703) 548-7792
Web site: www.homeopathic.org

National Dance Association
1900 Association Drive
Reston, VA 22091
Phone: (703) 476-3436
Web site: www.aahperd.org/nda.html

Sharp Institute for Human Potential and
Mind/Body Medicine
8010 Frost Street, Suite 300
San Diego, CA 92123
Phone: (800) 82-SHARP

CULTS

Cult Awareness Network (CAN)
1680 Vine St., #415
Los Angeles, CA 90028
Phone: (323) 468-0567
Fax: (323) 468-0562
Web site: www.cultawarenessnetwork.org

Cult Hotline and Clinic
1651 Third Avenue
New York, NY 10028
Phone: (212) 860-8533

Task Force on Cults
711 Third Avenue, 12th Floor
New York, NY 10017
Phone: (212) 983-4977

DENTAL FEARS

American Dental Association
211 East Chicago Avenue
Chicago, IL 60611
Phone: (312) 440-2500
Web site:
www.members.aol.com/adaa/index.html

DEPRESSION

Depression After Delivery
P.O. Box 1282
Morrisville, PA 19607
Phone: (800) 944-4773
Web site: www.infotrail.com/dad/dad.html

Depression and Related Affective Disorders
Association
The Johns Hopkins Hospital, Meyer 3-181
600 North Wolfe Street
Baltimore, MD 21287-7381
Phone: (410) 955-4647
Fax: (410) 614-3241
Web site: www.med.jhu.edu/drada
E-mail: drada@jhmi.edu

National Alliance for Research on Schizophrenia
and Depression
60 Cutter Mill Road, Suite 404
Great Neck, NY 11021
Phone: (800) 829-8289 or (516) 829-0091
Fax: (516) 487-6930
Web site: www.narsad.org

National Depressive and Manic-Depressive
Association
730 N. Franklin Street, Suite 501
Chicago, IL 60610-3526
Phone: (800) 826-3632
Fax: (312) 642-7243
Web site: www.ndmda.org

National Foundation for Depressive Illness
P.O. Box 2257
New York, NY 10116
Phone: (800) 239-1265
Web site: www.depression.org

DISSOCIATIVE DISORDERS

International Society for the Study of Dissociation
60 Revere Drive, Suite 500
Northbrook, IL 60062
Phone: (847) 480-0899
Fax: (847) 480-9282
Web site: www.issd.org

DOMESTIC VIOLENCE

Batterers Anonymous
1269 N.E. Street
San Bernardino, CA 92405
Phone: (714) 355-1100
E-mail: jmgoff@genesisnetwork.net

National Coalition Against Domestic Violence
(NCADV)
P.O. Box 18749
Denver, CO 80218-0749
Phone: (303) 839-1852
Fax: (303) 831-9251
Web site: www.ncadv.org

National Council on Child Abuse and
Family Violence
1155 Connecticut Avenue NW
Washington, D.C. 20036
Phone: (202) 429-6695
E-mail: nccafv@aol.com

DREAMS

Association for the Study of Dreams
6728 Old McLean Village Drive
McLean, VA 22101-3906
Phone: (703) 556-0618
Fax: (703) 556-8729
Web site: www.asdreams.org

Community Dream Sharing Network (CDN)
P.O. Box 8032
Hicksville, NY 11802
Phone: (516) 735-1969 or (516) 796-9455
Fax: (516) 796-9455
E-mail: comdream@aol.com

EATING DISORDERS

American Anorexia Bulimia Association
165 W. 46th Street, Suite 1008
New York, NY 10036
Phone: (212) 575-6200
Web site: www.aabainc.org

Anorexia Nervosa and Related Eating Disorders
P.O. Box 5102
Eugene, OR 97405
Phone: (503) 344-1144
Web site: www.anred.com

Bulimia Anorexia Self Help (BASH)
c/o Deaconess Hospital
6150 Oakland Avenue
St. Louis, MO 63139
Phone: (800) 762-3334

Eating Disorders Awareness and Prevention, Inc.
(EDAP)
603 Stewart Street, Suite 803
Seattle, WA 98101
Phone: (800) 931-2237 or (206) 382-3587
Fax: (206) 292-9890
Web site: www.edap.org
E-mail: info@edap.org

International Association of Eating Disorders
Professionals (IAEDP)
427 Center Pointe Circle, Suite 1819
Altamonte Springs, FL 32701
Phone: (800) 800-8126
Fax: (407) 831-7099
Web site: www.iaedp.com

National Association of Anorexia Nervosa and
Associated Disorders
P.O. Box 7
Highland Park, IL 60035
Phone: (847) 831-3438
Fax: (847) 433-4632
Web site: www.anad.org
E-mail: anad.20@aol.com

EYE MOVEMENT DESENSITIZATION AND REPROCESSING (EMDR)

Eye Movement Desensitization and Reprocessing
International Association (EMDRIA)
P.O. Box 141925
Austin, TX 78714-1925
Phone: (512) 451-5200
Fax: (512) 451-5256
Web site: www.emdria.org
E-mail: emdria@aol.com

FEAR OF FLYING

Fly Without Fear
211 E. 43rd Street
New York, NY 10017
Phone: (212) 697-7666

The Institute for Psychology of Air Travel
551 Boylston Street, Suite 202
Boston, MA 02116
Phone: (617) 437-1811
Web site: http://inspsyairt.com
E-mail: inspsyairt@aol.com

GRIEF

Bereavement and Loss Center of New York
170 E. 83rd Street
New York, NY 10028
Phone: (212) 879-5655

Elisabeth Kubler-Ross Center
So. Rte. 616
Head Waters, VA 24442
Phone: (703) 396-3441

Theos (groups in the U.S. and Canada for
    widowed people)
1301 Clark Building
717 Liberty Avenue
Pittsburgh, PA 15222
Phone: (412) 471-7779

HEADACHES

American Association for the Study
    of Headaches
19 Mantua Road
Mt. Royal, NJ 08061
Phone: (609) 423-0043
Web site: www.aash.org

National Headache Foundation
5252 N. Western Avenue
Chicago, IL 60625
Phone: (773) 878-7715
Web site: www.headaches.org

HOMELESSNESS

National Coalition for the Homeless
1012 14th Street NW, Suite 600
Washington, D.C. 20005-3406
Phone: (202) 737-6444
Fax: (202) 737-6445
Web site: http://nch.ari.net
E-mail: nch@ari.net

National Resource Center on Homelessness and
    Mental Illness Policy Research Associates, Inc.
262 Delaware Avenue
Delmar, NY 12054

Phone: (800) 444-7415
Fax: (518) 439-7612
Web site: www.prainc.com/nrc
E-mail: nrc@prainc.com

Projects for Assistance in Transition from
    Homelessness (PATH)
Technical Assistance Center
Advocates for Human Potential, Inc.
323 Boston Post Road
Sudbury, MA 01776
Phone: (978) 443-0055
Fax: (978) 443-4722

HUMOR

International Laughter Society
16000 Glen Una Drive
Los Gatos, CA 95030
Phone: (408) 354-3456

HYPNOSIS

American Psychotherapy and Medical
    Hypnosis Association
275 Hill Street, #302
Reno, NV 89501
Phone: (775) 786-5650
Web site: www.apmha.com

American Society of Clinical Hypnosis
2200 East Devon Avenue, Suite 291
Des Plaines, IL 60018
Phone: (847) 297-3317

Institute of Hypnotherapy
869 Yonge Street, Suite 101
Toronto, Ontario
Canada
M4W 2H2
Phone: (416) 921-4686

International Society for Medical and
    Psychological Hypnosis
1991 Broadway, 18B
New York, NY 10023
Phone: (212) 874-5290

LEARNING DISABILITIES

Learning Disabilities Association of America
4156 Library Road
Pittsburgh, PA 15234
Phone: (412) 341-1515
Web site: www.danatl.org

LEGAL ISSUES

Commission on Mental and Physical Disability Law
American Bar Association
740 15th Street NW
Washington, D.C. 20005
Phone: (202) 662-1570
Fax: (202) 662-1032
Web site: www.abanet.org/disability
E-mail: cmpdl@abanet.org

Judge David L. Bazelon Center for Mental Health Law
1101 15th Street NW, Suite 1212
Washington, D.C. 20005-5002
Phone: (202) 467-5730
Fax: (202) 223-0409
Web site: www.bazelon.org
E-mail: bazelon@nicom.com

National Association of Protection and Advocacy Systems
900 Second Street, NE, Suite 211
Washington, D.C. 20002
Phone: (202) 408-9514
Fax: (202) 408-9520
Web site: www.protectionandadvocacy.com
E-mail: napas@vipmail.earthlink.net

MARRIAGE AND FAMILY

American Association for Marriage and Family Therapy
1133 15th Street NW, Suite 300
Washington, D.C. 20005-2710
Phone: (202) 452-0109
Web site: www.aamft.org

Center for the Family
5725 Paradise Drive, #300B
Corte Madera, CA 94925-1218
Phone: (415) 924-5750

Stepfamily Association of America
215 Centennial Mall, Suite 212
Lincoln, NE 68508
Phone: (800) 735-0329

MENTAL HEALTH

American Group Psychotherapy Association
25 E. 21st Street, Sixth Floor
New York, NY 10010
Phone: (212) 477-2677
Fax: (212) 979-6627

Web site: www.agpa.org
E-mail: groupsinc@aol.com

American Mental Health Counselors Association
801 N. Fairfax, Street, Suite 304
Alexandria, VA 22314
Phone: (800) 326-2642 or (703) 548-6002
Fax: (703) 548-4775
Web site: www.amhca.org
E-mail: vmoore@amhca.org

American Psychiatric Association
1400 K Street NW
Washington, D.C. 20005
Phone: (202) 692-6850
Web site: http://www.psych.org
E-mail: apa@psych.org

American Psychological Association
750 First Street NE
Washington, D.C. 20002-4242
Phone: (800) 374-3120 or (202) 336-5700
Fax: (202) 336-5568
Web site: www.apa.org
E-mail: division@apa.org

Association for Advancement of Behavior Therapy
305 7th Avenue, 16th floor
New York, NY 10001-6008
Phone: (212) 647-1890
Fax: (212) 647-1865
Web site: www.aabt.org
E-mail: info@aabt.org

Beck Institute for Cognitive Therapy and Research
GSB Building
City Line and Belmont Avenues, Suite 700
Bala Cynwyd, PA 19004-1610
Phone: (610) 664-3020
Fax: (610) 664-4437
Web site: www.beckinstitute.org
E-mail: beckinst@gim.net

National Alliance for the Mentally Ill
200 N. Glebe Rd., Suite 1015
Arlington, VA 22203-3754
Phone: (703) 524-7600 or (800) 950-6264
Fax: (703) 524-9094
Web site: www.nami.org

National Association for the Advancement of Psychoanalysis
80 Eighth Avenue, Suite 1501
New York, NY 10011
Phone: (212) 741-0515

Fax: (212) 366-4347
Web site: www.naap.org
E-mail: naap72@aol.com

National Association of Cognitive-Behavioral
   Therapists
P.O. Box 2195
Weirton, WV 26062
Phone: (800) 853-1135
Fax: (304) 723-3982
Web site: www.nacbt.org
E-mail: nacbt@nacbt.org

National Institute of Mental Health
6001 Executive Boulevard, Room 8184
MSC 9663
Bethesda, MD 20892-9663
Phone: (800) 421-4211
Web site: www.nimh.nih.gov
E-mail: nimhinfo@nih.gov

National Mental Health Association
1021 Prince Street
Alexandria, VA 22314-2971
Phone: (703) 684-7722 or (800) 969-6642
Fax: (703) 684-5968
Web site: www.nmha.org
E-mail: infoctr@nmha.org

National Mental Illness Screening Project
1 Washington Street, Suite 304
Wellesley Hills, MA 02481
Phone: (800) 57304433
Fax: (781) 431-7447
Web site: www.nmisp.org

MENTAL HEALTH: CHILDREN AND ADOLESCENTS

American Academy of Child and
   Adolescent Psychiatry
3615 Wisconsin Avenue NW
Washington, D.C. 20016-3007
Phone: (202) 966-7300
Fax: (202) 966-2891
Web site: www.aacap.org

American Academy of Pediatrics
242 Northwest Point Boulevard
P.O. Box 927
Elk Grove Village, IL 60007
Phone: (847) 228-5005
Web site: www.aap.org

Federation of Families for Children's Mental Health
1021 Prince Street
Alexandria VA 22314-2971

Phone: (703) 684-7710
Fax: (703) 836-1040
Web site: www.ffcmh.org
E-mail: ffcmh@crosslink.net

MEN'S HEALTH

Men's Health Network
P.O. Box 75972
Washington, D.C. 20013
Hotline: (888) MEN-2-MEN
Web site: www.menshealthnetwork.org

MENTAL RETARDATION

American Association on Mental Deficiency
   (AAMD)
1719 Kalorama Road NW
Washington, D.C. 20009
Phone: (202) 387-1968

Association for Retarded Citizens (ARC)
P.O. Box 6109
Arlington, TX 76005
Phone: (817) 640-0204
E-mail: thearc@metronet.com

National Down Syndrome Society
141 5th Avenue
New York, NY 10010
Phone: (212) 460-9330
Web site: www.ndss.org

The ARC of the United States
1010 Wayne Avenue, Suite 650
Silver Spring, MD 20910
Phone: (301) 565-3842
Fax: (301) 565-5342
E-mail: info@thearc.org

OBSESSIVE-COMPULSIVE DISORDER

Obsessive-Compulsive Foundation
9 Depot Street
Milford, CT 06460-0070
Phone: (203) 878-5669
Web site: www.ocfoundation.org

PARKINSON'S DISEASE

American Parkinson's Disease Association
1250 Hylan Boulevard, Suite 4B
Staten Island, NY 10305

Phone: (718) 981-8001 or (800) 223-2732
E-mail: apda@admin.con2.com

United Parkinson Foundation
833 West Washington
Chicago, IL 60607
Phone: (312) 733-1893
E-mail:upf_itf@msn.com

PHOBIAS

Anxiety Disorders Association of America
11920 Parklawn Drive, Suite 100
Rockville, MD 20852
Phone: (301) 231-9350 or 231-92259
Web site: www.adaa.org

Phobics Anonymous
P.O. Box 1180
Palm Springs, CA 92263
Phone: (619) 322-COPE

National Mental Health Association
1021 Prince Street
Alexandria, VA 22314-2971
Phone: (703) 684-7722 or (800) 969-6642
Fax: (703) 684-5968
Web site: www.nmha.org
E-mail: infoctr@nmha.org

Special Interest Group on Phobias and Related
Anxiety Disorders (SIGPRA)
245 E. 87th Street
New York, NY 10028
Phone: (212) 860-5560
Web site: www.cyberpsych.org/anxsig.htm

POST-TRAUMATIC STRESS DISORDER

Anxiety Disorders Association of America
11900 Parklawn Drive, Suite 100
Rockville, MD 20852
Phone: (301) 231-9350
Web site: www.adaa.org

National Association of Veterans Administration
Chiefs of Psychiatry
54th Street and 48th Avenue
Minneapolis, MN 55417
Phone: (612) 725-6767

U.S. Veterans Administration
Mental Health and Behavioral Sciences Services
810 Vermont Avenue NW, Room 915
Washington, D.C. 20410
Phone: (202) 389-3416

SCHIZOPHRENIA

National Alliance for Research on Schizophrenia
and Depression
60 Cutter Mill Road, Suite 404
Great Neck, NY 11021
Phone: (516) 829-0091
Fax: (516) 487-6930
Web site: www.mhsource.com/narsdad.html

SELF-HELP AND SUPPORT GROUPS

National Self-Help Clearinghouse
25 W. 43rd Street, Room 620
New York, NY 10036
Phone: (212) 642-2944 or (212) 354-8525
Web site: www.selfhelpweb.org

Recovery, Inc.
802 N. Dearborn Street
Chicago, IL 60610
Phone: (312) 337-5661
Web site: www.recovery-inc.com

SEXUALLY TRANSMITTED DISEASES

American Academy of Dermatology
P.O. Box 4014
930 N. Meacham Road
Schaumburg, IL 60168-4014
Phone: (847) 330-0230 or (888) 362-DERM
Fax: (847) 330-0050
Web site: www.aad.org

American Social Health Association
P.O. Box 13827
Research Triangle Park, NC 27709
Phone: (919) 361-2742
Web site: www.sunsite.unc.edu/ASHA/

The Herpes, Resource Center
260 Sheridan Avenue, Suite 307
Palo Alto, CA 94306
Phone: (415) 328-7710 or (800) 227-8922

Sexual Function Health Council
American Foundation for Urologic Disease
300 West Pratt Street, Suite 401
Baltimore, MD 21201
Phone: (800) 242-2383
Web site: www.afud.org

Sexuality Information and Education Council
of the U.S. (SIECUS)
130 W. 42nd Street, Suite 2500
New York, NY 10036

Phone: (212) 819-9770
Web site: www.siecus.org

SLEEP

American Sleep Apnea Association
1424 K Street NW, Suite 302
Washington, D.C. 20005
Phone: (202) 293-3650
Web site: www.sleepapnea.org

American Sleep Disorders Association
6301 Bandel Road, Suite 101
Rochester, MN 55901
Phone: (507) 287-6006
Web site: www.asda.org

Narcolepsy Network
277 Fairfield Road, Suite 310B
Fairfield, NJ 07004
Phone: (973) 276-0115
Web site: www.websciences.org

National Sleep Foundation
729 15th Street NW, Floor 4
Washington, D.C. 20005
Phone: (202) 347-3471
Web site: www.sleepfoundation.org

SOCIAL PHOBIA/SOCIAL ANXIETY

Social Phobia/Social Anxiety Association
5025 N. Central Avenue, #421
Phoenix, AZ 85012
Phone: (602) 952-9846
Web site: www.socialphobia.org

SOCIAL WORKERS

National Association of Social Workers
750 First Street NE, Suite 700
Washington, D.C. 20002-4241

Phone: (800) 638-8799
Web site: www.socialworkers.org

SUICIDE

American Association of Suicidology
4201 Connecticut Avenue NW, Suite 310
Washington, D.C. 20008
Phone: (202) 237-2280
Fax: (202) 237-2282
Web site: www.suicidology.org

American Foundation for Suicide Prevention
120 Wall Street, 22nd floor
New York, NY 10005
Phone: (212) 363-3500 or (888) 333-AFSP
Fax: (212) 363-6237
Web site: www.afsp.org

Suicide Prevention Advocacy Network
5034 Odin's Way
Marietta, GA 30068
Phone: (888) 649-1366
Fax: (770) 642-1419
Web site: www.spanusa.org
E-mail: act@spanusa.org

VOLUNTEERISM

Volunteer Management Associates
320 South Cedar Brook Road
Boulder, CO 80304
Phone: (303) 447-0558 or (800) 944-1470

WOMEN'S HEALTH

National Women's Health Resource Center
120 Albany Street, Suite 820
New Brunswick, NJ 08901
Phone: (877) 986-9472
Web site: www.healthywomen.org

BIBLIOGRAPHY

Acquired Immunodeficiency Syndrome (AIDS)

Andre, Pierre. *People, Sex, HIV and AIDS: Social, Political, Philosophical and Moral Implications.* Huntington, W.Va.: University Press, 1995.

Andriote, John-Manuel. "Victory Deferred: How AIDS Changed Gay Life in America." Chicago: University of Chicago Press, 1999.

Banta, William F. *AIDS in the Workplace; Legal Questions and Practical Answers.* New York: Lexington Books, 1993.

Bartlett, John G. *The Guide to Living with HIV Infection.* Baltimore: Johns Hopkins University Press, 1988.

Check, William A. *AIDS.* Philadelphia: Chelsea House, 1999.

Devita, Vincent T. *AIDS: Etiology, Diagnosis, Treatment, Prevention,* 4th ed. Philadelphia: J. B. Lippincott, 1997.

Dispezio, Michael A. *The Science, Spread, and Therapy of HIV Disease: Everything You Need to Know but Had No Idea Who to Ask.* Shrewsbury, Mass.: ATL Press, 1998.

Donovan, Catherine A., and Elizabeth Stratton. "Changing Epidemiology of AIDS." *Canadian Family Physician* 40 (Aug. 1994).

Douglas, Paul Harding, and Laura Pinsky. *The Essential AIDS Fact Book.* New York: Pocket Books, 1996.

Epstein, Steven. *Impure Science: AIDS, Activism and the Politics of Knowledge.* Berkeley, Calif.: University of California Press, 1996.

Faison, Brenda S. *The AIDS Handbook: A Complete Guide to Education and Awareness.* Durham, N.C.: Designbase Publishing, 1991.

Gedatus, Gustav Mark. *HIV and AIDS.* Mankato, Minn.: Lifematters, 2000.

Gifford, Allen. *Living Well with HIV and AIDS.* Palo Alto, Calif.: Bull Publishers, 2000.

Goldfinger, Stephen E., ed. "AIDS: A Glimmer of Hope." *Harvard Health Letter* 20, no. 9 (July 1995).

Greif, Judith. *AIDS Care at Home: A Guide for Caregivers, Loved Ones and People with AIDS.* New York: Wiley, 1994.

Jenkins, Mark. *HIV/AIDS: Practical Medical, and Spiritual Guidelines for Daily Living When You're HIV-Positive.* Center City, Minn.: Haxelden Information & Educational Services, 2000.

Sirimarco, Elizabeth. *AIDS.* New York: Marshall Cavendish, 1994.

Storad, Conrad J. *Inside AIDS: HIV Attacks the Immune System.* Minneapolis: Lerner Publications, 1998.

Stewart, Gail. *People with AIDS.* San Diego: Lucent Books, 1996.

Ward, Darrell E. *The AmFAR AIDS Handbook: The Complete Guide to Understanding HIV and AIDS.* New York: W. W. Norton, 1999.

Addictions (see also ALCOHOLISM; SMOKING.)

Bepko, Claudia, ed. *Feminism and Addiction.* New York: Haworth Press, 1991.

Carroll, Marilyn. *Cocaine and Crack.* Hillside, N.J.: Enslow Publishers, 1994.

Chopra, Deepak. *Overcoming Addictions: The Spiritual Solution.* New York: Harmony Books, 1997.

Ganguli, H. G. L. "Meditation Subculture and Drug Use." *Human Relations* 38 (1985): 953.

Gorsuch, R. L., and M. C. Butler. "Initial Drug Abuse: A Review of Predisposing Social Psychological Factors." *Psychological Bulletin* 83 (1986): 120–137.

White, Robert K., and Deborah George Wright, eds. *Addiction Intervention: Strategies to Motivate.* New York: Haworth Press, 1998.

Mulry, J. T. "Drug Use in the Chemically Dependent." *Postgraduate Medicine* 83 (1988): 279–283.

Ruden, Ronald A. *The Craving Brain: The Biobalance to Controlling Addictions.* New York: HarperCollins, 1997.

Rounsaville, B. J. et al. *Evaluating and Treating Depression in Opiate Addicts.* Rockville, Md.: National Institute on Drug Abuse, 1985.

Adolescence and Mental Health

Bowring, M., and M. Kovacs. "Difficulties in Diagnostic Adolescents." *Journal of the American Academy of Child and Adolescent Psychiatry* 31 (1992): 611–614.

Clayton, R. R. and C. Ritter, "The Epidemiology of Alcohol and Drug Abuse among Adolescents." *Adv Alcohol Substance Abuse* 4 (1985): 69.

Costello, E. "Child Psychiatric Disorders and the Correlates: A Primary Care Pediatric Sample." *Journal of the American Academy of Child and Adolescent Psychiatry* 28 (1989): 851–855.

Dobson, James. C. *Preparing for Adolescence.* Santa Ana, Calif.: Vision House Publishers, 1978.

Ellickson, P. L., and K. A. McGuigan. "Early Predictors of Adolescent Violence." *American Journal of Public Health* 90, no. 4 (April 2000): 566–572.

Ferguson, Gary. *Shouting at the Sky: Troubled Teens and the Promise of the Wild.* New York: St. Martin's Press, 1999.

Geller, B. and J. Luby. "Child and Adolescent Bipolar Disorder: A Review of the Past 10 Years." *Journal of the American Academy of Child and Adolescent Psychiatry* 36 (1997): 1168–1176.

Hazell, P. L. et al. "Confirmation that the Child Behavior Checklist Clinical Scales Discriminate Juvenile Mania from Attention Deficit Hyperactivity Disorder." *Journal of Pediatric Child Health* 35, no. 2 (1999): 199–203.

Offer, D., E. Ostrov, and K. Howard. "The Mental Health Professional's Concept of the Normal Adolescent," *Archives of General Psychiatry* 38 (1981): 149–152.

Pipher, Mary Bray. *Reviving Ophelia: Saving the Selves of Adolescent Girls.* New York: Putnam, 1994.

Stepp, Laura Sessions. *Our Last Best Shot: Guiding Our Children through Early Adolescence.* New York: Riverhead Books, 2000.

Affective Disorders (see BIPOLAR DISORDER; DEPRESSION.)

Aggressive Behavior

Fawcett, J., ed. *Dynamics of Violence.* Chicago: American Medical Association, 1972.

Felthous, A. R., and S. R. Kellert. "Childhood Cruelty to Animals and Later Aggression Against People: A Review." *American Journal of Psychiatry* 144 (1987): 710.

Green, R. G., and E. I. Donnerstein, eds. *Aggression: Theoretical and Empirical Reviews,* vols. 1 and 2. New York: Academic Press, 1983.

Valzelli, L. *Psychobiology of Aggression and Violence.* New York: Raven Press, 1981.

Aging and Mental Health

Austad, Steven N. *Why We Age: What Science Is Discovering about the Body's Journey Through Life.* New York: John Wiley & Sons, 1997.

Baruch, Grace et al. *Lifeprints: New Patterns of Love and Work for Today's Woman.* New York: McGraw-Hill, 1983.

Brown, Judith K., and Virginia Kerns, eds. *In Her Prime: A New View of Middle-Aged Women.* South Hadley, Mass.: Bergin and Garvey, 1985.

DiGiovanna, Augustine Gaspar. *Human Aging: Biological Perspectives.* New York: McGraw-Hill, 1994.

Dychtwald, Ken. *Age Power: How the 21st Century Will Be Ruled By the New Old.* New York: J. P. Tarcher/Putnam, 1999.

Flint, Alastair J. "Anxiety Disorders in Late Life." *Canadian Family Physician* 45 (Nov. 1999): 2692–2679.

Friedan, Betty. *The Fountain of Age.* New York: Simon & Schuster, 1993.

Gittleman, Ann Louise. *How To Stay Young and Healthy in a Toxic World.* Los Angeles: Keats, 1999.

Grossberg, George T. "Understanding Anxiety and Its Treatment in the Elderly Population." *Anxiety Disorders Association of America Reporter* (winter 1998): 15–21.

Ilardo, Joseph A. *As Parents Age: A Psychological and Practical Guide.* Acton, Mass.: Vander Wyk & Burnham, 1998.

Lesnoff-Caravaglia, Gari. *Health Aspects of Aging: The Experience of Growing Old.* Springfield, Ill.: C. C. Thomas, 2000.

Loverde, Joy. *The Complete Eldercare Planner: Where to Start, Which Questions to Ask, and How to Find Help.* New York: Times Books, 2000.

Martz, Sandra Haldeman, ed. *When I Am an Old Woman I Shall Wear Purple.* Watsonville, Calif.: Papier-Mache Press, 1996.

Monte, Tom. *Staying Young: How to Prevent, Slow, or Reverse More than 60 Signs of Aging.* Emmaus, Pa.: Rodale Press, 1994.

Nash, Harold W. *Our Aging Brain: Changing and Growing.* Burlington, N.C.: Ontarolina, 1999.

Porcino, Jane. *Growing Older, Getting Better.* Reading, Mass.: Addison-Wesley, 1983.

Raj, Asholk. "The Spectrum of Panic Disorder in the Elderly." *Anxiety Disorders Association of America Reporter* (winter 1998): 13–19.

Ransohoff, Rita M. *Venus After Forty: Sexual Myths, Man's Fantasies, and Truths About Middle-Aged Women.* Far Hills, N.J.: New Horizon Press, 1987.

Wei, Jeanne Y. *Aging Well: The Complete Guide to Physical and Emotional Health.* New York: Wiley, 2000.

Agoraphobia (see also ANXIETY DISORDERS; PHOBIAS.)

Ballenger, James C., ed. *Biology of Agoraphobia.* Washington, D.C.: American Psychiatric Press, 1984.

Frampton, Muriel. *Agoraphobia: Coming to Terms with the World Outside.* Wellingstorough, U.K.: Turnstone Press, 1984.

Goldstein, Alan J. *Overcoming Agoraphobia: Conquering Fear of the Outside World.* New York: Viking, 1987.

Pace, Anita L., ed. *Life Isn't just a Panic: Stories of Hope by Recovering Agoraphobics.* Beaverton, Oreg.: Baby Steps Press, 1996.

Seagrave, Ann, and Faison Covington. *Free from Fears: New Help for Anxiety, Panic and Agoraphobia.* New York: Poseidon Press, 1987.

Scrignar, Chester R. *From Panic to Peace of Mind: Overcoming Panic and Agoraphobia.* New Orleans, La.: Brunn Press, 1991.

Seidenberg, Robert. *Women Who Marry Houses: Panic and Protest in Agoraphobia.* New York: McGraw-Hill, 1983.

Weekes, Claire. *Agoraphobia: Simple, Effective Treatment.* New York: Hawthorn Books, 1976.

Alcoholism

Barbour, Scott, ed. *Alcohol: Opposing Viewpoints.* San Diego: Greenhaven Press, 1998.

Berger, Gilda. *Alcoholism and the Family.* New York: Franklin Watts, 1993.

Cohen, M., J. C. Kern, and C. Hassett. "Identifying Alcoholism in Medical Patients." *Hospital and Community Psychiatry* 37 (1987): 399.

Cohen, S., and J. F. Callahan. *The Diagnosis and Treatment of Drug and Alcohol Abuse.* New York: Haworth Press, 1986.

Dick, R. *New Light on Alcoholism.* Corte Madera, Calif.: Good Book Publishing, 1994.

Fawcett, J. et al. "A Double-blind, Placebo Controlled Trial of Lithium Carbonate Therapy for Alcoholism." *Archives of General Psychiatry* 44 (1986): 248–258.

Goodwin, D. W. "Alcoholism and Genetics." *Archives of General Psychiatry* 42 (1985): 171–174.

Helzer, J.E. et al. "Alcoholism—North America and Asia: A Comparison of Population Surveys with the Diagnostic Interview Schedule." *Archives of General Psychiatry* 47 (1990): 313–319.

Holden, C. "Is Alcoholism Treatment Effective?" *Science* 236 (1987): 20–22.

Irwin, M., M. Schuckit, and T. L. Smith. "Clinical Importance of Age at Onset in Type I and Type II Primary Alcoholics." *Archives of General Psychiatry* 47 (1990): 320–324.

Ketchum, Katherine, and William F. Asbury. *Beyond the Influence: Understanding and Defeating Alcoholism.* New York: Bantam Books, 2000.

Liehelt, Robert A. *Straight Talk About Alcoholism.* New York: Pharos Books, 1992.

Light, W. J. H., *Psychodynamics of Alcoholism.* Springfield, Ill.: Charles C. Thomas, 1986.

O'Brien, Robert. *Encyclopedia of Understanding Alcohol and Other Drugs.* New York: Facts On File, 1999.

Powter, Susan. *Sober—and Staying That Way: The Missing Link in the Cure for Alcoholism.* New York: Simon & Schuster, 1997.

Rosenberg, Maxine B. *Not My Family: Sharing the Truth About Alcoholism.* New York: Bradbury Press, 1988.

St. Clair, Harvey R. *Recognizing Alcoholism and Its Effects: A Mini-Guide.* New York: Karger, 1991.

Torr, James D., ed. *Alcoholism (Current Controversies).* San Diego: Greenhaven Press, 2000.

Alternative Therapies (see COMPLEMENTARY THERAPIES)

Alzheimer's Disease

Bellenir, Karen, ed. *Alzheimer's Disease Sourcebook: Basic Consumer Health Information about Alzheimer's Disease, Related Disorders, and Other Dementias,* 2nd ed. Detroit, Mich.: Omnigraphics, 1999.

Davidson, Frena Gray. *Alzheimer's Disease: Frequently Asking Questions, Making Sense of the Journey.* Los Angeles: Contemporary Books, 1998.

Davies, Helen D. *Alzheimer's: The Answers You Need.* Forest Knolls, Calif.: Elder Books, 1998.

Given, C. W., C. E. Collins, and B. A. Givens. "Sources of Stress among Families Caring for Relatives with Alzheimer's Disease." *Nursing Clinics of North America* 23 (1988): 69–81.

Hall, Elizabeth T. *Caring for a Loved One with Alzheimer's Disease: A Christian Perspective.* New York: Haworth Pastoral Press, 2000.

Harmon, Dan. *Life Out of Focus: Alzheimer's Disease and Related Disorders.* Philadelphia: Chelsea House Publishers, 1999.

Medina, John. *What You Need to Know about Alzheimer's.* Oakland, Calif.: New Harbinger, 1999.

Reekum, Robert van, Martine Simard, and Karl Farcnik. "Diagnosis of Dementia and Treatment of Alzheimer's Disease." *Canadian Family Physician* 45 (April 1999): 945–952.

Warner, Mark L. *The Complete Guide to Alzheimer-Proofing Your Home.* West Lafayette, Ind.: Purdue University Press, 1998.

Anorexia Nervosa (see EATING DISORDERS)

Anxiety and Anxiety Disorders (see also OBSESSIVE-COMPULSIVE DISORDER; PHOBIAS; POST-TRAUMATIC STRESS DISORDER)

Agras, M. W. *Panic: Facing Fears, Phobias, and Anxiety.* New York: W. H. Freeman, 1985.

Barlow, D. H. *Anxiety and Its Disorders: The Nature and Treatment of Anxiety and Panic.* New York: The Guilford Press, 1988.

Barlow, D. H., and J. A. Cerny. *The Psychological Treatment of Panic.* New York: The Guilford Press, 1988.

Barlow, D. H., and Michael Craske. *Mastery of Your Anxiety and Panic II.* Albany, N.Y.: Graywind Publications, 1994.

Bassett, Lucinda. *From Panic to Power.* New York: HarperCollins, 1995.

Beck, Aaron. *Anxieties and Phobias.* New York: Basic Books, 1985.

Bloomfield, Harold H. *Healing Anxiety with Herbs.* New York: HarperCollins, 1998.

Bourne, Edmund J. *The Anxiety and Phobia Workbook.* Oakland, Calif.: New Harbinger, 1990.

Dattilio, Frank M., and Jesus A. Salas-Auvert. *Panic Disorder: Assessment and Treatment through a Wide-Angle Lens.* Phoenix, Ariz.: Zeig, Tucker & Co., 2000.

Doctor, Ronald M., and Ada P. Kahn. *Encyclopedia of Phobias, Fears, and Anxieties.* New York: Facts On File, 2000.

Feniger, Mani. *Journey from Anxiety to Freedom: Moving Beyond Panic and Phobias and Learning to Trust Yourself.* Rocklin, Calif.: Prima, 1997.

Freeman, Lynne. *Panic Free: Eliminate Anxiety/Panic Attacks without Drugs and Take Control of Your Life.* Sherman Oaks, Calif.: Arden Books, 1999.

Gardner, James. *Overcoming Anxiety, Panic, and Depression: New Ways to Regain Your Confidence.* Franklin Lakes, N.J.: Career Press, 2000.

Gorman, J. M., M. R. Leibowitz, and D. F. Klein. *Panic Disorders and Agoraphobia.* Kalamazoo, Mich.: Current Concepts in Medicine, 1984.

Goodwin, D. W. *Anxiety.* New York: Oxford University Press, 1986.

Gold, Mark S. *The Good News About Panic, Anxiety and Phobias.* New York: Bantam Books, 1990.

Marks, Isaac. *Living with Fear.* New York: McGraw-Hill, 1980.

————. *Fears, Phobias, and Rituals: Panic, Anxiety, and Their Disorders.* New York: Oxford University Press, 1987.

Nardo, Don. *Anxiety and Phobias.* New York: Chelsea House, 1992.

Ornstein, Robert, and David S. Sobel. "Calming Anxiety, Phobias and Panic." *Mental Medicine Update* III, no. 3 (1994).

Root, Benjamin A. *Understanding Panic and Other Anxiety Disorders.* Jackson, Miss.: University Press of Mississippi, 2000.

Ross, Jerilyn. *Triumph Over Fear: A Book of Help and Hope for People with Anxiety, Panic Attacks, and Phobias.* New York: Bantam Books, 1994.

Swedo, Susan, and H. L. Leonard. *It's Not All in Your Head: Now Women Can Discover the Real Causes of Their Most Commonly Misdiagnosed Health Problems.* New York: HarperCollins, 1996.

Trickett, Shirley. *Panic Attacks: A Natural Approach.* Berkeley, Calif.: Ulysses Press, 1999.

Warneke, Lorne. "Anxiety Disorders: Focus on Obsessive-Compulsive Disorder." *Canadian Family Physician* 39 (July 1993).

Wolman, Benjamin, and George Sticker. *Anxiety and Related Disorders: A Handbook.* New York: Wiley 1991.

Attention Deficit Hyperactivity Disorder

Barkley, Russell. *Attention Deficit Hyperactivity Disorder: A Handbook for Diagnosis and Treatment.* New York: Guilford Press, 1990.

Connelly, Elizabeth Russell. *Conduct Unbecoming: Hyperactivity, Attention Deficit, and Disruptive Behavior Disorders.* Philadelphia: Chelsea House Publishers, 1999.

Hallowell, Edward M., and J. J. Ratey. *Driven to Distraction.* New York: Pantheon, 1994.

————. *Answers to Distraction.* New York: Pantheon, 1995.

Ingersoll, Barbara D. *Daredevils and Daydreamers: New Perspectives on Attention Deficit/Hyperactivity Disorder.* New York: Doubleday, 1998.

LeFever, Gretchen B., Keila V. Dawson, and Ardythe L. Morrow. "The Extent of Drug Therapy for Attention Deficit-Hyperactivity Disorder among Children in Public Schools." *American Journal of Public Heath* 89, no. 9 (Sept. 1999): 1359–1364.

Mate, Gabor. "A New Perspective on Attention Deficit Disorder." *Canadian Family Physician* 46 (Feb. 2000): 408.

Sears, William. *The A.D.D. Book: New Understandings, New Approaches to Parenting Your Child.* Boston: Little, Brown, 1998.

Silver, Larry B. *Dr. Larry Silver's Advice to Parents on Attention Deficit Hyperactivity Disorder.* New York: Times Books, 1999.

Umansky, Warren. *ADD: Helping Your Child.* New York: Warner Books, 1994.

Behavior Therapy

Bellack, A. S., and M. Hersen, eds. *Dictionary of Behavioral Therapy Techniques.* New York: Pergamon Press, 1985.

Cantela, J. R., and A. Kearney. *The Covert Conditioning Handbook.* New York: Springer Publishing, 1986.

Hersen, M., ed. *Pharmacological and Behavioral Treatment: An Integrative Approach.* New York: Wiley, 1986.

Krug, R., and A. R. Cass. *Behavioral Sciences.* New York: Springer-Verlag, 1987.

Milne, D. *Training Behavior Therapists: Methods, Evaluation and Implication with Parents, Nurses and Teachers.* Cambridge, Mass: Brookline Books, 1986.

Body Image

Bauman, S. "Physical Aspects of the Self: A Review of Some Aspects of Body Image Development in Childhood." *Psychiatria Clinica North America* 4, no. 3 (1981): 455–470.

Brain, Robert. *The Decorated Body.* New York: Harper and Row, 1979.

Davis, Brangien. *What's Real, What's Ideal: Overcoming a Negative Body Image.* New York: Rosen, 1999.

Gillies, D. A. "Body Image Changes Following Illness and Injury." *Journal of Enterostomal Therapy* 11, no. 5 (1984): 186–189.

Janelli, L. M. "Body Image in Older Adults: A Review of the Literature." *Rehabilitation Nursing* 11, no. 4 (1986): 6–8.

Lasry, J. C. et al. "Depression and Body Image Following Mastectomy and Lumpectomy." *Journal of Chronic Diseases* 40, no. 6 (1987): 529–534.

Leon, G. et al. "Sexual, Body Image and Personality Attitudes in Anorexia Nervosa." *Journal of Abnormal Child Psychology* 13, no. 2 (1985): 245–258.

McFarland, Barbara. *Shame and Body Image: Culture and the Compulsive Eater.* Deerfield Beach, Fla.: Health Communications, 1990.

Moe, Barbara, A. *Understanding Negative Body Image.* New York: Rosen, 1999.

Boredom

Beckelman, Laurie. *Boredom.* Parsippany, N.J.: Crestwood House, 1995.

Csikszentmihalyi, Mihaly. *Beyond Boredom and Anxiety.* San Francisco: Josey-Bass Publishers, 1975.

Farmer, R., and N. Sundberg. "Boredom Proneness—the Development and Correlates of a New Scale." *Journal of Personality Assessment* 50, no. 1 (1986): 4–17.

Frick, S. "Diagnosing Boredom, Confusion, and Adaptation in School Children." *Journal of School Health* 55, no. 7 (1985): 254–257.

Leckart, B., and L. G. Weinberger. *Up from Boredom, Down from Fear.* New York: Richard Marek Publishers, 1980.

Morrant, J. C. A. "Boredom in Psychiatric Practice." *Canadian Journal of Psychiatry* 29 (1984): 431–434.

Rediger, G. L. *Lord, Don't Let Me Be Bored.* Philadelphia: Westminster Press, 1986.

Savitz, J., and M. Friedman. "Diagnosing Boredom and Confusion." *Nursing Research* 30, no. 1 (1981): 16–19.

Children and Mental Health

Campbell, M., W. H. Green, and S. I. Deutsch. *Child and Adolescent Psychopharmacology.* Beverly Hills, Calif.: Sage, 1985.

Eisen, Andrew R., Christopher A. Kearney, and Charles E. Schaefer. *Clinical Handbook of Anxiety Disorders in Children and Adolescents.* Northvale, N.J.: Jason Aronson, 1994.

Erikson, E. *Identity: Youth and Crisis.* New York: W. W. Norton, 1986.

Gittleman, R. *Anxiety Disorders of Childhood.* New York: Guilford, 1986.

Graham, P. *Child Psychiatry: A Developmental Approach.* New York: Oxford University Press, 1986.

Harris, P. L. *Children and Emotion: The Development of Psychological Understanding.* New York: Basil Blackwell, 1989.

Husain, Syed Arshad et al. "Stress Reactions of Children and Adolescents in War and Siege Conditions." *American Journal of Psychiatry* (Dec. 1998): 155–212.

King, Neville J., Viv Clowes-Hollins, and Thomas H. Ollendick. "The Etiology of Childhood Dog Phobia." *Behavior Research Therapy* 35, no. 1 (1997): 77.

Last, C. G., and C. C. Straus. "School Refusal and Anxiety-Disordered Children and Adolescence." *Journal of the American Academy of Childhood and Adolescent Psychology* 29 (1990): 31–35.

Muris, Peter, Harald Merckelbach and Ron Collaris. "Common Childhood Fears and Their Origins." *Behavior Research Therapy* 35, no. 10 (1997): 929–937.

Papolos, Dmitri and Janice Papolos. *The Bipolar Child.* New York: Broadway Books, 1999.

Selman, R., and A. Selman. "Children's Ideas About Friendship: A New Theory." *Psychology Today* 13 (1979): 70–80, 114.

Stewart, M., and J. Kelso. "A Two-year Follow-up of Boys with Aggressive Conduct Disorder." *Psychopathology* 20 (1987): 296–304.

Turecki, Stanley. *The Emotional Problems of Normal Children.* New York: Bantam, 1994.

Chronic Fatigue Syndrome

Brody, Jane E. "Chronic Fatigue Syndrome: How to Recognize It and What to Do about It." *New York Times,* 28 July 1988.

Fackelmann, K. A. "The Baffling Case of Chronic Fatigue Syndrome," *Science News* (Jan. 1989).

Feiden, Karyn. *Hope and Help for Chronic Fatigue Syndrome.* New York: Prentice Hall, 1990.

Hellinger, Dr. Walter C. et al. "Chronic Fatigue Syndrome and the Diagnostic Utility of Antibody to Epstein-Barr Virus Early Antigen." *Journal of American Medicine* (Aug. 19, 1988).

Manu, Dr. Peter et al. "The Frequency of the Chronic Fatigue Syndrome in Patients with Symptoms of Persistent Fatigue." *Annals of Internal Medicine* (Oct. 1, 1988).

Martin, A. W. *Steps to Fight Chronic Fatigue Syndrome for the Modern Woman.* Timmins, Ontario: R & T Press, 1999.

Patarca-Montero, Roberto, ed. *Chronic Fatigue Syndrome: Advances in Epidemiologic, Clinical, and Basic Science Research.* New York: Haworth Medical Press, 1999.

Straus, Dr. Stephen E. et al. "Acyclovir Treatment of the Chronic Fatigue Syndrome: Lack of Efficacy in a Placebo-Controlled Trial." *New England Journal of Medicine* 319, no. 26 (Dec. 29, 1988).

Tierney, Dr. Lawrence M. "Chronic Fatigue Syndrome: Current Recommendations for Diagnosis and Management." *Consultant* (March 1989).

Zoler, Mitchel L. "Chronic Fatigue: Taking the Syndrome Seriously" *Medical World News,* 12 December 1988.

Complementary Therapies (see also MIND/BODY CONNECTIONS)

Berman, Brian M. et al. "The Public Debate over Alternative Medicine: The Importance of Finding a Middle Ground." *Alternative Therapies* 6 no. 1 (Jan. 2000): 98–101.

Bloomfield, Frena. *Chinese Beliefs.* London: Arrow Books, 1983.

Butt, Gary, and Frena Bloomfield. *Harmony Rules.* London: Arrow Books, 1985.

Christi, Hakim. *The Traditional Healer's Handbook: A Classic Guide to the Medicine of Avicenna.* Rochester, Vt.: Healing Arts Press, 1991.

Eisenberg, D. et al. "Unconventional Medicine in the United States: Prevalence, Costs, and Patterns of Use." *New England Journal of Medicine* 328 (1993): 246–252.

———. *Encounters with Qi: Exploring Chinese Medicine.* New York: Norton, 1985.

Facklam, Howard. *Alternative Medicine: Cures or Myths?* New York: Twenty-First Century Books, 1996.

Feldenkrais, Moshe. *Awareness Through Movement.* New York: Harper & Row, 1977.

Fradet, Brian, ed. *The Natural Way of Healing: Stress, Anxiety and Depression.* New York: Dell Publishing, 1995.

Frawley, David. *Ayurvedic Healing: A Comprehensive Guide.* Salt Lake City, Utah: Passage Press, 1989.

Frawley, David and Vasant Lad. *The Yoga of Herbs: An Ayurvedic Guide to Herbal Medicine.* Santa Fe, N. Mex.: Lotus Press, 1986.

Gordon, James S. *Manifesto for a New Medicine: Your Guide to Healing Partnerships and Wise Use of Alternative Therapies.* Reading, Mass.: Addison-Wesley, 1996.

Heyn, Birgit. *Ayurveda: The Indian Art of Natural Medicine and Life Extension.* Rochester, Vt.: Healing Arts Press, 1990.

Kaminski, Patricia, and Richard Katz. *Flower Essence Repertory: A Comprehensive Guide to North American and English Flower Essences for Emotional and Spiritual Well-Being.* Nevada City, Calif.: The Flower Essence Society, 1994.

Lad, Dr. Vasant. *Ayurveda: The Science of Self-Healing—A Practical Guide.* Santa Fe, N.Mex.: Lotus Press, 1984.

McGill, Leonard. *The Chiropractor's Health Book: Simple Natural Exercises for Relieving Headaches, Tension and Back Pain.* New York: Crown, 1995.

Morrison, Judith M. *The Book of Ayurveda.* New York: Fireside, 1995.

Morton, Mary, and Michael Morton. *Five Steps to Selecting the Best Alternative Medicine.* Novato, Calif.: New World Library, 1996.

Moss, Charles A. "Five Element Acupuncture: Treating Body, Mind, and Spirit." *Alternative Therapies* 5, no. 5 (Sept. 1999): 52–61.

Reid, Daniel. *The Complete Book of Chinese Health and Healing.* Boston: Shambhala, 1994.

Rondberg, Terry A. *Chiropractic First: The Fastest Growing Healthcare Choice . . . Before Drugs or Surgery.* Chandler, Ariz.: The Chiropractic Journal, 1996.

Ryman, Danielle. *Aromatherapy. The Complete Guide to Plant and Flower Essences for Health and Beauty.* New York: Bantam Books, 1991.

Sachs, Judith. *Nature's Prozac: Natural Therapies and Techniques to Rid Yourself of Anxiety, Depression, Panic Attacks and Stress.* Englewood Cliffs, N.J.: Prentice Hall, 1997.

Stedman, Nancy. "You'd Better Shop Around." *Health* (Jan./Feb. 2000): 60–65.

Crisis Intervention

Aguilera, D. C., and J. M. Messick. *Crisis Intervention: Theory and Methodology,* 5th ed. St. Louis: CV Mosby, 1986.

Brownell, M. J. "The Concept of Crisis: Its Utility for Nursing." *Advances in Nursing Science* 6 (July 1984): 10–21.

Dixon, S. L. *Working with People in Crisis: Theory and Practice.* St. Louis: CV Mosby, 1979.

Everstine, D. S., and L. Everstine. *People in Crisis.* New York: Brunner/Mazel; 1983.

Schram P., and L. Burti. "Crisis Intervention Techniques Designed to Prevent Hospitalization." *Bulletin of the Meninger Clinic* 50, no. 2 (1986): 194–204.

Cross-Cultural Influences on Mental Health

Escobar, J. I. "Cross-Cultural Aspects of the Somatization Trait." *Hospital and Community Psychiatry* 38 (1987): 174–180.

Flaskerud, J. H. "The Effects of Culture-Compatible Intervention on the Utilization of Mental Health Services by Minority Clients." *Community Mental Health Journal* 22 (1986): 127–141.

Friedman, Steven. *Cultural Issues in the Treatment of Anxiety.* New York: The Guilford Press, 1997.

Jones, B. E., and B. A. Gray. "Problems in Diagnosing Schizophrenia and Affective Disorders Among Blacks." *Hospital and Community Psychiatry* 37 (1986): 61–65.

Koss, J. D. "Expectations and Outcomes for Patients Given Mental Health Care of Spiritist Healing in Puerto Rico." *American Journal of Psychiatry* 144 (1987): 56–61.

Leininger, M. M. "Transcultural Eating Patterns and Nutrition: Transcultural Nursing and Anthropological Perspectives." *Holistic Nursing Practice* 3 (1988): 16–25.

Littlewood, R., and M. Lipsedge. "The Butterfly and the Serpent: Culture, Psychopathology and Biomedicine." *Culture, Medicine and Psychiatry* 11 (1987): 289–335.

Matheson, L. "If You Are Not an Indian, How Do You Treat an Indian?" In *Cross-Cultural Training for Mental Health Professionals,* eds. H. P. Lefley and P. B. Pederson. Springfield, Ill.: Charles C. Thomas, 1986.

Mead, Margaret. *Sex and Temperament in Three Primitive Societies.* New York: William Morrow, 1963.

Murstein, Bernard I. "Qualities of Desired Spouse: A Cross-Cultural Comparison between French and American College Students." *Journal of Comparative Family Studies* 7, no. 3 (autumn 1976): 455–469.

Pachter, Lee M. "Culture and Clinical Care: Folk Illness Beliefs and Behaviors and Their Implications for Health Care Delivery." *JAMA* 271, no. 9 (March 2, 1994): 690–694.

Prince, R., and F. Tcheng-Laroche. "Culture-Bound Syndromes and International Disease Classifications." *Culture, Medicine and Psychiatry* 11 (1987): 3–19.

Dental Care and Mental Health

Getka, Eric J., and Carol R. Glass. "Behavioral and Cognitive-Behavioral Approaches to the Reduction of Dental Anxiety." *Behavior Therapy* 23 (1992): 433–448.

Jongh, Ad De et al. "One-session Cognitive Treatment of Dental Phobia: Preparing Dental Phobics for Treatment by Restructuring Negative Cognitions." *Behavior Research Therapy* 33, no. 8 (1995): 947–954, 1995.

Walker, Edward A. et al. "Assessing Abuse and Neglect and Dental Fear in Women." *JADA* 127 (April, 1998): 485–490.

Depression/Bipolar Disorder/Manic Depression

Baskin, Valerie D. *When Words Are Not Enough: The Women's Prescription for Depression and Anxiety.* New York: Broadway Books, 1997.

Bates, Tony. *Understanding and Overcoming Depression: A Common Sense Approach.* Freedom, Calif.: The Crossing Press, 2001.

Bloomfield, Harold H., and Peter McWilliams. *How to Heal Depression.* Los Angeles: Prelude Press, 1994.

Bohn, John, and James W. Jefferson, *Lithium and Manic Depression: A Guide,* rev. ed. Madison, Wis.: Lithium Information Center, University of Wisconsin, 1990.

———. "Antidepressants: Partial Response in Chronic Depression." *British Journal of Psychiatry* 165 (1994): 37–41.

———. "Overview of Mood Disorders: Diagnosis, Classification, and Management." *Clinical Chemistry* 40, no. 2 (1994): 273–278.

———. "The Morbidity and Mortality of Clinical Depression." *International Clinical Psychopharmacology.* 8 (1993): 217–220.

Fawcett, Jan, Nancy Rosenfeld, and Bernard Golden. *New Hope for People with Bipolar Disorder.* Roseville, Calif.: Prima, 2000.

Greist, John H., and James W. Jefferson. *Depression and Its Treatment: Help for the Nation's #1 Mental Problem,* rev. New York: Warner Books, 1992.

Healy, David. *The Anti-Depressant Era.* Cambridge, Mass.: Harvard University Press, 1997.

Kim, Henny H., ed. *Depression.* San Diego: Greenhaven Press, 1999.

Kramer, Peter D. *Listening to Prozac.* New York: Penguin Books, 1994.

Martin, Philip. *The Zen Path through Depression.* San Francisco: HarperSan Francisco, 1999.

Mondimore, Francis Mark. *Depression: The Mood Disease.* Baltimore: The Johns Hopkins University Press, 1993.

Muskianth, Dr. Susan. *Depression Matters.* Johannesburg, South Africa: Delta Books, 1997.

Packard, Helen C. *Prozac: The Controversial Cure.* New York: Rosen, 1998.

Quinn, Brian. *The Depression Sourcebook.* Los Angeles: Lowell House, 1997.

Reichenberg-Ullman, Judyth. *Prozac-free: Homeopathic Medications for Depression, Anxiety and Other Mental and Emotional Problems.* Rocklin, Calif.: Prima Health, 1999.

Robbins, Paul R. *Understanding Depression.* Jefferson, N.C.: McFarland, 1993.

Rosen, David H. *Transforming Depression.* New York: G.P. Putnam's Sons, 1993.

Sanders, Pete. *Depression and Mental Health.* Brookfield, Conn.: Copper Beech, 1998.

Stewart, Gail. *Teens and Depression.* San Diego: Lucent Books, 1998.

Turkington, Carol. *Making the Prozac Decision: A Guide to Antidepressants.* Los Angeles: Contemporary Books, 1997.

Whybrow, Peter C. *A Mood Apart: Depression, Mania and Other Afflictions of the Self.* New York: Basic Books, 1997.

Diagnosis and Classification of Mental Disorders

American Psychiatric Association. *Diagnostic and Statistical Manual of Mental Disorders,* 4th ed. Washington, D.C.: American Psychiatric Association, 1994.

King, L. S. *Medical Thinking: A Historical Preface.* Princeton, N.J.: Princeton University Press, 1989.

Divorce (see MARRIAGE AND DIVORCE)

Domestic Violence

Eisenstat, Stephanie, and Lundy Bancroft. "Domestic Violence." *New England Journal of Medicine* 341, no. 12 (Sept. 16, 1999): 886–892.

Limandri, B. J. "The Therapeutic Relationship with Abused Women." *Journal of Psychosocial Nursing and Mental Health Services* 25 (1987): 9–16.

Sonkin, D. J., D. Martin, and L. E. A. Walker. *The Male Batterer.* New York: Springer, 1985.

Walker, L. E. *The Battered Woman Syndrome.* New York: Springer, 1984.

Eating Disorders

Cassell, Dana K. *Encyclopedia of Obesity and Eating Disorders.* New York: Facts On File, 1994.

Devlin, M. J. et al. "Metabolic Abnormalities in Bulimia Nervosa." *Archives of General Psychiatry* 47 (1990): 144–148.

Drewnowski, A., S. A. Hopkins, and R. C. Kessler. "Prevalence of Bulimia Nervosa in the U.S. College Student Population." *American Journal of Public Health* 78 (1988): 1322–1325.

Fava, M. et al. "Neurochemical Abnormalities of Anorexia Nervosa and Bulimia Nervosa." *American Journal of Psychiatry* 146 (1989): 963–971.

Heater, Sandra Harvey. *Am I Still Visible?: A Woman's Triumph over Anorexia Nervosa.* White Hall, Va.: White Hall Books, 1983.

Hughes, T. L. et al. "Treating Bulimia with Desipramine." *Archives of General Psychiatry* 43 (1986): 182–186.

Kinoy, Barbara P., ed. *Eating Disorders: New Directions in Treatment and Recovery.* New York: Columbia University Press, 1994.

Lemberg, Raymond. *Eating Disorders: A Reference Sourcebook,* 2nd ed. Phoenix, Ariz.: Oryx Press, 1999.

Logue, C. M., R. R. Crowe, and J. A. Bean. "A Family Study of Anorexia Nervosa and Bulimia." *Comprehensive Psychiatry* 30 (1989): 179–188.

Mitchell, James E., ed. *Anorexia Nervosa and Bulimia: Diagnosis and Treatment.* Minneapolis, Minn.: University of Minnesota Press, 1985.

Mitchell, James E., R. L. Pyle, and E. D. Eckert. "A Comparison Study of Antidepressants in Structured, Intensive Group Psychotherapy in the Treatment of Bulimia Nervosa." *Archives of General Psychiatry* 47 (1990): 149–157.

Orbach, Susie. *Hunger Strike: an Anorexic's Struggle as a Metaphor for Our Age.* New York: Norton, 1986.

Romeo, Felicia F. *Understanding Anorexia Nervosa.* Springfield, Ill.: C.C. Thomas, 1986.

Sacker, Ira M. *Dying to Be Thin.* New York: Warner Books, 1987.

Sonder, Ben. *Eating Disorders: When Food Turns Against You.* New York: Franklin Watts, 1993.

Elderly and Mental Health

Berezin, M. A. "Psychotherapy of the Elderly: An Introduction." *Journal of Geriatric Psychiatry* 16, no. 3 (1983): 3–6.

Copstead, L. E., and S. Patterson. "Families of the Elderly." In *Nursing Management for the Elderly,* 2nd ed. eds. D. Carnevali and M. Patrick. Philadelphia: J. B. Lippincott, 1986.

Evans, L. K. "Sundown Syndrome in Institutionalized Elderly." *Journal of the American Geriatrics Society* 35 (1987): 101–108.

Hussian, R. A. *Geriatric Psychology: A Behavioral Perspective.* New York: Van Nostrand Reinhold, 1981.

Paulmeno, S. R. "Psychogeriatric Care: A Specialty within a Specialty." *Nursing Management* 2 (1987): 39–42.

Terry, R. D. *Aging and the Brain.* New York: Raven Press, 1988.

Faith and Spirituality

Fowler, J. W. *Stages of Faith: The Psychology of Human Development and the Quest for Meaning.* San Francisco: Harper & Row, 1981.

Frankl, V. *The Unconscious God.* New York: Washington Square Press, 1975.

Peck, M. S. *The Road Less Traveled: A New Psychology of Love, Traditional Values and Spiritual Growth.* New York: Simon & Schuster, 1978.

Tillich, P. *Dynamics of Faith.* New York: Harper & Row, 1957.

Family Interaction/Therapy

Carter, E. A., and M. McGoldrick, eds. *The Family Life Cycle: A Framework for Family Therapy.* New York: Gardner Press, 1980.

Combrinck-Graham, L. "A Developmental Model for Family Systems." *Family Process* 24 (1985): 139–150.

Gottlieb, B. H. "Social Support and the Study of Personal Relationships." *Journal of Social and Personal Relations* 2 (1985): 351.

Gray-Price, H., and S. Szczesny. "Crisis Intervention with Families of Cancer Patients: A Developmental Approach." *Topics in Clinical Nursing* 7 (1985): 58–70.

Seymour, R. J., and N. J. Dawson. "The Schizophrenic at Home." *Journal of Psychosocial Nursing* 26 (1986): 28–30.

Fantasy

Friday, Nancy. *Forbidden Flowers: More Women's Sexual Fantasies.* New York: Pocket Books, 1975.

———. *My Secret Garden: Women's Sexual Fantasies.* New York: Pocket Books, 1973.

Iwawaki, Saburo. "Sex Fantasies in Japan." *Personality Individual Differences* 4, no. 5 (1983): 543–545.

Feminist Viewpoints

Adams, Paul L. "The Mother Not the Father." *Journal of the American Academy of Psychoanalysis* 15, no. 4 (1987): 465–480.

Beauvoir, Simone de. *The Second Sex.* New York: Bantam Press, 1952.

Chicago, Judy. *The Dinner Party: A Symbol of Our Heritage.* Garden City, N.Y.: Anchor Press/Doubleday, 1979.

Friedan, Betty. *The Feminine Mystique.* New York: W. W. Norton, 1963.

Fuller, Margaret. *Woman in the Nineteenth Century.* New York: W. W. Norton, 1971.

Goldman, Emma. *Red Emma Speaks: Selected Writings and Speeches by Emma Goldman.* New York: Random House, 1972.

Greer, Germaine. *The Female Eunuch.* New York: McGraw-Hill, 1971.

Kraditor, Aileen. *Up From the Pedestal: Selected Writings in the History of American Feminism.* Chicago, Ill.: Quadrangle Books, 1968.

Millett, Kate. *Sexual Politics.* New York: Avon Books, 1971.

Morgan, Robin, ed. *Sisterhood is Powerful: An Anthology of Writings from the Woman's Liberation Movement.* New York: Vintage Books, 1970.

Rossi, Alice S., ed. *The Feminist Papers: From Adams to de Beauvoir.* New York: Bantam Books, 1988.

Spender, Dale, ed. *Feminist Theorists: Three Centuries of Key Women Thinkers.* New York: Pantheon Books, 1984.

Steinem, Gloria. *Outrageous Acts and Everyday Rebellions.* New York: Holt, Rinehart and Winston, 1983.

Woolf, Virginia. *A Room of One's Own.* New York: Harcourt, Brace, 1929.

Yllo, Kersti, and Michele Bograd. *Feminist Perspectives on Wife Abuse.* Newbury Park, Calif.: Sage Publications, 1988.

Grief

Collison, C., and S. Miller. "Using Images of the Future in Grief Work." *Image* 19 (1987): 9–11.

Johnson, S. E. *After a Child Dies: Counseling Bereaved Families.* New York: Springer, 1987.

Kubler-Ross, E. *On Death and Dying.* New York: Macmillan, 1969.

Lindemann, E. *Beyond Grief: Studies in Crisis Intervention.* New York: Aronson, 1979.

McCall, Junietta Baker. *Grief Education for Caregivers of the Elderly.* New York: Haworth Pastoral Press.

Osterweis, M., F. Solomon, and M. Green, eds. *Bereavement: Reactions, Consequences, and Care.* Washington, D.C.: National Academy Press, 1984.

Pollock, G. H. "The Mourning-Liberation Process in Health and Disease." *Psychiatria Clinica North America* 10 (1987): 345–354.

Stephenson, J. S. *Death, Grief, and Mourning: Individual and Social Realities.* New York: Macmillan, 1985.

Stewart, T., and C. R. Shields. "Grief in Chronic Illness: Assessment and Management." *Archives of Physical Medicine and Rehabilitation* 66 (1985): 447–450.

Vachon, M. L. S. "Unresolved Grief in Persons with Cancer Referred for Psychotherapy." *Psychiatria Clinica North America* 10 (1987): 467–486.

Van Praagh, James. *Health Grief: Reclaiming Life After Any Loss.* New York: Dutton, 2000.

Welshons, John E. *Awakening from Grief: Finding the Road Back to Joy.* Little Falls, N.J.: Open Heart Pub., 2000.

Worden, W. J. *Grief Counseling and Grief Therapy.* New York: Springer, 1982.

Guided Imagery (see also COMPLEMENTARY THERAPIES; MIND/BODY CONNECTIONS)

Achterberg, Jeanne. *Imagery in Healing: Shamanism and Modern Medicine.* San Francisco: Shambhala, 1985.

Burns, David. *Feeling Good: The New Mood Therapy.* New York: Avon Books, 1992.

Epstein, Gerald. *Healing Visualizations, Creating Healing through Imagery.* New York: Bantam, 1989.

Naparstek, Belleruth. *Staying Well with Guided Imagery.* New York: Warner Books, 1994.

Samuels, Michael. *Healing with the Mind's Eye.* New York: Random House, 1992.

Siegel, Bernie. *Love, Medicine and Miracles.* New York: Harper & Row, 1986.

———. *Peace, Love and Healing.* New York: Harper & Row, 1986.

Headaches

Blanchard, E. B. et al. "Placebo-controlled Evaluation of Abbreviated Progressive Muscle Relaxation and of Relaxation Combined with Cognitive Therapy in the Treatment of Tension Headache." *Journal of Consulting and Clinical Psychology* 58 (1990): 210–215.

———. "The Role of Regular Home Practice in the Relaxation Treatment of Tension Headache. *Journal of Consulting and Clinical Psychology* 59 (1991): 467–470.

Diamond, Seymour. *The Hormone Headache: New Ways to Prevent, Manage, and Treat Migraines and Other Headaches.* New York: Macmillan, 1995.

Finnigan, Jeffry. *Life Beyond Headaches.* Olympia, Wash.: Finnigan Clinic, 1999.

Hartnell, Agnes. *Migraine Headaches and the Foods You Eat: 200 Recipes for Relief.* Minneapolis: Chronimed, 1997.

Kahn, Ada P. *Headaches.* Chicago: Contemporary Books, 1983.

Inlander, Charles B., and Porter Shimer. *Headaches: 47 Ways to Stop the Pain.* New York: Walker and Company, 1995.

Maas, Paula, and Deborah Mitchell. *The Natural Health Guide To Headache Relief: The Definitive Handbook of Natural Remedies for Treating Every Kind of Headache Pain.* New York: Pocket Books, 1997.

Minirth, Frank B., with Sandy Dengler. *The Headache Book.* Nashville, Tenn.: Nelson Publishers, 1994.

Robbins, Lawrence D. *Headache Help: A Complete Guide to Understanding Headaches and the Medicines That Relieve Them.* Boston: Houghton Mifflin, 2000.

Solomon, Seymour, and Steven Fraccaro. *The Headache Book.* Yonkers, N.Y.: Consumer Reports Books, 1991.

Urbaniak, Eva. *Natural Healing for Headaches: High-Powered Cures for Ending Pain.* Gig Harbor, Wash.: Harbor Press, 2000.

Health and Well-being

Benson, Herbert. *The Wellness Book: The Complete Guide to Maintaining Health and Treating Stress-Related Illness.* Secaucus, N.J.: Carol Publishing, 1992.

Bohm, David. *Wholeness and the Implicate Order.* London: Ark, 1980.

Campbell, Joseph. *The Inner Reaches of Outer Space.* New York: Alfred Van Der Marck, 1985.

Capra, Fritjof. *The Turning Point.* New York: Bantam, 1982.

Castenada, Carlos. *The Art of Dreaming.* New York: HarperCollins, 1993.

Dubos, Rene. *Mirage of Health.* New York: Anchor Books, 1959.

Hoffer, Eric. *The True Believer.* New York: Harper & Row, 1951.

Illich, Ivan. *Medical Nemesis: The Expropriation of Health.* New York: Pantheon, 1982.

Ornstein, Robert, and David Sobel. *The Healing Brain: Breakthrough Discoveries About How the Brain Keeps Us Healthy.* New York: Simon & Schuster, 1987.

Pelletier, Kenneth R. *Sound Mind, Sound Body: A Model for Lifelong Health.* New York: Simon & Schuster, 1994.

Peterson, Christopher, and Lisa M. Bossio. *Health and Optimism.* New York: Macmillan, 1991.

Strasburg, Kate et al. *The Quest for Wholeness: An Annotated Bibliography in Patient-Centered Medicine.* Bolinas, Calif.: Commonwealth, 1991.

Stutz, David, and Bernard Feder. *The Savvy Patient: How to Be an Active Participant in Your Medical Care.* Yonkers, N.Y.: Consumer Reports Books, 1990.

Weil, Andrew. *Eight Weeks to Optimum Health: Proven Program for Taking Full Advantage of Your Body's Healing Power.* New York: Alfred A. Knopf, 1997.

Williams, R. W., and V. Williams. *Anger Kills: 17 Strategies for Controlling the Hostility That Can Harm Your Health.* New York: Times Books, 1993.

Wolinsky, Stephen. *Quantum Consciousness: The Guide to Experiencing Quantum Psychology.* Norfolk, Conn.: Bramble Books, 1993.

Homelessness

Bassuk, E. L. "The Homeless Problem." *Scientific American* 251, no. 1 (1984): 40–45.

Bassuk, E., and L. Rubin. "Homeless Children: A Neglected Population." *American Journal of Orthopsychiatry* 57 (1986): 2.

Bassuk, E. L., L. Rubin, and A. Lauriat. "Is Homelessness a Mental Health Problem?" *American Journal of Psychiatry* 141, no. 12 (1984): 1546–1550.

Bassuk, E. L., et al. "Characteristics of Sheltered Homeless Families." *American Journal of Public Health* 76 (1986): 9.

Marin, P. "Helping and Hating the Homeless." *Harper's* (Jan. 1987): 39–49.

Passaro, Joanne. *The Unequal Homeless: Men on the Streets, Women in Their Place.* New York: Routledge, 1996.

Stewart, Gail. *Homeless Teens*. San Diego, Calif.: Lucent Books, 1999.

Homosexuality/Lesbianism

Bozett, Frederick W. *Gay and Lesbian Parents*. New York: Praeger, 1987.

Clunis, D. Merilee, and G. Dorsey Green. *Lesbian Couples*. Seattle: Seal Press, 1988.

Curb, Rosemary, and Nancy Manahan, eds. *Lesbian Nuns: Breaking Silence*. Tallahassee, Fla.: Naiad Press, 1985.

Endersbe, Julie. *Homosexuality: What Does It Mean?* Mankato, Minn.: LifeMatters, 2000.

Faderman, Lillian. *Surpassing the Love of Men: Romantic Friendship and Love Between Women from the Renaissance to the Present*. New York: William Morrow, 1981.

Furnell, Peter J. "Lesbian and Gay Psychology: A Neglected Area of British Research." *Bulletin of the British Psychological Society* 39 (Feb. 1986): 41–47.

Gardner-Loulan, JoAnn. *Lesbian Sex*. San Francisco: Spinsters Ink, 1984.

Harris, Mary B., and Pauline Turner. "Gay and Lesbian Parents" *Journal of Homosexuality* 12, no. 2 (winter 1985–1986): 101–113.

Mondimore, Francis Mark. *A Natural History of Homosexuality*. Baltimore, Md.: Johns Hopkins University Press, 1996.

Owen, William F., Jr. "Medical Problems of the Homosexual Adolescent." *Journal of Adolescent Health Care* 6, no. 4 (July 1985): 278–285.

Polikoff, Nancy. "Lesbian Mothers, Lesbian Families: Legal Obstacles, Legal Challenges." *Review of Law and Social Change* 14 (1986): 907–914.

Spencer, Colin. *Homosexuality in History*. New York: Harcourt Brace, 1995.

Wyers, Norman L. "Homosexuality in the Family: Lesbian and Gay Spouses." *Social Work* 32, no. 2 (Mar.–Apr. 1987): 143–148.

Hypnosis

Bolduc, Henry Leo. *Self-Hypnosis: Scripts and Suggestions for Your Subconscious*. Palatine, Ill.: Mystical Mindscapes, 2000.

Callan, Jean. "Hypnosis: Trick or Treatment?" *Health* (May/June 1997).

Caprio, Frank Samuel. *Healing Yourself With Self-Hypnosis*. Paramus, N.J.: Prentice Hall, 1998.

Erickson, M. H., and E. L. Rossi. *Hypnotherapy: An Exploratory Casebook*. New York: Irvington, 1979.

Fisher, Stanley. *Discovering the Power of Self-Hypnosis: The Simple, Natural Mind/Body Approach to Change and Healing*. New York: Newmarket Press, 2000.

Hadley, Josie, and Carol Staudacher. *Hypnosis for Change*. Oakland, Calif.: New Harbinger Publications, 1996.

Haley, J. *Advanced Techniques of Hypnosis and Therapy: Selected Papers of Milton H. Erickson, M.D.* New York: Grune & Stratton, 1967.

Hewitt, William W. *Self-Hypnosis for a Better Life*. St. Paul, Minn.: Llewellyn Publications, 1997.

Rhue, J. W., S. J. Lynn, and I. Kirsch, eds. *Handbook of Clinical Hypnosis*. Washington, D.C.: American Psychological Association, 1993.

Rossi, E. L. *The Psychology of Mind-Body Healing: New Concepts of Therapeutic Hypnosis*. New York: Norton, 1993.

Stockwell, Shelley Lessin. *Hypnosis: How to Put a Smile on Your Face and Money in Your Pocket: The Stockwell System*. Rancho Palos Verdes, Calif.: Creatively Unlimited Press, 1998.

Immune System (See also PSYCHONEUROIMMUNOLOGY)

Borysenko, M. "The Immune system: An Overview." *Annals of Behavorial Medicine* 9 (1987): 3–10.

Cohen, S., D. A. J. Tyrrell, and A. P. Smith. "Psychological Stress and Susceptibility to the Common Cold." *New England Journal of Medicine* 325 (1991): 606–12.

Herbert, Tracy B. "Stress and the Immune System." *World Health* (Mar.–Apr. 1994).

Locke, Steven, and Douglas Colligan. *The Healer Within*, New York: New American Library, 1986.

Incest

Armstrong, Louise. *Kiss Daddy Goodnight: A Speak-Out on Incest*. New York: Pocket Books, 1979.

Brady, Katherine. *Father's Days: A True Story of Incest*. New York: Seaview Books, 1979.

Gelinas, D. J. "The Persisting Negative Effects of Incest." *Psychiatry* 46 (1983): 312–332.

Havelin, Kate. *Incest: Why Am I Afraid to Tell*. Mankato, Minn.: LifeMatters, 2000.

Miller, Deborah A., and Pat Kelly. *Coping With Incest*. New York: Rosen, 1992.

Russell, Diana E. H. *The Secret Trauma: Incest in the Lives of Girls and Women*. New York: Basic Books, 1986.

Ward, Elizabeth. *Father-Daughter Rape*. New York: Grove Press, 1985.

Legal Issues

Brakel, S. J., J. Parry and B. A. Waner. *The Mentally Disabled and the Law*, 3rd ed. Chicago: American Bar Foundation, 1985.

Sadoff, Robert L. *Legal Issues in the Care of Psychiatric Patients: A Guide for the Mental Health Professional*. New York: Springer, 1982.

Simon, J. T. *Clinical Psychiatry and the Law.* Washington, D.C.: American Psychiatric Press, 1987.

Weisstub, D. N., ed. *Law and Mental Health International Perspectives.* Toronto: Pergamon Press, 1986.

Loneliness

Hall, Radclyffe. *The Well of Loneliness.* New York: Anchor Books, 1990.

Lynch, James J. *A Cry Unheard: New Insights into the Medical Consequences of Loneliness.* Baltimore, Md.: Bancroft Press, 2000.

Moustakas, C. E. *Loneliness and Love.* Englewood Cliffs, N.J.: Prentice Hall, 1972.

Welt, S. R. "The Developmental Roots of Loneliness." *Archives Psychiatric Nursing* 1 (1987): 25–32.

Marriage and Divorce

Bray, James H. *Stepfamilies: Love, Marriage and Parenting in the First Decade.* New York: Broadway Books, 1998.

Briscoe, D. Stuart. *Marriage Matters!: Growing Through the Differences and Surprises of Life Together.* Wheaton, Ill.: H. Shaw Publishers, 1994.

Conover, Kris. *Marriage Made Simple: Fifty Hints for Building Long-Lasting Love.* New York: Plume, 1999.

David, Cynthia. *Women on the Brink of Divorce: A Guide to Self-Help Books.* Ft. Atkinson, Wis.: Highsmith Press, 1995.

Gottman, John Mordechai. *Why Marriages Succeed or Fail: What You Can Learn from the Breakthrough Research to Make Your Marriage Last.* New York: Simon & Schuster, 1994.

Heyn, Dalma. *Marriage Shock: The Transformation of Women into Wives.* New York: Villard, 1997.

Roleff, Tamara L., and Mary E. Williams, eds. *Marriage and Divorce.* San Diego: Greenhaven Press, 1997.

Raffel, Lee. *Should I Stay or Go?: How Controlled Separation Can Save Your Marriage.* Lincolnwood, Ill.: Contemporary Books, 1999.

Simpson, Eileen B. *Late Love: A Celebration of Marriage After Fifty.* Boston: Houghton Mifflin, 1994.

Meditation (see also MINDFULNESS MEDITATION)

Benson, Herbert. *The Relaxation Response.* New York: Avon Books, 1975.

———. *Beyond the Relaxation Response.* New York: Berkeley Press, 1985.

Borysenko, Joan, and J. Duscher. *On Wings of Light: Meditations for Awakening to the Source.* New York: Warner, 1992.

Chopra, Deepak. *Quantum Healing.* New York: Bantam, 1989.

———. *Creating Health: How to Wake Up the Body's Intelligence.* Boston: Houghton Mifflin, 1991.

———. *Unconditional Life.* New York: Bantam, 1992.

———. *Ageless Body, Timeless Mind.* New York: Crown, 1993.

———. *Creating Affluence: Wealth Consciousness in the Field of All Possibilities.* San Rafael, Calif.: New World Library, 1993.

Connor, Danny, with Michael Tse. *Qigong: Chinese Movement and Meditation for Health.* York Beach, Maine: Samuel Weiser, 1992.

Cousins, Norman. *The Healing Heart.* New York: Norton, 1983.

Denniston, Denish, and Peter McWilliams. *The TM Book: Transcendental Meditation, How to Enjoy the Rest of Your Life.* Allen Park, Mich.: Versemonger Press, 1975.

Dossey, L. *Space, Time and Medicine.* Boston: Shambhala, 1982.

———. *Meaning and Medicine: A Doctor's Tales of Breakthrough and Healing.* New York: Bantam, 1991.

———. *Recovering the Soul.* New York: Bantam, 1989.

Dychtwald, K. *Bodymind.* Los Angeles: Tarcher, 1986.

Levey, Joel. *Simple Meditation and Relaxation.* Berkeley, Calif.: Conari Press, 1999.

Mahesh Yogi, Maharishi. *Science of Being and Art of Living: Transcendental Meditation.* New York: Meridian, 1995.

Paulson, Genevieve Lewis. *Energy-Focused Meditation: Body, Mind, Spirit.* St. Paul, Minn.: Llewellyn, 2000.

Thondup, Tulku. *Boundless Healing: Meditation Exercises to Enlighten the Mind and Heal the Body.* Boston: Shambhala, 2000.

Memory

Baas, L. "Memory Error." *Nursing Clinics of North America* 20 (1985): 731–743.

Baddeley, Alan D. *Your Memory: A User's Guide.* London: Prion, 1993.

Galizia, V. "Pharmacotherapy of Memory Loss in the Geriatric Patient." *Drug Intelligence and Clinical Pharmacy* 18 (1984): 784–790.

Gillis, D. "Patients Suffering from Memory Loss Can Be Taught Self-Care." *Geriatric Nursing.* (Sept./Oct. 1986): 257–261.

Klatzky, R. L. *Human Memory: Structure and Processes.* New York: W. H. Freeman, 1980.

Kurland, Michael. *The Complete Idiot's Guide to Improving Your Memory.* New York: Alpha Books, 1999.

Larson, E., A. Larue, and D. Wyma. "Memory Loss: Is It Reversible?" *Patient Care* (April 30, 1987): 54–66.

Markson, E. "Gender Roles and Memory Loss in Old Age: An Exploration of Linkages." *International Jour-*

nal of Aging and Human Development 22, no. 3 (1985–86): 205–214.

Moss, M. et al. "Differential Patterns of Memory Loss Among Patients with Alzheimer's Disease, Huntington's Disease, and Alcoholic Korsakoff's Syndrome." Archives of Neurology, 43 (1986): 239–246.

Rupp, Rebecca. How We Remember and Why We Forget. New York: Three Rivers Press, 1998.

Sargeant, Delys. Remembering Well: How Memory Works, and What to Do When it Doesn't. North Carlton, Cand.: Allen & Unwin, 1998.

Squire, L. R. Memory and Brain. New York: Oxford University Press, 1987.

Thompson, R. F. "The Neurobiology of Learning and Memory." Science 233 (1986): 941–947.

Winter, Arthur. Brain Workout: Easy Ways to Power Up Your Memory, Sensory Perception, and Intelligence. New York: St. Martin's Griffin, 1997.

Men and Mental Health

Bednarik, Karl. The Male in Crisis. New York: Alfred A. Knopf, 1970.

Farrell, Warren. Why Men Are the Way They Are. New York: McGraw-Hill, 1986.

Mailer, Norman. The Prisoner of Sex. New York: New American Library, 1971.

Rogers, Katherine M. The Troublesome Helpmate: A History of Misogyny in Literature. Seattle, Wash.: University of Washington Press, 1966.

Mental Health Promotion

Greiner, P. A. "Nursing and Worksite Wellness: Missing the Boat." Holistic Nursing Practice 2 (1987): 53–60.

Marlatt, G. A., and J. R. Gordon. Relapse Prevention. New York: Guilford, 1985.

McBride, A. B. "Mental Health Effects of Women's Multiple Roles." Image 20 (1988): 41–47.

Nemcek, M. A. "Research Trends in the Health Promotion of Well Adults." American Association of Occupational Health Nurses Journal 34 (1986): 470–475.

Mental Retardation

Akesson, H. O. "The Biological Origin of Mild Mental Retardation." Acta Psychiatrica Scandinavida, 74 (1986): 3–7.

Beavers, J., R. B. Hampson, Y. F. Hulgus, and W. R. Beavers. "Coping in Families with a Retarded Child." Family Process 25 (1986): 365–377.

Dunbar, Robert E. Mental Retardation. New York: Franklin Watts, 1991.

Levy, Robert M. The Rights of People with Mental Disabilities: The Authoritative ACLU Guide to the Rights of People with Mental Illness and Mental Retardation. Carbondale, Ill.: Southern Illinois University Press, 1996.

Lubetsky, M. "The Psychiatrist's Role in the Assessment and Treatment of the Retarded Child." Child Psychiatry and Human Development 16 (1987): 261–271.

Matson, J., and C. Frame. Psychopathology Among Mentally Retarded Children and Adolescents. Beverly Hills, Calif.: Sage Publications, 1986.

Munro, J. D. "Epidemiology and the Extent of Mental Retardation." Psychiatria Clinica North America 9 (1986): 591–624.

Payton, J. B., J. E. Burkhart, M. Hersen, and W. J. Helsel. "Treatment of ADHD in Mentally Retarded Children: A Preliminary Study." Journal of American Academic Child Adolescent Psychiatry 28 (1989): 761–767.

Reiss, A. L., and L. F. Freund. "Fragile X Syndrome." Biological Psychiatry 27 (1990): 223–240.

Mind/Body Connections (see also COMPLEMENTARY THERAPIES; PSYCHONEUROIMMUNOLOGY)

Benson, Herbert. The Relaxation Response. New York: Avon Books, 1975.

———. Beyond the Relaxation Response. New York: Berkeley Press, 1985.

Borysenko, Joan. Minding the Body, Mending the Mind. New York: Bantam, 1988.

———. Guilt is the Teacher, Love is the Lesson. New York: Warner, 1991.

Chopra, Deepak. Perfect Health. New York: Harmony Books, 1990.

———. Quantum Healing: Exploring the Frontiers of Mind/Body Medicine. New York: Bantam Books, 1989.

Cousins, Norman. Head First: The Biology of Hope and the Healing Power of the Human Spirit. New York: Viking Penguin, 1990.

———. Anatomy of an Illness as Perceived by the Patient. New York: Norton, 1979.

———. The Healing Heart. New York: Norton, 1983.

Dienstfrey, Harris. Where the Mind Meets the Body. New York: HarperCollins, 1991.

Dossey, Larry. Space, Time and Medicine. Boston: Shambhala, 1982.

Goleman, Daniel, and Joel Gurin, eds. Mind Body Medicine: How to Use Your Mind For Better Health. Yonkers, N.Y.: Consumer Reports Books, 1993.

Gordon, James S. et al. Mind, Body and Health: Toward an Integral Medicine. New York: Human Sciences Press, 1984.

Locke, Steven E., and Douglas Colligan. The Healer Within: The New Medicine of Mind and Body. New York: Dutton, 1986.

Moyers, B. *Healing and the Mind.* New York: Doubleday, 1993.

Ornstein, Robert, and David Sobel. *The Healing Brain.* New York: Simon & Schuster, 1988.

Pelletier, Kenneth R. *Mind as Healer, Mind as Slayer,* rev. ed. New York: Delacorte, 1992.

———. *Sound Mind, Sound Body: A New Model for Lifelong Health.* New York: Simon & Schuster, 1994.

———. *Holistic Medicine: From Stress to Optimum Health.* Magnolia, Mass: Peter Smith, 1984.

Siegel, Bernie. *Love, Medicine and Miracles.* New York: Harper and Row, 1986.

———. *Peace, Love and Healing.* New York: Harper and Row, 1989.

Mindfulness Meditation (insight meditation)

Goldstein, Joseph, and Jack Kornfield. *Seeking the Heart of Wisdom: The Path of Insight Meditation.* Boston: Shambhala, 1987.

Hanh, Thich Nhat. *Being Peace.* Berkeley: Parallax Press, 1987.

———. *The Miracle of Mindfulness: A Manual of Meditation.* Boston: Beacon, Press, 1976.

———. *The Sun My Heart.* Berkeley: Parallax Press, 1988.

Kabat-Zinn, Jon. *Full Catastrophe Living: Using the Wisdom of Your Body and Mind to Face Stress, Pain and Illness.* New York: Delacorte Press, 1991.

———. *Wherever You Go, There You Are.* New York, Hyperion, 1994.

Levine, Stephen. *A Gradual Awakening.* Garden City, N.Y.: Anchor/Doubleday, 1979.

Suzuki, Shunryu. *Zen Mind, Beginner's Mind.* New York: Weatherhill, 1986.

Neurobiology

Andreasen, N. C. "Brain Imaging: Applications in Psychiatry" *Science* 239 (1988): 1381–1388.

Andreasen, N. C., ed. *Brain Imaging: Applications in Psychiatry.* Washington, D.C.: American Psychiatric Press, 1989.

Baron, M. et al. "Genetic Linkage Between X-Chromosome Markers and Bipolar Affective Illness." *Nature* 326 (1987): 289–292.

Carlton, P., and P. Manowitz. "Dopamine and Schizophrenia: An Analysis of the Theory." *Neuroscience and Biobehavioral Review* 8 (1984): 137–151.

Cooper, J. R., F. E. Bloom, R. H. Roth. *The Biochemical Basis of Neuropharmacology,* 5th ed. New York: Oxford University Press, 1987.

Doane, B. K., and K. F. Livingston. *The Limbic System: Functional Organization and Clinical Disorders.* New York: Raven, 1986.

Fuster, J. M. *The Prefrontal Cortex: Anatomy, Physiology, and Neuropsychology of the Frontal Lobe,* 2nd ed. New York: Raven, 1989.

Gold, P., F. Goodwin, and G. Chrousos. "Clinical and Biochemical Manifestations of Depression: Relation to the Neurobiology of Stress, Part 1." *New England Journal of Medicine* 319 (1988): 348–353.

Seeman, P. et al. "Elevation of Brain Neuroleptic/Dopamine Receptors in Schizophrenia," in *Perspectives in Schizophrenia Research,* eds. C. Baxter and T. Melnechuk. New York: Raven Press, 1980.

Watson, J. D., J. Tooze, and D. T. Kurtz. *Recombinant DNA: A Short Course.* New York: W. H. Freeman, 1983.

Nutrition for Better Mental Health

Brody, Jane. *Jane Brody's Nutrition Book.* New York: W.W. Norton, 1981.

Brown, Judith E. *Everywoman's Guide to Nutrition.* Minneapolis: University of Minnesota Press, 1991.

Finn, Susan Calvert, and Linda Stern. *The Real Life Nutrition Book: Making the Right Food Choices without Changing Your Life-Style.* New York: Penguin Books, 1992.

Haas, Robert. *Eat Smart, Think Smart: How to Use Nutrients and Supplements to Achieve Maximum Mental and Physical Performance.* New York: HarperCollins, 1994.

Kotsanis, Frank N., and Maureen A. Mackey, eds. *Nutrition in the '90s: Current Controversies and Analysis,* vol. 2. New York: M. Dekker, 1994.

Quillan, Patrick. *Beating Cancer with Nutrition.* Tulsa, Okla.: Nutrition Times Press, 1994.

Werbach, Melvyn. *Healing Through Nutrition: A Natural Approach to Treating 50 Common Illnesses with Diet and Nutrients.* New York: HarperCollins, 1993.

Obsessive-Compulsive Disorder
(see also ANXIETY DISORDERS)

Alper, Gerald. *The Puppeteers: Studies of Obsessive Control.* New York: Fromm International Publishing, 1994.

Chansky, Tamar Ellsas. *Freeing Your Child From Obsessive-Compulsive Disorder: A Powerful, Practical Program for Parents of Children and Adolescents.* New York: Times Books, 2000.

DeSilva, Padmal. *Obsessive-Compulsive Disorder: The Facts.* New York: Oxford University Press, 1998.

Gravitz, Herbert L. *Obsessive-Compulsive Disorder: New Help for the Family.* Santa Barbara, Calif.: Healing Visions Press, 1998.

Livingston, B. *Learning to Live With Obsessive-Compulsive Disorder*. Milford, Conn.: OCD Foundation, 1989.

Rappaport, Judith. *The Boy Who Couldn't Stop Washing: The Experience and Treatment of Obsessive-Compulsive Disorder*. New York: Dutton, 1989.

Reyes, Karen. "Obsessive-Compulsive Disorder: There is Help." *Modern Maturity* (Nov.–Dec. 1995).

Waltz, Mitzi. *Obsessive Compulsive Disorder: Help for Children and Adolescents*. Cambridge, Mass.: O'Reilly, 2000.

Pain

Bogin, Meg. *The Path of Pain Control*. Boston: Houghton, Mifflin, 1982.

Corey, David, with Stan Solomon. *Pain: Free Yourself for Life*. New York: Dutton, 1989.

Hardy, Paul A. J. *Chronic Pain Management: The Essentials*. London: Greenwich Medical Media, 1997.

Rowh, Mark. "Coping With Pain." *The Rotarian* (June 2000): 27–28.

Singh Khalsa, Dharma. *The Pain Cure: The Proven Medical Program That Helps End Your Chronic Pain*. New York: Warner Books, 1999.

Stacy, Charles B. et al. *The Fight Against Pain*. Yonkers, N.Y.: Consumer Reports Books, 1992.

Panic Attacks and Panic Disorder (see anxiety and anxiety disorders)

Performance Anxiety

Dunkel, Stuart Edward. *The Audition Process: Anxiety Management and Coping Strategies*. Stuyvesant, N.Y.: Pendragon Press, 1989.

Moss, Robert. "Stage Fright Is Actors' Eternal Nemesis," *New York Times*, 6 January 1992, 2 (E).

Salmon, P. G. "A Psychological Perspective on Musical Performance Anxiety: A Review of the Literature." *Medical Problems of Performing Arists* (March 1990): 2–11.

Salmon, Paul. *Notes From the Green Room: Coping With Stress and Anxiety in Musical Performance*. New York: Lexington Books, 1992.

Steptoe, A., and H. Fidler. "Stage Fright and Orchestral Musicians: A Study of Cognitive Behavioral Strategies and Performance Anxiety." *British Journal of Psychology* 78 (1987): 241–49.

Wesner, R. B., R. Noyes, Jr., and T. L. Davis. "The Occurrence of Performance Anxiety Among Musicians." *Journal of Affective Disorders* 18 (1990): 177–85.

Pharmacological Approach for Mental Health Concerns

Appleton, William S. *Prozac and the New Antidepressants: What You Need to Know About Prozac, Zoloft, Paxil, Luvox, Wellbutrin, Effexor, Serzone, and More*. New York: Plume, 1997.

Davidson, J. R. T., S. M. Ford, R. D. Smith, and N. L. S. Potts. "Long-term Treatment of Social Phobia Clonazapam." *Journal of Clinical Psychiatry* 52, no. 11 (1991): 16–20.

Fieve, Ronald R. *Prozac*. New York: Avon, 1994.

Liebowitz, M. R. et al. "Treatment of Social Phobia with Drugs Other Than Benzodiazepines." *Journal of Clinical Psychiatry* 52 (1991): 10–15.

Monroe, Judy. *Antidepressants*. Springfield, N.J.: Enslow Publishers, 1997.

Turkington, Carol. *Making the Prozac Decision: A Guide to Antidepressants*. Los Angeles: Lowell House, 1997.

Wilkinson, Beth. *Drugs and Depression*. New York: Rosen, 1994.

Phobias (see also ANXIETY DISORDERS)

Bourne, Edmund J. *The Anxiety & Phobia Workbook*. Oakland, Calif.: New Harbinger Publications, 1995.

Cheek, J. *Conquering Shyness*. New York: Dell, 1989.

Doctor, Ronald M., and Ada P. Kahn. *Encyclopedia of Phobias, Fears and Anxieties*. New York: Facts On File, 2000.

DuPont, Robert L. *Phobia: A Comprehensive Summary of Modern Treatments*. New York: Brunner/Mazel, 1982.

Jampolsky, Gerald. *Love Is Letting Go of Fear*. New York: Bantam Books, 1979.

Marks, Isaac M. *Living with Fear*. New York: McGraw-Hill, 1980.

———. *Fears, Phobias, and Rituals*. New York: Oxford University Press, 1987.

Marshall, John R. *Social Phobia: From Shyness to Stage Fright*. New York: Basic Books, 1994.

Markway, B. G. et al. *Dying of Embarrassment: Help for Social Anxiety and Phobias*. Oakland, Calif.: New Harbinger, 1992.

Monroe, Judy. *Phobias: Everything You Wanted to Know, but Were Afraid to Ask*. Springfield, N.J.: Enslow Publishers, 1996.

Nardo, Don. *Anxiety and Phobias*. New York: Chelsea House, 1992.

Uhde, T. W., M. E. Tancer, B. Black, and T. M. Brown. "Phenomenology and Neurobiology of Social Phobias: Comparison with Panic Disorder." *Journal of Clinical Psychology* 52 (November 1991): 31–40.

Zane, Manuel D., and Harry Milt. *Your Phobia*. Washington, D.C.: American Psychiatric Press, 1984.

Post-Traumatic Stress Disorder (PTSD)
(see also ANXIETY DISORDERS)

Catherall, Donald Roy. *Back from the Brink: A Family Guide to Overcoming Traumatic Stress.* New York: Bantam Books, 1992.

Egendorf, A. *Healing from the War: Trauma and Transformation After Vietnam.* New York: Houghton Mifflin, 1985.

Eitinger, Leo, and Robert Krell, with Miriam Rieck. *The Psychological and Medical Effects of Concentration Camps and Related Persecutions on Survivors of the Holocaust.* Vancouver: University of British Columbia Press, 1985.

Eth, S., and R. S. Pynoos. *Post-Traumatic Stress Disorder in Children.* Washington, D.C.: American Psychiatric Press, 1985.

Herman, Judith. *Trauma and Recovery.* New York: Basic Books, 1992.

Lindy, Jacob D. *Vietnam: A Casebook.* New York: Brunner/Mazel, 1987.

Peterson, Kirtland C., Maurice F. Prout, and Robert A. Schwartz. *Post-Traumatic Stress Disorder: A Clinician's Guide.* New York: Plenum Press, 1991.

Porterfield, Kay Marie. *Straight Talk About Post-Traumatic Stress Disorder: Coping with the Aftermath of Trauma.* New York: Facts On File, 1996.

Sonnenberg, S. M., A. S. Blank, and J. A. Talbott, eds. *The Trauma of War: Stress and Recovery in Vietnam Veterans.* Washington, D.C.: American Psychiatric Press, 1985.

Van der Kolk, B. A., ed. *Post-Traumatic Stress Disorder: Psychological and Biological Sequelae.* Washington, D.C.: American Psychiatric Press, 1996.

Psychology, Contemporary (see also
COMPLEMENTARY THERAPIES; MIND/BODY CONNECTIONS; PSYCHONEUROIMMUNOLOGY)

Berne, Eric. *Games People Play.* New York: Grove Press, 1964.

Borysenko, Joan. *Guilt Is the Teacher, Love Is the Lesson.* New York: Warner Books, 1990.

Bradshaw, John. *Bradshaw On: The Family.* Deerfield Beach, Fla.: Health Communications, 1988.

———. *Healing the Shame That Binds You.* Deerfield Beach, Fla.: Health Communications, 1988.

Cousins, Norman. *The Healing Heart.* New York: Avon Books, 1984.

Csikzentmihalyi, Mihaly. *Flow: The Psychology of Optimal Experience.* New York: HarperCollins, 1991.

Peck, M. Scott. *The Road Less Traveled.* New York: Simon & Schuster, 1978.

Wolinsky, Stephen H. *Trances People Live: Healing Approaches in Quantum Psychology.* Norfolk, Conn.: Bramble, 1991.

Psychoneuroimmunology

Ader, Robert, D. Felton, and N. Cohen, eds. *Psychoneuroimmunology,* 2nd ed. San Diego: Academic Press, 1990.

Bohm, David. *Wholeness and the Implicate Order.* London: Routledge and Kegan Paul, 1980.

Cousins, Norman. *Anatomy of an Illness.* New York: Bantam Books, 1981.

Kiecolt-Glaser, J. K., and R. Glaser. "Psychoneuroimmunology: Can Psychological Interventions Modulate Immunity?" *Journal of Consulting and Clinical Psychology* 60 (1992): 569–575.

Relaxation

Agras, W. S., C. B. Taylor, H. C. Kraemer, M. A. Southam, and J. A. Schneider. "Relaxation Training for Essential Hypertension at the Worksite: II. The Poorly Controlled Hypertensive." *Psychosomatic Medicine* 49 (1987): 264–273.

Benson, Herbert. *The Relaxation Response.* New York: Avon Books, 1975.

———. *Beyond the Relaxation Response.* New York: Berkeley Press, 1985.

———. *Your Maximum Mind.* New York: Times Books, 1987.

Benson, Herbert, Eileen M. Stuart, and staff of the Mind/Body Medical Institute. *The Wellness Book: The Comprehensive Guide to Maintaining Health and Treating Stress-Related Illness.* New York: Carol, 1992.

Blumenfeld, Larry, ed. *The Big Book of Relaxation: Simple Techniques to Control the Excess Stress in Your Life.* Roslyn, N.Y.: Relaxation Company, 1994.

Davis, Martha, Elizabeth Robbins Eshelman, and Matthew McKay. *The Relaxation and Stress Reduction Workbook.* Oakland, Calif.: New Harbinger Publications, 1995.

Schizophrenia

Andreasen, N. C. "The Diagnosis of Schizophrenia." *Schizophrenia Bulletin* 13 (1987): 9–22.

Baron, M. "Genetics of Schizophrenia." *Biological Psychiatry* 21 (1986): 1051–1066.

Black, D. W., and T. J. Boffeli. "Simple Schizophrenia: Past, Present, and Future." *American Journal of Psychiatry* 146 (1989): 1267–1273.

Breier, A., and B. M. Astrachan. "Characterization of Schizophrenic Patients Who Commit Suicide." *American Journal of Psychiatry* 141 (1984): 206–209.

Casanova, M. F., and J. E. Kleinman. "The Neuropathology of Schizophrenia: A Critical Assessment of Research Methodologies." *Biological Psychiatry* 27 (1990): 353–362.

Freedman, R. et al. "Neurobiological Studies of Sensory Gating in Schizophrenia." *Schizophrenia Bulletin* 13 (1987): 669–678.

Friedman, Michelle S. *Everything You Need to Know About Schizophrenia.* New York: Rosen, 2000.

Geyer, M. A., and D. L. Braff. "Startle Habituation and Sensorimotor Gating in Schizophrenia and Related Animal Models." *Schizophrenia Bulletin* 13 (1987): 643–668.

Hare, E. H. "Epidemiology of Schizophrenia and Affective Psychoses." *British Medical Bulletin* 43 (1987): 514.

Harmon, Daniel E. *Schizophrenia: Losing Touch With Reality.* Philadelphia: Chelsea House, 2000.

Hyde, Alexander P. *Living With Schizophrenia.* Chicago: Contemporary Books, 1980.

Kane, J. et al. "Clozapine for the Treatment of Resistant Schizophrenia." *Archives of General Psychiatry* 45 (1988): 789–796.

Leete, E. "The Treatment of Schizophrenia: A Patient's Perspective." *Hospital and Community Psychiatry* 38 (1987): 5.

Levitt, J. J., and M. T. Tsuang. "The Heterogeneity of Schizoaffective Disorder: Implications for Treatment." *American Journal of Psychiatry* 145 (1988): 926–936.

Parker, G., P. Johnston, and L. Hayward. "Parental 'Expressed Emotion' as a Predictor of Schizophrenic Relapse." *Archives of General Psychiatry* 45 (1988): 806.

Tsuang, Ming T. *Schizophrenia: The Facts.* New York: Oxford University Press, 1997.

Self-Esteem

Dobson, James C. *The New Hide and Seek: Building Self-Esteem in Your Child.* Grand Rapids, Mich.: Fleming H. Revell, 1999.

Hazelton, Deborah M. *Solving the Self-Esteem Puzzle.* Deerfield Beach, Fla.: 1991.

Hillman, Carolynn. *Recovery of Your Self-Esteem.* New York: Simon & Schuster, 1992.

Johnson, Carol. *Self-Esteem Comes In All Sizes.* New York: Doubleday, 1995.

Kahn, Ada P., and Sheila Kimmel. *Empower Yourself: Every Woman's Guide to Self-Esteem.* New York: Avon Books, 1997.

Lindenfield, Gael. *Self-Esteem.* New York: HarperPaperbacks, 1997.

McKay, Matthew. *The Self-Esteem Companion: Simple Exercises to Help You Challenge Your Inner Critic and Celebrate Your Personal Strengths.* Oakland, Calif.: New Harbinger Publications, 1999.

Minchinton, Jerry. *Maximum Self-Esteem: The Handbook for Reclaiming Your Sense of Self-Worth.* Yanzant, Miss.: Arnford House, 1993.

Prato, Louis. *Be Your Own Best Friend: How to Achieve Greater Self-Esteem, Health, and Happiness.* New York: Berkley Books, 1994.

Steinem, Gloria. *Revolution From Within: A Book of Self-Esteem.* Boston: Little, Brown, 1992.

Sexually Transmitted Diseases

Breitman, Patti. *How to Persuade Your Lover to Use a Condom and Why You Should.* Rocklin, Calif.: Prime, 1987.

Curran, Christine Perdan. *Sexually Transmitted Diseases.* Springfield, N.J.: Enslow Publishers, 1998.

Dudley, William, ed. *Sexually Transmitted Diseases.* San Diego: Greenhaven Press, 1999.

Endersbe, Julie. *Sexually Transmitted Diseases: How Are They Prevented?* Mankato, Minn.: LifeMatters, 2000.

Kilby, Donald. *A Manual of Safe Sex: Intimacy without Fear.* Toronto: B. C. Decker, 1986.

Little, Marjorie. *Sexually Transmitted Diseases.* Philadelphia: Chelsea House, 2000.

Lumiere, Richard and Stephen Cook. *Healthy Sex. . . . And Keeping It That Way: A Complete Guide to Sexual Infections.* New York: Simon & Schuster, 1983.

Marr, Lisa. *Sexually Transmitted Diseases: A Physician Tells You What You Need to Know.* Baltimore, Md.: Johns Hopkins University Press, 1998.

Sleep

Caldwell, J. Paul. *Sleep: Everything You Need to Know.* Willowdale, Ontario: Firefly Books, 1997.

Dee, Nerys. *Your Dreams and What They Mean: How to Understand the Secret Language of Sleep.* San Bernardino, Calif.: R. Reginald/Borgo Press, 1990.

Dement, William C., and Christopher Vaughan. *The Promise of Sleep.* New York: Delacorte Press, 1999.

Ernst, E. *Sleep: Practical Ways to Restore Health Using Complementary Medicine.* New York: Sterling, 1999.

Inlander, Charles B. *67 Ways to Good Sleep.* New York: Walker, 1995.

Lamberg, Lynne. *The American Medical Association Guide to Better Sleep.* New York: Random House, 1984.

Silverstein, Alvin, Virginia Silverstein, and Laura Silverstein Nunn. *Sleep.* Danbury, Conn.: Franklin Watts, 2000.

Smoking (see also ADDICTIONS)

Buckley, Christopher. *Thank You For Not Smoking.* New York: Random House, 1994.

Hammond, S. Katharine. "Environmental Tobacco Smoke Presents Substantial Risk in Workplaces." *The*

Journal of the American Medical Association (Sept. 26, 1995).

Hirschfelder, Arlene B. *Encyclopedia of Smoking and Tobacco.* Phoenix, Ariz.: Oryz Press, 1999.

Liesges, Robert C., and Margaret DeBon. *How Women Can Finally Stop Smoking.* Alameda, Calif.: Hunter House, 1994.

Rogers, Jacquelyn. *You Can Stop Smoking.* New York: Pocket Books, 1995.

Sanders, Pete and Steve Myers. *Smoking.* Brookfield, Conn.: Copper Beech Books, 1996.

Pietrusza, David. *Smoking.* San Diego: Lucent Books, 1997.

Social Phobias (see ANXIETY AND ANXIETY DISORDERS; PHOBIAS)

Social Support, Support Groups, and Self-help

Kahn, Ada P. "Psychosocial Support Influences Survival of Cancer Patients." *Psychiatric News* (Oct. 1991).

Kreiner, Anna. *Everything You Need to Know About Creating Your Own Support System.* New York: Rosen, 1996.

Pilisuk, Marc, and Susan H. Parks. *The Healing Web: Social Networks and Human Survival.* Hanover, N.H.: University Press of New England, 1986.

Spiegel, David. *Living Beyond Limits.* New York: Times Books, 1993.

White, Barbara J., and Edward J. Madara. *The Self-Help Sourcebook: Finding and Forming Mutual Aid Self-Help Groups.* Denville, N.J.: American Self-Help Clearinghouse, St. Clares-Riverside Medical Center, 1992.

Stress and Stress Management

Brammer, L. M., *How to Cope with Life Transitions: The Challenge of Personal Change.* New York: Hemisphere Publishing, 1991.

Bridges, W. *Managing Transitions: Making the Most of Change.* Reading, Mass.: Wesley, 1991.

Colin, Stacey. "How to Find Your Stress Hot Spots." *McCalls* (Sept. 1994).

Eliot, Robert S. *From Stress to Strength: How to Lighten Your Load and Save Your Life.* New York: Bantam Books, 1994.

Evans, Karin. "Is Stress Wrecking Your Mood?" *Health* (April 2000): 119–124.

Feder, Barnaby J., "A Spreading Pain, and Cries for Justice," *New York Times,* 5 June 1994.

Gordon, James S. *Stress Management.* New York: Chelsea House, 1990.

Hafen, B. Q., K. J. Frandsen, K. J. Karren, and K. R. Hooker. *The Health Effects of Attitudes, Emotions and Relationships.* Provo, Utah: EMS Associates, 1992.

Kahn, Ada P. *Stress A to Z: A Sourcebook for Facing Everyday Challenges.* New York: Facts On File, 2000.

Lark, Susan M. *Anxiety and Stress: A Self-Help Program.* Los Altos, Calif.: Westchester Publishing, 1993.

Lehrer, Paul M., and Robert L. Woolfolk, eds. *Principles and Practice of Stress Management,* 2nd ed. New York: The Guilford Press, 1993.

Maddi, Salvatore, and Suzanne Kobasa. *The Hardy Executive: Health under Stress.* Homewood, Ill.: Dow Jones-Irwin, 1984.

Miller, Lyle H., and Alma Dell Smith. *The Stress Solution: An Action Plan to Manage the Stress in Your Life.* New York: Pocket Books, 1993.

Ornish, Dean. *Stress, Diet, and Your Heart.* New York: Holt, Rinehart and Winston, 1983.

Padus, Emrika, ed. *The Complete Guide to Your Emotions and Your Health.* Emmaus, Pa.: Rodale, 1992.

Patel, Chandra. *The Complete Guide to Stress Management.* New York: Plenum Press, 1991.

Sapolsky, Robert M. *Why Zebras Don't Get Ulcers.* New York: W. H. Freeman, 1994.

Selye, Hans. *Stress Without Distress.* New York: J. B. Lippincott, 1974.

———. *The Stress of Life,* rev. ed. New York: McGraw-Hill, 1978.

Seaward, Brian Luke. *Stressed is Desserts Spelled Backwards: Rising above Life's Challenges with Humor, Hope, and Courage.* Berkeley, Calif.: Conari Press, 1999.

Suicide

Asberg, M., P. Nordstrom, and L. Traskman-Benz. "Biological Factors in Suicide." In *Suicide,* ed. A. Roy. Washington, D.C.: American Psychiatric Association, 1987.

Bonger, B. *The Suicidal Patient: Clinical and Legal Standards of Care.* Washington, D.C.: American Psychological Association, 1992.

Bouknight, R. R. "Suicide Attempt by Drug Overdose." *American Family Physician* 33 (1986): 4.

Boyd, J. H., and E. K. Moscicki. "Firearms and Youth Suicide." *American Journal of Public Health* 76 (1986): 1240–1242.

Brent, D. A. et al. "Risk Factors for Adolescent Suicide." *Archives of General Psychiatry* 45 (1988): 581–588.

Bunney, W. E., and J. A. Fawcett. "Biochemical Research in Depression and Suicide." In *Suicidal Behaviors,* ed. H. L. P. Resnik. Boston: Little, Brown, 1968.

———. "Possibility of a Biochemical Test for Suicide Potential." *Archives of General Psychiatry* 13 (1965): 212.

Busch, Katie A. et al. "Clinical Features of Inpatient Suicide." *Psychiatric Annals* 23, no. 5 (May 1993): 256–262.

Chamberlain, Paul. *Final Wishes: A Cautionary Tale on Death, Dignity and Physician-Assisted Suicide.* Downers Grove, Ill.: Intervarsity Press, 2000.

Donnelly, John, ed. *Suicide: Right or Wrong?* Buffalo, N.Y.: Prometheus Books, 1990.

Fawcett, Jan. "Suicide Risk Factors in Depressive and in Panic Disorder." *Journal of Clinical Psychiatry* 53, no. 3 (March 1992): 9–13.

———. "Suicide: The Consequences of Anxiety in Clinical Depression." *Primary Psychiatry* (May 1997): 35–42.

Fawcett, Jan, David C. Clark, and Katie A. Busch. "Assessing and Treating the Patient at Risk for Suicide." *Psychiatric Annals* 23, no. 5 (May 1993): 244–255.

Fawcett, T. J. et al. "Clinical Predictors of Suicide in Patients with Major Affective Disorders: A Controlled Prospective Study." *American Journal of Psychiatry* 144 (1987): 35–40.

Hawton, K. *Suicide and Attempted Suicide Among Children and Adolescents.* Beverly Hills, Calif.: Sage Publications, 1986.

Jacobs, Douglas G. *Harvard Medical School Guide to Suicide Assessment and Intervention.* San Francisco, Calif.: Jossey-Bass, 1999.

Links, Paul S. et al. "Preventing Recurrent Suicidal Behavior." *Canadian Family Physician* 45 (Nov. 1999): 2656–2660.

Maris, R. et al. *Assessment and Prediction of Suicide.* New York: Guilford, 1992.

Mullis, M. R., and P. H. Byers. "Social Support in Suicidal Patients." *Journal of Psychosocial Nursing and Mental Health Services* 25, no. 4 (1987): 16.

Murphy, G. E. "Suicide in Alcoholism." In *Suicide,* ed. A. Roy. Baltimore, Md.: Williams & Wilkins, 1986.

Murphy, G. E., and R. D. Wetzel. "The Lifetime Risk of Suicide and Alcoholism." *Archives of General Psychiatry* 47 (1990): 383–392.

Phillips, D. P., and L. L. Carstonson. "Clustering of Teenage Suicides After Television News Stories About Suicide." *New England Journal of Medicine* 55 (1986): 685–689.

Quinnett, Paul G. *The Forever Decision: For Those Thinking about Suicide and for Those Who Know, Love, or Counsel Them.* New York: Continuum, 1992.

Roy, A. "Suicide in Schizophrenia." In *Suicide,* ed. A. Roy. Baltimore, Md.: Williams & Wilkins, 1986.

Sainsbury, P. "The Epidemiology of Suicide." In *Suicide,* ed. A. Roy. Baltimore, Md.: Williams & Wilkins, 1986.

Woog, Adam. *Suicide.* San Diego: Lucent Books, 1997.

Wrobleski, Adina. *Suicide Why?: 85 Questions and Answers About Suicide.* Minneapolis: Afterwords, 1995.

Zeinert, Karen. *Suicide: Tragic Choice.* Berkeley Heights, N.J.: Enslow Publishers, 1999.

Tourette Syndrome

Cohen, D., R. Bruun, and J. Leckman. *Tourette's Syndrome.* New York: Wiley, 1991.

Pauls, D. L., and J. F. Leckman. "The Inheritance of Gilles de la Tourette's Syndrome and Associated Behaviors." *New England Journal of Medicine* 315 (1986): 993–997.

Visualization (see GUIDED IMAGERY)

Women and Mental Health

Berg, Barbara J. *The Crisis of the Working Mother.* New York: Summit Books, 1986.

Freudenberger, Herbert, and Gail North. *Women's Burnout: How to Spot It, How to Reverse It, and How to Prevent It.* Garden City, N.Y.: Doubleday, 1985.

Kahn, Ada P. "Women and Stress." *Sacramento Medicine* (Sep. 1995).

Lerner, Harriet Goldhor. *The Dance of Anger.* New York: Harper & Row, 1985.

———. *The Dance of Intimacy.* New York: Harper & Row, 1989.

Long, B. C., and C. J. Haney. "Coping Strategies for Working Women: Aerobic Exercise and Relaxation Interventions." *Behavior Therapy* 19 (1988): 75–83.

Powell, J. Robin. *The Working Woman's Guide to Managing Stress.* Englewood Cliffs, N.J.: Prentice Hall, 1994.

Siress, Ruth Hermann. *Working Women's Communications Survival Guide: How to Present Your Ideas with Impact, Clarity, and Power and Get the Recognition You Deserve.* Englewood Cliffs, N.J.: Prentice Hall, 1994.

Weinstock, Lorna, and Eleanor Gilman. *Overcoming Panic Disorder: A Woman's Guide.* Chicago: Contemporary Books, 1998.

Witkin, Georgia. *The Female Stress Syndrome: How to Become Stress-Wise in the '90s.* New York, 1991.

Workplace and Mental Health

Adams, Scott. *The Dilbert Principle: A Cubicle's-Eye View of Bosses, Meetings, Management Fads and Other Workplace Afflictions.* New York: HarperBusiness, 1997.

Arrobe, Tanya. "Reducing the Cost of Stress: An Organizational Model." *Personnel Review* 19 (winter 1990).

Brown, Stephanie. *The Hand Book: Preventing Computer Injury.* New York: Ergonomne, 1993.

Frankenhaeuser, Marianne. "The Psychophysiology of Workload, Stress, and Health: Comparison Between the Sexes." *Annals of Behavioral Medicine* 13, no. 4: 197–204.

Karasek, Robert, and Tores Theorell. *Health Work: Stress, Productivity, and the Reconstruction of Working Life.* New York: Basic Books, 1990.

Leana, Carrie R., and Daniel C. Feldman. *Coping with Job Loss: How Individuals, Organizations and Communities Respond to Layoffs.* New York: Lexington Books, 1992.

Meyer, G. J. *Executive Blues: Down and Out in Corporate America.* New York: Franklin Square Press, 1997.

Murphy, Lawrence R. "Stress Management in Work Settings: A Critical Review of the Health Effects." *American Journal of Health Promotion* 11, no. 2 (Nov./Dec. 1996).

Paulsen, Barbara. "Work and Play: A Nation Out of Balance." *Health* (Oct. 1994).

Peterson, Michael. "Work, Corporate Culture, and Stress: Implications for Worksite Health Promotion." *American Journal of Health Behavior* 21, no. 4 (1997): 243–252.

Repetti, Rena, Karen Matthews, and Ingrid Waldron. "Employment and Women's Health Effect of Paid Employment on Women's Mental and Physical Health." *American Psychologist* 44, no. 11: 1394–1401.

Rosch, Paul J. "Measuring Job Stress: Some Comments on Potential Pitfalls." *American Journal of Health Promotion* 11, no. 6 (July/Aug. 1997).

Schor, Juliet. *The Overworked American: The Unexpected Decline of Leisure.* New York: Basic Books, 1991.

Shalowitz, Deborah. "Another Health Care Headache: Job Stress Could Strain Corporate Budgets." *Business Insurance* 25 (May 20, 1991).

Snyder, Don J. *The Cliff Walk: A Memoir of a Job Lost and a Life Found.* Boston: Little, Brown, 1997.

Walker, Cathy. "Workplace Stress." *Canadian Dimension* 27 (Aug. 1993).

Worry

Hallowell, Edward M. *Worry: Controlling It and Using It Wisely.* New York: Random House, 1997.

Yoga

Devananda, Swami Vishnu. *The Swivananda Companion to Yoga.* New York: Fireside/Simon & Schuster, 1983.

Groves, Dawn. *Yoga For Busy People: Increase Energy and Reduce Stress in Minutes a Day.* Emeryville, Calif.: New World Library, 1995.

Iyengar, Geeta S., *Yoga: A Gem for Women.* Palo Alto, Calif.: Timeless Books, 1990.

Lad, Vasant, and David Frawley. *The Yoga of Herbs.* Santa Fe, N.Mex.: Lotus Press, 1986.

Taylor, Louise. *A Woman's Book of Yoga: A Journal for Health and Self-Discovery.* Boston: Charles F. Tuttle, 1993.

Terkel, Susan Neiburg. *Yoga is for Me.* Minneapolis: Lerner Publications, 1987.

Vishnudevananda, Swami. *The Complete Illustrated Book of Yoga.* New York: Crown Publishers, 1995.

INDEX

NAMT *See* National Association for Music Therapy
narcissism
  body **71**
  codependency in 98, **272**
  criticism and 117
  self-esteem in 348
narcolepsy 139, 260, **272**, 361
narcotic drugs **272**
Nardil 22, 38, **273**, 303
NARSAD *See* National Alliance for Research on Schizophrenia and Depression
NASW *See* National Association of Social Workers
National Advisory Council on Adult Education 218
National Alliance for the Mentally Ill 24, 137, **273**, 343, 381
National Alliance for Research on Schizophrenia and Depression (NARSAD) **273**, 343
National Association to Aid Fat Americans 282
National Association of Anorexia Nervosa and Associated Disorders (ANAD) 153
National Association of Black Social Workers 11
National Association for Music Therapy (NAMT) 270
National Association of Social Workers (NASW) 367
National Association of Veterans Administration Chiefs of Psychiatry 309
National Cancer Institute 364
National Center for Complementary and Alternative Medicine 106
National Center for Health Statistics 68
National Center for Homeopathy 204
National Chronic Fatigue Syndrome Association 92
National Coalition Against Domestic Violence 146
National Coalition Against the Misuse of Pesticides 162
National Commission for the Certification of Acupuncturists 8
National Committee for Adoption 10
National Council on the Aging 18
National Council on Child Abuse and Family Violence 146
National Council on Compulsive Gambling 181
National Council on Problem Gambling 182
National Depressive and Manic-Depressive Association (NDMDA) 137, **273**, 381
National Down Syndrome Congress 259

National Fitness Foundation 167
National Foundation for Depressive Illness **273–274**
National Gay Task Force 238
National Headache Foundation 193, 196
National Heart, Lung and Blood Institute 199, 201
National Information Center for Children and Youth with Disabilities 141
National Institute on Alcohol Abuse and Alcoholism (NIAAA) 139, 173
National Institute on Drug Abuse (NIDA) 139, **274**
National Institute of Mental Health (NIMH) 44, 137, 139, 185, 273, **274**, 304, 309, 312
National Institutes of Health 91, 201
National Mental Health Association 24, 137, **274**, 292, 305, 343
National Organization of Social Security Claimants' Representatives (NOSSCR) 366
National Organization for Women 408
National Pesticide Telecommunications Network 162
National Safety Council 162
National Safe Workplace Institute 162
National Self-Help Clearinghouse 348
National Survey of Family Growth 68
National Women's Political Caucus 408
natural childbirth 87–88
naturopathy **274**
nausea **274–275**
  in hangover 192
  in motion sickness 268
  in nervousness 276
  in pregnancy 310
  relieving 298
  in stage fright 368
NDMDA *See* National Depressive and Manic-Depressive Association
near-death experiences **275**
necrophilia 293
nefazodone 38, 346, 350
negative attitude 54
negative imagery 411
negative reinforcement 330
nerves, cranial 114
nervous **275–276**
nervous breakdown **276**
nervous habits **276**
"nervous stomach" 82, 276
nervous system
  autonomic **55**
  central *See* central nervous system

  parasympathetic 55
  sympathetic 55, **384**
neurasthenias 275
neurobiologic theories 299
neuroendocrine transducers 207
neurohormones 207
neuroleptic **276**
neuroleptic malignant syndrome 392
neurological examination **276**
neurology **276–277**
neuromyasthenia **277**
neuron **277**
neuropsychiatry **277**
neuropsychological testing **277**
neurosis **277**, 320
  vs. psychosis 322
neurosurgery **277–278**
neurosyphilis 278
neurotransmitters 278
neurotransmitter theory 134
newborn(s) *See* infant(s)
New England Journal of Medicine 105, 380
A New Guide To Rational Living (Ellis) 73
NIAAA *See* National Institute on Alcohol Abuse and Alcoholism
niacin deficiency 280
nicotine dependence 3, 223, **278**, 363, 394
NIDA *See* National Institute on Drug Abuse
nightmare **278**, 294, 308
night terror **278–279**
NIMH *See* National Institute of Mental Health
Nishiyama, Katsuo 231–232
nitroglycerin 36
Nocturnal Penile Tumescence (NPT) Test 220
noncompliance **279**
Noncompliance Institute of Los Angeles 279
nonrapid-eye-movement sleep (NREM) 362
nonsteroidal anti-inflammatory drug (NSAID) 173, 289
nonverbal communication 232, 240
noradrenaline *See* norepinephrine
norepinephrine 12, 74, **279**, 393
  and affective disorders 15
  beta-adrenergic-blocking drugs and 55
  and depression 38, 278
  and dopamine 146
  gamma-aminobutyric acid and 182
  music therapy and 271
  and thyroid-releasing hormone 67
Norpramin 138, **279**
North American Society of Teachers of the Alexander Technique 72

nortriptylene 38, 56, **279**, 290
NOSSCR *See* National Organization of Social Security Claimants' Representatives
nostalgia **279–280**
NREM *See* nonrapid-eye-movement sleep
NSAID *See* nonsteroidal anti-inflammatory drug
numbness 187, 294
Numorphan 286
nutrition 200, **280**
nutritional disorders 280
nymphomania **280–281**

O

obesity **282**
  and high blood pressure 200
  self-esteem and 282, 347
  and snoring 365
  stimulants for 260
object relations **282**
obscenity **282**
obsession(s) 283
  in agoraphobia 21
  culture and 118
  with perfection 297
obsessional worries, about AIDS 5
obsessive-compulsive disorder (OCD) 46–47, 190, **282–284**
  alienation in 27
  checking in 87
  and depression 283
  hostility in 209
  positron emission tomography in 307
  rumination in 337
  shopaholism in 357
  vs. Tourette syndrome 395
  treatment of 96, 239, 283–284
Obsessive-Compulsive Disorder Foundation 190, 284
obstructive sleep apnea syndrome (OSAS) 365
OCD *See* obsessive-compulsive disorder
O'Connor, Sandra Day 409
Oedipus complex 85, 106, 176, **284**, 322
O'Guinn, Thomas C. 357
ohashiatsu **284**
Ohl, Dana A. 221
olanzapine 41, 343, 415
older adult(s) *See* elderly
Older Women's League 84
O'Neil, George 248
O'Neil, Nena 248
oneirophobia 148
only children 68, 242, **284–285**
oophorectomy 85
open adoption 10
open marriage 248, **285–286**
operant conditioning 62, 107–108
operant shaping 108